Hematology in Practice

SECOND EDITION

Betty Ciesla, MS, MT(ASCP)SH^{CM}
Faculty, Medical Technology Program
Morgan State University
Baltimore, Maryland
Assistant Professor Medical Technology Program
Stevenson University
Stevenson, Maryland

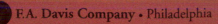
F.A. Davis Company • Philadelphia

F. A. Davis Company
1915 Arch Street
Philadelphia, PA 19103
www.fadavis.com

Copyright © 2012 by F. A. Davis Company

Printed in the United States of America

Last digit indicates print number: 10 9 8 7 6 5 4

Acquisitions Editor: Christa Fratantoro
Manager of Content Development: George W. Lang
Developmental Editor: Karen Williams
Art and Design Manager: Carolyn O'Brien

As new scientific information becomes available through basic and clinical research, recommended treatments and drug therapies undergo changes. The author(s) and publisher have done everything possible to make this book accurate, up to date, and in accord with accepted standards at the time of publication. The author(s), editors, and publisher are not responsible for errors or omissions or for consequences from application of the book, and make no warranty, expressed or implied, in regard to the contents of the book. Any practice described in this book should be applied by the reader in accordance with professional standards of care used in regard to the unique circumstances that may apply in each situation. The reader is advised always to check product information (package inserts) for changes and new information regarding dose and contraindications before administering any drug. Caution is especially urged when using new or infrequently ordered drugs.

Library of Congress Cataloging-in-Publication Data

Ciesla, Betty.
  Hematology in practice / Betty Ciesla. — 2nd ed.
     p. ; cm.
  Includes bibliographical references and index.
  ISBN-13: 978-0-8036-2561-7
  ISBN-10: 0-8036-2561-8
  1. Blood—Diseases. 2. Hematology. I. Title.
  [DNLM: 1. Hematologic Diseases—Case Reports. 2. Hematologic Tests—methods—Case Reports. WH 120]
  RB145.C525 2012
  616.1'5—dc22

                              2011000734

For my daughters, who changed my life
For my husband, whom I cherish
For my mother and sisters, who challenged my imagination

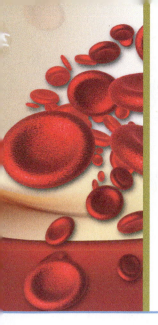

Preface to the Second Edition

I am delighted to have the opportunity to do a second edition of this textbook. The first edition was well received, and I have made every effort to include the "vision" of those who wrote to me with corrections and suggestions. I extend my heartfelt thanks. With the assistance of so many capable contributors and reviewers, I have made changes that can only benefit students studying hematology. More questions have been added to each chapter, and updates have been made to the cases and content of each chapter where appropriate. The acute leukemia and myeloproliferative chapters reflect the current World Health Organization (WHO) categories, and Chapter 20 has been significantly expanded. This new edition includes a glossary, updated power points, animations, and embedded student assists. All chapters have been updated, and case studies have been reviewed for applicability and accuracy.

As an academic subject, hematology is difficult to learn, retain, and master. My hope is that you enjoy this second edition and find it even more appealing than the first. Having a textbook that is user-friendly, portable, and useful is essential, and that is what I have aimed to create, with your help and suggestions. As you continue in your career as a laboratory professional, may this textbook have a place in your library or on your desk. I welcome your comments at beciesla@msn.com and look forward to your assistance in this endeavor.

Betty Ciesla MS, MT(ASCP)SH^{CM}

PREFACE TO THE FIRST EDITION

In its most fundamental form, hematology is the study of blood in health and in disease. Blood is the window to the body; it is the predictor of vitality and long life. In ancient times, blood was worshipped. Men were bled to obtain a cure and blood was studied for its mystical powers. It was an elevated body fluid. The discipline of hematology was an outgrowth of this fascination with blood. As we practice it in the clinical laboratory today, this discipline encompasses skill, art and instinct.

Hematology is about relationships—the relationships of the bone marrow to the systemic circulation, the relationship of the plasma environment to the red cell life span, and the relationship of hemoglobin to the red cell. In this textbook, you, the student, are a vital part of this relationship. I have queried many students over my two decades of teaching and asked them what it is *they* want to see in a textbook. I have asked: What helps? What gets in the way? What makes you feel more comfortable? Students answered honestly and in great detail, and I even managed to have one of my students review each chapter, so that the student perspective would not be minimized.

Hematology is a difficult subject to master because it forces students to think in an unnatural way. Educators are always asking why, well before students can cross the intellectual bridge between the marrow and the peripheral smear. Many students begin a hematology course with little foundation in blood cell morphology, physiology, or medical terminology. With this is mind, I have built several helpful strategies within this text. Each chapter contains readable text that engages the students to learn, master, and then apply the critical concepts in hematology. Medical terminology is absorbed through a designated Word Key section, defining terms to which student may not have been exposed. End of chapter summaries and multiple levels of case studies illustrate the key principles of each chapter. Additionally, there are unique troubleshooting cases in each chapter which encourages each student to role play as a working professional to develop and refine problem solving skills *in practice*. A test bank and a digital resource disk round out the pedagogy presented in this exciting text.

I hope that this text travels with you as you continue your career in the laboratory professions and I hope that the information motivates you and arouses your intellectual curiosity. Two year and four year students can benefit from the chosen topics within the text and perhaps it may even find a home on the shelves of working laboratories nationally and internationally. I welcome your comments (beciesla@msn .com) and encourage you to assist me in creating a memorable textbook.

Betty Ciesla, MS, MT (ASCP)SH

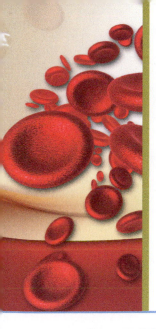

Contributors

Barbara Caldwell, MS, MT(ASCP)SH^{CM}
Administrative Director, Clinical Laboratory Services
Montgomery General Hospital
Olney, Maryland

Donna D. Castellone, MS, MT(ASCP)SH
Clinical Projects Manager, Hemostasis/Hematology
Medical, Clinical, and Statistical Affairs
Siemens Healthcare Diagnostics
Tarrytown, New York

Betty Ciesla, MS, MT(ASCP)SH^{CM}
Faculty, Medical Technology Program
Morgan State University
Baltimore, Maryland
Assistant Professor Medical Technology Program
Stevenson University
Stevenson, Maryland

Kathleen Finnegan, MS, MT(ASCP)SH^{CM}
Clinical Associate Professor
Chair, Clinical Laboratory Sciences Program
State University of New York at Stony Brook
Stony Brook, New York

Lori Lentowski, BS, MT(ASCP)
St. Joseph's Medical Center
Towson, Maryland

Mitra Taghizadeh, MS, MT(ASCP)
Former Assistant Professor
Department of Medical and Research Technology
University of Maryland School of Medicine
Baltimore, Maryland

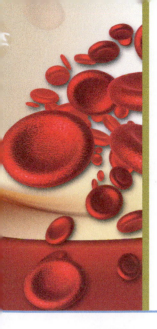

Reviewers

Lisa Countryman-Jones,
BS, MT(ASCP) CLS, CPT(NCA), ACCE
Faculty Member, Clinical Practice Coordinator
Medical Laboratory Technology Program
Portland Community College
Portland, Oregon

Andrea G. Gordon, MT(ASCP)SH
Vice President of Academic Affairs
River Valley Community College
Claremont, New Hampshire

Shirley R. Hagan, MS, MT(ASCP)
Adjunct Instructor
Medical Laboratory Technology Program
Grayson County College
Health Science Division
Denison, Texas

Elizabeth Jones, MT, ABHI (CHT), ASPT (CPT)
Instructor
Medical Laboratory Program
Community Technical and Adult Education Center
Allied Health Department
Ocala, Florida

Natalie E. Lyter, BS, MT(ASCP)SH
Instructor
Medical Laboratory Technician Program
Harrisburg Area Community College
Health Career Department
Harrisburg, Pennsylvania

Bernardino D. Madsen, MT (ASCP)
Instructor
Medical Laboratory Technology Program
Casper College
School of Health Science
Casper, Wyoming

Sueanne Seegers, MT
Faculty
Medical Laboratory Technology Program
Shoreline Community College
Health Occupations and PE Division
Shoreline, Washington

Jamie Titus, BS, MLT(ASCP)
Adjunct Instructor
Medical Laboratory Technology Program
Seward County Community College/Area Technical School
Allied Health Department
Liberal, Kansas

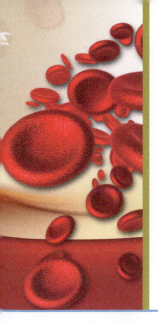

Acknowledgments

I am indebted to Christa Fratantoro, my acquisitions editor at F.A. Davis, and to Karen Williams, my developmental editor. Both women offered me patience, professionalism, and friendship. Additionally, my great thanks to Dino Masden at Casper College in Wyoming for his artistic eye in taking more digital photos for me and to Kathleen Finnegan for her additions to Chapter 20. Finally, a heartfelt debt of thanks to Megan Zadra, who labored on the PowerPoints with great success and acumen.

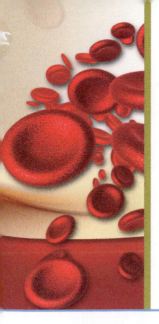

Contents

Part I

Basic Hematology Principles

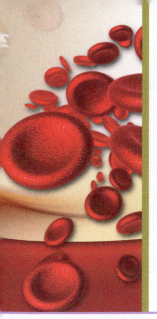

Chapter 1

Introduction to Hematology and Basic Laboratory Practice

Betty Ciesla

Objectives

After completing this chapter, the student will be able to:

1. Describe the significance of the field of hematology in relation to sickness and health.

2. List the basic parts of the compound microscope.

3. Discuss the function and magnification of each of the microscope objectives.

4. Identify appropriate corrective actions when encountering routine problems with the operation of a microscope.

5. Define *standard precautions* as related to biologic hazards.

6. Describe safe work practices for personal protective equipment and disposal of biologic hazards.

7. Describe the components of quality assurance in the hematology laboratory.

8. Define the terms *preanalytic and postanalytic variables, delta checks, accuracy, precision, reproducibility*, and *reference intervals*.

9. Formulate a plan of action based on the troubleshooting scenarios presented in the text.

INTRODUCTION TO HEMATOLOGY

In its most fundamental form, hematology is the study of blood in health and in pathologic conditions. Blood is the window to the body; it is a predictor of vitality—of long life. In ancient times, blood was worshipped. Men were bled to obtain a cure, and blood was studied for its mystical powers. It was a venerated bodily fluid. The discipline of hematology was an outgrowth of this fascination with blood.

As we practice hematology in the clinical laboratory today, this discipline encompasses skill, art, and instinct. For those of us who are passionate about this subject, it is the art of hematology that so intrigues us. To view a peripheral smear and have the knowledge not only to identify the patient's hematologic condition correctly but also to predict how the bone marrow may have contributed to that condition is an awesome feeling. Hematology is about relationships: the relationship of the bone marrow to the systemic circulation, the relationship of the plasma environment to the red blood cell life span, and the relationship of the hemoglobin to the red blood cell. For most students, hematology is a difficult subject to master because it forces students to think in an unnatural way. Instructors usually ask *why, what,* and *how.* Why does this cell appear in the peripheral smear? What relationship does it have to the bone marrow? How was it formed? Many students begin a hematology course with little foundation in blood cell morphology. They have no real grasp of medical terminology and few facts concerning blood diseases. They are not equipped to answer *why, what,* and *how.* The instructor's goal is to guide the student toward an appreciation of his or her role as a clinical laboratorian in hematology. Instructors can help the student to develop the morphologic and analytic skills necessary for adept practice in the hematology laboratory. Yet to be truly notable in this field, keen instincts concerning a set of results, a particular cell, or a patient's history play a defining role.

Blood has always been a fascinating subject for authors, poets, scholars, and scientists. References to blood appear in hieroglyphics, in the Bible, on ancient pottery, and in literature. Hippocrates laid the foundation for hematology with his theory of the body's four humors—blood, phlegm, black bile, and yellow bile—and his concept that all blood ailments resulted from a disorder in the balance of these humors. These principles remained unchallenged for 1400 years. Gradually, scientists such as Galen, Harvey, van Leeuwenhoek, Virchow, and Ehrlich were able to elevate hematology into a discipline of medicine with basic morphologic observations that can be traced to a distinct **pathophysiology**. We owe a huge debt of gratitude to these men. Although they had little in the way of advanced technology, their inventions and observations helped describe and quantify cells, cellular structure, and function. Much of what has been learned concerning the etiology of hematologic disease has been discovered since the 1920s; therefore, hematology, as a distinct branch of medicine, is in its early stages.[1]

THE MICROSCOPE

The binocular microscope is an essential tool to the hematology laboratory professional. It is a piece of equipment that is stylistically simple in design, yet extraordinarily complex in its ability to magnify an image, provide visual details of that image, and make the image visible to the human eye.[2] Most commonly used today are compound binocular microscopes, which use two lens systems to magnify the image. The ocular devices on the microscope provide an initial 10× magnification; additional magnification is obtained through the use of three or four different powered objectives.[3] A light source is located under the microscope stage. Light is beamed to the image directly or through filters that vary the wavelength. In addition, a diaphragm apparatus is usually located in the base of the microscope. Opening or closing the diaphragm can increase or reduce the volume of light directed toward the image.[4] This is most useful when examining cellular structures in the nucleus that need more light to be properly visualized. Following is a *brief* description of the most significant parts of the microscope.

Significant Parts of the Microscope

The *eyepieces,* or *oculars,* are located laterally to the microscope base (Fig. 1.1) and function as an additional magnification component to the objective magnification. Most microscopes are binocular and contain two eyepieces, each of which magnifies the diameter of an object placed on the stage to the power of the eyepiece, usually 10×.

The *objectives* of the compound microscope are 10×, 40×, and 100×. Often, a 50× (oil) magnification is incorporated in a hematology microscope. Each objective has three numbers inscribed on it: a magnification number, an aperture number (NA), and a tube length number. The NA refers to the resolution power of the objective, which is the ability of the objective to gather light and distinguish objects in close proximity to each other. The higher the NA number, the higher

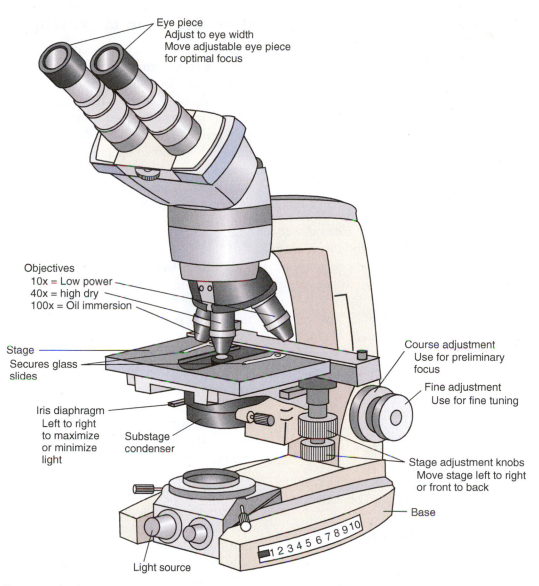

Figure 1.1 Compound microscope.

the resolution. Tube length refers to the distance from the eyepiece to the objective. Magnification refers to how large the image can appear and how much of the viewing field can be observed. Objectives on modern microscopes are composed of many lenses and prisms that produce an extremely high quality of optical performance.

The *iris diaphragm,* located below the microscope stage, increases or decreases light from the microscope light source. If the diaphragm is opened to its full capacity, the cell or structure is viewed with maximum light. If the diaphragm is minimally opened, the cell or structure is much less illuminated, which may be desirable depending on the source of the sample (i.e., stained versus unstained material).

The *stage* is a flat surface with an opening created for light to pass through. Two flat metal clips have been mounted in which to secure the glass slide. Below the stage surface are two control knobs that move the slide horizontally or vertically.

Coarse and *fine adjustment knobs* are located on either side of the microscope base. These adjustment knobs bring the image into focus through movement of the stage, which is either raised or lowered according to the degree of focus needed.

Care of the Microscope

The microscope is an essential piece of equipment to the practice of hematology and must be handled with care and respect. Hematology instructors need to teach the care and maintenance of the microscope in the hope that these "best practices" will be adopted and practiced in the workplace. The microscope should rest on a level, vibration-free surface. When lifting it from a storage cabinet and moving it to another location, the microscope must be secured on the bottom by one hand and held by the arm with the other hand. Additionally, users must be instructed on how to move objectives from one position to another without dragging non-oil objectives into oil from a slide left on the stage. The high-dry objective must never be used with oil, only with slides with cover slips. Objectives are easily scratched or damaged by careless handlers; consequently, they must be cleaned with lens paper after each use. Oil objectives should be wiped free of oil when not in use, and eyepieces must be cleaned with lens paper of dust, dirt, or cosmetic debris with each viewing. When stored, cords should never be wrapped around the objectives or oculars, which are easily scratched or damaged.

Good microscopy habits should always be cultivated, practiced, and communicated. Microscopy guidelines should be posted in each area where microscopes are used. The guidelines should include the following:

- General use of the microscope
- Instructions for transporting the microscope
- Instructions for proper cleaning of the microscope
- Storage guidelines that include proper position of microscope cords, stage, and objectives

Corrective Actions in Light Microscopy

Many problems that are encountered when using a microscope can be easily corrected by using common sense. Some of the most common "problems" in light microscopy are as follows:

- Image cannot be seen at any power: Try turning the slide over; perhaps the wrong side of the slide has been placed on the microscope stage.
- Fine details cannot be detected in immature cells: For immature cells, use the $100\times$ lens and open up diaphragms to the maximum width for maximum light.
- The $40\times$ objective is blurred: Try wiping off the $100\times$ lens; perhaps the $100\times$ lens was oil-filled and was dragged across the slide.
- Particles appear on the slide that are not large enough to be platelets: Perhaps mascara has been left on the eyepiece; use lens cleaner to clean the eyepieces.

Innovations in Microscopy

Digital microscopes are becoming routine pieces of equipment in hematology laboratories. These microscopes scan blood smears for cells, identify them, calculate a white blood cell differential count, and store the cellular images of the cells for future review. Slides are then reviewed for red blood cell morphology and abnormalities by a trained operator.[5] Although the initial purchase cost of a digital microscope is expensive, its speed, sensitivity, and reduced technologist time make it an attractive option for larger laboratories.

STANDARD PRECAUTIONS

The clinical laboratory presents an environment with many potential risks ranging from biologic hazards to chemical or fire hazards. Safety training has become a mandatory part of responsible employee practice and training not only for employees but also for their colleagues. Safety training sessions are an essential part of employee training. These sessions represent a lifeline toward optimal behavior should an employee encounter an unexpected hazard. Biologic hazards constitute a major risk area, and this section focuses specifically on this area. Chemical and environmental hazards are briefly summarized. The website of the U.S. Occupational Safety and Health Administration (www.OSHA.gov) provides a ready source of information about such hazards.

Most patient samples used in the hematology laboratory are derived from human body fluids (e.g., blood, organ or joint fluids, stools, urine, semen). Each of these is a potential source of bacterial, fungal, or viral infection; consequently, each sample is potentially hazardous. Laboratorians must protect themselves from contamination by observing practices that prevent direct contact with body fluids or a contaminated surface, contamination, or inhalation. In 1996, the U.S. Centers for Disease Control and Prevention issued a set of standard precautions aimed at creating a safe working environment for laboratory practice. These standard precautions combine principles of body substance isolation and universal precautions.

Personal Protective Equipment

The main features of standard precautions that relate to safe hematology laboratory practice include personal protective equipment (PPE) and safety features other than PPE.[6] PPE includes gloves, eye and face shields, countertop shields, and fluid-resistant gowns or laboratory coats.

Gloves

Gloves must be worn during any activity with potential for contact with bodily fluids. Gloves must be changed immediately if they become contaminated or damaged. When patient contact is initiated, gloves must be changed with each patient. Gloves are removed before exiting the laboratory for any purpose (Fig. 1.2).

Gowns and Laboratory Coats

Gowns and laboratory coats must be fluid-resistant, with long sleeves and wrist cuffs. They may not be worn outside of the laboratory and must be changed if they become contaminated or torn. Disposable coats are treated as biohazardous material and discarded; cloth coats are laundered by the employer's service.

Splash Shields (Face, Eye, Surface)

Goggles, face shields, masks, and Plexiglas countertop shields are used to minimize the risks of aerosol and specimen splashes. Many automated instruments have cap-piercing mechanisms that reduce the risk of aerosol production during routine procedures. Personal protective equipment is vital to employee safety (Figs. 1.3 through 1.5; Table 1.1).

Safety Features Other Than Personal Protective Equipment

1. **Handwashing:** This is a basic yet most effective tool to prevent contamination. Soap and water must be used, and the handwashing procedure should include the wrists and at least a 10- to 15-second soap application

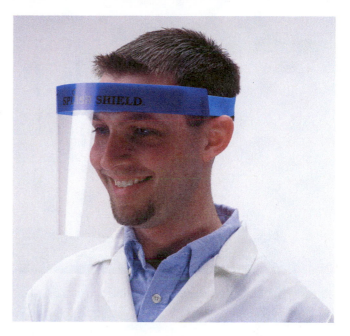

Figure 1.3   Face shield.   From MarketLab, Kentwood, MI, with permission.

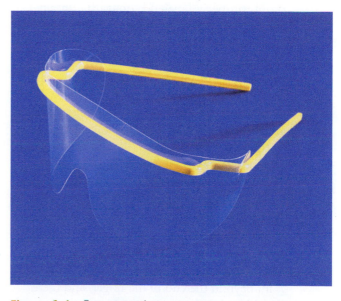

Figure 1.4   Eye protection.   From MarketLab, Kentwood, MI, with permission.

with warm water; this represents significantly more time than most individuals spend in handwashing. It cannot be stressed enough that proper handwashing using the recommended times is the first step in the decontamination **protocol**. Germicidal soaps are suggested. Hands must be washed with every patient contact, after gloves are removed, and if gloved or ungloved hands have been contaminated with a bodily fluid sample.

2. **Puncture-resistant containers:** Care must be taken with contaminated sharps. Needles,

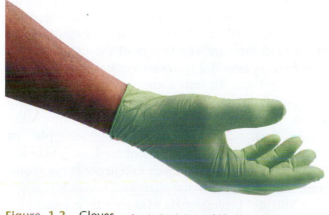

Figure 1.2   Gloves.   From MarketLab, Kentwood, MI, with permission.

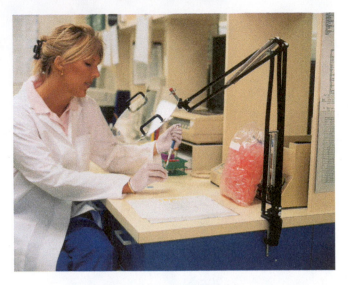

Figure 1.5 Biohazard shield with flexible arm. From MarketLab, Kentwood, MI, with permission.

blades, pipettes, syringes, and glass slides must be placed in a leak-proof, puncture-proof, properly labeled biohazard container.

3. **Mechanical pipetting device:** Mouth pipetting is never permitted, and other objects (e.g., pens, pencils) should be kept away from the mouth and mucous membranes.

4. **Eating, drinking, and smoking:** These activities are strictly forbidden in the laboratory area. Food or drink items should not be kept in the laboratory.

5. **Notebooks, textbooks, and loose papers:** These are not allowed in the laboratory work area.

6. **Personal hygiene:** Regarding issues of personal hygiene, **long hair** must be tied back, **beards** must be trimmed to no more than 1 in. in length, **fingernails** must be no longer than $\frac{1}{4}$ in. beyond the end of the finger, and there should no **jewelry** ornamentation of the fingers.

Table 1.1 ◉ Personal Protective Equipment

- Gloves
- Fluid-resistant gowns
- Laboratory coats
- Goggles
- Face shield
- Mask
- Plexiglas countertop shield

7. **Dangling jewelry:** Earrings and necklaces and other dangling jewelry are not allowed.
8. **Cosmetics:** Laboratory employees may not use **cosmetics** or **lip balm**.

Chemical and Environmental Hazards

The clinical laboratory is an area in which chemicals are handled and maintained. Clothing, body parts, and surface areas are all potential spill areas for hazardous chemicals. Each employee should understand and adhere to the chemical spill action plan. Additionally, employees who routinely handle chemicals should wear goggles, avoid splashing, and stringently follow mixing guidelines. Environmental hazards include fire hazards, electrical hazards, radioactive hazards, and physical hazards. The details of hazards are as follows:

- Fire hazards: Be familiar with the fire evacuation route, fire blanket location, and fire extinguisher location.
- Electrical hazards: Be aware of frayed cords, unsafe practices such as wet hands on electrical sockets, and whether all electrical equipment is grounded.
- Radioactive hazards: Persons in areas in the laboratory where radioactive materials are used should wear a radioactive badge.
- Physical hazards: Dangling jewelry should be avoided, hair should be pulled back and contained, and close-toed shoes must be worn.

BASIC CONCEPTS OF QUALITY ASSURANCE PLANS IN THE HEMATOLOGY LABORATORY

Quality assurance is a comprehensive and systematic process that strives to ensure reliable patient results. This process includes every level of laboratory operation.[7] Phlebotomy services, competency testing, error analysis, standard protocols, PPE, quality control, and turnaround time are key factors in the quality assurance system. Table 1.2 provides a more complete set of indicators. From the time a sample arrives in the laboratory until the results are reported, a rigorous quality assurance system is the key feature in ensuring quality results. Each part of the quality assurance plan or process should be analyzed, monitored, and reconfigured as necessary to emphasize excellence at every outcome. Although many hospitals and research facilities have "quality" professionals who provide oversight for quality assurance plans for their facilities, an elemental understanding of terms related to the total quality

Table 1.2 ● Short List of Quality Assurance Indicators

- Number of patient redraws
- Labeling errors
- Patient and specimens properly identified
- Critical values called
- Pass rate on competency testing
- Test cancellation
- Integrity of send-out samples
- Employee productivity
- Errors in data entry
- Testing turnaround times
- Delays caused by equipment failures or maintenance
- Performance on proficiency testing

assurance plan is required of all staff technologists and students.

Quality control is a large part of the quality assurance program at most facilities. Students will be introduced to the term *quality control* early and often. It is an essential function in the clinical laboratory. Following is a brief overview of the quality control procedures used in promoting quality assurance in the hematology laboratory. This overview is not intended to be comprehensive but rather introduces terminology and concepts pertinent to the entry-level professional.

Quality Control Monitoring in the Hematology Laboratory

The analytic component, or the actual measurement of an analyte in body fluids, is monitored in the laboratory by quality control, a component of the laboratory quality assurance plan. The analytic method in the hematology laboratory primarily includes instrumentation and reagents. *Standards,* or *calibrators,* are solutions that have a known amount of an analyte and are used to calibrate the method or instrument.[7] For example, the hemoglobin standard is 12 g/100 mL, meaning that there is exactly 12 g of hemoglobin in 100 mL of solution. The system is calibrated from this standard. Conversely, controls, or control materials, are used to monitor the performance of a method after calibration. Control materials are assayed concurrently with patient samples. The analyte value for the controls is calculated from the calibration data in the same manner as the unknown or patient's results are calculated.[7]

The measured values of control materials are compared with their expected values, or target range. Reporting unknown patient sample results is dependent on this evaluation process.

A **statistical quality control system** is used to establish the target range for the analyte. The procedure involves obtaining at least 20 control values for the analyte to be measured. Ideally, the repeated control results should be the same; however, there will always be variability in the assay. The concept of clustering of the data points around one value is known as central tendency. The mean, mode, and median are statistical parameters used to measure the central tendency. The mean is the arithmetic average of a group of data points, the mode is the value occurring most frequently, and the median is the middle value of a dataset. If the mean, mode, and median are nearly the same for the control values, the data have a normal distribution.[7]

The standard deviation and coefficient of variation are measures of the spread of the data within the distribution about the mean. Standard deviation is a precision measurement that describes the average "distance" of each data point from the mean in a normal distribution. This measurement is mathematically calculated for a group of numbers. If the measured control values follow a normal distribution curve, 68.6% of the measured values fall within the mean and one standard deviation (SD) from the mean, 95.5% fall within the mean and two standard deviations (2SD) from the mean, and 99.7% fall within the mean and three standard deviations (3SD) from the mean. The 95.5% confidence interval is the accepted limit for the clinical laboratory.

Coefficient of variation (CV) is the standard deviation expressed as a percentage. The lower the CV, the more precise are the data. The usual CV for laboratory results is less than 5%, which indicates that the distribution is tighter around the mean value.[8]

Clarifying *accuracy* and *precision* is usually a troublesome task because these terms are often used interchangeably. When a test result is accurate, it means that it has come closest to the correct value if the reference or correct value is known. In most cases, when a methodology has been established for a particular analysis, standard or reference material is run to establish a reference interval. Accuracy is defined as the result closest to the true value.[9]

Precision relates to reproducibility and repeatability of test samples using the same methodology. Theoretically, patient results should be repeatable if analyzed numerous times using the same method. If there is great variability of results around a target value, the precision is compromised (Fig. 1.6).[8]

Normal, or Reference, Intervals

Normal, or reference, intervals are values that have been established for a particular analyte, method, or instrument and a particular patient population. To establish a reference interval, the size of the sample must be at least 25 and should represent healthy male and female adults and children. When the test samples have been analyzed under predetermined conditions, a set reference value is determined from which reference limits and reference intervals may be established according to statistical methods. Subsequent patient samples are compared with the reference interval to determine if they are normal or outside of the reference interval.[10]

Delta Checks

Delta checks are a function of the laboratory information system. This function allows the operator to perform a historical check on the sample from the previous results. If the variation in patient sample exceeds the established standard set for delta checks, results are flagged in some way, and a cause may be identified before the results are released. Preanalytic problems, misidentified samples, analytic errors, or changes in the patient condition may contribute to erratic delta checks.

Reflex Testing

If automated complete blood count (CBC) results present a flagging signal, the technologist must perform operations to validate the results. Usually flags are displayed next to a specific result. For example, an "H" indicates high results, whereas an "L" indicates low results. Multiple flags may be generated for the entire CBC. Manual methods may be needed, or additional tests (e.g., adding a differential count or manual slide review) may need to be performed on the sample to provide accurate test results. Technologists should be vigilant when hematologic data are flagged because it almost always means that the sample has some abnormality.

Preanalytic Variables

Preanalytic variables refer to any factors that may affect the sample before testing. Some issues to be considered include whether the sample was properly identified, properly collected (inverted 6× to 8× if anticoagulated) in the correct **anticoagulant**, and delivered to the testing facility in a timely fashion. (Table 1.3) lists preanalytic variables.

Postanalytic Variables

Postanalytic variables refer to operations that occur after sample testing. These variables affect the integrity of sample results. Examples are proper documentation of test results, timely reporting of results to a designated individual if a critical value was observed, and proper handling of samples that may involve calculations or dilutions. Table 1.4 lists postanalytic variables.

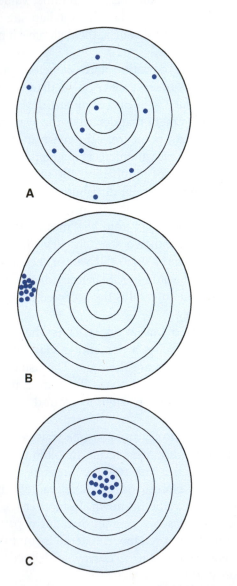

Figure 1.6   Is it accurate or precise? (A) Shots are neither accurate nor precise. (B) Shots are precise but miss the mark, not accurate. (C) Shots are accurate and precise.

Table 1.3 ○ Preanalytic Variables

- Proper patient identification
- Properly labeled tubes
- Proper anticoagulant
- Proper mixing of sample
- Timely delivery to laboratory
- Tubes checked for clots
- Medications administered to the patient
- Previous blood transfusions
- Intravenous line contamination
- Blood sample properly collected (proper tube, proper anticoagulant)

Table 1.4 ○ Postanalytic Variables

- Delta checks
- Results released
- Critical results called
- Reflex testing initiated
- Specimen check for clots

Critical Values

Critical values are results that exceed or are markedly decreased from the reference range or the patient's history of results. These results are usually flagged by the automated instrument. It is essential that either the physician or the appropriate designee be notified immediately by a member of the reporting laboratory because many critical results involve immediate medical or patient care decisions.

○ *Summary Points*

- Hematology is the study of blood in health and disease.
- Morphologic, analytic, and microscopy skills are needed in the practice of hematology.
- Compound microscopes have a two-lens system to magnify the image.
- The objectives of the microscope are 10×, 40×, and 100×; a 50× oil immersion lens may be added.

- Proper care of the microscope is essential for maintaining microscopic quality.
- Standard precautions and procedures are policies designed to prevent the spread of infection and disease.
- PPE includes gloves, eyewear, laboratory coats, face shields, and fluid-resistant gowns.
- Handwashing is the most important element of standard precautions.
- Quality assurance is a set of laboratory practices that ensure reliable outcomes for patient results.
- Quality control is part of the quality assurance plan and consists of standards, controls, normal distribution, and statistical parameters.
- Accuracy and precision are measured by the mean standard deviation around a set of data points.
- Patient identification is the essential first step in ensuring the quality of laboratory results.
- Preanalytic variables refer to events or circumstances that occur to the unknown sample before analysis.
- Postanalytic variables refer to laboratory practice after the sample has been analyzed.
- Critical results are results that exceed or are markedly decreased from the reference interval.

CONDENSED CASE

A purple top tube was received from the emergency department on a 24-year-old man with a possible gastrointestinal bleed. A hemoglobin and hematocrit were ordered. When the sample was run through the automated instrumentation, a clot was detected. A redrawn sample was ordered, and the same thing occurred again—a clotted sample. *Name three reasons for a clotted sample.*

Answer
Clotted samples may occur if (A) the phlebotomy was difficult, (B) the sample was not inverted at least six to eight times, or (C) the tube was expired.

CASE STUDY

A technologist in the hematology laboratory has been observed wearing blood-spattered gloves. Her colleagues in the laboratory are uncomfortable working with her, and they have confronted her on this issue. Her explanation for her behavior is that gloves are expensive and that frequent changing leads to excessive spending on gloves and other disposables. Her colleagues are concerned for their safety, and because they have been unsuccessful in changing her behavior, they consult the hematology supervisor for guidance. *How should this employee be counseled?*

Insights to the Case Study

The employee is jeopardizing the health of her co-workers because of her noncompliance. Standard laboratory precautions clearly state that she is to remove soiled or contaminated gloves and replace them with clean gloves. She should be counseled as such. Although her concern for the laboratory budget is commendable, issues of finances are under the auspices of administration and not a matter for her concern. The employee should review the safety manual, a mandatory requirement she has already signed stating that she understands and will comply with all of the safety requirements of the laboratory.

Review Questions

1. Standard precautions involve
   a. Behavior that prevents contact with virally infected patients.
   b. Behavior that prevents direct contact with bodily fluids or contaminated surfaces.
   c. Behavior that prevents contact with pediatric patients.
   d. Behavior that prevents contact with terminally ill patients.

2. Which one of the following is considered personal protective equipment?
   a. Operating room attire
   b. Head nets
   c. Laboratory coats
   d. White shoes

3. What types of samples are used primarily in the clinical laboratory?
   a. Blood and bodily fluids
   b. Solid organs
   c. Bone
   d. Skin

4. Which part(s) on the microscope is (are) used for focusing?
   a. Oculars
   b. Stage
   c. Diaphragm
   d. Coarse and fine adjustments

5. Which one of the following is a postanalytic factor?
   a. Calling results when a critical value is obtained
   b. Tube checked for clots
   c. Patient identification
   d. Sample mixing

6. The proper definition for a *standard* is
   a. Materials used to calibrate a method.
   b. A normal distribution curve.
   c. A target range.
   d. Solutions with a known amount of the analyte.

7. Which of the following is the definition of a reference interval?
   a. A solution of a known amount of analyte
   b. Materials analyzed concurrently with unknown samples
   c. Values established for a particular analyte, given a method, instrument, or patient population
   d. Validation techniques on flagged samples

8. Which of the following is *not* considered a postanalytic variable?
   a. Delta checks
   b. Proper anticoagulant used
   c. Specimen check for clots
   d. Critical results called

9. Error analysis, standard protocols, and turn-around time all are part of the
   a. Quality assurance system.
   b. Quality control program.
   c. Reference standards.
   d. Delta check protocol.

10. The average of a group of data points is defined as the
    a. Mean.
    b. Mode.
    c. Median.
    d. Modicum.

◉ TROUBLESHOOTING

What Do I Do When the Results Fail the Delta Check?

A sample was received into the laboratory on a patient who had been admitted 48 hours earlier. Several results on the patient, a man, had changed dramatically since the last CBC results were evaluated in the hematology laboratory. The results in question are marked by an asterisk. A delta check is an historical check on blood results that are stored in the automated hematology instrument. If there is great variability in results from one time to the next, the results are flagged, and some corrective action needs to be taken.

Test	Saturday	Sunday	Unit of Measure	Reference Range
WBC	18.1*	13.7	$\times 10^9/L$	4.8–10.8
RBC	3.55*	4.94	$\times 10^{12}/L$	4.7–6.1
Hgb	11.4*	15.4	g/dL	14–18
Hct	32.1*	44.5	%	42–52

The parameters that are marked with an asterisk (*) have failed the delta check. What can account for the variation in the patient's results in a 24-hour period? An investigation was begun. There are two likely possibilities. *Is there a medical explanation for the change in results, or is this a preanalytic variable (mislabeling, i.e., wrong patient's results)?* The white blood cell count, red blood cell count, hemoglobin, and hematocrit have changed dramatically from Saturday to Sunday. A frequent explanation for this situation is that the patient has undergone blood transfusions causing an increase in red blood cell count, hemoglobin, and hematocrit. This patient had no transfusion history, however, and so this is not considered a factor in the dramatically increased values. The next consideration is a mislabeled sample. On a hunch, the technologist requested that the blood bank ABO type both samples. Both samples typed as O positive. No new information was obtained from this procedure. The laboratory then began another line of investigation. The floor was called, and the laboratory was informed that the patient whose laboratory results were being called (the Sunday sample) had been discharged the previous day. The sample in question (the Sunday sample) was incorrectly identified. How could the mislabeling take place? The discharged patient's name had **not** been removed from the room or from the computer system. The sample labeling had not been done at the bedside, with voice confirmation by the patient. Instead, the sample had been labeled based on the room number alone. Because of the diligence of the laboratory staff, the mistakes were identified, and any further adverse complications were prevented. The sample that the laboratory received was actually the blood from the new patient who now occupied the room. The Sunday sample results were nullified.

W O R D   K E Y

Anticoagulant • Agent that prevents or delays blood coagulation

Pathophysiology • Study of how normal processes are altered by disease

Protocol • Formal idea, plan, or scheme concerning patient care, bench work, administration, or research

References

1. Wintrobe M. Milestones on the path of progress. In: Wintrobe M, ed. Blood, Pure and Eloquent. New York: McGraw-Hill, 1980; 1–27.
2. Abramowitz M. Microscope: Basic and Beyond. Vol. 1. Melville, NY: Olympus America Inc, 2003; 1.25.
3. Wallace MA. Care and use of the microscope. In: Rodak B, ed. Hematology: Clinical Principles and Applications, 2nd ed. Philadelphia: WB Saunders, 2002; 32–34.
4. Strasinger SA, Di Lorenzo MS. Use of the microscope. In: Strasinger SA, Di Lorenzo MS, eds. Urinalysis and Body Fluids, 4th ed. Philadelphia: FA Davis, 2001; 73.
5. Patton M. Advances in microscopy. ADVANCE for Medical Laboratory Professionals 15:21–23, 2003.
6. Strasinger SA, Di Lorenzo MS. Safety in the clinical laboratory. In: Strasinger SA, Di Lorenzo MS, eds. Urinalysis and Bodily Fluids, 4th ed. Philadelphia: FA Davis, 2001; 2–5.
7. Koepke JA. Quality control and quality assurance. In Steine-Martin FA, Lotspeich-Steininger CA, Koepke JA, eds. Clinical Hematology: Principles, Procedures and Correlation, 2nd ed. Philadelphia: Lippincott, 1998; 567.
8. Finch SA. Safety in the hematology laboratory. In: Rodak BF, ed. Hematology: Clinical Principles and Applications, 2nd ed. Philadelphia: WB Saunders, 2003; 4–5.
9. Kellogg MD. Quality assurance. In: Anderson SK, Cockayne S, eds. Clinical Chemistry: Concepts and Applications. New York: McGraw-Hill, 2003; 47–49.
10. Sasse EA. Reference intervals and clinical decisions limits. In: Kaplan LA, Pesce AH, eds. Clinical Chemistry: Theory, Analysis and Correlations, 3rd ed. St. Louis: Mosby, 1996; 366–368.

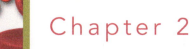

Chapter 2

From Hematopoiesis to the Complete Blood Count

Betty Ciesla

Objectives

After completing this chapter, the student will be able to:

1. Define the components of hematopoiesis.

2. Describe the organs used for hematopoiesis throughout fetal and adult life.

3. Define the microenvironment and the factors affecting differentiation of the pluripotent stem cell (PSC).

4. Describe the four functions of the spleen.

5. Differentiate between intramedullary and extramedullary hematopoiesis.

6. Define the myeloid:erythroid ratio.

7. Review the bone marrow procedure, the methods and materials, and the technologist's role in ensuring that bone marrow was recovered.

8. List the components of the complete blood count (CBC).

9. Calculate red blood cell indices.

10. Describe clinical conditions that cause valid shifts in the mean corpuscular volume.

11. Recognize normal and critical values in an automated CBC.

12. Describe ineffective and effective erythropoiesis.

13. Define the importance of correlation checks in a CBC.

14. Describe the clinical conditions that may produce polychromatophilic cells and elevate the reticulocyte count.

15. Define the morphologic classification of anemias.

16. Summarize the symptoms of anemia.

HEMATOPOIESIS: THE ORIGIN OF CELL DEVELOPMENT

Hematopoiesis is defined as the production, development, differentiation, and maturation of all blood cells. Within these four functions is cellular machinery that outstrips most high-scale manufacturers in terms of production quotas, customs specifications, and quality of final product. When one considers that the bone marrow is able to produce 3 billion red blood cells, 1.5 billion white blood cells, and 2.5 billion platelets per day per body weight,[1] the enormity of this task in terms of output is almost incomprehensible. Within the basic bone marrow structure lies the mechanisms to do the following:

1. Supply the peripheral circulation constantly with mature cells
2. Mobilize the bone marrow to increase production if hematologic conditions warrant
3. Compensate for decreased hematopoiesis by providing for hematopoietic sites outside of the bone marrow (non–bone marrow sites, liver, and spleen)

The bone marrow is extremely versatile and serves the body well by supplying life-giving cells with a multiplicity of functions. Various organs serve a role in hematopoiesis, and these organs differ from fetal to adult development. The yolk sac, liver, and spleen are the focal organs in fetal development. From 2 weeks until 2 months in fetal life, most erythropoiesis occurs in the fetal yolk sac. This period of development, known as the mesoblastic period, produces primitive erythroblasts and embryonic hemoglobins (Hgbs) such as Hgb Gower I and Gower II and Hgb Portland. These hemoglobins are constructed as tetramers with two alpha chains combined with either epsilon or zeta chains. As embryonic hemoglobins, they do not survive into adult life or participate in oxygen delivery. During the hepatic period, which continues from 2 months through 7 months of fetal life, the liver and spleen take over the hematopoietic role (Fig. 2.1). White blood cells and megakaryocytes begin to appear in small numbers. The liver serves primarily as an erythroid-producing organ but also gives rise to fetal hemoglobin, which consists of alpha and gamma chains. The spleen, thymus, and lymph nodes also become hematopoietically active during this stage, producing red blood cells and lymphocytes; however, from 7 months until birth, the bone marrow assumes the primary role in hematopoiesis, a role that continues into adult life. Additionally, Hgb A, the majority adult hemoglobin (alpha 2, beta 2), begins to form. The full complement of Hgb A is not realized until 3 to 6 months postpartum, as gamma chains from Hgb F

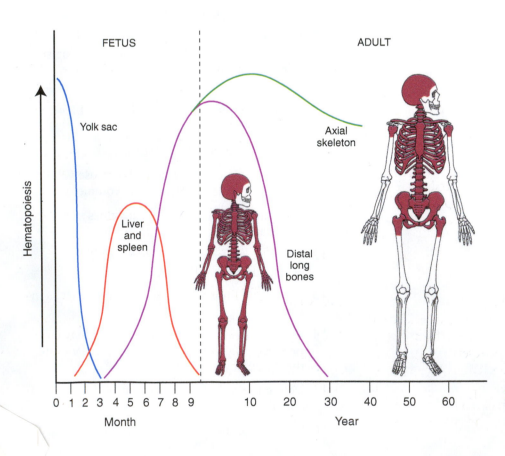

Figure 2.1 Marrow formation in fetus *(left)* versus the adult *(right)*.

are diminished and beta chains increase. In a normal individual 6 months old or older, 95% to 98% of the total hemoglobin is Hgb A, 2% to 5% is Hgb A_2, and less than 2% is Hgb F.

Hematopoiesis within the bone marrow is termed *intramedullary hematopoiesis*. The term *extramedullary hematopoiesis* describes hematopoiesis outside the bone marrow environment, primarily in the liver and spleen. Because these organs play major roles in early fetal hematopoiesis, they retain their hematopoietic memory and capability. The liver and spleen can function as organs of hematopoiesis if needed in adult life. Several circumstances within the bone marrow (e.g., infiltration of leukemic cells, tumor) may diminish the normal hematopoietic capability of the bone marrow and force these organs to perform again as primary or fetal organs of hematopoiesis. If extramedullary hematopoiesis develops, the liver and spleen become enlarged, a condition known as **hepatosplenomegaly**. Physical evidence of hepatosplenomegaly is present in an individual who looks puffy and protrusive in the left upper and slightly right upper abdominal area. Hepatosplenomegaly is always an indicator that hematologic health is compromised.

THE SPLEEN AS AN INDICATOR ORGAN OF HEMATOPOIETIC HEALTH

Few organs can match the versatility of the spleen. This small but forgotten organ, previously dismissed as inconsequential, is a powerhouse of prominent red blood cell activity such as filtration, production, and cellular immunity. Under normal circumstances, the organ cannot be felt or palpated on physical examination. Located on the left side of the body under the rib cage, the spleen is a fist-shaped organ that weighs about 8 oz, is soft in texture, and receives 5% of the cardiac output per minute. The spleen is a blood-filled organ that consists of red pulp, white pulp, and the marginal zone. The function of the red pulp is primarily red blood cell filtration, the white pulp deals with lymphocyte processing, and the marginal zone stores white blood cells and platelets.

Functions of the Spleen

There are four main tasks of the spleen that relate to red blood cell viability and the immunologic capability of the spleen. The first function is the reservoir, or storage, activity of the spleen. The spleen harbors one-third of the circulating mass of platelets and one-third of the granulocyte mass and may be able to mobilize platelets into the peripheral circulation as necessary. In the event of splenic rupture or trauma, large numbers of platelets may be spilled into the peripheral circulation. This event may predispose to unwanted clotting events because platelets serve as catalysts for hemostasis. The second function of the spleen is the filtration capacity. The spleen has a unique inspection mechanism and examines each red blood cell and platelet for abnormalities and inclusions. Older red blood cells may lose their elasticity and deformability in the last days of their 120-day life span and are culled from the circulation by splenic phagocytes. Bilirubin, iron, and globin by-products released through the culling process are recycled through the plasma and circulation.

Red blood cells that are filled with inclusions (e.g., Howell-Jolly bodies, Heinz bodies, Pappenheimer bodies) are selectively reviewed and cleared from the cells. Inclusions are "pitted" and pulled from the red blood cell without destroying the cellular integrity, and red blood cells are left to continue their journey through the circulation.[2] Antibody-coated red blood cells have their antibodies removed and usually reappear in the peripheral circulation as spherocytes, a smaller, more compact red blood cell structure with a shortened life span. One of the least appreciated roles of the spleen is the immunologic role. As the largest secondary lymphoid organ, the spleen plays a valuable role in promoting phagocytic activity for encapsulated organisms such as *Haemophilus influenzae, Streptococcus pneumoniae,* or *Neisseria meningitidis.* The spleen provides opsonizing antibodies, substances that strip the capsule from the bacterial surface. When this is accomplished, the unencapsulated bacteria are more vulnerable to the phagocytic **reticuloendothelial system (RES)**[3] and less able to mount an infection to the host system. Without a functioning spleen, this important function is negated and can lead to serious consequences, including fatality, for the infected individual. The final function of the spleen is its hematopoietic function, discussed earlier in this chapter.

Potential Risks of Splenectomy

Enlarged, infarcted, or minimally functioning spleens can cause difficulty for patients; these conditions are discussed in later chapters. Traditionally, the spleen was seen as an inconsequential and easily discarded organ that was not necessary to life function. Although the splenectomy procedure may provide hematologic benefit to patients who have problems with their spleen, individuals who do not have spleens have additional risks, as mentioned earlier. There have been reports in the literature of overwhelming postsplenectomy infections (OPSIs) that may occur years after the spleen has been removed. In most cases, these infections occur within 3 years, but some have been reported 25 years after the splenectomy. Many individuals die of OPSIs or at the very least have multiorgan involvement. As an organ of the hematopoietic system, the spleen has immense capability and provides a high value and versatility (Table 2.1). If the decision is made to remove the spleen, the surgeon should leave some splenic tissue in place and carefully manage the asplenic patient. Asplenic individuals represent a more vulnerable population.

BONE MARROW AND MYELOID: ERYTHROID RATIO

The bone marrow is one of the largest organs of the body, encompassing 3% to 6% of body weight and weighing 1500 g in an adult.[4] It is hard to conceptualize the bone marrow as an organ because it is not a solid organ that one can touch, measure, or weigh easily. Because bone marrow tissue is spread throughout the body, one can visualize it only in that context. It is composed of yellow marrow, red marrow, and an intricate supply of nutrients and blood vessels. Within this structure are erythroid cells (red blood cells), myeloid cells (white blood cells), and megakaryocytes (platelets) in various stages of maturation, along with osteoclasts, stroma, and fatty tissue.[5] Mature cells enter the peripheral circulation via the bone marrow sinuses, a central structure lined with endothelial cells that provide passage for mature cells from extravascular sites to the circulation (Fig. 2.2). The cause and effect of hematologic disease are usually rooted in the bone marrow, the central factory for production of all adult hematopoietic cells. In the first 18 years of life, bone marrow is spread throughout all of the major

bones of the skeleton, especially the long bones. As the body develops, the marrow is gradually replaced by fat until the prime locations for bone marrow in an adult become the iliac crest (located in the pelvic area) and the sternum (located in the chest area).

In terms of cellularity, there is a unique ratio in the bone marrow termed the *myeloid:erythroid (M:E)* ratio. This numerical designation provides an approximation of the myeloid elements in the marrow and their precursor cells and the erythroid elements in the marrow and their precursor cells. The normal ratio of 3:1 to 4:1 reflects the relationship between production and life span of the various cell types. White blood cells have a much shorter life span than red blood cells—6 to 10 hours for neutrophils as opposed to 120 days for erythrocytes[5]—and must be produced at a much higher rate for normal hematopoiesis.

ALTERATIONS IN MYELOID: ERYTHROID RATIO

The M:E ratio is sensitive to hematologic factors that may impair red blood cell life span, inhibit overall production, or cause dramatic increases in a particular cell line. Each of these conditions reflects bone marrow

Table 2.1 ⊙ Functions of the Spleen
Hematopoietic function Can produce white blood cells, red blood cells, and platelets if necessary
Reservoir function One-third of platelets and granulocytes are stored in the spleen
Filtration function Aging red blood cells are destroyed; spleen removes inclusion from red blood cells; if red blood cell membrane is less deformable or antibody-coated, spleen presents a hostile environment leading to production of spherocytes
Immunologic function Opsonizing antibodies are produced, trapping and processing antigens from encapsulated organs

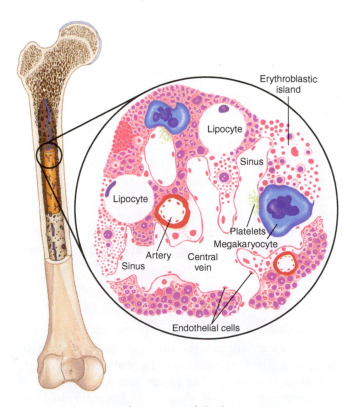

Figure 2.2 Internal structure of the bone marrow. Adapted from Glassy E. Color Atlas of Hematology: An Illustrated Guide Based on Proficiency Testing. Northfield, IL: College of American Pathologists, 1998, with permission.

dynamics through alterations of the M:E ratio. Many observations in the peripheral smear can be traced back to the pathophysiologic events at the level of bone marrow. A perfect example of this is the response of the bone marrow to anemia. As anemia develops and becomes more severe, the patient becomes symptomatic, and the kidney senses **hypoxia** secondary to a decreased hemoglobin level. Tissue hypoxia stimulates an increased release of erythropoietin (EPO), a red blood cell–stimulating hormone, from the kidney. EPO travels through the circulation and binds with a receptor on the youngest of bone marrow precursor cells, the pronormoblast (see Chapter 3). Bone marrow has the capacity to expand production six to eight times in response to an anemic event.[6] Consequently, the bone marrow delivers reticulocytes and nucleated red blood cells to the peripheral circulation prematurely if the kidney senses hypoxic stress. What is observed in the peripheral blood smear is polychromasia (stress reticulocytes, large polychromatophilic red blood cells) and nucleated red blood cells. Both of these cell types indicate that the bone marrow is regenerating in response to an event, a dynamic that represents the harmony between bone marrow and peripheral circulation.

ROLE OF STEM CELLS AND CYTOKINES

A unique feature of the bone marrow microenvironment is the presence of stem cells. These multipotential cells resemble lymphocytes and are available in the bone marrow in the ratio of one stem cell for every 1,000 non–stem cell elements.[1] Stem cells were demonstrated in the classic experiment of Till and McCullugh in 1961. These investigators irradiated the spleens and bone marrows of mice, rendering them acellular, and then injected them with bone marrow cells. Within days, colonies appeared on the spleens of the mice and were referred to as colony-forming units–spleen (CFU-S), with cells capable of regenerating into mature hematopoietic cells. In present-day terminology, CFU-S are pluripotential stem cells (Fig. 2.3). Multipotential stem cells are capable of differentiation into nonlymphoid or lymphoid precursor committed cells.[7]

Nonlymphoid committed cells develop into the entire white blood cell, red blood cell, or megakaryocytic family (CFU-GEMM). Lymphocytic committed cells (LSCs) develop into T cells or B cells, which are of different origins. T cells are responsible for cellular immunity (cell-to-cell communication), whereas B cells are responsible for humoral immunity, the production of circulating antibodies directed by plasma cells. Each of these committed cells evolves into its adult form

through proliferation, differentiation, and maturation. Chemical signals such as cytokines and interleukins are uniquely responsible for promoting a specific lineage of cell. Most of these substances are glycoproteins that target specific cell stages. They control replication and clonal or lineage selection and are responsible for maturation rate and growth inhibition of stem cells.[8] Many cytokines are available as pharmaceutical products. Recombinant technology has made it possible to purify and produce cytokines such as interleukins, EPO, granulocyte colony-stimulating factor (G-CSF), and granulocyte-macrophage colony-stimulating factor (GM-CSF). These products are used to stimulate a specific cell production to yield therapeutic benefit for patients. Specific conditions in which recombinant cytokines have been useful are as follows:[9]

1. Recovery from neutropenia resulting from **myelotoxic** therapy
2. Treatment of graft-versus-host disease after bone marrow transplant therapy
3. Increasing white blood cell counts in patients with AIDS on antiretroviral therapy
4. Stimulation of red blood cell production for chronically anemic patient and chemotherapy patients

Table 2.2 provides an abbreviated list of cytokines and the cell lines they stimulate.

ERYTHROPOIETIN

The cytokine EPO is a hormone produced by the kidneys that functions as a targeted erythroid growth factor.

Table 2.2 ⊙ Abbreviated List of Cytokines and Growth Factors	
Cytokine	**Cell Modifier**
IL-2	T cells, B cells, NK cells
IL-3	Multilineage stimulating factor
IL-4	B cells, T cells, mast cells
IL-6	Stem cells, B cells
IL-7	Pre-B cells, T cells, early granulocytes
IL-11	Megakaryocytes
GM-CSF	Granulocytes, macrophages, fibroblasts, endothelial cells
EPO	Red blood cell progenitor cells

IL, interleukin; GM, granulocyte-monocyte; CSF, colony-stimulating factor; EPO, erythropoietin; NK, natural killer; fibroblast, connective tissue support cell; endothelial cells, lining cells of blood vessels.

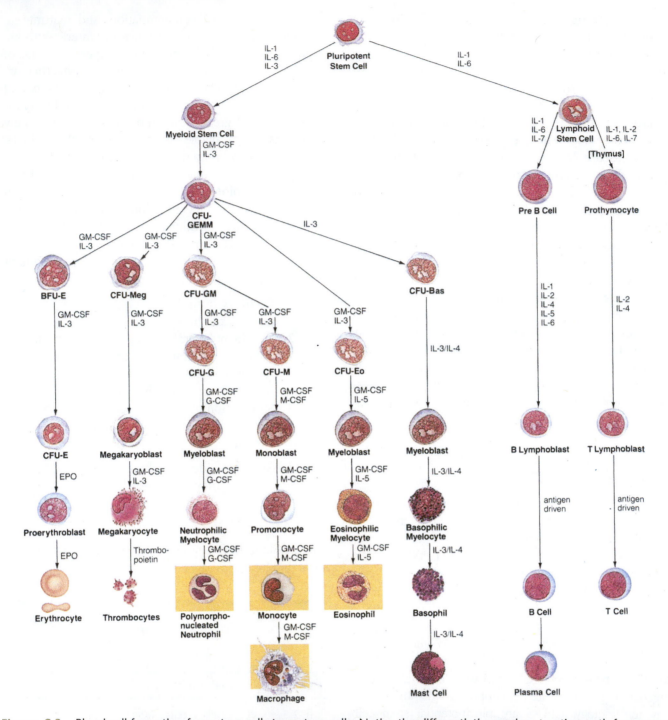

Figure 2.3 Blood cell formation from stem cells to mature cells. Notice the differentiation and maturation path from stem cells, through the CFU-GEMM to the LSC, terminating in mature cells into the peripheral circulation. CFU, colony-forming unit; GEMM, granulocyte, erythrocyte, monocyte, macrophage; IL, interleukin; LSC, lymphoid stem cell. Reproduced from Sandoz Pharmaceuticals Corporation and Schering-Plough.

This hormone has the ability to stimulate red blood cell production through a receptor on the pronormoblast, the youngest red blood cell precursor in the bone marrow. EPO is secreted on a daily basis in small amounts and functions to balance red blood cell production.[10] If the body becomes anemic, and hemoglobin levels decline, the kidney senses tissue hypoxia and secretes more EPO; consequently, red blood cell production accelerates, and younger red blood cells are released prematurely. Normal red blood cell maturation from the precursor cell, the pronormoblast, takes 5 days; with accelerated erythropoiesis, maturation decreases to 3 to 4 days. Human recombinant erythropoietin (r-HuEPO) is available as a pharmaceutical product and can be used for individuals experiencing renal disease, individuals who have become anemic as a result of **chemotherapy**, or individuals who refuse whole blood products for religious reasons.

ROLE OF THE LABORATORY PROFESSIONAL IN THE BONE MARROW PROCEDURE

Obtaining a bone marrow aspirate or biopsy specimen is an invasive and potentially painful procedure, and for this reason, this procedure is carefully evaluated before proceeding. The laboratory professional has multiple roles in the bone marrow aspirate or biopsy procedure. Fundamentally, the laboratorian may act as an assistant to the pathologist or hematologist in the preparation of materials for the procedure. Next, the technologist informs the pathologist or hematologist if the sample is acceptable or unacceptable. This judgment of the laboratory professional determines whether the procedure is repeated or completed. There are few anemias for which a bone marrow procedure is necessary for diagnostic purposes. Diagnosing white blood cell disorders such as leukemia or lymphoma, however, relies on a baseline bone marrow evaluation.

BONE MARROW PROCEDURE

In an adult patient, the iliac crest of the pelvic girdle is the site of choice, and the patient is usually face down while the physician chooses an appropriate area. The area is anesthetized with local anesthesia for the requisite amount of time, and the physician proceeds to advance the aspirate needle into the crest with a twisting, downward motion (Fig. 2.4).[11] When the needle has seeded into the marrow, its position is solid and not movable. The stylus is removed, and a syringe is placed at the end of the needle. With a quick motion, the syringe plunger is pulled back, and a small amount (approximately 1 mL) of bloody fluid and marrow spicule material is aspirated into the syringe. The laboratory professional assesses the sample for the presence of bone marrow spicules; communicates to the physician whether marrow is observed; and then proceeds to prepare slides from the aspirate material, fishing out bone marrow spicules with a microbiologic loop or pipette. If a biopsy sample is requested, the cutting blade is introduced into the bore of the needle and advanced until it enters the medullary cavity. A very small core of bone (¾ in.) is obtained. After withdrawing the cutting blade, the biopsy sample is removed by inserting a stylus and then pushing it to remove the biopsy sample. The procedure terminates as the physician withdraws the needle and applies pressure to the area. The technologist makes touch preparation of the core biopsy, using sterile tweezers to apply the biopsy sample gently to several cover slips. The remaining aspirate and biopsy material are placed in a 5% Zenker's

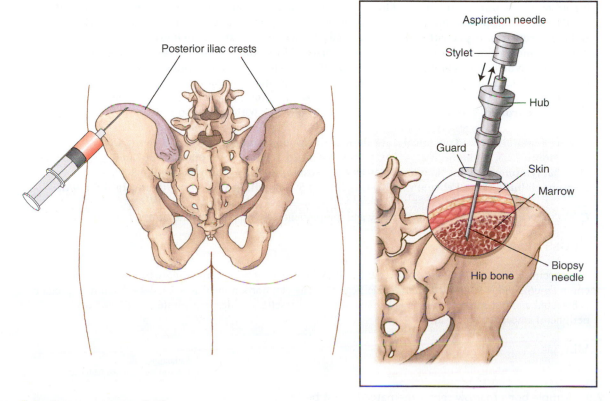

Figure 2.4 Bone marrow aspiration.

fixative and processed in the histology laboratory. The patient should remain in bed for the next hour so that pressure is applied to the aspirate location. Patients with decreased platelet counts may need to be monitored more closely and have pressure exerted on the biopsy site for longer periods after the procedure is completed.

BONE MARROW REPORT

When the slides from the biopsy or aspirate material are stained, the physician evaluates the bone marrow for overall cellularity, M:E ratio (300 to 500 cells are scanned), maturation of each cell line, marrow-to-fat

ratio, and presence of abnormal or tumor cells. The bone marrow iron store is evaluated using Prussian blue stain, and the marrow architecture is observed for abnormalities in the stromal structure (e.g., necrosis, fibrosis).[12] Combined with the patient's complete blood count (CBC), these results enable the physician to reach a diagnosis. A copy of a sample bone marrow report is included in Figure 2.5.

COMPLETE BLOOD COUNT

The CBC is one of the most frequently ordered and most time-honored laboratory tests in the hematology

---

Patient :

Pathology No. :

Med. Record No. :   **405004**
Sex : F   Age :   70
Date of Birth :   6/10/33
Location: General Hospital

Date Collected : 2/4/04
Date Received :   2/5/04
Physicians :

Specimen(s): . Bone marrow biopsy

PATHOLOGIC DIAGNOSIS:

BONE MARROW BIOPSY, ASPIRATE SMEAR AND PERIPHERAL: MYELOMA.

MICROSCOPIC DESCRIPTION:

The bone marrow is variably cellular ranging from 50 to 95 % and shows sheets of plasma cells including many immature forms. The residual bone marrow shows trilineage hematopoiesis with an ME ratio of approximately 3:1. Megakaryocytes are present and structurally unremarkable. Bone marrow iron is present and not increased. Reticulin stain shows no increase of fibrosis. Aspirate smears show adequate marrow cellularity. Maturation of both myeloid and erythroid elements is synchronous and progressive. Megakaryocytes are present and structurally unremarkable. Storage iron is present. Multiple aggregates of plasma cells including immature forms and binuclear cells are present. Peripheral smear shows Rouleaux phenomenon. Red cells are normochromic. There is anisocytosis and poikilocytosis with tear drop cells.

Recent hematologic and chemical data show white blood count 6.0, red blood count 4.66, hemoglobin 12.3, hematocrit 26.4, MCV 78.1, MCH 26.3, RDW 15.6, platelets 367,000, granulocytes 80. 3 %, lymphocytes 8.9 %, monocytes 10.1 %, eosinophil 0.4 %, and basophil 0.3 %. Immunoglobulin from February 3, 2004: IgG total 596 mg/dl, IgA 3,664 mg/dl and IgM 9 mg/dl.

COMMENT: Bone marrow morphology and immunochemistry are diagnostic of myeloma.

GROSS DESCRIPTION:

The specimen labeled "BONE MARROW BIOPSY" consists of bone marrow core biopsy measuring 2 cm in length, and is submitted after decalcification. The clot portion measures 2 x 2 x 0.8 cm in aggregate is bisected and the entire specimen is submitted in one cassette. 4 slides of aspirate smears and one peripheral smear are received.

MEH:jak

Pathologist
Electronically signed 02/06/2004

Figure 2.5 Sample bone marrow report (hematocrit must be 36.4).

laboratory. This evaluation consists of nine components and offers the clinician various hematologic data to interpret and review that directly relate to the health of the bone marrow, represented by the numbers and types of cells in the peripheral circulation. The nine components of the CBC (Fig. 2.6) are the white blood cell count (WBC), red blood cell count (RBC), hemoglobin (Hgb), hematocrit (Hct), mean corpuscular volume (MCV), mean corpuscular hemoglobin (MCH), mean corpuscular hemoglobin content (MCHC), platelet count, and red blood cell distribution width (RDW).

Depending on the type of automated instrumentation used, some of these parameters are read directly from the instrument, and some are calculated. Generally, most automated instruments directly read the WBC, RBC, Hgb, and MCV. The Hct is a calculated parameter. Correlation checks between the hemoglobin and hematocrit are a significant part of quality assurance for the CBC and are known as the "rule of three." The formulas for correlation checks/rule of three are as follows: RBC × 3 = Hgb and Hgb × 3 = Hct ± 3. As a matter of practice, each operator of any

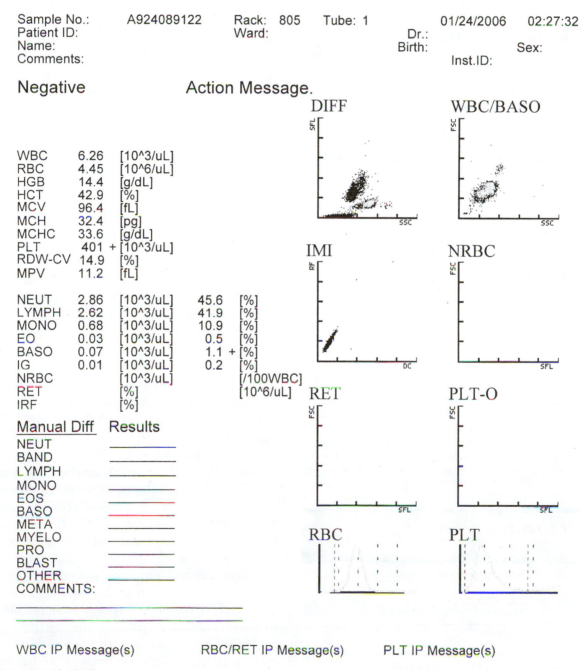

Figure 2.6   Sample CBC.

automated instrumentation should be able to establish quickly and accurately a correlation check for each sample. Failure to fall within the correlation check is usually the first indicator of postanalytic error and may indicate corrective actions, such as reviewing a peripheral smear, tracing the origin of the samples, or other investigation. Additionally, each instrument presents a pictorial representation of the hematologic data registered as either a histogram or a scatterplot, and most now offer an automated reticulocyte count. This is discussed in the procedure section. Table 2.3 presents normal values for a CBC from an adult, and Table 2.4 presents selected red blood cell values for a newborn. These data are also presented on the inside cover of this book.

Not all data on the CBC are viewed with equal importance or usefulness. In an informal study conducted by Dr. Linda Sandhaus (Director, Core Laboratory for Hematology, 2004) at the University of Cleveland, most physicians reported that the preferred information was the hemoglobin, hematocrit, platelet count, and WBC. The MCV was generally viewed as important by primary care physicians. The RDW and automated reticulocyte count were used primarily by "newer" clinicians.

MORPHOLOGIC CLASSIFICATION OF ANEMIAS

Anemias are generally classified either morphologically or according to pathophysiologic cause. The pathophysiologic approach refers to the cause of anemias—whether an anemia is caused by excessive destruction or diminished production of red blood cells. Although this is a respected approach, more clinicians are familiar with the morphologic classification of anemias that relies on the red blood cell indices: MCV, MCH, MCHC. This classification is readily available using CBC data and can be acted on fairly quickly as a means to begin an investigation into cause. There are three morphologic classifications of anemia:

- Normochromic, normocytic anemia
- Microcytic, hypochromic anemia
- Macrocytic, normochromic anemia

A *normocytic, normochromic anemia* implies a normal red blood cell MCV (80 to 100 fL) and normal hemoglobin content of red blood cells (MCHC of 32% to 36%). Although the red blood cell and hemoglobin values may be reduced, the size and hemoglobin content per cell are in the normal range. Red blood cells are normal size with a normal hemoglobin content. A *microcytic, hypochromic anemia* implies MCV of less than 80 fL with MCHC of less than 32%. In this blood picture, the red blood cells are smaller and lack hemoglobin, having an area of central pallor much greater than the usual 3-μm area. A *macrocytic, normochromic anemia* implies MCV of greater than 100 fL. Red blood cells are larger than 8 μm with hemoglobin content in the normal range. If an anemia is suspected and confirmed by a CBC, the peripheral smear picture should reflect the morphologic classification generated by automated results. For example, a patient sample with MCV of 67 fL and MCHC of 30% should have red blood cells that are small and pale. If the peripheral smear results do not correlate with the automated results, an investigation should be initiated to determine the cause of the discrepancy. A detailed explanation of

Table 2.3 ⊙ Normal Values Using SI Units	
WBC	$4.8–10.8 \times 10^9$/L
RBC	Males $4.7–6.1 \times 10^{12}$/L
	Females $4.2–5.4 \times 10^{12}$/L
Hgb	Males 14–18 g/dL
	Females 12–16 g/dL
Hct	Males 42%–52%
	Females 37%–47%
MCV	80–100 fL
MCH	27–31 pg
MCHC	32%–36%
RDW	11.5%–14.5%
Platelet count	$150–450 \times 10^9$/L

Hct, hematocrit; Hgb, hemoglobin; MCH, mean corpuscular hemoglobin; MCHC, mean corpuscular hemoglobin content; MCV, mean corpuscular volume; RBC, red blood cell count; RDW, red blood cell distribution width; WBC, white blood cell count.

Table 2.4 ⊙ Selected Red Blood Cell Values for Newborns	
RBC	$4.0–6.0 \times 10^{12}$/L
Hgb	17–23 g/dL
Hct	53%–65%
MCV	98–118 fL

Hct, hematocrit; Hgb, hemoglobin; MCV, mean corpuscular volume; RBC, red blood cell count.

anemias under each morphologic classification is provided in the subsequent chapters.

CALCULATING RED BLOOD CELL INDICES AND THEIR ROLE IN SAMPLE INTEGRITY

The red blood cell indices provide information concerning the size and hemoglobin content of red blood cells by providing the MCV, MCH, and MCHC. The MCV is one of the most stable parameters in the CBC, with little variability (less than 1%) over time.[13] For this reason, the MCV plays an extremely valuable role in monitoring the preanalytic and analytic qualities of the sample. The MCV either is directly read by the instrumentation method or is a calculated value. If it is calculated, the formula is as follows:

$$MCV = (Hct \div RBC) \times 10$$

The normal value is 80 to 100 fL and implies a red blood cell that has a size of 6 to 8 μm. Explanations for a shift in MCV include the presence of cold agglutinins (red blood cells coated with cold antibody, causing a false increase in size), transfusion therapy (newly transfused cells are larger), and reticulocytosis (presence of polychromatophilic macrocytes). Specimen or preanalytic factors that may account for a shifting MCV include the following:[14,15]

1. Contamination by drawing through the intravenous lines or indwelling catheters
2. Specimens from hyperglycemic patients
3. Specimens from patients on some chemotherapy drugs or zidovudine (AZT) therapy

Any shift in MCV that cannot be explained as a result of the previously listed circumstances should prompt the laboratory to investigate a possible sample mismatch or misidentification. As a delta check parameter, the MCV has a high value when determining sample integrity. See Table 2.5 for causes of MCV shifts.

Table 2.5 ◉ Conditions Relating to Shifts in Mean Corpuscular Volume
• Cold agglutinins (false increase)
• Transfusions
• Chemotherapy—not all drugs
• AZT (zidovudine) therapy
• Hyperglycemia—transient shifts

The MCH and MCHC provide information concerning red blood cell hemoglobin load. The MCH can be calculated by the following formula:

$$MCH = (Hgb \div RBC) \times 10$$

The normal value is 27 to 31 pg, which implies that the average weight of hemoglobin per RBC in a given amount of red blood cells is in the appropriate range. The MCHC content can be calculated using the following formula (expressed in percentage):

$$MCHC = (Hgb \div Hct) \times 100$$

The normal value is 32% to 36%, which implies that the concentration of hemoglobin per red blood cell is in the appropriate proportion.

VALUE OF THE RED BLOOD CELL DISTRIBUTION WIDTH

The eighth parameter of the CBC is the RDW, a mathematical calculation that gives insight into the amount of anisocytosis (variation in size) and, to some degree, poikilocytosis (variation in shape) in a peripheral smear. The RDW is derived as follows:

$$(\text{Standard deviation of RBC volume} \div \text{mean MCV}) \times 100$$

The normal value for RDW is 11.5% to 14.5%. The standard deviation of red blood cell volume is derived from size histogram data that plot red blood cell size after a large number of red blood cells have been analyzed by the instrument. The RDW is useful because in many cases the RDW becomes abnormal earlier in the anemia process, whereas the MCV is not affected until later in the anemic process. Because many anemias (e.g., iron deficiency anemias) develop over time, this parameter may provide a sensitive indicator of red blood cell size change[16] before the red blood cell indices become overtly abnormal.

The final item in the CBC is a platelet count. Platelet estimates and platelet morphology are discussed in Chapter 20.

CRITICAL VALUES

As mentioned in Chapter 1, critical values are values that are outside the reference range and that demand immediate action by the operator or technologist. Table 2.6 provides a list of critical values. If a patient presents with a critical value on a CBC, the physician or unit must be notified immediately. Records of this communication are essential and are a major part of quality assurance. All technologists should realize the importance and urgency of acting appropriately when a critical value has been obtained.

Table 2.6 ● Sample Critical Values

WBC
Low 3.0×10^9/L

High 25.0×10^9/L

Hgb
Low 7.0 g/dL

High 19.0 g/dL

Platelets
Low 20.0×10^9/L

High 1000×10^9/L

Hgb, hemoglobin; WBC, white blood cell count.

CLINICAL APPROACH TO ANEMIAS

Anemia is defined as a reduction in hemoglobin, RBC, and hematocrit in a given age group and gender where reference ranges have been established. Many anemias develop secondary to other conditions, but some result primarily from diseased red blood cells. Establishing a diagnosis of anemia requires a careful history and physical examination and an assessment of the patient's symptoms. A thorough family history can provide information on diet, ethnicity, history of bleeding or anemia, and medical history of relatives. Patients with moderate anemias, having hemoglobin of 7 to 10 g/dL, may show few physical symptoms because of the compensatory nature of the bone marrow. When the hemoglobin decreases to less than 7 g/dL, symptoms invariably develop. Pallor, fatigue, **tachycardia**, **syncope**, and hypotension are some of the most common signs of anemia. Pallor and hypotension are associated with decreased blood volume, fatigue and syncope are associated with decreased oxygen transport, and tachycardia and heart murmur are associated with increased cardiac output (Table 2.7).

Table 2.7 ● Symptoms of Anemia Linked to Pathophysiology

- Decreased oxygen transport leads to fatigue, **dyspnea, angina pectoris**, and syncope
- Decreased blood volume leads to pallor, **postural hypotension**, and shock
- Increased cardiac output leads to **palpitation**, strong pulse, and heart murmurs

● *Summary Points*

- Hematopoiesis is defined as the production, development, and maturation of all blood cells.
- Erythropoiesis in the fetus occurs in the yolk sac, spleen, and liver.
- Erythropoiesis in the adult occurs primarily in the bone marrow.
- Hematopoiesis within the bone marrow is termed *intramedullary hematopoiesis*; outside the bone marrow, it is termed *extramedullary hematopoiesis*.
- The bone marrow is one of the largest nonsolid organs of the body.
- The M:E ratio (3:1 to 4:1) reflects the amount of myeloid elements in the bone marrow compared with the erythroid elements in the bone marrow.
- Multipotential stem cells are capable of differentiating into nonlymphoid or lymphoid precursor committed cells.
- EPO is a hormone produced by the kidneys that regulates erythroid production.
- Bone marrow aspirate and biopsy are invasive procedures usually performed at the location of the iliac crest in adults.
- The CBC consists of nine parameters: WBC, RBC, Hgb, Hct, MCV, MCH, MCHC, RDW, and platelet count.
- The MCV is one of the most stable CBC parameters over time.
- Increases in MCV can occur as a result of transfusion, reticulocytosis, hyperglycemia, and methotrexate.
- The RDW may be an early indicator of an anemia.
- Critical values are values that are outside the reference range and that need to be immediately reported and acted on.
- The reticulocyte count is the most effective means of assessing red blood cell regeneration in response to anemic stress.
- Red blood cell production is effective when the bone marrow responds to anemic stress by producing an increased number of reticulocytes and nucleated red blood cells.
- Ineffective red blood cell production is described as death of red blood cell precursors in the bone marrow before they can be delivered to the peripheral circulation.
- Morphologic classification of anemias is determined by the red blood cell indices.

- Microcytic, hypochromic anemias are characterized by MCV of less than 80 fL and MCHC of less than 32%.
- Macrocytic, normochromic anemias are characterized by MCV of greater than 100 fL.

- Normocytic, normochromic anemias are characterized by MCV of 80 to 100 fL and MCHC of 32% to 36%.
- Normal red blood cells are disk-shaped flexible sacs filled with hemoglobin and having a size of 6 to 8 μm.

Review Questions

1. What are the organs of hematopoiesis in fetal life?
   a. Bone marrow
   b. Thymus and thyroid gland
   c. Spleen and liver
   d. Pancreas and kidneys

2. How does the bone marrow respond to anemic stress?
   a. Production is expanded, and red blood cells are released to the circulation prematurely
   b. Production is expanded, and platelets are rushed into circulation
   c. Production is diminished, and the M:E ratio is increased
   d. Production is diminished, and the M:E ratio is unaffected

3. Which chemical substances are responsible for differentiation and replication of the pluripotent stem cell?
   a. Cytokines
   b. Insulin
   c. Thyroxine
   d. Oxygen

4. A hormone released from the kidney that is unique for erythroid regeneration is
   a. Estrogen.
   b. Erythropoietin.
   c. Progestin.
   d. Testosterone.

5. In an adult, the usual location for obtaining a bone marrow aspirate is the
   a. Sternum.
   b. Iliac crest.
   c. Long bones.
   d. Lower lumbar spine.

6. What is the most stable parameter of the CBC?
   a. WBC
   b. MCV
   c. RDW
   d. Platelet count

7. Which one of the red blood cell indices reflects the concentration of hemoglobin per individual red blood cell?
   a. Hgb
   b. MCV
   c. MCHC
   d. MCH

8. Of the following formulas, which formula indicates the correlation check between hemoglobin and hematocrit?
   a. (Hgb ÷ Hct) × 100
   b. Hgb × 3 = Hct
   c. Hct = MCV × RBC
   d. (Hgb ÷ RBC) × 100

9. Which of the following CBC parameters may provide an indication of anemia before the MCV indicates an overt size change?
   a. RDW
   b. MCH
   c. WBC
   d. MCHC

10. Which of the following tests is the most effective means of assessing red blood cell generation in response to anemia?
    a. RDW
    b. Reticulocyte count
    c. Platelet count
    d. CBC

CASE STUDY

When a 50-year-old woman was referred to a hematologist for recurring pancytopenia, her WBC was 2.5×10^9/L; RBC, 2.1×10^{12}/L; Hgb, 9.0 g/dL; Hct, 30%; platelet count, 40×10^9/L; MCV, 70 fL; MCH, 26 pg; and MCHC, 30.5%. In addition to pancytopenia, she had been experiencing shortness of breath and fatigue for the past 3 weeks, and lately these symptoms had gotten worse. Her family history was unremarkable, but she explained that she has had excessive menstrual bleeding for the past 4 months. A CBC, differential, and a bone marrow examination were ordered. *What is the likely cause for this patient's pancytopenia?*

Insights to the Case Study

This patient has a microcytic, hypochromic anemia characterized by small cells lacking hemoglobin. The MCV and MCHC are outside of the normal range and have decreased. Additional studies such as serum iron, total iron binding capacity, and serum ferritin need to be initiated to determine the cause of her anemia, but with a history of menorrhagia for approximately 3 weeks, iron deficiency anemia is the most likely diagnosis. No specific diagnostic cause for the decrease in WBC was determined, and the patient will be followed with a CBC every 3 months.

○ TROUBLESHOOTING

What Do I Do When the Red Blood Cell Indices Are Extremely Elevated?

The clinical laboratory received a specimen from a 36-year-old man with a history of HIV infection. The patient had a history of multiple admissions and was being admitted this time for hyponatremia and severe anemia. The initial results are as follows:

WBC	2.3×10^9/L
RBC	142×10^{12}/L
Hgb	8.6 g/dL
Hct	18.2%
MCV	126.0 fL*
MCH	60.5 pg*
MCHC	48%*
RDW	14.5%
Platelets	85×10^6/L

In this sample, the Hgb and Hct have failed the correlation check, and the red blood cell indices in this patient are astronomically high and have been flagged by the automated instrument. The most likely explanation for these results is the development of a strong cold agglutinin in the patient's sample. Cold agglutinins or cold antibodies were first described by Landsteiner in 1903 and are usually IgM in origin. These agglutinins may occur as a primary anemia or a secondary development to a primary disorder. Individuals who have cold agglutinin disease are usually elderly and have a chronic hemolytic anemia combined with extreme sensitivity to cold temperatures leading to Raynaud's syndrome. These individuals may bind complement at colder temperature and hemolyze, causing a decreased Hgb and Hct. Agglutination in the digits and extremities may cause vascular obstruction and lead to **acrocyanosis**. In many cases, relocation to a warmer climate results in far fewer hemolytic episodes. Secondary cold agglutinins are observed in individuals with infectious mononucleosis, anti-*Mycoplasma* antibodies, cytomegalovirus antibodies, malaria, anti-hepatitis antibodies, and HIV antibodies. In each of these cases, the immune system is compromised and sets the conditions for the development of an autoantibody against the patient's cells. The resolution of the CBC is to warm the sample in a 37°C water bath for a prescribed amount of time according to laboratory protocol. The sample is then recycled through the automated instrument, and the results are compared and reported. If the cold agglutinin persists, the sample may need to be warmed for a second time to allow the results to equilibrate within reportable range. The CBC results show the patient's results after a 30-minute warming:

WBC	2.2×10^9/L
RBC	2.69×10^{12}/L
Hgb	8.6 g/dL
Hct	25.8%
MCV	95.9 fL
MCH	31.9 pg
MCHC	33.3%
RDW	20.4%
Platelets	87×10^6/L

(*Refer to reference values on front inside cover of this book.)

WORD KEY

Acrocyanosis • Blue or purple mottled discoloration of the fingers, toes, or nose (or all three)

Angina pectoris • Oppressive pain or pressure in the chest

Chemotherapy • Drug therapy used to treat infections, cancers, and other diseases

Dyspnea • Shortness of breath

Hepatosplenomegaly • Enlargement of liver and spleen

Hypoxia • Decreased oxygen

Myelotoxic • Chemicals that destroy white blood cells

Palpitation • Sensation of rapid or irregular beating of the heart

Postural hypotension • Change in blood pressure from sitting to standing

RES system • Reticuloendothelial system, the mononuclear phagocytic system

Syncope • Fainting

Tachycardia • Fast and hard heartbeat

References

1. Wallace MS. Hematopoietic theory. In: Rodak B, ed. Hematology: Clinical Procedure and Applications, 2nd ed. Philadelphia: WB Saunders, 2002; 73.
2. Tablin F, Chamberlain JK, Weiss L. The microanatomy of the mammalian spleen. In: Bowdler AJ, ed. The Complete Spleen: Structure, Function and Clinical Disorders, 2nd ed. Totowa, NJ: Humana Press, 2002; 18–20.
3. Dailey MO. The immune function of the spleen. In: Bowdler AJ, ed. The Complete Spleen: Structure, Function and Clinical Disorders, 2nd ed. Totowa, NJ: Humana Press, 2001; 54–56.
4. Singer SJ, Nicholson L. The fluid mosaic of the structure of cell membranes. Annu Rev Biochem 43:805, 1974.
5. Eshan A. Bone marrow. In: Harmening D. Clinical Hematology and Fundamentals of Hemostasis, 4th ed. Philadelphia: FA Davis, 2002.
6. Crosby WH, Akeroyd JH. The limit of hemoglobin synthesis in hereditary hemolytic anemia. Am J Med 13:273–283, 1952.
7. Herzog EL, Chai L, Krause DS. Plasticity of marrow derived stem cells. Blood 102:3483–3493, 2003.
8. Roath S, Laver J, Lawman JP, et al. Biologic control mechanism. In: Gross S, Roath S, eds. Hematology: A Problem-Oriented Approach. Baltimore: Williams & Wilkins, 1996; 7.
9. Bell A. Morphology of human blood and marrow cells. In: Harmening D, ed. Clinical Hematology and Fundamentals of Hemostasis, 4th ed. Philadelphia: FA Davis, 2002; 30–32.
10. Lappin TRJ, Rich IN. Erythropoietin: The first 90 years. Clin Lab Hematol 18:137, 1996.
11. Jamshidi K, Swaim WR. Bone marrow biopsy with unaltered architecture: A new biopsy device. J Lab Clin Med 77:335, 1971.
12. Krause J. Bone marrow overview. In: Rodak B, ed. Hematology: Clinical Procedures and Applications, 2nd ed. Philadelphia: WB Saunders, 2002; 188–195.
13. Lombarts AJPF, Leijsne B. Outdated blood and redundant buffy-coats as sources for the preparation of multiparameter controls for Coulter-type (resistive-particle) hemocytometry. Clin Chim Acta 143:7–15, 1984.
14. Savage RA, Hoffman GC. Clinical significance of osmotic matrix errors in automated hematology: The frequency of hyperglycemic osmotic matrix errors producing spurious macrocytosis. Am J Clin Pathol 80:861–865, 1983.
15. Pauler DK, Laird NM. Non-linear hierarchical models for monitoring compliance. Stat Med 21:219–229, 2002.
16. Adams-Graves P. Approach to anemia. In: Ling F, Duff P, eds. Obstetrics and Gynecology: Principles for Practice. New York: McGraw-Hill, 2001.

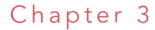

Chapter 3

Red Blood Cell Production, Function, and Relevant Red Blood Cell Morphology

Betty Ciesla

Objectives

After completing this chapter, the student will be able to:

1. Outline erythropoietic production from origin to maturation with emphasis on stages of red blood cell development.

2. Describe immature red blood cells with regard to nucleus:cytoplasm ratio, cytoplasm color, nuclear structure, and size.

3. Clarify the role of erythropoietin in health and disease.

4. Differentiate between American Society of Clinical Pathology and College of American Pathologists terminology for the red blood cell series.

5. Identify the three major red blood cell metabolism pathways essential for red blood cell energy needs.

6. Describe the composition of the red blood cell membrane with regard to key proteins and lipids.

7. Describe the components necessary for maintaining a normal red blood cell life span.

8. Outline the plasma factors that affect red blood cell life span.

9. Define anisocytosis and poikilocytosis.

10. Differentiate between microcyte and macrocyte.

11. Indicate the clinical conditions in which variations in size are seen.

12. Indicate the clinical conditions in which the variations in hemoglobin content are seen.

13. Describe the clinical conditions that show polychromatophilic cells.

14. Identify the pathophysiology and the clinical conditions that may lead to target cells, spherocytes, ovalocytes and elliptocytes, sickle cells, and fragmented cells.

15. List the most common red blood cell inclusions and the disease states in which they are observed.

BASIC RED BLOOD CELL PRODUCTION

Red blood cell production is a dynamic process that originates from pluripotent stem cells; stem cells are phenomenal structures that can give rise to many tissues, including skin, bone, and nerve cells. Next to the mapping of the human genome, the use of stem cells as therapeutic agents is one of the paramount discoveries of the 20th century. What makes stem cells so appealing is their versatility. They respond to a programmed chemical environment in bone marrow or in cell culture, replicating and eventually producing the tissue that corresponds to their chemical menu. Red blood cells derive from the committed stem cell, the CFU-GEMM described in Chapter 2. This cell, derived from the pluripotential stem cell, is under the influence of chemical signals, the cytokines that orchestrate the differentiation and maturation of the cell to a committed pathway. Red blood cells are controlled by erythropoietin (EPO), a low-molecular-weight hormone produced by the kidneys and dedicated to red blood cell regeneration. EPO travels through the circulation and locks onto a receptor on the pronormoblast, the youngest red blood cell precursor, stimulating the production of 16 mature red blood cells from every pronormoblast precursor cell (pluripotent stem cell) (Fig. 3.1).[1]

RED BLOOD CELL MATURATION

Mature red blood cells are one of the few cellular structures in the human body that begin as nucleated cells and become anucleate. This remarkable development occurs in the bone marrow over 5 days as each precursor cell goes through three successive divisions, yielding smaller and more compact red blood cells.[1] Several features of the red blood cell change dramatically: cell size decreases, the nucleus:cytoplasm (N:C) ratio decreases, nuclear chromatin becomes more condensed, and the cytoplasm color is altered during hemoglobin production (Table 3.1). A unique hormone, EPO is secreted by the kidneys and stimulates red blood cell production via a receptor on the pronormoblast (the mother red blood cell). The kidney acts as a gauge of tissue hypoxia, secreting more EPO when necessary to increase red blood cell production. In the bone marrow, erythrocytes at various stages of maturation seem to cluster in specific areas, the so-called erythroblastic island, which is easily identified in the bone marrow aspirate by the tell-tale morphologic clues of erythropoiesis—extremely round nuclear material combined with basophilic cytoplasm. The main site of erythropoiesis in adults is the bone marrow located in the sternum and iliac crest; in children, erythropoiesis takes place in the long bones and sternum.

RED BLOOD CELL TERMINOLOGY

Several nomenclatures describe the maturation stages of the red blood cell. They are presented here because many textbooks use them interchangeably. There seems to be little advantage in using one terminology over the other; however, the original intent of creating the terminologies was to clarify the terms created in the 1800s to describe

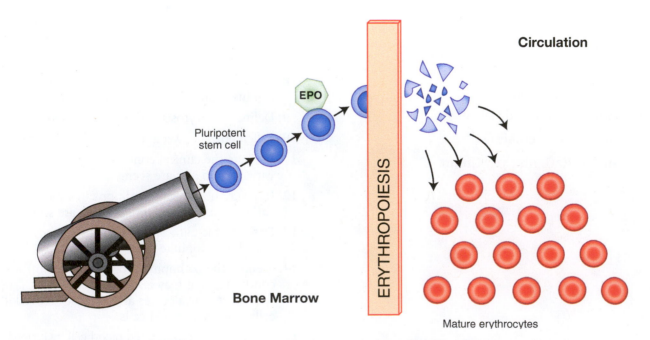

Figure 3.1 Through the erythropoietic process, a single pluripotent stem cell yields 16 mature erythrocytes.

Table 3.1 ⊙	Key Features of Red Blood Cell Development

- Nuclei are always "baseball" round
- Basophilia of cytoplasm is an indicator of immaturity
- Cell size reduces with maturity
- As hemoglobin develops, cytoplasm becomes more orange-red
- N:C ratio decreases as cell matures
- Cytoplasm of red blood cell does not contain granules
- Nuclear chromatin becomes more condensed with age
- Nucleated red blood cells are not a physiologic component of normal peripheral smear

red blood cell maturation and make the stages of maturation easier to remember and master. The College of American Pathologists (CAP) uses the word "blast" in the description of maturation stages, whereas the American Society of Clinical Pathologists (ASCP) incorporates "rubri" into the first four maturation stages (Table 3.2). CAP terminology is used throughout this textbook.[2]

MATURATION STAGES OF THE RED BLOOD CELL

There are six stages of maturation in the red blood cell series: pronormoblast, basophilic normoblast, polychromatophilic normoblast, orthochromic normoblast, reticulocyte, and mature red blood cell. In general, several morphologic clues mark the red blood cell maturation series, as follows:

- When the red blood cell is nucleated, the nucleus is "baseball" round.

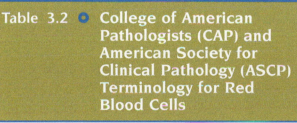

Table 3.2 ⊙ College of American Pathologists (CAP) and American Society for Clinical Pathology (ASCP) Terminology for Red Blood Cells	
CAP	**ASCP**
Pronormoblast	Rubriblast
Basophilic normoblast	Prorubricyte
Polychromatophilic normoblast	Rubricyte
Orthochromic normoblast	Metarubricyte
Reticulocyte	Reticulocyte
Erythrocyte	Erythrocyte

- There are no granules in the cytoplasm of red blood cells.
- The cytoplasm in younger cells is extremely basophilic and becomes more lavender-tinged as hemoglobin is synthesized.
- Size decreases as the cell matures.
- Nuclear chromatin material becomes more condensed in preparation for extrusion from the nucleus.
- The N:C ratio decreases as the nuclear material becomes more condensed and smaller in relationship to the entire red blood cell.

In the bone marrow and in the peripheral smear, each of these clues is helpful in enabling the technologist to stage a particular red blood cell. Identification of immature red blood cells should be systematic and based on reliable morphologic criteria. Each red blood cell maturation stage is described using size, N:C ratio, nuclear chromatin characteristics, and cytoplasm descriptions. N:C ratio is the amount of nucleus to the amount of cytoplasm present; the higher the N:C ratio, the more immature the cell. Nuclear chromatin is described with respect to chromatin distribution, chromatin texture, and color.

Pronormoblast (Fig. 3.2)

Size: 18 to 20 μm, the largest and most immature, the "mother cell"

N:C ratio: 6:1

Nuclear chromatin: Round nucleus with a densely packed chromatin, evenly distributed, fine texture with deep violet color, nucleoli may be present but are hard to visualize

Cytoplasm: Dark marine blue definitive areas of clearing

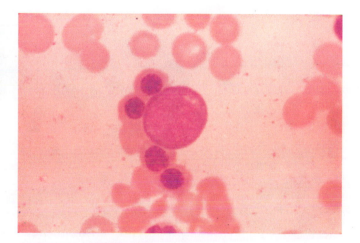

Figure 3.2 Pronormoblast. © 1967 American Society of Clinical Pathologists. Reprinted with permission.

Basophilic Normoblast (Fig. 3.3)

Size: 16 μm

N:C ratio: 6:1

Nuclear chromatin: Round nucleus with crystalline chromatin appearance, parachromatin underlayer may be visible, red-purple color to chromatin

Cytoplasm: Cornflower blue with indistinct areas of clearing

Polychromatophilic Normoblast (Fig. 3.4)

Size: 13 μm

N:C ratio: 4:1

Nuclear chromatin: Condensed, moderately compacted

Cytoplasm: Color mixture, blue layered with tinges of orange-red, "the dawn of hemoglobinization" as hemoglobin begins to be synthesized

Orthochromic Normoblast (Fig. 3.5)

Size: 8 μm

N:C ratio: 1:1

Nuclear chromatin: Dense, velvet-appearing homogeneous chromatin

Cytoplasm: Increased volume, with orange-red color tinges with slight blue tone

Reticulocyte (Polychromatic Macrocyte) (Fig. 3.6)

Size: 8 μm

Appearance: Remnant of RNA visualized as reticulum, filamentous structure in chains or as a single dotted structure in new methylene blue stain, seen in Wright's stain as large bluish red cells, polychromatophilic macrocytes

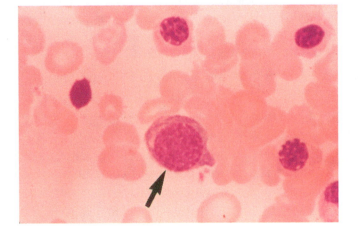

Figure 3.3 Basophilic normoblast. © 1967 American Society of Clinical Pathologists. Reprinted with permission.

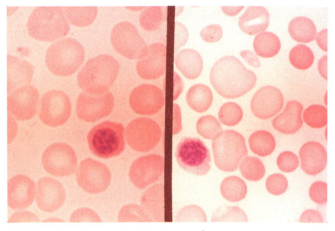

Figure 3.5 Orthochromic normoblast. © 1967 American Society of Clinical Pathologists. Reprinted with permission.

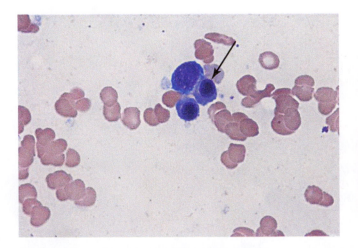

Figure 3.4 Polychromatophilic normoblast. Courtesy of Bernardino Madsen, Casper College, Wyoming.

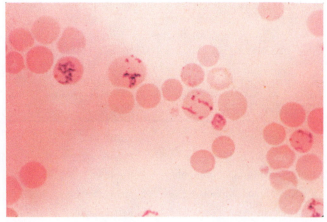

Figure 3.6 Reticulocyte. © 1967 American Society of Clinical Pathologists. Reprinted with permission.

Mature Red Blood Cell (Fig. 3.7)

Size: 6 to 8 µm

Appearance: Disk-shaped cell filled with hemoglobin, having an area of central **pallor of 1 to 3 µm**

RED BLOOD CELL MEMBRANE DEVELOPMENT AND FUNCTION

The mature red blood cell is a magnificently designed instrument for hemoglobin delivery. As a hemoglobin-filled sac, the red blood cell travels more than 300 miles through the peripheral circulation, submitting itself to the swift waters of the circulatory system, squeezing through the threadlike splenic sinuses, and bathing in the plasma microenvironment. Cellular and environmental factors contribute to red blood cell survival. For the red blood cell to survive for its 120-day life cycle, the following conditions are necessary:

- The red blood cell membrane must be deformable.
- Hemoglobin structure and function must be adequate.
- The red blood cell must maintain osmotic balance and permeability.

The mature red blood cell is an anucleate structure with no capacity to synthesize protein, but it is capable of a limited metabolism that enables it to survive for 120 days.[3] An intact, competent, and fully functioning red blood cell membrane is an essential ingredient to a successful red blood cell life span. The

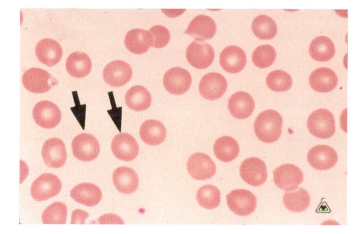

Figure 3.7 Normal red blood cell. Note discocyte shape and small area of central pallor. From The College of American Pathologists, with permission.

membrane of the red blood cell is a trilaminar and three-dimensional structure containing glycolipids and glycoproteins on the outermost layer directly beneath the red blood cell membrane surface. Cholesterol and phospholipids form the central layer, and the inner layer, the **cytoskeleton**, contains the specific membrane protein, spectrin, and ankyrin (Fig. 3.8).

Composition of Lipids in the Interior and Exterior Layers

Fifty percent of the red blood cell membrane is protein, 40% is lipid, and the remaining 10% is cholesterol. The lipid fraction is a two-dimensional interactive fluid that serves as a barrier to most water-soluble

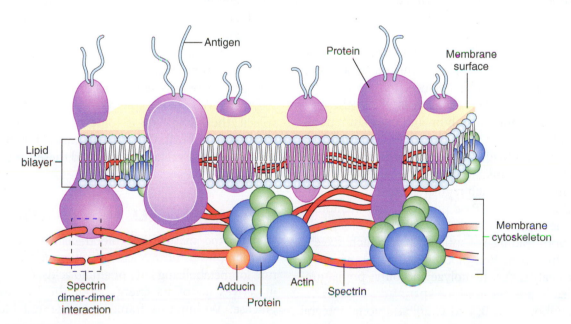

Figure 3.8 Red blood cell membrane. Note placement of integral proteins (glycophorins—in purple) versus peripheral protein (spectrin).

molecules. Cholesterol is equally distributed through the red blood cell membrane and constitutes 25% of the membrane lipid; however, plasma cholesterol and membrane cholesterol are in constant exchange. Cholesterol may accumulate on the surface of the red blood cell membrane in response to excessive accumulation in the plasma. Increased plasma cholesterol causes increased deposition of cholesterol on the red blood cell surface. The red blood cell becomes heavier and thicker, causing rearrangement of hemoglobin. This may be one pathway to the formation of target cells and acanthocytes, red blood cell morphologies that exhibit decreased red blood cell survival. Acanthocytes may also develop subsequent to cholesterol depositions in patients with liver disease and lecithin cholesterol acetyltransferase (LCAT) deficiency.

Composition of Proteins in the Lipid Bilayers: Integral Proteins

The protein matrix of the red blood cell membrane is supported by two types of protein. The **integral** proteins start from the cytoskeleton and expand through the membrane to penetrate the other edge of the red blood cell surface. **Peripheral** proteins are confined to the red blood cell cytoskeleton. The integral proteins provide the backbone for the active and passive transport of the red blood cell and provide supporting structure for more than 30 red blood cell antigens.[3] Ions and gases move across the red blood cell membrane in an organized and harmonious fashion. Water (H_2O), chloride (Cl), and bicarbonate (HCO_3) diffuse freely across the red blood cell membrane as a result of specialized channels, such as aquaphorins. Other ions such as sodium (Na^+), potassium (K^+), and calcium (Ca^{2+}) are more highly regulated by a careful intracellular-to-extracellular balance. For sodium, the ratio is 1:12, and for potassium, it is 25:1[4]; the ratio represents the amount of sodium and potassium transport in and out of the cell. This ratio is the optimal ratio for red blood cell survival and is controlled by cationic energy pumps requiring ATP for Na^+ and K^+ and by calmodulin, which regulates calcium migration through the calcium-ATPase pumps. If the membrane becomes more permeable to Na^+, rigid red blood cells may develop leading to spherocytes, which have a decreased life span. Red blood cells, which are more water permeable, may hemolyze and burst prematurely, again leading to reduced life span.

Glycophorins A, B, and C are additional integral membrane proteins, containing 60% carbohydrates and most of the membrane sialic acid, which imparts a net negative charge to the red blood cell surface. Many red blood cell antigens are located on this portion of the membrane. Red blood cell antigens M and N are located on glycophorin A, whereas red blood cell antigens S and s are located on glycophorin B. Glycophorin C provides a point of attachment to the cytoskeleton or inner layer of the red blood cell membrane.

Cytoskeleton: Peripheral Proteins

The cytoskeleton is an interlocking network of proteins that play a significant role in the deformability and elasticity of the red blood cell membrane. The third layer of the red blood cell membrane supports the lipid bilayer and supplies the peripheral proteins. Spectrin and ankyrin are peripheral proteins that are responsible for the deformability properties of the red blood cell. Deformability and elasticity are crucial properties to red blood cells because the red blood cell with an average diameter of 6 to 8 μm must maneuver through vascular apertures such as the splenic cords and capillary arterioles, which have diameters of 1 to 3 μm. The intact and deformable red blood cell can stretch 117% of its surface area as it weathers the turmoil of circulation, squeezing through small spaces.

Inherited abnormalities of spectrin can lead to the production of spherocytes, a more compact red blood cell with a reduced life span. Spectrin-deficient red blood cells are normal in size; they are shaped after they exit the bone marrow. It is only when they are pushed into the systemic circulation and subjected to the rigors of the spleen that the outer layer of the red blood cell membrane is shaved, leading to the more compact and damaged cell, the spherocyte. This particular spherocyte mechanism, which occurs in hereditary spherocytosis, best illustrates the progressive loss of membrane that occurs in hereditary spherocytosis. When the spherocyte is reviewed by the spleen, the membrane is removed, leaving a remodeled red blood cell. Other mechanisms for the formation of spherocytes may occur, and these are discussed later.

RED BLOOD CELL METABOLISM

Because the mature red blood cell is an anucleate structure, it has no nuclear or mitochondrial architecture for metabolizing fatty or amino acids. Consequently, it derives all of its energy from the breakdown of glucose. Within this framework, the red blood cell must maintain its shape, keep hemoglobin in the reduced (Fe^{2+}) state, and move electrolytes across the membrane. Three metabolic pathways are essential for red blood cell function, as follows:

1. The Embden-Meyerhof pathway provides 90% of cellular ATP because red blood cell metabolism is essentially **anaerobic.** The functions of ATP are multifactorial and include maintenance of membrane integrity, regulation of the intracellular and extracellular pumps, maintenance of hemoglobin function, and replacement of membrane lipids.[5] This pathway also generates NAD$^+$ from NADH, an important structure in the formation of 2,3-diphosphoglycerate, a key element to oxygen loading and unloading.

2. The phosphogluconate pathway provides 5% to 10% of the ATP necessary so that reduced NADPH is produced and globin chains are not degraded when subjected to oxidative stress and the accumulation of hydrogen peroxide. If this pathway is deficient, globin chains may precipitate, forming Heinz body inclusions in the red blood cell. Heinz body inclusions lead to the formation of bite cells in the peripheral blood as Heinz bodies are pitted from the cell by the spleen.

3. The methemoglobin reductase pathway, which maintains hemoglobin iron in the reduced ferrous state (Fe^{2+}) so that oxygen can be delivered to the tissues, is dependent on the reduction of NAD to NADPH (Fig. 3.9). If NADPH is absent, methemoglobin accumulates in the red blood cells. Oxygen transport capabilities are seriously impaired because methemoglobin cannot combine with oxygen.

ABNORMAL RED BLOOD CELL MORPHOLOGY

Automated instrumentation in hematology has redefined the level of practice in most hematology laboratories. Along with the complete blood count (CBC), most instruments offer an automated differential count. When values from the differential or CBC are out of the reference range, results are flagged. If a result is flagged, the operator or technologist must make a decision either to perform reflex testing or to pull a peripheral smear for review or complete differential to resolve the abnormal result. The smears that are scanned or reviewed are from patients who are more seriously ill, however, and may have illness with multiple **pathologies**. For this reason, proficiency in identifying normal and abnormal red blood cells is a desirable skill, one that must be practiced as a student and an employee. This section concentrates on defining abnormal red blood cell morphology and the pathologies that cause that morphology. Automated cell counting and differential counters have not yet replaced the well-trained eye with respect to the subtleties of red blood cell morphology.

There is no substitute for a well-distributed, well-stained peripheral smear when assessing red blood cell morphology. When it is established that the peripheral smear is well distributed and well stained, two principal questions must be asked when an abnormal morphology is observed:

1. Is the morphology in every field?
2. Is the morphology artificial or pathologic?

Technologists review approximately 10 well-stained and well-distributed fields in a peripheral smear and then make a judgment about whether anisocytosis (variation in size) and poikilocytosis (variation in shape) are present. If these are present, technologists proceed to record and quantitate the size and shape changes. A numerical scale or qualitative remarks are used to grade the specific morphology. Numeric procedures for assessing red blood cell morphology are explained in Chapter 20. What is most important in the assessment of red blood cell morphology is the discovery of the physiologic cause for the creation of that morphology so that the patient can be treated and his or her hematologic health restored.

Variations in Red Blood Cell Size

A normal red blood cell is a disk-shaped structure that is approximately 6 to 8 μm and has a mean corpuscular volume (MCV) of 80 to 100 fL and a mean corpuscular hemoglobin content (MCHC) of 32% to 36%. Variations in size are seen as microcytes (less than 6 μm) or macrocytes (greater than 9 μm). Microcytic cells result from four main clinical conditions: iron deficiency anemia, thalassemic syndromes, iron overload conditions, and anemia of chronic disorders.

Microcytic cells are part of the clinical picture in iron deficiency anemia and result from impaired iron metabolism caused by either deficient iron intake or defective iron absorption.[6] Iron is an essential element to the formation of the hemoglobin molecule. The heme portion of hemoglobin is formed from having four iron atoms surrounded by the protoporphyrin

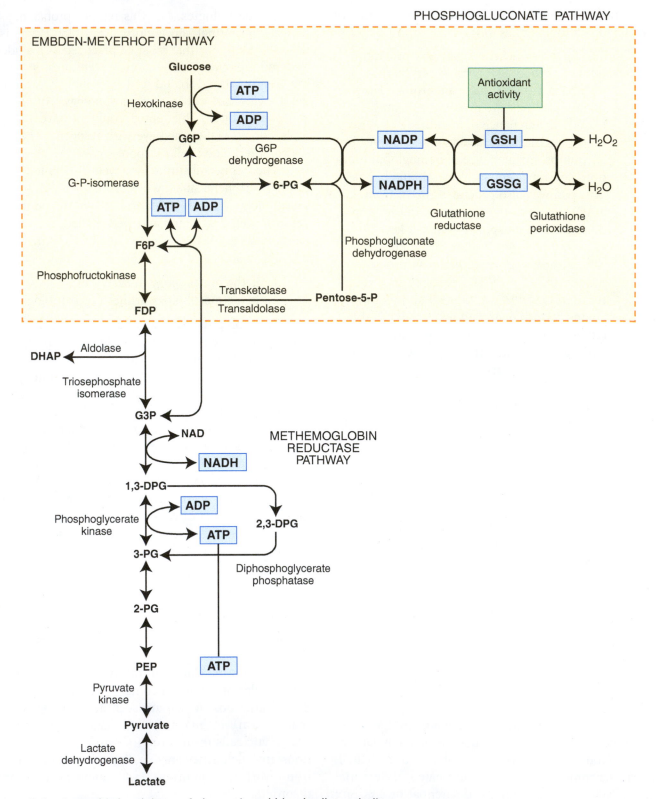

Figure 3.9   Anaerobic breakdown of glucose in red blood cell metabolism.   Adapted from Hillman RF, Finch CA. Red Cell Manual, ed 7. Philadelphia: FA Davis, 1996; 15, with permission.

ring. Two pairs of globin chains are assembled onto the molecule, with the heme structure lodged in the pockets of the globin chains. Iron needs to be incorporated into the four heme structures of each hemoglobin molecule and needs to be absorbed from the bloodstream and transferred, via transferrin, to the pronormoblasts of the bone marrow for incorporation into the heme structure. Iron-starved red blood cells divide more rapidly than normal red blood cells, searching for iron, and are smaller because of these rapid divisions.

The thalassemic conditions give rise to microcytes owing to decreased or absent globin synthesis. When either alpha or beta chains are missing or diminished, normal adult hemoglobin is not synthesized, and hemoglobin configuration is impaired, leading to microcytic cells that have an increased central pallor, known as hypochromia. The third microcytic mechanism occurs in red blood cells from individuals who have iron overload disorders, such as hereditary hemochromatosis. These individuals show a dimorphic blood smear—some microcytes mixed with macrocytes, some red blood cells exhibiting normal hemoglobin levels, and some showing hypochromia. The final microcytic mechanism is from individuals who have the anemia of inflammation. Approximately 10% of these individuals, who have the anemia of inflammation arising from renal failure or thyroid dysfunction, also show microcytic red blood cells in their peripheral smear because iron delivery to the reticuloendothelial system is impaired.

All immature red blood cells are nucleated structures, and nuclear synthesis depends on vitamin B_{12} and folic acid. If either of these vitamins is unavailable or cannot be absorbed through the gastrointestinal system, a macrocytic cell evolves. More information concerning vitamin B_{12} and folic acid is available in Chapter 6. Macrocytic red blood cells have a diminished life span, and a megaloblastic anemia develops with MCV that exceeds 110 fL. In the bone marrow, erythropoiesis is ineffective because the red blood cell precursors are prematurely destroyed before they are released into the peripheral circulation.[7] Additionally, an **asynchrony** develops between the nuclear structure and the cytoplasm, as nuclear development and hemoglobin development become unbalanced. The nuclear age appears to be out of sync with the cytoplasm development. A pancytopenia is noted in the CBC, and hypersegmented neutrophils and macroovalocytes are also part of the megaloblastic picture. In individuals who have borderline increased MCV, large cells may be generated subsequent to alcoholism and liver disease, or the increase in MCV may result from high reticulocyte counts where polychromatophilic macrocytes are seen in the peripheral smear (Fig. 3.10).

Variations in Red Blood Cell Color

Color variations in red blood cells are observed as polychromasia or hypochromia. Polychromasia occurs subsequent to excessive production of red blood cell precursors in response to anemic stress. When the bone marrow responds to anemic stress, it

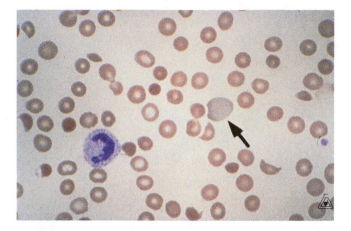

Figure 3.10   Polychromatophilic macrocyte.   From The College of American Pathologists, with permission.

releases reticulocytes and, sometimes, orthochromic normoblasts (nucleated red blood cells [nRBCs]) prematurely. In the peripheral smear, increased polychromasia, red blood cells that are gray-blue and larger than normal, is seen. Polychromatophilic macrocytes are actually reticulocytes; however, the reticulum can be visualized only when these cells are stained with supravital stain. The presence of polychromasia is an excellent indicator of bone marrow health. Polychromasia is observed in the following situations:

- When the bone marrow is responding to anemia
- When therapy is instituted for iron deficiency anemia or megaloblastic anemia
- When the bone marrow is being stimulated as a result of a chronic hematologic condition, such as thalassemia or sickle cell disorders

Hypochromic red blood cells exhibit a larger than normal area of central pallor (greater than 3 µm) and are usually seen in conditions in which hemoglobin synthesis is impaired. Most hypochromic cells have an MCHC of less than 32%. The development of hypochromia is usually a gradual process and can be seen on the peripheral smear as a delicately shaded area of hemoglobin within the red blood cell structure. Any starkly defined area of red blood cell pallor is usually artifactual and not true hypochromia. Not all hypochromic cells are microcytic, but all microcytic cells are hypochromic. Hypochromia of varying degrees can be seen in iron deficiency anemia, in thalassemic conditions, and in the sideroblastic processes (Fig. 3.11).

Variations in Red Blood Cell Shape

Variations in the shape of the red blood cell are always linked to a red blood cell pathophysiology. Abnormal

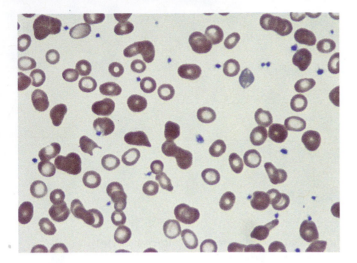

Figure 3.11 Hypochromia.   Courtesy of Kathleen Finnegan, Stony Brook University, New York.

red blood cell morphology presents the morphologist with visual clues for what might be the source of the patient's hematologic problems, whether it is decreased red blood cell production, increased destruction, or defective splenic function. Five distinct morphologies are discussed. Although these are not all-inclusive, they represent most abnormalities seen in a metropolitan population.

Spherocytes

Spherocytes are compact red blood cells with a near-normal MCV and an elevated MCHC, usually greater than 36%. They are easily recognized among the rest of the red blood cell background on the peripheral smear because they are dense, dark, and small (Fig. 3.12). Spherocytes arrive in the peripheral circulation via three distinct mechanisms.

The first mechanism involves individuals who have hereditary spherocytosis (HS), which results from inherited spectrin abnormalities. Mature red blood cells in patients with HS arrive in the peripheral circulation with a normal appearance, but as the cells try to negotiate the splenic sinuses, the spleen senses the membrane imperfections and shears the exterior membrane, leaving a more compact but osmotically fragile structure—the spherocyte. The restructured red blood cell has a reduced life span, and the patient has a life-long moderate anemia. Second, aging red blood cells lose pieces of membrane during senescence. Because red blood cells pass through the spleen hundreds of times during their 120-day life cycle, older and less perfect red blood cells are trapped by this organ and rendered as spherocytes, where they are eventually removed by the reticuloendothelial system. The final pathophysiology producing a spherocyte involves the formation of antibody-coated red blood cells, which occurs subsequent to an autoimmune or immune process. As antibody-coated cells percolate through the spleen, the antibody coating is removed, and small amounts of red blood cell membrane are lost. The cell that is left to traverse the circulation—the spherocyte—is smaller, denser, and more fragile in its microenvironment.

Sickle Cells

Sickle cells are a highly recognizable red blood cell morphology, with a crescent shape and pointed projections at one of the terminal ends of the red blood cell (Fig. 3.13). Individuals with sickle cells have sickle hemoglobin as one component of their adult hemoglobin complement. Sickle hemoglobin (Hgb S) is an abnormal hemoglobin. Red blood cells containing Hgb S homozygously have a dramatically reduced life span owing to the fact that sickle hemoglobin is intractable and forms tactoids under conditions of hypoxic stress. When red blood cells containing Hgb S try to maneuver through the spleen and the kidney, the hemoglobin

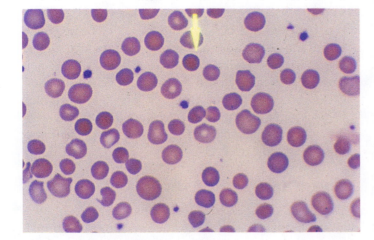

Figure 3.12 Spherocyte. Note the density of spherocytes compared with the red blood cell background.
From The College of American Pathologists, with permission.

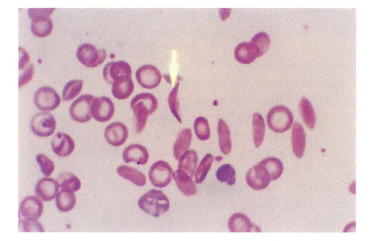

Figure 3.13   Sickle cell. Note pointed projection.   From The College of American Pathologists, with permission.

lines up in stiff bundles. This makes the red blood cell less elastic and unable to squeeze through the micro-circulation of the spleen. The cell deforms, takes the sickle shape, and is permanently harmed. Many sickle cells may revert to normal disk shape on oxygenation, but approximately 10% are unable to revert; these are labeled as irreversible sickle cells. Reversible sickle cells appear in the peripheral smear as thicker, more round-ed, half-moon–shaped cells with no pointed projec-tions. When properly oxygenated, they resume the nor-mal disk-shaped structure of the red blood cells. Sickle cells may appear in combination with other disorders, such as hemoglobin SC and hemoglobin S–thalassemia.

Stomatocytes

Stomatocytes appear with elongated areas of central pallor approximately three-fourths the diameter of the red blood cells. Several chemical agents, such as phenothiazine and chlorpromazine, can induce this morphology. The osmotic fragility of these cells

increases owing to elevated sodium intake through the red blood cell membrane. Stomatocytes are often induced artifactually and can be distinguished from true stomatocytes by their more defined outline. Genuine stomatocytes are shaded within the hemoglo-bin of the red blood cell. Stomatocytes can be seen in the Rh null phenotype, in hereditary stomatocytosis (rare), and in some alcoholic conditions (Fig. 3.14).

Ovalocytes and Elliptocytes

Ovalocytes and elliptocytes are red blood cell mor-phologies that are often used interchangeably, yet these two distinct morphologies have several recognizable differences (Fig. 3.15). Ovalocytes are egg-shaped and capable of many variations of hemoglobin distribution. These cells may appear macrocytic, hypochromic, or normochromic. Ovalocytes—more specifically, macro-ovalocytes—may be observed in the megaloblastic process. Normochromic ovalocytes are typically seen in thalassemic syndromes.

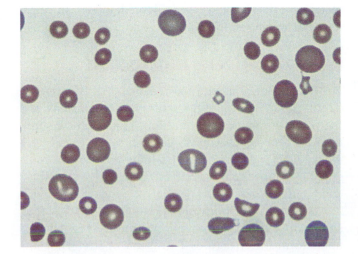

Figure 3.14   Stomatocyte. Note central red blood cell with slitlike hypochromia.   Courtesy of Bernardino Madsen, Casper College, Wyoming.

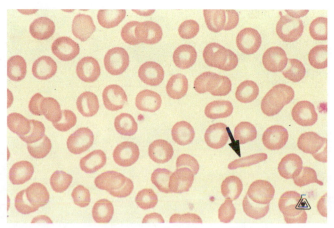

Figure 3.15   Elliptocyte.   From The College of American Pathologists, with permission.

Elliptocytes are a distinct morphology derived from abnormal spectrin and protein 4.1 component, both red blood cell membrane proteins. In the primary condition, hereditary elliptocytosis, elliptocytes are the predominant morphology, yet this condition is fairly benign with little consequence to the red blood cell. The other two genotypes of this disorder, hereditary pyropoikilocytosis and spherocytic hereditary elliptocytosis, are a much more serious morphology, with severe anemia. They are discussed in Chapter 7. Elliptocytes may also be present in the peripheral smear of iron-deficient individuals and in patients with idiopathic myelofibrosis.

Target Cells

Target cells appear in the peripheral smear as a bull's eye–shaped cell. They are seen in the peripheral blood owing to three mechanisms: (1) as an artifact, (2) because of decreased volume secondary to loss of hemoglobin, and (3) because of increased red blood cell surface membrane (Fig. 3.16). As cholesterol increases in the plasma, the red blood cell surface expands, resulting in increased surface area. Target cells appear as hypochromic, with a volume of hemoglobin rimming the cells and a thin layer of hemoglobin located centrally, eccentrically, or as a thick band. As a morphology, target cells appear in iron deficiency anemia, hemoglobin C disease and associated conditions, liver disease, and after **splenectomy**. When hemoglobin is affected qualitatively, target cells appear. Figure 3.17 shows a schematic of target cell formation.

Acanthocytes

Acanthocytes represent a peculiar red blood cell morphology that is marked by smaller size because they are surrounded by uneven, thornlike spicules

projecting from the red blood cell surface (Fig. 3.18). Spicules can range in number from three to nine and must be distinguished from the burr cell, in which even projections arise from the red blood cell surface. Excess cholesterol, increased surface area, and decreased lecithin are features of acanthocytes. Consequently, acanthocytes may appear in liver disease, autoimmune hemolytic anemia, McLeod syndrome (lack of Kell antigens), and LCAT deficiency. High numbers of acanthocytes appear in congenital abetalipoproteinemia.

Fragmented Cells

Fragmented cells represent a group of variant morphologies ranging from schistocytes to helmet cells. Regardless of the pathophysiology, these cells appear fragmented; pieces of the red blood cell membranes have been sheared, and hemoglobin leaks through the membranes, causing anemia. Physiologic events that may cause this situation include the formation of large inclusions (Heinz bodies) or the predispositions of **thrombi**. Heinz bodies are large inclusions that form in the red blood cell because of oxidative stress, usually in patients with glucose-6-phosphate dehydrogenase deficiency (see Chapter 7). As the inclusion-rich red blood cells try to negotiate the spleen, the inclusion-rich cell is pitted, leaving a helmet cell (Fig. 3.19). Schistocytes may be encountered because of shear stress from systemic thrombin disposition resulting from **disseminated intravascular coagulation** or thrombotic thrombocytopenic purpura.[8] They may also occur in burn patients or patients who have undergone heart valve surgery. Burr cells are usually seen in conditions of uremia or dehydration, conditions that result from a change in tonicity of circulating fluids (Fig. 3.20). Additionally, burr cells may occur in blood smears that have been forced to dry through repeated waving in the air. See Table 3.3.

RED BLOOD CELL INCLUSIONS

The cytoplasm of all normal red blood cells is free of debris, granules, or other structures. Inclusions are the result of distinctive conditions. This section summarizes four of the most common red blood cell inclusions (Table 3.4): Howell-Jolly bodies, siderotic granules/Pappenheimer bodies, basophilic stippling, and Heinz bodies.

Howell-Jolly bodies are remnants of DNA that appear in the red blood cell as round, deep purple, nondeformable structures 1 to 2 μm in size. They are eccentrically located in the cytoplasm and seen when erythropoiesis is rushed. Howell-Jolly bodies are

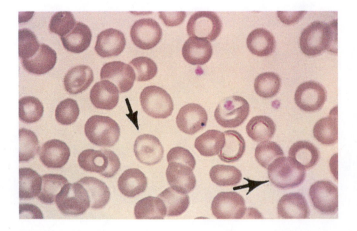

Figure 3.16 **Target cell.** From The College of American Pathologists, with permission.

How Target Cells Are Formed

As a result of artifacts, air-drying, and hemoglobin precipitation:
Examples: High humidity, slow drying, and hemoglobin C

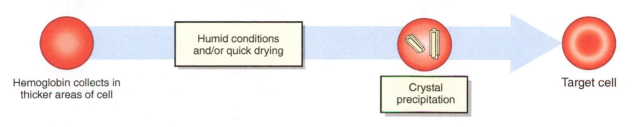

Hemoglobin collects in thicker areas of cell

Humid conditions and/or quick drying

Crystal precipitation

Target cell

As a result of decreased volume:
Examples: Iron deficiency, thalassemia, and hemoglobinopathies (Hb S, E)

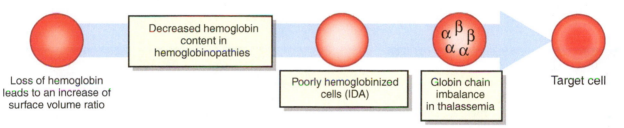

Loss of hemoglobin leads to an increase of surface volume ratio

Decreased hemoglobin content in hemoglobinopathies

Poorly hemoglobinized cells (IDA)

Globin chain imbalance in thalassemia

Target cell

As a result of increased surface membrane:
Examples: Liver disease (obstructive jaundice), LCAT deficiency, and asplenism

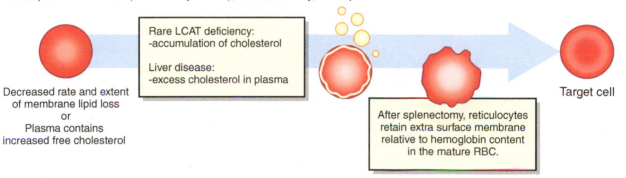

Decreased rate and extent of membrane lipid loss
or
Plasma contains increased free cholesterol

Rare LCAT deficiency:
-accumulation of cholesterol

Liver disease:
-excess cholesterol in plasma

After splenectomy, reticulocytes retain extra surface membrane relative to hemoglobin content in the mature RBC.

Target cell

Figure 3.17 Three possibilities for target cell formation. Adapted from Glassy E. Color Atlas of Hematology: An Illustrated Guide Based on Proficiency Testing. Northfield, IL: College of American Pathologists, 1998, with permission.

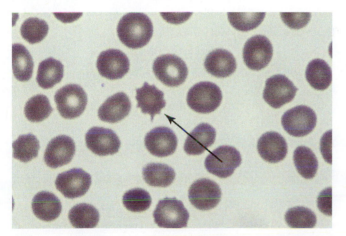

Figure 3.18 Acanthocytes. Note uneven thorny projections.
Courtesy of Bernardino Madsen, Casper College, Wyoming.

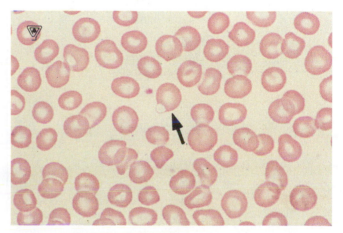

Figure 3.19 Bite cells (helmet cells). From The College of American Pathologists, with permission.

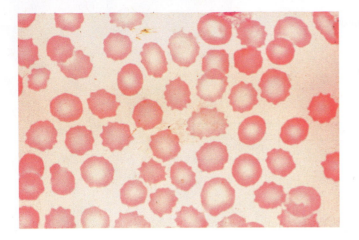

Figure 3.20   Burr cells.   © 1967 American Society of Clinical Pathologists.
Reprinted with permission.

thought to represent remnants of the orthochromic normoblast nucleus as it is extruded from the cytoplasm. The spleen usually pits these inclusions from the cytoplasm, but when the bone marrow responds to anemic conditions the spleen cannot keep pace with Howell-Jolly body formation. Numerous Howell-Jolly bodies may be observed in postsplenectomy, patients; however, because the spleen is unavailable to inspect and remove them from the cell cytoplasm (Fig. 3.21).

Siderotic granules/Pappenheimer bodies are seen in the iron loading processes such as hereditary hemochromatosis and iron loading anemias after transfusion therapy. They appear as small, light purple, beaded inclusions, located along the periphery of the red blood cells. Prussian blue staining is confirmatory

Table 3.3 ○ Red Blood Cell Morphologies Matched to Clinical Conditions

Red Blood Cell Morphology	Relative Clinical Conditions	Red Blood Cell Morphology	Relative Clinical Conditions
Schistocytes	Burns and heart valve implants	Ovalocytes/ Elliptocytes	Hereditary ovalocytosis
	Disseminated intravascular coagulation (DIC)		Iron deficiency anemia
	Hemolytic uremic syndrome (HUS)		Megaloblastic anemia
	Thrombotic thrombocytopenic purpura (TTP)		Pernicious anemia
	Bite cells—G6PD deficiency		Iron deficiency anemia
	Renal transplant patients	Sickle cells	Sickle cell anemia
Microcytes	Iron deficiency	Spherocytes	ABO incompatibility
	Thalassemic conditions		DIC
Macrocytes	Megaloblastic anemias (vitamin B_{12} deficiency and folic acid deficiency)		Bacterial toxins
			Autoimmune hemolytic anemias
	Pernicious anemia		Blood transfusion reactions
	Increased reticulocytes		Hereditary spherocytosis
Acanthocytes	Abetalipoproteinemia	Stomatocyte	Alcoholism
	Neonatal hepatitis		Hereditary spherocytosis
	Postsplenectomy		Malignancies
	Vitamin E deficiency		Rh null syndrome
	Cirrhosis of liver with associated hemolytic anemia	Target cells	Hemoglobinopathies
			Sickle cell thalassemia
	McLeod syndrome		Hemolytic anemias
Burr cells	Burns		Iron deficiency
	Gastric carcinoma		Liver disease including cirrhosis
	Peptic ulcers		Postsplenectomy
	Renal insufficiency	Teardrops	Myeloproliferative syndromes
	Uremia		Severe anemias
	Pyruvate kinase deficiency		

Table 3.4 ⊙ Summary of Inclusions	
Inclusion	**Composition**
Howell-Jolly body	DNA in origin
Basophilic stippling	RNA remnants
Siderotic granules/ Pappenheimer bodies	Iron
Heinz bodies	Denatured hemoglobin

in determining whether these inclusions are iron in origin; consequently, these inclusions are termed siderotic granules in Prussian blue staining and Pappenheimer bodies in Wright's stain. Siderotic granules may also be viewed in thalassemic conditions and in postsplenectomy patients (Fig. 3.22).

Basophilic stippling is a result of RNA and mitochondrial remnants. These remnants appear as diffusely basophilic granules located throughout the cytoplasm and are either dustlike or coarse in appearance. They are difficult to visualize in the peripheral smear without fine focusing, but red blood cell–containing basophilic stippling often is polychromatophilic. Whenever erythropoiesis is accelerated, basophilic stippling is likely to be found as well in individuals with lead poisoning (Fig. 3.23).

Heinz bodies result from denatured hemoglobin and are defined as large structures approximately 1 to 3 μm in diameter located toward the periphery of the red blood cell membrane (Fig. 3.24). Although they cannot be visualized by Wright's stain, bite cells in the peripheral smear are evidence that a Heinz body has been formed and removed by the spleen. Staining with a supravital stain such as brilliant cresyl blue or crystal violet may be necessary to visualize the actual Heinz body inclusion. Heinz bodies are seen in glucose-6-phosphate dehydrogenase deficiency and in any unstable hemoglobinopathy such as hemoglobin Zurich (Fig. 3.24). See Figure 3.25 for a schematic representation of Heinz body formation. See also Table 3.5.

VALUE OF THE RETICULOCYTE COUNT

The reticulocyte count is the most effective means of assessing red blood cell generation or response to anemia. Reticulocytes are non-nucleated red blood cells that contain remnant RNA material, or reticulum. Reticulum usually *cannot* be visualized by Wright's stain; counting and evaluating reticulocytes requires staining with supravital stains such as new methylene blue or brilliant cresyl blue. On Wright's stain, reticulocytes are seen as polychromatophilic macrocytes, or large bluish cells. The normal reticulocyte rate is 0.5% to 2.0% in adults and 2.0% to 6.0% in newborns. Because the bone marrow is

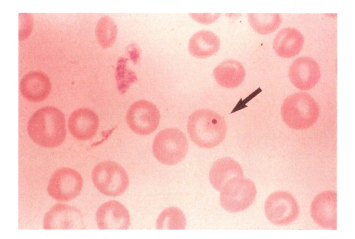

Figure 3.21 Howell-Jolly bodies.   © 1967 American Society of Clinical
Pathologists. Reprinted with permission.

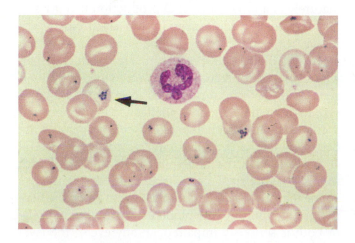

Figure 3.22 Siderotic granules.   © 1982 American Society of Clinical
Pathologists. Reprinted with permission.

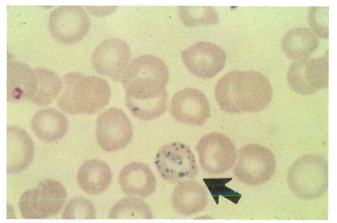

Figure 3.23 Basophilic stippling.   From The College of American
Pathologists, with permission.

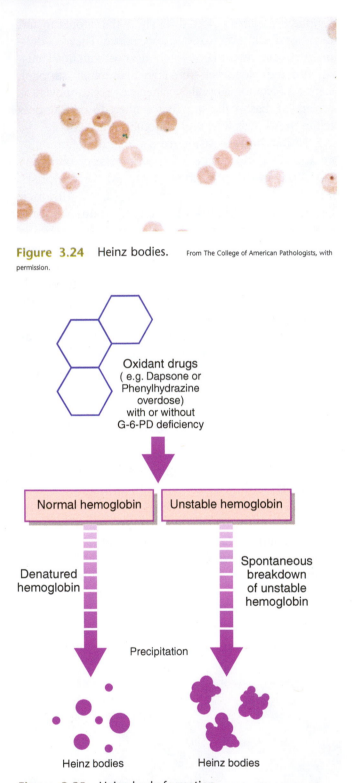

Figure 3.24 Heinz bodies. From The College of American Pathologists, with permission.

Figure 3.25 Heinz body formation. Adapted from Glassy E. Color Atlas of Hematology: An Illustrated Guide Based on Proficiency Testing. Northfield, IL: College of American Pathologists, 1998, with permission.

Table 3.5 ◉ Inclusion Matched to Disease	
Red Blood Cell/ White Blood Cell Inclusion	**Disease Association**
Auer rods	Acute myeloid, monocytic leukemias
Basophilic stippling	Lead poisoning
	Arsenic poisoning
	Thalassemia syndromes
	Accelerated erythropoiesis
	Pyrimidine 5'-nucleotidase deficiency
Cabot rings	Postsplenectomy
	Pernicious anemia
Döhle bodies	Infection
	Burn patients
Hemoglobin C	Hemoglobin C disease (Hgb SC crystals take a gloved-hand shape)
Heinz bodies	G6PD deficiency*
Howell-Jolly bodies	Hemolytic anemias
	Postsplenectomy
	Megaloblastic anemia
Pappenheimer bodies	Acquired iron loading anemias
	Postsplenectomy
	Thalassemia
	Hereditary hemochromatosis
Toxic granulation	Infections
	Burn patients
	Drug therapy

*G6PD, glucose-6-phosphate dehydrogenase.

red blood cells may be visualized in the peripheral smear as the bone marrow races to deliver cells prematurely at a rapid rate. EPO production increases in response to hypoxia (anemia), and erythroid hyperplasia in the bone marrow (the condition in which more red blood cell precursors are produced than white blood cell precursors) is clear evidence of rapid generation. Failure to produce the expected reticulocyte increase may occur in ineffective erythropoiesis, a condition in which red blood cell precursors are destroyed before they are delivered to the peripheral circulation, or if the bone marrow is infiltrated with tumor or abnormal cells. A decreased reticulocyte count may also be seen in aplastic conditions, where the production of white blood cells or red blood cells or both is seriously impaired. In any event, the level or lack of reticulocyte response is an important indicator of bone marrow function.

capable of expanding its production seven times the normal rate, an elevated reticulocyte count or reticulocytosis is the *appropriate* response in anemic stress. Reticulocytes are seen in the peripheral smear as polychromatophilic macrocytes; additionally, nucleated

CONDENSED CASE

At a local physician office laboratory (POL), one technologist was assigned to do complete differentials or to review smears depending on the automated count. She noticed that in every smear she reviewed, burr cells were a prominent part of the red blood cell morphology. She began to get suspicious and considered the possibility that the burr cells were artifactual. *What are the potential causes for artifactually induced burr cells?*

Answer

Burr cells can be artifactual if (1) the blood smears that are made are forced to air-dry through repeated shaking or (2) the buffer used in staining is not at the proper pH.

○ Summary Points

- Red blood cell production is controlled by EPO, a hormone released from the kidney.

- The main sites of adult erythropoiesis are the sternum and iliac crest.

- Each pronormoblast produces 16 mature red blood cells.

- As they mature, red blood cells decrease in size, become less basophilic in their cytoplasm, develop the orange tinge of hemoglobin, and lose their nucleus.

- The most common NRBC seen in the peripheral smear is an orthochromic normoblast.

- The red blood cell membrane is a trilaminar structure containing glycolipids, glycoproteins, cholesterol, and proteins that anchor the cell and provide deformability such as spectrin and ankyrin.

- Integral proteins start from the cytoskeleton and expand through the entire red blood cell membrane.

- Peripheral proteins are confined to the red blood cell cytoskeleton.

- Sodium and potassium migrate from the plasma across the red blood cell membranes in an organized fashion controlled by cationic pumps.

- Deformability and elasticity are crucial properties of the red blood cell membrane, which must be able to extend its surface area up to 117% to accommodate its passage through arterioles and capillary space.

- The Embden-Meyerhof pathway provides 90% of cellular ATP necessary for anaerobic red blood cell metabolism.

- Microcytes and macrocytes represent size changes in the red blood cells determined by abnormal pathologies.

- Microcytes are seen in iron deficiency anemia, in thalassemic conditions, in iron loading processes, and with the anemia of inflammation in some individuals.

- Macrocytes are associated with megaloblastic processes, liver disease, high reticulocyte counts, and chemotherapy.

- The observation of polychromasia on a peripheral blood smear indicates accelerated erythropoiesis.

- Hypochromia is a color variation in the red blood cell determined by lack of hemoglobin synthesis.

- Sickle cells are observed when Hgb S is part of the hemoglobin component; there are two types of sickle cells: irreversible and reversible or oat-shaped sickle cells.

- Spherocytes are seen in hereditary spherocytosis, in autoimmune hemolytic anemias, or as a part of red blood cell senescence.

- Target cells are seen in any condition affecting hemoglobin function and in liver disease or other processes where cholesterol is loaded in the circulation.

- Fragmented cells occur as a result of membrane loss and may be seen in heart valve disease, in burns, or in conditions where there is a predisposition of thrombi.

- Ovalocytes can be seen in thalassemic processes and in megaloblastic anemias in which macro-ovalocytes are seen.

- Elliptocytes are seen in iron deficiency anemia, hereditary elliptocytosis, and idiopathic myelofibrosis.

- Acanthocytes are red blood cells that are smaller and possess uneven, thorny projections.

- Howell-Jolly bodies are DNA in origin and seen in conditions of accelerated erythropoiesis; basophilic stippling is RNA in origin and is seen in lead poisoning and accelerated erythropoiesis.

- Heinz bodies are formed from denatured hemoglobin, usually from patients with glucose-6-phosphate dehydrogenase deficiency.

- Pappenheimer bodies/siderotic granules are iron in origin and seen in iron loading processes or in patients who are hypertransfused.

CASE STUDY

A 55-year-old woman complained to her physician that her fingers and toes became blue during cold weather. When she warmed them up, her digits became painful. She also noted that she has been feeling extremely fatigued, with tachycardia and dyspnea. There was no family history of anemia or any other inherited hematologic condition, but there has been a history of vascular disease on her paternal side. A CBC and differential were ordered with the following results: WBC, 8.0×10^9/L; RBC, 2.04×10^{12}/L; Hgb, 9.0 g/dL; Hct, 24.0%; MCV, 117 fL; MCH, 44.1 pg; and MCHC 37.5%. A reticulocyte count was ordered after the CBC was performed. *Which anemic condition can lead to this patient's unusual symptoms?*

Insights to the Case Study

This patient is showing signs of anemia with a low RBC, Hgb, and Hct. Additionally, she is showing the physical symptoms of anemia, which include shortness of breath (dyspnea), heart palpitations (tachycardia), and fatigue. Her symptoms related to her fingers and toes suggest Raynaud's syndrome, and her physician proceeded to order a direct antiglobulin test battery using all three anti–human globulin reagents. This test was positive with agglutination in the complement anti–human globulin reagent, indicating complement coating of the red blood cells. Her physician diagnosed cold agglutinin syndrome in the early stages. Cold agglutinin syndrome is a hemolytic anemia most often associated with cold reactive autoantibodies, which are complement binding. This syndrome accounts for approximately 16% to 23% of all cases of immune hemolytic processes. Patients experience hemolysis and hemoglobinuria at cold temperatures and the physical symptoms indicated in this case. Many individuals move to warmer climates to prevent hemolytic episodes or if symptoms exacerbate. In addition, this patient's peripheral blood smear showed occasional spherocytes and moderate polychromasia, and her reticulocyte count was 3.0% (normal value, 0.5% to 2.0%).

Review Questions

1. What is a significant morphologic difference between irreversibly sickled cells and reversible sickled cells?
   a. Puddled hemoglobin
   b. Crystal formation central to the sickle cells
   c. Pointed projections to the sickle cell
   d. Fragmentation of the red blood cell membrane

2. What are two integral proteins in the red blood cell structure that house red blood cell antigens?
   a. Glycoproteins and glycolipids
   b. Glycophorin A and glycophorin B
   c. Cholesterol and spectrin
   d. Sodium and potassium

3. All of the following are characteristic of the red blood cell in stages of development *except*
   a. Nuclei are "baseball" round.
   b. Immature cells are larger.
   c. N:C ratio decreases as the cell matures.
   d. Distinct granulation in the cytoplasm.

4. Which red blood cell inclusions originate as a result of denatured hemoglobin?
   a. Howell-Jolly bodies
   b. Heinz bodies
   c. Pappenheimer bodies
   d. Malarial parasites

5. In which conditions can you see elliptocytes?
   a. Iron loading processes
   b. Aplastic anemia
   c. Iron deficiency anemia
   d. Hereditary spherocitosis

6. Which red blood cell morphology may form as a result of excess cholesterol taken on the red blood cell membrane?
   a. Macrocytes
   b. Target cells
   c. Schistocytes
   d. Ovalocytes

7. Hypochromia is used to define
   a. Color change in the red blood cell.
   b. Variation in shape of the red blood cell.
   c. Variation in size of the red blood cell.
   d. Decrease in hemoglobin content of the red blood cell.

8. The erythrocyte stage that marks the beginning of hemoglobinization is called
   a. Basophilic normoblast.
   b. Polychromatophilic normoblast.
   c. Orthochromic normoblast.
   d. Pronormoblast.

9. A key morphologic feature of the nucleated red blood cell stages is
   a. Basophilic cytoplasm through every stage of maturation.
   b. Granules in the cytoplasm.
   c. "Baseball" round nucleus.
   d. Increase in size as the cell matures.

10. The red blood cell protein that is responsible for deformability and flexibility of the red blood cell is
   a. Spectrin.
   b. Glycophorin.
   c. Glycine.
   d. EPO.

⦿ TROUBLESHOOTING

What Do I Do When There Is a Drastic Change in a Patient's Differential Results During the Same Shift?

A 47-year-old man recovering from bacterial meningitis was having his blood drawn on a daily basis for CBC. His sample was received in the morning with the morning draw at 8 a.m. (see the chart). Later in the day, the technologist received another request for a CBC on the same patient and noticed quite a difference in the automated differential. The RBC, Hgb, Hct, MCV, and RDW all resembled the first sample from the a.m. draw. The technologist suspected that the second sample had been mislabeled. She retrieved both samples and asked the blood bank to perform ABO grouping on the samples. Results are as follows.

8 a.m. Draw		2 p.m. Draw	
CBC	**Differential**	**CBC**	**Differential**
WBC 11.1	Neutrophils 86%	WBC 12.4	Neutrophils 66%
RBC 3.97	Lymphocytes 8%	RBC 3.82	Lymphocytes 20%
Hgb 12.7	Monocytes 5%	Hgb 12.5	Monocytes 12%
Hct 38.0	Eosinophils 1	Hct 36.0	Eosinophils 2%
MCV 95.6	Basophils 0	MCV 94.3	Basophils 0%
MCH 32.0		MCH 32.7	
MCHC 33.5		MCHC 34.7	
RDW 13.9		RDW 12.6	
Platelets 224		Platelets 313	

Blood Banking Report

8 a.m. sample: O pos

2 p.m. sample: A pos

The CBCs of both samples were fairly equal with no cause for alarm; however, there were some disparities in the differential of the two samples. Even though both sets of results were acceptable and no result was flagged, the technologist had a nagging suspicion that the second sample was mislabeled. She took both samples, the a.m. and p.m. samples, to the blood bank to be ABO typed. The blood types on these samples did not match, but the patient has a history of type O blood from blood bank files. The floor was notified that the sample was mislabeled, the sample was discarded, and the afternoon results on that patient were negated. Putting all of the pieces of this puzzle together led to a confirmation of the technologist's original suspicions about the patient's p.m. sample. Rather than verify the p.m. results, the technologist chose to investigate the possibility of a mislabeled sample. Discovering an error in patient sample collection provides an opportunity for the laboratory to remind hospital units that proper sample collection and identification procedures are tantamount to accurate patient results.

W O R D   K E Y

Anaerobic • Able to live without oxygen

Asynchrony • Failure of event to occur at the same time

Cytoskeleton • Internal structural framework of the cell

Disseminated intravascular coagulation • Pathologic condition in which the coagulation pathways are hyperstimulated—either excessive fibrin disposition or excess plasmin production

Pathology • Study of the nature and cause of disease that involves changes in structure and function

Splenectomy • Removal of the spleen

Thrombi • Plural of thrombus; a blood clot that obstructs a blood vessel or a cavity of the heart

References

1. Bell A. Morphology of human blood and marrow cells. In: Harmening D, ed. Clinical Hematology and Fundamentals of Hemostasis, 4th ed. Philadelphia: FA Davis, 2002; 10.
2. Schwabbauer M. Normal erythrocyte production, physiology and destruction. In: Steine-Martin E, Lotspeich-Steininger C, Koeple JA, eds. Clinical Hematology: Principles, Procedures and Correlations, 2nd ed. Philadelphia: Lippincott, 1998; 61.
3. Hubbard JD. A concise review of clinical laboratory sciences. Baltimore, MD: Williams & Wilkins, 1997; 139–140.
4. Harmening D, Hughes V, Del Toro C. The red cell: Structure and function. In: Harmening D, ed. Clinical Hematology and Fundamentals of Hemostasis, 4th ed. Philadelphia: FA Davis, 2002; 62.
5. Besa E. Hemolytic anemia. In Besa E, Catalano P, Kant JA, eds. Hematology. Philadelphia: Harwal Publishing, 1992; 98–99.
6. Hussong JW. Iron metabolism and hypochromic anemias. In Harmening D, ed. Clinical Hematology and Fundamentals of Hemostasis, 4th ed. Philadelphia: FA Davis, 2002; 105.
7. Ciesla B. Pondering red cell morphology. ADVANCE for Medical Laboratory Professionals 15:10–11, 2003.
8. Womack EP. Treating thrombotic thrombocytopenic purpura with plasma exchange. Lab Med 30:279, 1999.

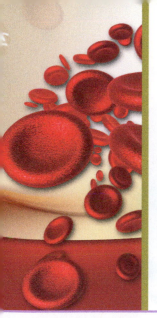

Chapter 4

Hemoglobin Function and Principles of Hemolysis

Betty Ciesla

Objectives

After completing this chapter, the student will be able to:

1. Identify the components of hemoglobin.

2. Define the normal structural elements related to hemoglobin synthesis.

3. Describe hemoglobin function.

4. Describe the origin of hemoglobin synthesis in erythroid precursors.

5. List the normal adult hemoglobins.

6. Describe the chemical configuration and percentages of the normal adult hemoglobins, Hgb A, Hgb A2, and Hgb F.

7. Relate the shift from fetal hemoglobin to adult hemoglobin in terms of fetal to adult development.

8. Outline the steps involved in oxygen delivery and the elimination of carbon dioxide.

9. Describe the oxygen dissociation curve in general terms.

10. Differentiate the abnormal hemoglobins in terms of toxicity and oxygen capacity.

11. Describe hemolysis in terms of its effect on the bone marrow, blood smear, and blood chemistry.

12. Define extravascular hemolysis with respect to organ of origin and laboratory diagnosis.

13. Define intravascular hemolysis with respect to organs affected and laboratory diagnosis.

14. Recall the terminologies used to classify the hemolytic anemias.

HEMOGLOBIN STRUCTURE AND SYNTHESIS

Hemoglobin is the life-giving substance of every red blood cell, the oxygen-carrying component of the red blood cell. Each red blood cell is nothing more than a fluid-filled sac, with the fluid being hemoglobin. Every organ in the human body depends on oxygenation for growth and function, and this process is ultimately controlled by hemoglobin. In 4 months (120 days), red blood cells with normal hemoglobin content submit to the rigors of circulation. Red blood cells are stretched, twisted, pummeled, and squeezed as they make their way through the circulatory watershed. The hemoglobin molecule consists of two primary structures:

- *Heme portion*: This structure involves four iron atoms in the ferrous state (Fe^{2+}), because iron in the ferric state (Fe^{3+}) cannot bind oxygen, surrounded by protoporphyrin IX, or the porphyrin ring, a structure formed in the nucleated red blood cells. Protoporphyrin IX is the final product in the synthesis of the heme molecule. It results from the interaction of succinyl coenzyme A and delta-aminolevulinic acid in the mitochondria of the nucleated red blood cells. Several intermediate by-products are formed, including porphobilinogen, uroporphyrinogen, and coproporphyrin. When iron is incorporated, it combines with protoporphyrin to form the complete heme molecule. Defects in any of the intermediate products can impair hemoglobin function.
- *Globin portion*: This structure consists of **amino acids** linked together to form a polypeptide chain, a bracelet of amino acids. The most predominant chains for adult hemoglobins are the alpha and beta chains. Alpha chains have 141 amino acids in a unique arrangement, and beta chains have 146 amino acids in a unique arrangement. The heme and globin portions of the hemoglobin molecule are linked together by chemical bonds.
- *2,3-Diphosphoglycerate (2,3-DPG)*: 2,3-DPG is a substance produced via the Embden-Meyerhof pathway during anaerobic glycolysis.[1] This structure is intimately related to oxygen affinity of hemoglobin and is explained in that section.

Each hemoglobin molecule consists of four heme molecules with iron at the center and two pairs of globin chains (Fig. 4.1). The heme structure sits lodged in

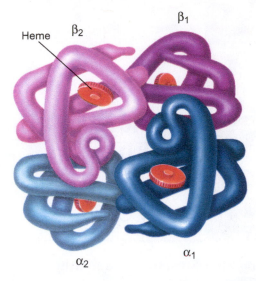

Figure 4.1 Hemoglobin molecule: note four heme molecules tucked inside globin chains.

the pocket of the globin chains. Hemoglobin begins to be synthesized at the polychromatic normoblast stage of red blood cell development. This synthesis is visualized by the change in cytoplasmic color from a deep blue to a lavender-tinged cytoplasmic color. Of hemoglobin, 65% is synthesized before the red blood cell nucleus is extruded, with an additional 35% synthesized by the reticulocyte stage.[2] Normal mature red blood cells have a full complement of hemoglobin, which occupies a little less than one-half of the surface area of the red blood cell.

Genetics and Chain Formation of Hemoglobin

Three types of hemoglobin are synthesized: embryonic hemoglobins, fetal hemoglobin, and adult hemoglobins. Each of these types of hemoglobins has a specific arrangement of globin chains, and each globin chain is under the influence of a specific chromosome. Chromosome 11 contains the genes for the production of epsilon, beta, gamma, and delta chains. Each parent contributes one gene for the production of each of these chains. Each individual has two genes for the production of any of these chains, one from the mother and one from the father. Chromosome 16 is responsible for the alpha and zeta genes. There are two genes on the chromosome for the production of alpha chains and one gene for the production of zeta chains (Fig. 4.2). Each parent contributes two genes for the production of alpha chains and one gene for the production of zeta chains. Each individual has four genes for the production of alpha chains (two from each parent) and two for zeta chains (one from each parent).

Alpha chains are a constant component of each adult hemoglobin (Hgb A, A_2, F); each hemoglobin has two obligatory alpha chains as part of its chemical configuration. The epsilon and zeta chains are reserved for the production of embryonic hemoglobins. As the embryo develops, Hgb Gower I (α_2, ε_2) and Hgb Portland ($\gamma_2\zeta_2$) are synthesized and remain in the embryo for 3 months. These hemoglobins do not participate in oxygen delivery. Hgb F ($\alpha_2\gamma_2$), fetal hemoglobin, begins to be synthesized at approximately 3 months in fetal development and remains as the majority hemoglobin at birth. The amount of gamma chains declines and the amount of beta chains increases 3 to 6 months after delivery, making Hgb A ($\alpha_2\beta_2$) the majority adult hemoglobin (95% to 98%). Hgb A_2 ($\alpha_2\delta_2$; 3% to 5%) and Hgb F (less than 1%) are also part of the normal adult hemoglobin **complement**. The unique position of amino acids in each chain and the specificity of the amino acid itself are essential to the normal function of the hemoglobin molecule. Synthetic or structural abnormalities of the protein chains may lead to hemoglobin defects.

Hemoglobin Function

Oxygen delivery is the principal purpose of the hemoglobin molecule. Additionally, the hemoglobin molecule is a structure capable of pulling CO_2 away from the tissues and keeping the blood in a balanced pH. The hemoglobin molecule loads oxygen on a one-to-one basis, one molecule of oxygen to one molecule of heme in the oxygen-rich environment of the alveoli of the lungs. Hemoglobin becomes saturated with oxygen, forming oxyhemoglobin, and has a high affinity for oxygen in this pulmonary environment. The network of capillaries in the lungs makes the diffusion of oxygen a rapid process. As the oxyhemoglobin molecule transits through the circulation, it transports oxygen, unloading it to the tissues in areas of low oxygen affinity. As hemoglobin goes through the loading and unloading process, changes appear in the molecule. These changes are **allosteric** changes; the term allosteric relates to the way hemoglobin is able to rotate on its axis, determine the action of salt bridges between the globin structures, and dictate the movement of 2,3-DPG. The hemoglobin molecule appears in a tense and a relaxed form.[3] When tense, hemoglobin is not oxygenated, 2,3-DPG is at the center of the molecule, and the salt bridges between the globin chains are in place. When oxygenated, the relaxed form is in place; 2,3-DPG is expelled, salt bridges are broken, and the molecule is capable of fully loading oxygen.

Oxygen Dissociation Curve

The binding and release of oxygen from the hemoglobin molecule is defined by the oxygen dissociation (OD) curve (Fig. 4.3). This curve is represented as a sigmoid shape (an "S" shape), not the straight-line shape familiar to most students. The curve is designed to illustrate the unique qualities of oxygen dissociation and to attempt to demonstrate graphically how the hemoglobin molecule and oxygen respond to normal and abnormal physiologies.[4] What is essential when considering the hemoglobin molecule is that when the molecule is fully saturated, it has all of the oxygen it can hold and a high level of oxygen tension. As it travels from the pulmonary circulation to the venous circulation, it has more of an inclination to give up its oxygen in response to the oxygen needs of

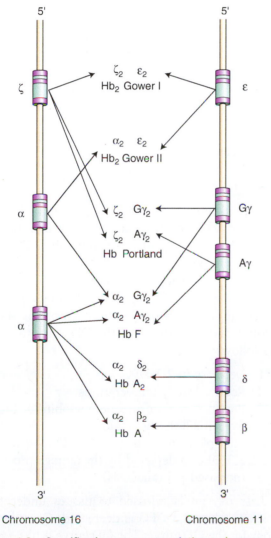

Chromosome 16   Chromosome 11

Figure 4.2 Specific chromosomes relative to human hemoglobin formation.

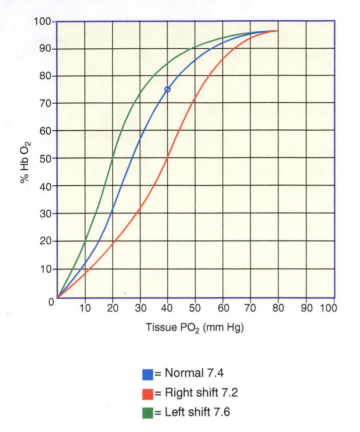

= Normal 7.4

= Right shift 7.2

= Left shift 7.6

Figure 4.3   Oxygen dissociation curve. In the normal curve (blue) at 40 mm Hg, 75% of the hemoglobin molecule is saturated with oxygen, leaving 25% capable of being released to tissue. Note the right shifted curve (red). At 40 mm Hg, hemoglobin is 50% saturated but willing to give up 50% of its oxygen to the tissues. Note the left shifted curve (green). At 40 mm Hg, hemoglobin is 85% saturated but willing to release only 12% to the tissues.

the tissue it is serving. Figure 4.3 demonstrates the following:[5]

1. There is a progressive increase in the percentage of the hemoglobin that is bound with oxygen as the blood P_{O_2} increases.
2. In the lungs, in which the blood P_{O_2} is 100 mm Hg, hemoglobin is 97% saturated with oxygen.
3. In venous circulation, in which the P_{O_2} is 40 mm Hg, 75% of the hemoglobin molecule is saturated with oxygen, and 25% of the oxygen is capable of being released when the hemoglobin level is normal.

Two possibilities are demonstrated by this relationship: depending on the need of tissues for oxygen, the hemoglobin molecule either holds onto oxygen (oxygen affinity) or releases more oxygen as physiologic circumstances dictate.

*   When referring to the OD curve, we speak about it in terms of having a "shift to the right" or a "shift to the left."

*   Shifting the curve means that physiologic conditions are present in the body that affect the relationship of oxygen and hemoglobin. In most cases, the hemoglobin molecule compensates by holding or delivering oxygen depending on tissue need. This compensatory mechanism can be demonstrated through the OD curve.
*   When the curve is right shifted, hemoglobin has less attraction for oxygen and is more willing to release oxygen to the tissues. In a right-shifted OD curve at 40 mm Hg, hemoglobin is 50% saturated but willing to give up 50% of its oxygen to the tissue because of need.
*   When the curve is left shifted, hemoglobin has more of an attraction for oxygen and is less willing to release it to the tissues. In a left-shifted OD curve at 40 mm Hg, hemoglobin is 75% saturated but willing to release only 12% to the tissues.

Conditions That Shift the Oxygen Dissociation Curve

Physiologic conditions that shift the curve to the right include the following:

1. Anemia
2. Decreased pH (**acidosis**)
3. Increase in 2,3-DPG
4. Elevated body temperature (fever)

In the anemic state, the cells act more efficiently to deliver oxygen to the tissues even though there are fewer red blood cells and less hemoglobin. The compensatory mechanism of the OD curve works adequately if the hemoglobin level is 8 to 12 g/dL. For the most part, it is only when the hemoglobin level decreases to less than 8 g/dL that symptoms start to develop. Conditions that shift the OD curve to the left are as follows:

1. Decrease in 2,3-DPG
2. Reduced body temperatures
3. Presence of abnormal hemoglobins or high oxygen affinity hemoglobins
4. Multiple transfusions of stored blood where 2,3-DPG is depleted by the storage process
5. Increased pH (**alkalosis**)

Less oxygen is released to tissues under these conditions when 2,3-DPG is decreased. Consider this analogy for the OD curve: The OD curve is like a roller coaster. As you start up the incline, you hold on tight; as you roll down the hill, you are more willing to throw your arms up in the air and release or relax your grip. So it is with the right shifted OD curve.

Abnormal Hemoglobins

Normal hemoglobin is a highly stable protein that can be converted to cyanmethemoglobin, a colored pigment. Hemoglobins that are physiologically abnormal have a higher oxygen affinity and produce conditions that are usually toxic to the human body.

Three abnormal hemoglobins are methemoglobin, sulfhemoglobin, and carboxyhemoglobin. Increasing the amounts of any of these abnormal hemoglobins in the bloodstream can be potentially fatal. Often, the production of abnormal hemoglobins results from accidental or purposeful ingestion or absorption of substances, or drugs, that are harmful. Abnormal hemoglobins sometimes are produced as a result of inherited defects.

- In the abnormal hemoglobin methemoglobin, iron has been oxidized to the Fe^{3+} state, which is no longer capable of binding oxygen. Methemoglobin builds up in the circulation; if the level is greater than 10%, individuals appear **cyanotic** (having a blue color), especially in the lips and fingers.[6] Aniline drugs and some antimalarial treatments may induce a methemoglobinemia in individuals who are unable to reduce methemoglobin. Hemoglobin M, an inherited condition arising from an amino acid substitution, may also result in cyanotic conditions.
- Carboxyhemoglobin levels increase in smokers and certain industrial workers. Hemoglobin has an affinity for carbon monoxide that is 200 times greater than its affinity for oxygen; therefore, no oxygen is delivered to the tissues. For this reason, carbon monoxide poisoning, whether deliberate or accidental, is efficient and relatively painless. This process is reversible, however, if caught in time.
- Sulfhemoglobin can be formed on exposure to agents such as sulfonamides or sulfa-containing drugs. The affinity of sulfhemoglobin for oxygen is 100 times lower than that of normal hemoglobin. It may be toxic at a very low level (Table 4.1).

Table 4.1 ⊙ **Abnormal Hemoglobins**
• Sulfhemoglobin
• Carboxyhemoglobin
• Methemoglobin

HEMOLYTIC PROCESS

Red blood cell senescence or death is a natural process for red blood cells at the end of their 120-day life span. As a natural by-product, the contents of the red blood cell are released and returned to various parts of the circulation to be recycled in the process of red blood cell regeneration. When red blood cell death occurs in an orderly fashion, the hematologic balance is maintained. Hemoglobin is kept at normal levels, and the bone marrow maintains a steady production of red blood cells. If premature cell death or hemolysis occurs, a series of events begin to cascade, providing laboratory evidence that cells are dying faster than their normal 120-day life cycle (Table 4.2). When this happens, the body's peripheral circulation begins its intervention process. There is evidence for hemolysis in the bone marrow, in the peripheral circulation, and in the blood plasma. The bone marrow shows erythroid **hyperplasia**, meaning an increase in red blood cell precursors and premature release of reticulocytes and young red blood cells. The normal myeloid:erythroid (M:E) ratio of 3:1 to 4:1 is shifted toward an increase in red blood cell precursors, giving a ratio of perhaps 1:2. The peripheral smear provides visual clues of hemolysis by showing an increase in **polychromasia** and the possible presence of nucleated red blood cells and possibly spherocytes. Spherocytes may appear in the peripheral circulation if red blood cells become coated with antibody. As antibody-coated red blood cells travel through the spleen, the spleen subsequently shears off the antibody as the red blood cell percolates through this organ.[7] None of these visual indicators is likely to be observed in a *normal* peripheral smear. They are seen in a peripheral smear in *response* to a hemolytic event. Plasma changes are discussed later in the chapter.

Types of Hemolysis

Hemolysis can be an extravascular or an intravascular process. Of all hemolysis, 90% is extravascular and occurs in the spleen, liver, lymph nodes, and bone

Table 4.2 ⊙ **Relationship of Hemolysis and Clinical Events**	
Clinical Events	**Physical Symptoms**
↓ RBC, Hgb, Hct	Symptoms of anemia: pallor, fatigue, tachycardia
↑ Bilirubin	Jaundice
Hemoglobinemia	Blood-tinged plasma
Hemoglobinuria	Blood-tinged urine

marrow, the organs of the reticuloendothelial system. Red blood cells are destroyed, and their contents are phagocytized with hemoglobin released into the macrophages. Extravascular hemolysis is a well-established pathway in which red blood cell breakdown leads to the release of the internal products of hemoglobin, primarily heme and globin (Fig. 4.4). The amino acids of the globin chains are recycled into the amino acid pool, and the products of heme are taken through different pathways. Iron is transported via transferrin, the transport protein to the bone marrow or storage sites to be used in erythropoiesis, while the rest of the hemoglobin molecule reacts with hemoxygenase, yielding a by-product biliverdin, which is reduced to unconjugated bilirubin. This bilirubin product attaches to albumin and is transported to the liver.

Ten percent of hemolysis is intravascular, and it occurs as red blood cells are lysed directly in the blood vessel. Hemoglobin is released into the plasma (Fig. 4.5). Hemoglobinemia, red-tinged plasma, is observed after the blood sample is centrifuged. This unusual finding is seen only in intravascular lysis. Hemoglobinuria, blood in the urine, may also be a

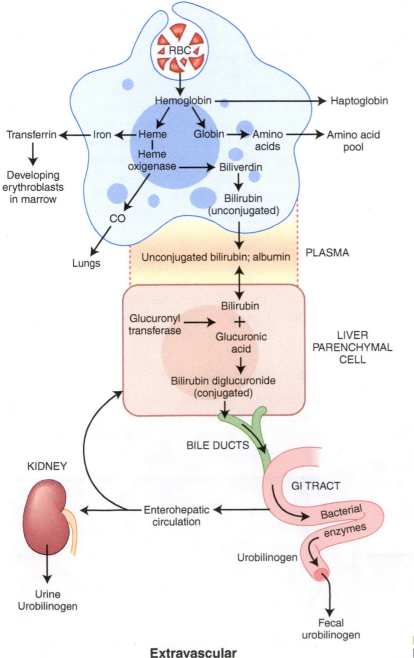

Extravascular

Figure 4.4 Extravascular hemolysis: increased bilirubin, decreased haptoglobin.

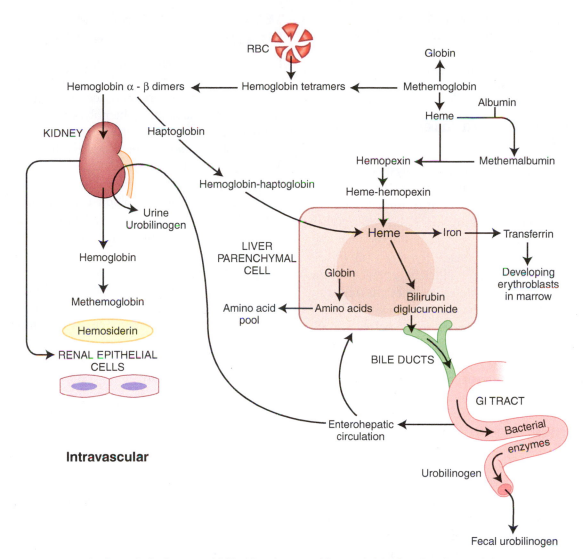

Figure 4.5 Intravascular hemolysis: increased bilirubin, decreased haptoglobin, but free hemoglobin present.

by-product of direct intravascular lysis that may be complement mediated. If complement is activated as in the case of ABO transfusion reaction, proteins are introduced that cause additional damage to the red blood cell membrane.[8] Evidence of intravascular lysis indicates a serious condition that must be addressed promptly.

Laboratory Evidence of Hemolysis

Hemolysis can be distinguished in the laboratory by various methods. Most of these measurements are obtained in the hematology and chemistry laboratories by routine laboratory procedures. The first consideration is to establish whether the patient has hemolysis, as evidenced by increased reticulocyte count, increased polychromasia, and possible nucleated red blood cells in the peripheral smear. The second consideration is to

establish the cause and type of hemolysis. If the patient is experiencing *intravascular* lysis, the following conditions are present:

- Hemoglobin, hematocrit, and red blood cell count are decreased.
- Serum bilirubin is elevated.
- Serum haptoglobin is markedly decreased.
- Hemoglobinemia (free hemoglobin in plasma) may be present.
- Hemoglobinuria (hemoglobin in urine) may be present.
- Reticulocyte count is elevated.
- Lactate dehydrogenase (LDH) is elevated.

Under conditions of *extravascular* lysis, the following conditions are present:

- Hemoglobin, hematocrit, and red blood cell count are decreased.

- Serum bilirubin is elevated.
- Reticulocyte count is elevated.
- Haptoglobin is low.
- Hepatosplenomegaly may be seen.
- LDH is elevated.

Physiology of Intravascular Hemolysis

Intravascular and extravascular hemolysis can be distinguished by paying careful attention to laboratory data. It is imperative for a student to understand why each of these events is taking place, however. When considering intravascular lysis, conditions that may predispose to rapid and volatile lysis within vessels may activate complement, an efficient accessory to the hemolytic process. Red blood cells burst, releasing their contents, and the alpha and beta dimers of hemoglobin protein chains are released immediately into the plasma. From the plasma, they are bound to haptoglobin. The hemoglobin-haptoglobin complex is too large to be filtered by the kidneys, so it is not excreted, but rather transported to the liver, where it is destroyed and broken down. The actual haptoglobin measurement of the plasma is lower in a hemolytic event, indicating that there are no sites left for this molecule to be bound with hemoglobin. The complete blood count (CBC) shows reduced hemoglobin, hematocrit, and RBC in response to excessive red blood cell destruction, and the reticulocyte count is elevated in response to the erythroid hyperplasia of the bone marrow. Reticulocytes are released prematurely in response to the red blood cell need in anemic conditions; therefore, the reticulocyte count is almost always elevated. Additionally, LDH is increased. LDH is a red blood cell enzyme that increases in the plasma as red blood cells are lysed prematurely. Hemoglobinemia may appear as red-tinged plasma because the red blood cells have burst directly inside the vessels; consequently, centrifuged blood samples may have a red-tinged or pink-tinged plasma component. Hemoglobinuria is a direct representation of free hemoglobin being filtered by the kidney into the urine; therefore, urine samples may be blood-tinged.

Intravascular events may take 48 hours to manifest through laboratory results. Many of the same laboratory findings that occur in intravascular events may occur in extravascular hemolysis, with the exception of hemoglobinuria and hemoglobinemia. Additionally, the spleen may become enlarged in extravascular hemolysis because damaged red blood cells may become sequestered in this organ.

TERMINOLOGY RELEVANT TO THE HEMOLYTIC ANEMIAS

The hemolytic anemias are classified according to many different schemes. In this chapter, we have classified the hemolytic anemias according to the site of hemolysis by classifying hemolytic events as either extravascular or intravascular. Many textbooks discuss the hemolytic anemias in terms of those that result from intrinsic defects of the red blood cell versus those that result from extrinsic events that are not related to the structure of the red blood cell but affect its life span. Intrinsic defects of the red blood cell relate to inherited deficiencies of the red blood cell membrane, hemoglobin structure or synthesis, or biochemical components. Extrinsic defects relate to events that are secondary to red blood cell structure and function but may still result in a hemolytic event. Regardless of the classification, it is paramount that the hemolytic anemias be recognized, evaluated, and managed so that life-threatening sequelae do not arise.[9] See Table 4.3 for a modified list of anemias classified by intrinsic or extrinsic defects.

○ *Summary Points*

- Hemoglobin has two main components: heme and globin.
- Heme consists of iron and the protoporphyrin ring.
- Globin consists of amino acid chains of specific lengths and specific amino acids; alpha and beta chains are the two most significant amino acid chains.

Table 4.3 ○ Hemolytic Anemias Classified by Intrinsic or Extrinsic Defects (Modified List)	
Intrinsic Red Blood Cell Defects Leading to Hemolysis	**Extrinsic Defects Leading to Hemolysis**
Hemoglobinopathies: structural and synthetic	Autoimmune hemolytic anemia
Red blood cell membrane defects	Parasitic infection
Red blood cell enzyme defects	Microangiopathic hemolytic anemia
Stem cell defects	Environmental agents, including venoms and chemical agents

CONDENSED CASE

An 80-year-old woman visited the emergency department at 9 p.m. with complaints of dizziness of 3 days' duration and right-sided abdominal pain. In the treatment room, three tubes of blood were drawn from the patient: a purple top, a blue top, and a tiger top. The samples were not inverted, and they remained unlabeled in the treatment room for at least 1 hour, sitting in an emesis basin. The patient was subsequently admitted to the hospital at 3 a.m., and all of her blood work was redrawn. *What was the probable cause for the second blood draw?*

Answer

This scenario represents two important breakdowns of phlebotomy protocol—lack of inversion of anticoagulated tubes and lack of labeling. Tubes that are anticoagulated should be inverted no less than six times for proper mixing of blood and anticoagulant. Failure to do so could easily result in clotted tubes. Proper labeling of tubes should occur at the bedside, immediately after the sample has been drawn. The patient should identify himself or herself verbally, and this identification should be verified through the identification bracelet. Rigorous efforts must be taken for proper patient identification.

- Alpha chains have 141 amino acids, and beta chains have 146 amino acids.
- Hgb Gower and Hgb Portland are embryonic hemoglobins; Hgb F is fetal hemoglobin; and the adult hemoglobins are Hgb A, Hgb A_2, and Hgb F.
- Oxygen delivery is the primary purpose of the hemoglobin molecule.
- 2,3-DPG is intimately related to the oxygen affinity of hemoglobin.
- The OD curve schematically represents the saturation of hemoglobin with oxygen and the release of oxygen from the hemoglobin molecule under normal and abnormal physiologic conditions.

- Hemolysis is the premature destruction of the red blood cell before its 120-day life cycle.
- Hemolysis may be classified as intravascular or extravascular, which relates to the site of hemolysis.
- Intravascular hemolysis occurs inside the blood vessels; extravascular hemolysis occurs outside the blood vessels, primarily in the reticuloendothelial system.
- Hemolytic anemias may be classified by intrinsic defects of the red blood cell or extrinsic defects that affect the red blood cell.

CASE STUDY

Eight-year-old twin boys were brought into the emergency department with complaints of intermittent fevers and lethargy. The boys had not been feeling well for the last 2 weeks. They had recently returned from a trip to Nigeria with their parents. All members of the family had been treated with antimalarial medication before the trip. Neither parent exhibited any of the symptoms of the children. A CBC with differential and a peripheral smear for malarial parasites were ordered. The children were slightly anemic, with hematocrits at 33%, and both boys had elevated WBCs of around $15.0 \times 10^9/L$.

Insights to the Case Study

Both of these boys had malaria, and ring forms were observed in the thin preparation on the peripheral smear. *Plasmodium falciparum* was identified. Additionally, they had begun to show slight hemolysis as evidenced by their slightly decreased hematocrits. Drug-resistant strains of malaria are becoming increasingly common throughout the world, and cases of malaria are increasing not only in endemic areas in Africa, but also in countries such as Peru and Tajikistan, areas where malaria infections are not endemic and the occurrence of drug resistance is unlikely. When one considers that malaria still kills 1.1 million individuals a year and is infecting up to a half-billion people a year,[10] this health situation is of major importance. Hardest hit are the most vulnerable populations, such as young children

Continued

in remote villages who may not have access to vaccine or treatment. Death or life-changing neurologic manifestations are common in this population. Many strains of the malaria parasite have also become resistant to chloroquine, previously the panacea for malarial protection. Factors such as noncompliance with drug protocol (not taking the drug as long as is necessary) and the indiscriminant use of this drug have led the malarial parasite to adapt to the drug and become resistant to the more common remedies. Our patients were thought to have a drug-resistant strain of malaria, were placed on sulfadoxine/pyrimethamine (Fansidar) and made a good recovery.

Review Questions

1. Which of these hemoglobins is an embryonic hemoglobin?
   a. Hgb A
   b. Hgb Gower
   c. Hgb F
   d. Hgb A_2

2. How many total genes does a person possess for the production of alpha chains?
   a. One
   b. Two
   c. Four
   d. Three

3. Name one condition that may shift the OD curve to the left.
   a. Inheriting a high oxygen affinity hemoglobin
   b. Metabolic acidosis
   c. Anemia
   d. Increased hemoglobin concentration

4. If polychromasia is increased in the peripheral smear, the _____ should be elevated.
   a. WBC
   b. RBC
   c. Reticulocyte count
   d. Basophil count

5. If 2,3-DPG increases, the hemoglobin molecule releases more oxygen. This is known as a _____OD curve.
   a. Left-shifted
   b. Normal physiologic
   c. Right-shifted
   d. Neutral

6. Which of the following statements regarding 2,3-DPG is correct?
   a. It catalyzes porphyrin synthesis
   b. It controls hemoglobin affinity for oxygen
   c. It prevents oxidative penetration of hemoglobin
   d. It converts methemoglobin to oxyhemoglobin

7. When the iron in the hemoglobin molecule is in the ferric (Fe^{3+}) state, hemoglobin is termed
   a. Carboxyhemoglobin.
   b. Methemoglobin.
   c. Ferrihemoglobin.
   d. Sulfhemoglobin.

8. What percent of hemoglobin is synthesized in the reticulocyte stage?
   a. 65%
   b. 95%
   c. 35%
   d. 45%

9. Epsilon and zeta chains are part of which of the following hemoglobins?
   a. Hgb Portland
   b. Hgb F
   c. Hgb A
   d. Hgb A_2

10. Fetal hemoglobin consists of which of the following chains?
    a. $\alpha_2\beta_2$
    b. $\alpha_2\gamma_2$
    c. $\alpha_2\delta_2$
    d. $\alpha_2\varepsilon_2$

○ TROUBLESHOOTING

What Do I Do When There Is a Discrepancy in the Hemoglobin Value?

A 50-year-old man presented to the emergency department with chest pain, shortness of breath, and tightness in the chest area. He was immediately moved to the treatment room, where cardiac enzymes, troponin, CBC, cholesterol, and triglycerides were ordered. For illustrative purposes, only the results of the CBC are given, as follows:

WBC	12.0×10^9/L
RBC	4.83×10^{12}/L
Hgb	15.0 g/dL
Hct	39.0%
MCV	81 fL
MCH	31 pg
MCHC	39%
Platelet	$340,000 \times 10^9$/L

While the other results were pending, the CBC was run on automated instrumentation. The operator noticed that the hemoglobin and hematocrit failed the correlation check by not adhering to the rule of three: hemoglobin $\times$ 3 = hematocrit $\pm$3%. Because the hemoglobin was significantly elevated compared with the hematocrit, the hemoglobin value was suspect. The patient sample was spun and observed for lipemia. The plasma was cloudy and grossly lipemic, and when remixed, a milky appearance could be seen in the mixed sample. Lipemia interferes with the optical measurement of hemoglobin, giving a false elevation of hemoglobin, and all subsequent measurements that depend on a hemoglobin value in the calculation—MCH and MCHC. It became clear that corrective action needed to be taken to provide valid results. Corrections for lipemia can occur via one of two methods: the plasma blank correction method or the plasma by dilution replacement method. The most frequently encountered method is the plasma blank correction method, in which the sample is spun, a plasma aliquot is removed, and then the spun plasma is recycled through the instrument. This plasma value is used in the following formula to correct the hemoglobin result:

Corrected hemoglobin = Initial whole blood hemoglobin – (Plasma hemoglobin blank $\times$ [1 – Initial whole blood hematocrit/100])

When our plasma blank was run, we obtained a value of 3.0.

Therefore, our correction would be as follows:
= 15.5 – (3.0 $\times$ [1 – 0.39])
= 15.5 – 1.83
= 13.7

This hemoglobin value is now used in the calculation for MCH and MCHC, to yield corrected MCH and MCHC results of 28.3 and 35.1.

The second corrective method is the diluent replacement method. When the whole blood has been cycled through the automated instrument, an aliquot of the sample is removed and spun. The plasma from the spun sample is carefully removed and replaced by an equal amount of saline or other diluent. The removal of plasma and replacement with saline are critical in this procedure. If this step has been done accurately, there would be little difference in the RBC, and this would serve as a quality control for the accuracy of pipetting in this method. Too wide a variation in the RBCs would indicate poor pipetting. When an accurate replacement has been established, the saline sample is cycled, and the hemoglobin can be reported directly from this sample and used to recalculate indices.

Either of these methods involves labor-intensive, yet essential, steps in reporting an accurate CBC. The operator first must recognize the discrepancy between hemoglobin and hematocrit and then be familiar with the corrective steps that need to be taken to provide a reliable CBC.[11]

(Refer to normal values in Chapter 2.)

WORD KEY

Acidosis • Increase in the acidity of blood (as in diabetic acidosis) caused by an excessive loss of bicarbonate (as in renal disease)

Alkalosis • Increase in blood alkalinity caused by an accumulation of alkaline or reduction in acid

Allosteric • Shape change

Amino acid • One of a large group of organic compounds marked by the presence of an amino group ($NH2$) and a carboxyl group ($COOH$), the building blocks of protein and the end products of protein digestion

Complement • Group of proteins in the blood that play a vital role in the body's immune defenses through a cascade of interaction

Cyanosis • Blue tinge to the extremities (lips, fingers, toes)

Hyperplasia • Excessive proliferation of normal cells in the normal tissue of an organ

Polychromasia • Blue tinge to the red blood cells indicating premature release

References

1. Brown BA. Hematology: Principles and Procedures, 6th ed. Philadelphia: Lippincott Williams & Wilkins, 2003; 42–43.
2. Turgeon ML. Normal erythrocyte lifecycle and physiology. In: Turgeon ML, ed. Clinical Hematology: Theory and Procedures, 3rd ed. Philadelphia: Lippincott Williams & Wilkins, 1999; 66.
3. Ludvigsen FB. Hemoglobin synthesis and function. In: Steine-Martin EA, Lotspeich-Steininger CA, Koepke JA, eds. Clinical Hematology: Principles, Procedures and Correlations, 2nd ed. Philadelphia: Lippincott, 1998; 75.
4. Hillman RS, Finch CA. General characteristics of the erythron. In: Hillman R, Finch C, eds. Red Cell Manual, 7th ed. Philadelphia: FA Davis, 1996; 17–19.
5. Harmening DM, Hughes VC, DelToro C. The red blood cell: Structure and function. In: Harmening D, ed. Clinical Hematology and Fundamentals of Hemostasis, 4th ed. Philadelphia: FA Davis, 2002; 66–67.
6. Bunn HF. Human hemoglobins: Normal and abnormal: Methemoglobinemia. In: Nathan SH, Oski A, eds. Hematology of Infancy and Childhood, 4th ed. Philadelphia: WB Saunders, 1993; 720–723.
7. Wright MS, Smith LA. Laboratory investigation of autoimmune hemolytic anemias. Clin Lab Sci 12:119–122, 1999.
8. Nemchik L. Introduction to anemias of increased erythrocyte destruction. In: Steine-Martin EA, Lotspeich-Steininger CA, Koepke JA, eds. Clinical Hematology: Principles, Procedures and Correlations, 2nd ed. Philadelphia: Lippincott, 1998; 245.
9. Ucar K. Clinical presentation and management of hemolytic anemias. Oncology 10:163–170, 2002.
10. Birch D. Malaria: Quest for a vaccine. Baltimore Sun, June 18, 2000.
11. Lemery L, Ciesla B. Why Did This Sample Fail the Correlation Checks? Chicago: American Society of Clinical Pathologists Tech Sample, 1997; G-12.

Part II

Red Blood Cell Disorders

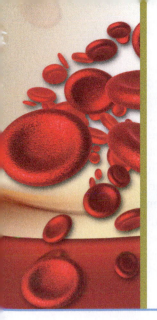

Chapter 5

The Microcytic Anemias

Betty Ciesla

Objectives

After completing this chapter, the student will be able to:

1. Describe the red blood cell indices related to the microcytic anemias.
2. List the microcytic anemias considered in a differential diagnosis of microcytic processes.
3. Describe iron transport from ingestion to incorporation in hemoglobin.
4. List the three stages of iron deficiency.
5. Describe the physical symptoms of a patient with iron deficiency anemia.
6. Identify the iron needs of children and adults.
7. Identify the laboratory tests used in the diagnosis of iron deficiency anemia.
8. Describe the iron overload conditions.
9. Define the pathophysiology of hereditary hemochromatosis.
10. Outline the symptoms of patients with hereditary hemochromatosis.
11. Describe the diagnosis and clinical management of patients with hereditary hemochromatosis.
12. Describe the basic pathophysiologic defect in the thalassemia syndromes.
13. Describe the alpha thalassemic conditions with regard to gene deletions and clinical symptoms.
14. List the three types of beta thalassemia.
15. Discuss the clinical manifestations of the beta thalassemias with regard to bone marrow changes, splenic changes, skeletal changes, and hematologic changes.
16. Correlate the morphologic changes in the red blood cell with the defect in the alpha and beta thalassemias.
17. Describe the major hemoglobin in each of the thalassemic states.
18. Describe the transfusion protocols of patients with thalassemia major and the contraindications.

Anemia is a significant health issue in the world population, affecting every ethnic class and social strata. The clinical laboratory plays a decisive role in supplying the physician with clinical data in defining the cause and determining the treatment of this condition. Broadly defined, individuals become *anemic* when their red blood cells are no longer able to supply oxygen to their body tissues. Anemias may be classified according to their physiology or their morphology. The morphologic classification is based on red blood cell indices, whereas the physiologic classification is based on symptoms and bone marrow response. This chapter stresses the morphologic classification of anemias.

Normal red blood cell indices are mean corpuscular volume (MCV) of 80 to 100 fL; mean corpuscular hemoglobin (MCH) of 27 to 31 pg, and mean corpuscular hemoglobin content (MCHC) of 32% to 36%. If a microcytic, hypochromic anemia develops, hemoglobin synthesis is disrupted, and the MCV is less than 80 fL and the MCHC is less than 32%. The red blood cells are termed microcytic, hypochromic and appear as small cells, deficient in hemoglobin. The laboratorian can be instrumental in helping the physician recognize that a microcytic anemic process is occurring, determining the cause, and deciding on a management or therapeutic plan. The microcytic anemias include iron deficiency anemia (IDA), sideroblastic anemias (acquired and inherited), the thalassemias, and a percentage of anemias of inflammation or chronic disease that transcend into IDA.

IRON INTAKE AND IRON ABSORPTION

Iron is one of the most abundant metals in the world, yet IDA continues to be one of the most prominent nutritional disorders worldwide.[1] Iron balance is regulated by several conditions including the following:

- Amount of iron ingested
- Amount of iron absorbed
- Red blood cell formation using recycled and new iron
- Iron stores
- Iron loss through blood loss or other sources (Fig. 5.1.)

The amount of iron that must be obtained through the diet varies according to age and gender. Men and infants should absorb about 1 mg/day, premenopausal women about 0.2 to 2.0 mg/day, and children about 0.5 mg/day.[2] For perspective, if a man eats a 2500-calorie diet, he ingests about 15 mg of iron, of which only 10% is absorbed, giving him 1.5 mg/day of iron that can be used for red blood cell production or stored in the reticuloendothelial system (RES).[3] Iron in the diet is available as heme iron through meats or as nonheme/nonmeat iron. Table 5.1 lists iron sources. For an infant, iron-fortified formulas and breast milk are major sources of iron. As an infant develops and rapidly gains weight, there is a high demand for iron. Most infants and young children need some dietary supplementation to maintain iron balance (see Table 5.7).

When ingested, iron is absorbed in the gastrointestinal (GI) tract and then transported into the circulation. The main portion of the GI tract involved in this process is the duodenum and jejunum of the small intestine, which on average absorbs only about 10% of ingested iron. This absorption rate is not static; it decreases or increases relative to iron stores and the body's needs. When iron is absorbed, stomach acid converts the iron molecule from the Fe^{3+} (ferric) to the Fe^{2+} (ferrous) state, and iron molecules are transported through the circulation to the bone marrow via transferrin. Transferrin, the transport vehicle, is a plasma protein formed in the liver that assists iron delivery to erythroblasts in the bone marrow. Transferrin receptors on the pronormoblast bind iron so that iron molecules can immediately begin incorporation into the heme molecule during erythropoiesis. The ability of the transferrin receptor to bind iron is influenced by the iron being delivered; the pH of the body; and, on the molecular level, the influence of an iron regulatory factor, ferritin repressor protein.[4] An essential ingredient for seamless iron absorption and transport is a healthy GI tract. Procedures such as **gastrectomy** or gastric bypass, atrophic gastritis, and celiac disease may compromise iron absorption.[5] There are dietary substances that enhance or diminish the absorption of iron from the diet (Tables 5.2 and 5.3) and foods with a high iron value (Table 5.4).

IRON STORAGE AND RECYCLED IRON

Ferritin and hemosiderin are the primary storage forms of iron. These compounds are harbored in the liver, spleen, bone marrow, and skeletal muscle. Ferritin can be measured in plasma, whereas hemosiderin is more often identified in the urine or stained through bone marrow slides. In men, iron stores are generally 1.0 to 1.4 g of body iron; in women, iron stores are generally 0.2 to 0.4 g. Given these figures and with the realization that the iron absorption requirement is on average 1 mg/day, it is easy to understand why anemia may take years to develop in adults with iron-poor diets.

The Iron Cycle: Ingestion, Absorption, Storage

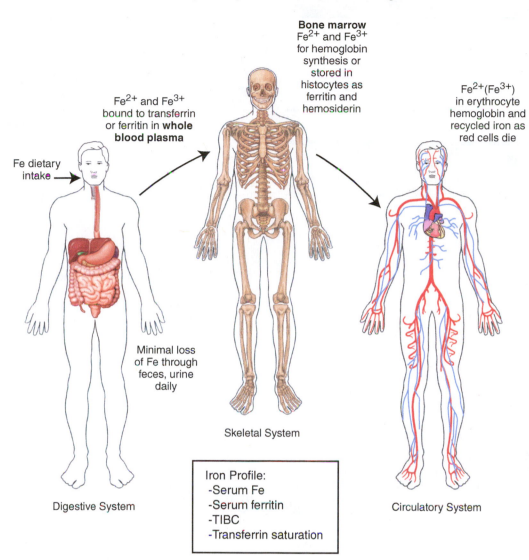

Bone marrow
Fe^{2+} and Fe^{3+}
for hemoglobin
synthesis or
stored in
histocytes as
ferritin and
hemosiderin

Fe^{2+} and Fe^{3+}
bound to transferrin
or ferritin in **whole
blood plasma**

$Fe^{2+}(Fe^{3+})$
in erythrocyte
hemoglobin and
recycled iron as
red cells die

Fe dietary
intake

Minimal loss
of Fe through
feces, urine
daily

Skeletal System

Iron Profile:
-Serum Fe
-Serum ferritin
-TIBC
-Transferrin saturation

Digestive System

Circulatory System

Figure 5.1   The iron cycle: Ingestion, absorption, and storage.

Table 5.1 ⊙ Multiple Forms of Iron in the Body

Iron in food

Heme sources: Meat

Nonheme sources: Beans, clams, vegetables

Iron in storage

Ferritin: Found in liver, spleen, skeletal muscle, bone marrow

Hemosiderin: Found in excreted urine

Iron in circulation

Iron and globin are recycled as a result of red blood cell senescence

Table 5.2 ⊙ Enhancers of Iron Absorption

• Orange juice
• Vitamin C
• Pickles
• Soy sauce
• Vinegar
• Alcohol

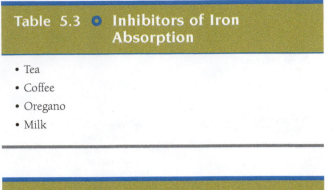

Table 5.3 ⊙ Inhibitors of Iron Absorption

- Tea
- Coffee
- Oregano
- Milk

Table 5.4 ⊙ Foods With High Iron Value

- Clams
- Soybeans
- Lentils
- Pinto beans
- Liver
- Garbanzo beans
- Tofu
- Packaged oatmeal

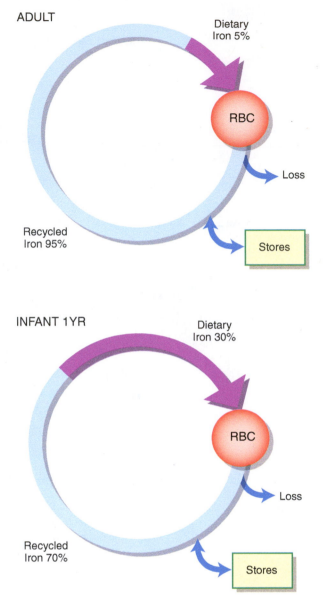

Figure 5.2 Iron need versus amount of recycled iron available.

Specifically, body stores in men of 1 g would last 3 to 4 years before iron depletion occurs.[6] Most cases of iron deficiency relate directly to external blood loss, especially **menorrhagia** or slow GI bleed. Blood lost outside the body has no chance of being recycled into the usable by-product of heme and globin.

The recycling of iron from heme and amino acids from globin after the lysis of aged red blood cells is a very efficient process. Heme is returned to the bone marrow, and the amino acids of the globin chain are returned to the amino acid pool. Each of these products later is recruited for hemoglobin formation and red blood cell production. In an adult, approximately 95% of recycled iron is used for red blood cell production, whereas in an infant, only 70% is used for this purpose (Fig. 5.2). Because of this relationship, it is easy to understand the significance of adequate iron sources during the early years of development.

IRON DEFICIENCY ANEMIA

Pathophysiology and Symptoms

IDA can be a secondary condition resulting from blood loss or inadequate iron intake. It may also be a secondary condition caused by a disease process or conditions that deplete iron stores, such as GI bleed or pregnancy. In either case, IDA manifests as a microcytic, hypochromic process, in which the red blood cells are small and deficient in hemoglobin (Table 5.5). Iron-starved red blood cells divide more rapidly as they search for iron. The red blood cells are smaller because of excess red blood cell divisions. The complete blood count (CBC) is characterized by a decreased red blood cell count (RBC), hemoglobin, hematocrit, MCV, and MCHC and increased red blood cell distribution width (RDW). The development of IDA is a three-stage process:

- *Stage I*: Continuum of iron depletion from the marrow (Prussian blue stain shows absence of iron)
- *Stage II*: Iron-deficient erythropoiesis and slight microcytic, hypochromic picture
- *Stage III*: Frank case of IDA in the peripheral circulation, microcytes, and hypochromia

Table 5.5 ⊙	Stages of Iron Deficiency Anemia Matched to Diagnostic Signals

Stage 1: Iron stores depleted; test for
Absence of stainable bone marrow iron

Decreased serum ferritin level

Increased TIBC

Stage 2: Iron-deficient erythropoiesis; test for
Slight microcytosis

Slight decreased hemoglobin

Decreased transferrin saturation

Stage 3: Iron deficiency anemia; test for
Decreased serum iron

Decreased serum ferritin

Increased TIBC

Decreased transferrin saturation

In most cases, the patient does not present with overt symptoms until anemia develops (stage III); however, **serum ferritin** decreases at every stage. The physician may use diagnostic laboratory tests such as serum iron and serum ferritin to diagnose IDA well before the patient develops anemia. Individuals in high-risk groups should be monitored periodically for iron status (Table 5.6).

There are many symptoms that mark an individual as being iron deficient. Some of these symptoms are unique to iron deficiency, and some are general symptoms of anemia. Clinically, a patient with anemia may present with the following:

- Fatigue
- Pallor

Table 5.6 ⊙	Causes of Iron Deficiency Anemia

Related to increased iron demands
Growth spurts in infants and children

Pregnancy and nursing

Related to lack of iron intake
Poor diet

Conditions that diminish absorption

Related to blood loss
Menorrhagia

Gastrointestinal bleeding (GI bleed)

Hemolysis

Other physical causes of bleeding

- Vertigo
- Dyspnea
- Cold intolerance
- Lethargy

Additionally, patients may experience cardiac problems such as palpitations and angina (see Table 2.7). Symptoms *unique* to a patient with IDA include pica (abnormal craving for unusual substances such as dirt, ice, or clay), cheilitis (inflammation around the lips), and koilonychias (spooning of the nail beds) (Fig. 5.3). Additionally, evidence suggests that iron deficiency in infants may result in developmental delays and behavioral disturbances.[7] In pregnant women, iron deficiency in the first two trimesters may lead to an increase in preterm delivery and an increased likelihood of delivering a low-birth-weight child.[7] Anemia affects 3.5 million individuals in the United States, with approximately 50% of these cases being IDA.[1] Sensitivity to the possibility of iron deficiency, backed by good diagnostic data, is the best weapon for eliminating IDA in the Western world.

Tests Used to Help Diagnose Iron Deficiency

From a clinical standpoint, if iron deficiency is suspected, testing for iron deficiency must analyze the patient's *red blood cell status* and *iron status*. In terms of the CBC, all parameters except the white blood cell count (WBC) and platelet count are less than the normal reference range (see Table 2.3). In some cases (e.g., if a patient is actively bleeding), the platelet count is elevated. MCV and MCHC are markedly lower than normal, RDW may be mildly elevated, and peripheral smear shows small red blood cells that are deficient in hemoglobin. Target cells and elliptocytes may occasionally be seen (Fig. 5.4). The reticulocyte count is

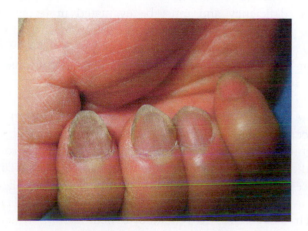

Figure 5.3   Koilonychia.

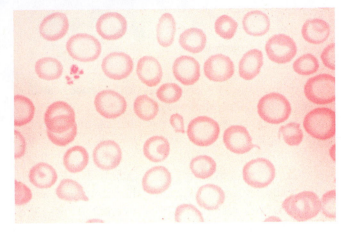

Figure 5.4   Microcytic, hypochromic red blood cells.
© 1967 American Society of Clinical Pathologists. Reprinted with permission.

decreased compared with the level of anemia, indicating slightly ineffective erythropoiesis.

Tests that assess a patient's iron status include serum iron, serum ferritin, transferrin or total iron binding capacity (TIBC), and transferrin saturation. Serum iron is a measure of the total amount of iron in the serum with a normal value of 50 to 150 μg/L. Serum ferritin is one of the most sensitive indicators of iron stores, with a normal value of 20 to 250 μg/L for men and 10 to 120 μg/L for women. Ferritin is an acute phase reactant, and conditions such as chronic inflammation or chronic infection may falsely elevate the serum ferritin level. In these cases, an accurate assessment of iron stores is difficult. TIBC measures the availability of iron binding sites on the transferrin molecule. If an individual is iron deficient, there are many binding sites available searching for iron, and the TIBC value increases. This value is elevated in iron-deficient patients (reference range 250 to 450 μg/L) but subject to fluctuations in patients who use oral contraceptives or have liver disease, chronic infections, or nephrotic syndrome. TIBC is less sensitive to iron deficiency and must be evaluated in terms of the patient's other health issues. Transferrin saturation (% saturation) is derived as the product of the serum iron concentration divided by the TIBC and multiplied by 100. The normal value is 20% to 50%.

Additional but lesser known tests that are available to measure iron status are the serum transferrin receptor (sTfr) assay and the reticulocyte hemoglobin content (CHr) assay. sTfr is an early indication of iron deficiency that measures the number of transferrin receptors on the red blood cell surface.[8] The number of available receptors increases as iron is depleted. The CHr assay refers to reticulocyte hemoglobin, which increases if reticulocytes circulate longer in response to

anemia.[9] sTfr and CHr are not widely available outside the reference laboratory setting.

Occasionally, a diagnosis of IDA is made too casually and is based on a patient's age group, gender, or vague complaints. Young women who give a history of fatigue or menstrual problems are often simply given a trial of iron therapy with no supporting laboratory workup. A diagnosis of IDA should be made *only* with supporting laboratory data that reflect the patient's red blood cell and iron status. The patient should insist that this work be done before therapy is initiated, as unnecessary iron use has the potential for serious consequences.

Causes of Iron Deficiency

Many populations are vulnerable to IDA. Infants and pregnant or nursing women may have nutritional deficiency, young children may develop IDA when their growth and development rate outstrip their iron intake, and young women who have increased iron need due to menstruation may develop IDA (see Table 5.6). The primary cause of iron deficiency in the Western world is GI bleeding for men and excessive menses for women. External blood loss presents a significant challenge to the body because millions of shed red blood cells can never be used for recycling new red blood cells. Slow GI bleeds and dysfunctional uterine bleeding over time lead to a depletion of iron stores, and IDA results. Storage iron, represented by ferritin, represents a primary reservoir of iron that can be used as other iron sources are depleted. The average ferritin concentrations are 135 μg/L in men, 43 μg/L in women, and 30 μg/L in children.[10] Barring any other external loss of blood, iron deficiency solely resulting from lack of dietary sources would develop over a protracted period.

Treatment for Iron Deficiency

Treatment for iron deficiency is given orally in the form of drops (good for infants and children) or tablets. Iron preparations are in the form of ferrous sulfate, ferrous gluconate, and ferrous fumerate at 325 mg and are readily available over-the-counter in most places.[10] Side effects from oral iron therapy include constipation, stomach discomfort, and diarrhea. Most side effects can be overcome with consultation from the pharmacist for a gentler preparation. It is essential to remain compliant and to continue on iron therapy despite side effects. Laboratory evaluations such as CBC and reticulocyte count should show marked improvement in a few weeks. Additionally, microcytosis and hypochromia seen in the peripheral smear eventually are replaced by normocytic and normochromic red blood cells. Although oral iron normalizes the hematologic picture, an investigation should begin as to the source of the anemia and whether there are any underlying causes that are contributory. Table 5.7 provides recommendations to prevent and control iron deficiency in the United States.

ANEMIA OF CHRONIC DISEASE AND INFLAMMATION: PATHOPHYSIOLOGY, DIAGNOSIS, AND TREATMENT

The anemia of chronic disease, or the anemia of inflammation, is one of the most common anemias in hospital populations and second only to iron deficiency in terms of frequency. Many individuals with chronic

Table 5.7 ◉ Recommendations to Prevent and Control Iron Deficiency in the United States

Infants (0–12 mo) and children (1–5 yr)
• Encourage breastfeeding *or*
• Iron-fortified formula
• Provide one feeding of fruits, vegetables, juice by 6 mo
• Screen children for anemia every 6 mo

School-age children (5–12 yr) and adolescent boys (12–18 yr)
• Screen only those with history of IDA or low iron intake groups

Adolescent girls (12–18 yr) and nonpregnant women of childbearing age
• Encourage intake of iron-rich food and foods that increase iron absorption
• Screen nonpregnant women every 5–10 years through childbearing years

Pregnant women
• Start oral doses of iron at first prenatal visit
• Screen for anemia at first prenatal visit
• If hemoglobin is less than 9 g/dL, provide further medical attention

Postpartum women
• Risk factors include continued anemia, excessive blood loss, and multiple births

Men older than 18 years and postmenopausal women
• No routine screening recommended

Modified from Centers for Disease Control and Prevention. Recommendations to Prevent and Control Iron Deficiency in the United States. April 1998. Available at: http://www.cdc.gov/mmnr/preview/mmwrhtml/100051880.htm. Accessed September 24, 2006.

disorders such as **collagen vascular disease**, chronic kidney disease, thyroid disorders, and malignancies may have an anemia that eventually develops into a microcytic anemia (Table 5.8). When this occurs, most physicians order laboratory testing to establish whether there is also an iron deficiency process; this is termed *differential diagnosis*. Differential diagnosis is a process by which a physician examines a group of laboratory values and symptoms and tries to correlate them to a particular physiology.

Patients with the anemia of chronic disease show borderline low red blood cell count, hemoglobin, and hematocrit; slightly low MCV; and normal MCHC. The peripheral smear is essentially normal with slight variation in size and chroma. Serum iron is low, serum ferritin is normal or increased, and serum TIBC is decreased. Although this is *not* the profile for a patient with IDA, the patient has a low serum iron in both conditions. Several theories account for these data. In the anemias of inflammation, iron is blocked from reaching erythroid precursors because of impaired release from macrophages, there is impaired EPO production, and the pronormoblasts are not as responsive to EPO from patients with chronic disease.[11] Few individuals require a blood transfusion for treatment of anemia. Usually, when the underlying disease is successfully managed, symptoms of anemia seem to resolve. Hepcidin, a hormone produced by the liver, regulates iron transit,[12] and its production is greatly influenced by iron overload and anemia of inflammation. Hepcidin increases as iron levels increase. The expanding role of hepcidin in iron metabolism will undoubtedly have exciting testing implications in the future.[13]

THE SIDEROBLASTIC ANEMIAS

The disorders in this category of anemias are related to mitochondrial overload. They are either inherited or

Table 5.8 ◉ Conditions Leading to Anemia of Inflammation or Anemia of Chronic Disease

• Rheumatoid arthritis
• Chronic renal disease
• Thyroid disorders
• Malignancies
• Inflammatory bowel disease

acquired. This iron accumulation leads to the presence of iron deposits in the red blood cell precursors in the marrow, called ringed sideroblasts (Fig. 5.5); a dimorphic blood picture; and increased serum ferritin. If the sideroblastic anemia is inherited, it can be a congenital sex-linked or autosomal recessive condition. A mutation in delta amino levulinic acid leads to this linked condition. Additionally, secondary acquired iron loading may occur as a result of alcoholism, lead poisoning, isoniazid, or chloramphenicol use. Inherited sideroblastic anemias are the result of inherited abnormal genes, which is discussed later in the chapter.

In any case, the patient's peripheral smear shows a microcytic process, with dimorphism (some microcytes and some normal cells, some hypochromic and some normochromic) (Fig. 5.6) and the presence of Pappenheimer bodies (Fig. 5.7), red blood cells with precipitated iron inclusions that look like grape clusters in the periphery of the red blood cell. An iron

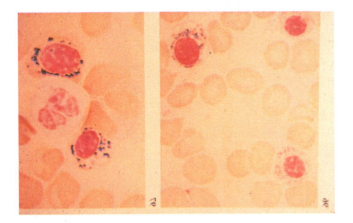

Figure 5.5 Ringed sideroblast in the bone marrow. From The College of American Pathologists, with permission.

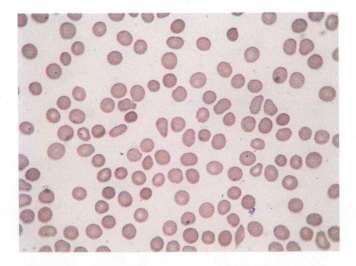

Figure 5.6 Dimorphism in the red blood cells: Two cell populations and different levels of hypochromia. Courtesy of Kathleen Finnegan, Stony Brook University, New York.

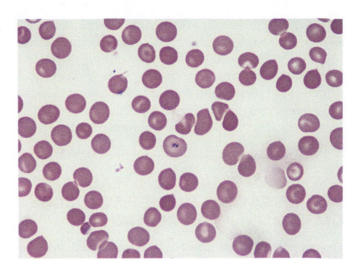

Figure 5.7 Pappenheimer bodies. Courtesy of Bernardino Madsen, Casper College, Wyoming.

profile reveals increased serum ferritin and increased serum iron. As can be expected, when the underlying condition is successfully managed, the iron overload conditions are resolved. Table 5.9 compares the microcytic disorders.

Hereditary Hemochromatosis

Hereditary hemochromatosis (HH) is one of the most common genetic disorders in persons with European ancestry and a major disorder. More than 1 million people are affected in the United States.[14] Caucasians, African Americans, and Hispanics are particularly at risk. This disorder has a low profile relative to other blood disorders, however, partially because it is almost always a diagnosis of exclusion. HH is an autosomal recessive disorder carried on chromosome 6 that is closely linked to HLA-A3. It may be inherited homozygously or heterozygously with homozygotes more prone to iron overload. Signs of excessive iron loading, however, are also present in 10% of heterozygotes.[15] Because of this inheritance, individuals with HH begin to load iron excessively from a young age and continue iron loading with every decade.

The diagnosis of HH is made accidentally in most individuals as a result of blood screening for an unrelated issue. In these individuals, the customary process of iron absorption and storage becomes unbalanced because of the inheritance of *HFE,* an abnormal gene that regulates the amount of iron absorbed from the diet. Two mutations, C282Y and H63D, have been described.[15] Although the complete role of these mutant variations in the *HFE* gene is not fully understood, it is known that the normal product of these genes does not bind to the transferrin receptor in the normal iron delivery process. As a result of this faulty

Table 5.9 ● Differential Diagnosis of Microcytic Disorders

Diagnosis	Serum Iron	TIBC	% Saturation	Ferritin
AOI/ACD	↓	↓	↓	↑
HH	↑	↓	↑	↑
IDA	↓	↑	↓	↓
SA	↑	↓	↑	↑
Thalassemia minor	↑/N	N	N	N

AOI/ACD, anemia of inflammation/anemia of chronic disease; HH, hereditary hemochromatosis; IDA, iron deficiency anemia; SA, sideroblastic anemia.

mechanism, iron is constantly loaded into the storage sites and leads to multiorgan damage and symptoms over decades.[16] Iron accumulation is a multifactorial event, starting from iron excess with few symptoms and progressing to full-blown iron accumulation in tissues and tissue damage.

Symptoms and Laboratory Diagnosis of Hereditary Hemochromatosis

HH is a great impersonator and has myriad symptoms that usually serve to confuse rather than lead to a direct diagnosis (Table 5.10). The more common symptoms include the following:

- Chronic fatigue and weakness
- Cirrhosis of the liver
- Hyperpigmentation
- Diabetes
- Impotence
- Sterility
- Cardiac arrhythmias
- Tender swollen joints

Table 5.10 ● Confusing Symptoms of Hereditary Hemochromatosis

Symptom	Possible Other Cause
Chronic fatigue, weakness	Could be seen in IDA
Cirrhosis of the liver	Could be seen in alcoholism
Cardiac arrhythmias	Could be seen in valve problems, congestive heart failure
Tender swollen joints	Could be seen in collagen vascular diseases
Hair loss, hyperpigmentation	Could be seen in endocrine disorders

- Hair loss
- Abdominal symptoms

Each of the previously listed symptoms alone could point a physician in a direction other than HH, yet when these symptoms are combined with a microcytic process, a screening for iron status provides relevant information. As has already been indicated, screening for iron status includes the following:

- Serum iron
- Serum transferrin level
- TIBC
- Possibly transferrin saturation

In patients with HH, serum iron, serum ferritin, and transferrin saturation are elevated, whereas TIBC and transferrin fall in the normal reference range. Symptoms may not be seen and blood values may not be elevated in younger individuals. Serum ferritin levels greater than 150 µg/L and transferrin saturation levels greater than 45% are indicative of HH. Genetic testing would be appropriate for these individuals to establish if they possess the C282Y and the H63D mutation present in 80% to 95% of patients with HH, but this testing is expensive and should be ordered judiciously. The laboratory is critical in the diagnosis of HH, and its value cannot be underestimated in providing definitive data for this crucial diagnosis.

Treatment for Hereditary Hemochromatosis

Untreated HH can be fatal, and advanced iron overload frequently leads to liver cancer (Fig. 5.8). The treatment of choice for individuals with a diagnosis of HH is aggressive therapeutic phlebotomy, or bloodletting, as it used to be termed. The goal of this procedure is to reduce the serum ferritin level to less than 10 µg/dL and keep the patient's hematocrit at around 35%. For most patients, one or two phlebotomies are performed per week as long as the patient can tolerate the procedure. When the patient's serum ferritin has returned to near

12- to 16-hour infusion pump. Patients usually use a subcutaneous injection site for infusion and infuse during the nighttime hours. Excess iron is chelated and then excreted in the urine. Infusion sites must be rotated often to avoid infections and irritation (Fig. 5.9). Patients who are noncompliant in ridding themselves of iron through either phlebotomy or Desferal significantly shorten their life span. Early diagnosis of HH can easily be accomplished by adding blood tests such as serum ferritin and transferrin saturation to the menu of tests offered during yearly physical examinations. The medical community is slowly becoming aware of this "silent killer" as individual consumers become more knowledgeable about this disease and as organizations such as the Iron Overload Disease Association (www.ironoverload.org) become more aggressive in outreach and education. The complications of HH are *preventable*, but the efforts of many individuals—nutritionists, physicians, laboratory personnel, and patients—are needed to raise awareness and expand educational outreach.

THALASSEMIA SYNDROMES
Brief History and Demographics

More than 2 million Americans carry the gene for thalassemia,[17] but most have never heard the word *thalassemia*, which comes from the Greek word *thalassa* and means "from the sea." Relatively few individuals develop severe forms of thalassemia, but those who do

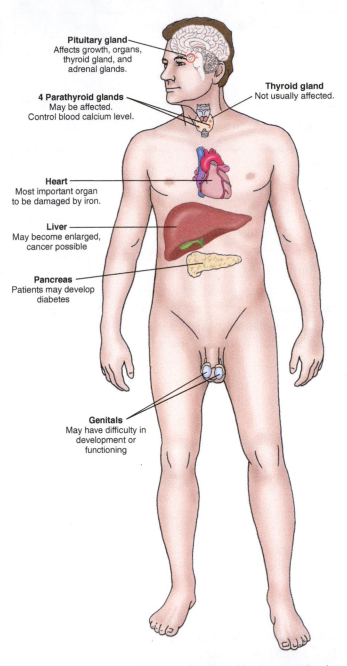

Pituitary gland
Affects growth, organs, thyroid gland, and adrenal glands.

4 Parathyroid glands
May be affected. Control blood calcium level.

Thyroid gland
Not usually affected.

Heart
Most important organ to be damaged by iron.

Liver
May become enlarged, cancer possible

Pancreas
Patients may develop diabetes

Genitals
May have difficulty in development or functioning

Figure 5.8 Organs of the body damaged by iron overload.

normal, phlebotomies are performed three or four times a year to keep the serum ferritin in range. Symptoms lessen and in some cases disappear completely when the iron level is reduced. Excess iron depresses the immune system, and it has been suggested that iron overload causes a significant amount of diabetes.

For patients who cannot tolerate phlebotomies or are unwilling to go through the procedure, deferrioxamine (Desferal), an iron-**chelating** agent, can be used. In this procedure, a dose of Desferal is matched to body weight and delivered through a continuous

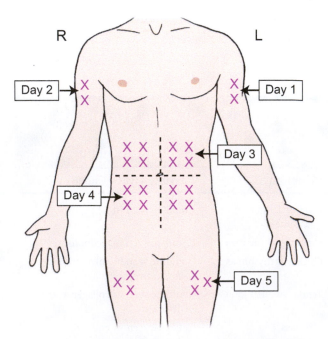

R   L

Day 2   Day 1

Day 3

Day 4

Day 5

Figure 5.9 Rotation chart for subcutaneous injections.
Adapted from Cooley's Anemia Foundation, with permission.

face a lifetime of transfusions and medical management of multiorgan problems. The thalassemic gene is ubiquitous, yet it has a particular penetration in Mediterranean areas and in Middle Eastern, Northern African, Indian, Asian, and Caribbean populations. More cases are being seen and treated in the United States as more diverse populations enter the country. Laboratory professionals seem to be more aware of the possibility of thalassemic conditions when faced with a patient who presents with a microcytic process and normal iron status. Physicians and medical students, interns, and residents often fail to consider the thalassemias as reasons for a microcytic process, most likely as a result of lack of in-depth training or exposure. A respectful relationship between the laboratory and medical staff can be tremendously beneficial in diagnosing and treating new cases of thalassemia.

Dr. Thomas Cooley and Dr. Pearl Lee described the first cases of thalassemia disease in North America in 1925. Clustering five cases together, these clinicians described four children who had anemia, hepatosplenomegaly, skin discoloration, jaundice, and peculiar facial features and bone changes. Their bone marrows showed erythroid hyperplasia (Fig. 5.10), and their peripheral smears showed many nucleated red blood cells, target cells, and microcytes (Fig. 5.11). Not much has changed in the initial presentation of an individual with thalassemia disease or thalassemia major. Although Dr. N. W. Valentine described the mode of inheritance for this disorder in 1944, and genetic interactions and cloning of the thalassemic genes have been accomplished since 1960, there still is no cure.

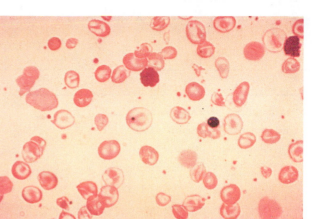

Figure 5.11   Thalassemia major, showing a high degree of poikilocytosis and nucleated red blood cells.   From The College of American Pathologists, with permission.

Pathophysiology of the Thalassemias

In contrast to the other microcytic processes discussed, the thalassemias have *nothing* to do with iron. The thalassemias are globin chain disorders that involve the lack of production of alpha or beta globin chains. The thalassemias are defects of hemoglobin synthesis. Failure to synthesize either the alpha or the beta chain impairs production of the normal physiologic adult hemoglobin, Hgb A ($\alpha_2\beta_2$), Hgb A$_2$ ($\alpha_2\delta_2$), and Hgb F ($\alpha_2\gamma_2$). The construction of each of these normal hemoglobins depends on alpha and beta chains being synthesized as part of their normal tetramer. When this synthesis is impaired, hemoglobins form as a result of the unbalanced chain production that negatively affects the life span of the red blood cell. Additionally, there are multiorgan complications, the development of a microcytic anemia, and a peripheral smear with many red blood cell morphologic abnormalities.

There are two major types of thalassemias: alpha thalassemia and beta thalassemia. Put simply, the alpha thalassemias result from gene deletions. Each individual inherits four alpha genes, two maternal and two paternal. Each of the four clinical presentations of alpha thalassemia results from the deletion of one or more of the alpha genes. The beta thalassemias revolve around the inheritance of a defective beta gene, either from one parent (heterozygously) or from both parents (homozygously). To date, 200 beta gene mutations have been described, and these mutations have been broadly divided into the B^0 or B$^+$ gene. In B^0 individuals, there is a complete lack of synthesis of the beta chain, and in B$^{+ pt}$ individuals, a limited amount of the beta chain is synthesized. Both of these mutations affect specific populations (Table 5.11). On the

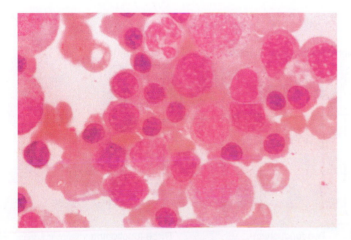

Figure 5.10   Erythroid hyperplasia—the bone marrow's response to anemic stress.   © 1982 American Society of Clinical Pathologists. Reprinted with permission.

Table 5.11 ⦿	Gene Expression in Population
B⁰	**B⁺**
Northern Italy	Mediterranean region
Greece	Southeast Asia
Algeria	Middle East
Saudi Arabia	Indian subcontinent
	West Africa

molecular level, beta chain defects result from faulty transcription of messenger RNA.

Alpha Thalassemias

Incidence and Pathophysiology

The alpha thalassemias have a high incidence in Asian populations (e.g., Thailand, Vietnam, Cambodia, Indonesia, and Laos).[18] They also occur in Saudi Arabian and Filipino populations. The alpha chain is the critical building block for construction of all normal adult physiologic hemoglobins because each adult hemoglobin depends on the production of the alpha chain. The alpha chain is also crucial in the development of fetal hemoglobin; without alpha chain development, Hgb F does not form. There are four clinical states of alpha thalassemia that are related to the number of alpha genes deleted (Fig. 5.12).

Clinical Conditions of Alpha Thalassemias

- The most severe state is Bart's hydrops fetalis, which is characterized by a total absence of alpha chain synthesis. No Hgb A is formed, only Hgb Bart's (γ_4), which is a high oxygen affinity hemoglobin. Because this hemoglobin is an abnormal tetramer and oxygen-loving (Hgb Bart's holds onto oxygen and resists delivering oxygen to the tissues), the anemia that develops is severe and usually leads to stillbirth or spontaneous abortion.

- Hgb H disease is the next most severe condition. There is only one functional alpha gene;

Normal chromosome 16

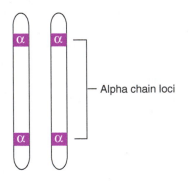

Alpha chain loci

Clinical Conditions of Alpha Thalassemia

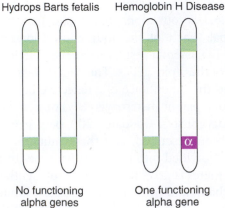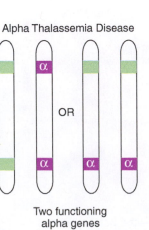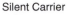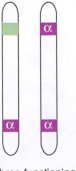

Hydrops Barts fetalis — No functioning alpha genes

Hemoglobin H Disease — One functioning alpha gene

Alpha Thalassemia Disease — Two functioning alpha genes — OR

Silent Carrier — Three functioning alpha genes

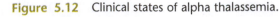

Figure 5.12 Clinical states of alpha thalassemia.

the other three genes are deleted. Little Hgb A is produced; instead, a new Hgb H is formed, which is also a fairly unstable tetramer (β_4) and represents 5% to 40% on alkaline electrophoresis (see Chapter 8). Hemoglobin levels are less than 10 g/dL (average 6 to 8 g/dL), and reticulocyte counts are 5% to 10%. Microcytosis and hypochromia are observed in the peripheral smear with red blood cell fragments (Fig. 5.13). An unusual inclusion, Hgb H inclusion, is formed. On supravital staining with brilliant cresyl blue or crystal violet, this inclusion looks like a pitted golf ball (Fig. 5.14). In the peripheral circulation, Hgb H is usually pitted from the red blood cell by the spleen, leaving the cell more fragile and less elastic, with a shortened life span. Individuals with Hgb H disease have lifelong anemia with variable splenomegaly and bone changes.

The final two clinical conditions are less severe: the two-gene deletion state (alpha thalassemia trait) and the one-gene deletion state, the silent carrier. An individual with the alpha thalassemia trait possesses only two viable Hgb A genes and may have only mild anemia with many microcytic, hypochromic cells. Some Hgb Bart's is formed. A silent carrier is hematologically normal or slightly microcytic, and the patient may be unaware of his or her alpha gene status. Diagnosis in patients from both of these alpha thalassemia subsets (alpha thalassemia trait and silent carrier) may be difficult; however, the presence of elliptocytes and target cells in peripheral smears can present a high predictive value if smears are carefully reviewed for these findings.[19] See Table 5.12 for a list of diagnostic aids.

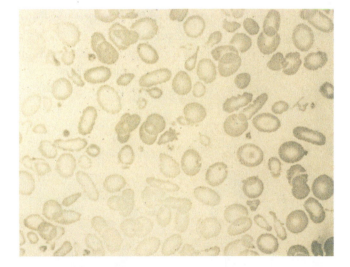

Figure 5.13 Peripheral smear from an individual with Hgb H. From The College of American Pathologists, with permission.

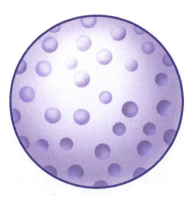

H Bodies in mature red cell

Figure 5.14 Hgb H inclusions as seen after brilliant cresyl blue staining. Adapted from Glassy E. Color Atlas of Hematology: An Illustrated Guide Based on Proficiency Testing. Northfield, IL: College of American Pathologists, 1998, with permission.

Table 5.12 ● Alpha Thalassemias

Condition	Genes Deleted	Clinical Expression	Hemoglobin Electrophoresis
Bart's hydrops fetalis	4	Stillborn, hydrops	Hgb Bart's (γ_4)
Hgb H disease	3	Microcytic, hypochromic, Hgb H inclusions, high reticulocytes	Hgb H (β_4) 5%–40% Hgb A approximately 60%
Alpha thalassemia trait	2	Mild anemia, microcytic, hypochromic, elliptocytes, targets	Small levels of Hgb Bart's 5%–10%
Silent carrier	1	Normal hematologically, but few elliptocytes, targets	Normal

Diagnosis and Treatment

If the most severe alpha thalassemic condition is suspected, especially in pregnancy, amniocentesis fluid or chronic villi sampling may be obtained and examined for the presence of alpha genes through molecular diagnostic procedures. In the case of Bart's hydrops fetalis, most pregnancies are terminated or individuals deliver severely edematous fetuses that are not viable. Cord blood is usually tested for hemoglobin electrophoresis, which usually shows a high percentage of Hgb Bart's. Genetic counseling is strongly advised for these individuals and for individuals in high-risk ethnic groups. Hgb H may be suspected if CBC shows slightly elevated RBC combined with extremely low MCV (less than 60 fL) and RDW results that are extremely elevated (normal value 11% to 15%) owing to the misshapen red blood cells and fragments compared with the more homogeneous microcytic, hypochromic population seen in IDA. Although Hgb H may be present at 5% to 40%, failure to show an abnormal hemoglobin band by electrophoresis should not eliminate suspicion.[20] Hgb H, a fast-moving hemoglobin on alkaline electrophoresis, may be missed by traditional methods. The final two conditions—alpha thalassemia trait and the silent carrier condition—may not be recognized on peripheral smear analysis because their hematologic pictures are not that abnormal.

Treatment for Hgb H disease is supportive, and transfusions are given only if necessary. Iron deficiency must be eliminated as a reason for the microcytic indices so that the patient is not given iron unnecessarily.

Beta Thalassemia Major: Cooley's Anemia, Mediterranean Anemia

Beta thalassemia major is an inherited blood disorder that affects million of individuals worldwide. In the United States, more than 2 million individuals are carriers of the thalassemic gene, resulting in significant penetrance of this gene, which often results in disease. In beta thalassemia major, little or no beta chain is synthesized; consequently, no (or very little) Hgb A is synthesized. This condition results from a union between two carriers, and mendelian genetics indicate a one-in-four chance of producing a severely affected individual (Fig. 5.15). The other offspring may be carriers. Beta thalassemia major is a serious genetic blood disorder, affecting multiple organs, quality of life, and longevity. Most infants born with thalassemia major are not ill for the first 6 months because fetal hemoglobin is the majority hemoglobin at birth. In the normal sequence of events, gamma chains are silenced, and beta chains increase, forming Hgb A between 3 and 6 months. In

thalassemia major, there are no beta chains to combine with the alpha chains, and Hgb F production continues; however, there is an imbalance of alpha chains. When alpha chains cannot combine, they are unpaired and precipitate inside the red blood cell, causing a markedly decreased life span (7 to 22 days). Between 2 and 4 years of age, most young children with beta thalassemia major begin to show a failure to thrive, irritability, enlarged spleens, symptoms of anemia, **jaundice**, and transfusion requirement.

Living With Thalassemia Major

Patients and families with thalassemia major balance multiple health issues on a daily basis as they struggle to maintain a normal life. Medical management of this disease is continuous, frustrating, and disruptive for children who have the disease and parents who are caregivers and carriers. Severe anemia underlies most of the other complications; although variable, hemoglobin values are often 6 to 9 g/dL, about one-half the normal level. The patient's peripheral smear shows a severe microcytic, hypochromic process with a high number of nucleated red blood cells, marked polychromasia, and a high degree of red blood cell morphology (see Fig. 5.11).

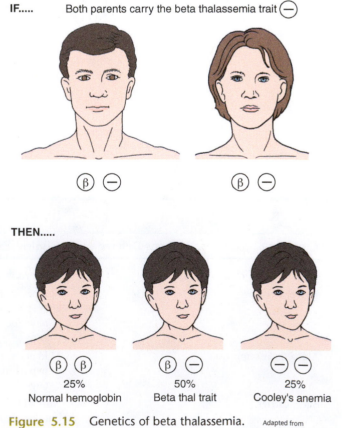

Figure 5.15 Genetics of beta thalassemia. Adapted from Cooley's Anemia Foundation, with permission.

Because this chronic anemic state has led to chronic overexpansion of the capable bone marrow (the bone marrow increases its output up to 20 times), the quality of bone that is laid down is thin and fragile. Pathologic fractures and bony changes in the facial structure (thalassemic facies) and skull are normally seen and give a thalassemic individual a strange look. Bossing, or protrusion, of the skull is prominent, as is orthodontic misalignment. The spleen reaches enormous proportions because abnormal red blood cells have been harbored and sequestered on a daily basis. Enlarged spleens cause excessive hemolysis and discomfort. Many patients have splenectomies, and this surgery *does* ameliorate some of the anemia issues. Splenectomy presents the patient with other challenges, however, because it is not a benign procedure (see Chapter 2).

One of the gravest problems is iron overload. Patients with beta thalassemia major absorb more iron through diet because of increased erythropoiesis, and they accumulate iron because they take in an additional 200 mg of iron with each transfusion of packed red blood cells.[21] Patients with thalassemia major in the United States have an average transfusion regimen of blood once every 2 to 5 weeks, so iron accumulation is expected and must be medically monitored and managed. For more information, please refer to the Cooley's Anemia Foundation (www.CAF.org).

Treating and Managing Thalassemia Major

Patients with thalassemia major are on either a low-transfusion or a high-transfusion protocol. A low-transfusion protocol treats the patient symptomatically, administering transfusion when symptoms warrant. A high-transfusion protocol aims to keep the patient's hemoglobin level close to 10 g/dL, and the patient is transfused every 2 to 5 weeks. There are good arguments for both protocols, bearing in mind that transfusion exposes the individual not only to excess iron but also to foreign red blood cell antigens and other blood-borne diseases. A high-transfusion protocol gives the patient the best hope for a normal quality of life by increasing his or her hemoglobin and providing better bone quality, better growth, less iron, and near-normal spleen size. Iron overload looms as a major outcome of the high-transfusion protocol, however, and is the major focus of clinical management.

Patients must be assessed for liver, pancreatic, endocrine, and cardiac iron. Although noninvasive procedures are available, they are specialized and not available at every clinical facility. Iron overload poses significant risk to cardiac function and leads to hepatic and endocrine complications. Iron chelation is recommended when the serum ferritin level has reached about 1,000 µg/L; this usually correlates with about 10 to 20 transfusions from the onset of diagnosis.[22] The procedure for chelation with Desferal was explained earlier in this chapter. Compliance is crucial in patients with thalassemia major and becomes difficult to maintain as the patient moves from childhood to adolescence and becomes less willing to be hooked up to the infusion pump. In late 2005, an oral chelating agent, deferasirox (Exjade or ICL670; Novartis, East Hanover, New Jersey), became available. Despite compliance with chelating therapy, cardiac complications continue to be the leading cause of death in patients with thalassemia major.

Therapeutic modalities for severely thalassemic patients include bone marrow transplantation and stem cell transplantation. For patients considering bone marrow transplant, finding a compatible donor is the necessary first step. If this can be accomplished, bone marrow transplant should be considered early, before the patient develops too many complications of thalassemia. The transplant procedure itself is rigorous and risky. Stem cell transplantation, although a viable alternative, takes much forethought and often is limited by the fact that stem cells have not been collected from the umbilical cord after delivery.

Thalassemia Intermedia and Beta Thalassemia Trait

Individuals with thalassemia intermedia are not a well-defined subset of thalassemia major patients. As a clinical group, they develop problems later in life than patients with thalassemia major, and they may *not* need transfusions. They develop larger spleens, but their transfusion requirements, if present, are less frequent. Bone changes may be present, but they are mild. Patients with thalassemia intermedia may require iron depletion with Desferal therapy but much less frequently than patients with thalassemia major.

Beta thalassemia trait is the heterozygous condition in which only one abnormal beta gene is inherited from the parent. This condition mimics IDA with individuals presenting with microcytic, hypochromic indices and moderately low hemoglobin and hematocrit values.[23] Hgb A_2 increases to approximately 5% to 10%. Beta thalassemia minor has often been confused with IDA (Fig. 5.16), but close examination of the CBC shows an increased RBC. Above all other values, the increased RBC is significant in this condition because it represents that the bone marrow is compensating for having only one-half the complement of beta chains. This change, although subtle, is often unrecognized by

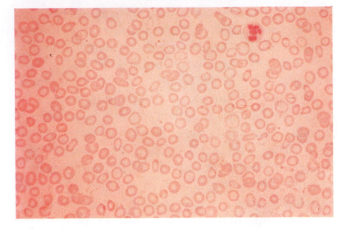

Figure 5.16 Microcytic, hypochromic blood smear in thalassemia minor. From The College of American Pathologists, with permission.

clinicians, and for this reason many patients with beta thalassemia minor have been put on iron protocols that offer no therapeutic value. Iron is *not* the problem in beta thalassemia minor (see Table 5.9). Although a therapeutic trial of iron may not harm the patient in the long run, it is not good medical management. Patients who have microcytic indices may represent the largest number of anemia patients. A careful diagnosis that considers broader possibilities for a microcytic presentation is in the best interest of the patient and the health-care system as a whole (Table 5.13).

⊙ Summary Points

- An anemia classified as microcytic, hypochromic means that there is decreased MCV and decreased MCHC.

- The most common microcytic anemias are IDA, sideroblastic anemias, hereditary hemochromatosis, and anemia of chronic disease.

- Iron is ingested, absorbed from the duodenum and jejunum, and then moved to the bone marrow by transferrin, the transport protein.

Table 5.13 ⊙ Diagnostic Clues for the Thalassemic Conditions

If you suspect the two- or three-gene deletion alpha thalassemic state
- MCV much lower than in IDA
- RDW much more severe in alpha thalassemias

If you suspect the silent carrier alpha thalassemic state
- MCV in normal or low-normal range
- Presence of elliptocytes on the smear an indicator

If you suspect beta thalassemia major state
- MCV low
- High numbers of nucleated red blood cells on smear
- Presence of targets, fragments on smear
- Microcytosis and hypochromia
- Hgb F major hemoglobin on electrophoresis

If you suspect beta thalassemia minor state
- MCV is lower than in IDA
- RBC elevated
- Microcytosis and hypochromia
- May see basophilic stippling, targets on smear
- Hgb A_2 elevated

- Individuals with IDA experience symptoms of anemia and perhaps cheilitis, koilonychia, or pica.

- Individuals with iron deficiency have decreased serum iron and serum ferritin and increased TIBC.

- The anemia of chronic disease or the anemia of inflammation is one of the most common anemias in the hospital population.

- HH is an inherited iron loading anemia.

- Multiple organs are affected in HH because individuals with HH have been iron loading for decades.

- The serum iron and serum ferritin are high in HH.

CONDENSED CASE

A South Vietnamese adolescent girl is seen in the student health clinic for complaints of shortness of breath. Her laboratory results reveal WBC = 9.0 × 10⁹/L, Hgb = 80.0 g/dL, Hct = 26%, MCV = 62 fL, and MCHC = 30.7. Peripheral smear revealed moderate target cells, microcytes, hypochromia, and some fragments. Hemoglobin electrophoresis at pH 8.6 indicates three bands: a heavy band in the A position, a lighter band in the F position, and a moderate band that is faster than Hgb A. *What is your clinical impression?*

Answer

This patient most likely has Hgb H disease and is showing signs of anemia. She has done a good job of compensating and probably never needed transfusion. Her peripheral smear abnormalities combined and her electrophoresis results are fairly conclusive for this alpha thalassemia.

- Therapeutic phlebotomy is the therapy of choice for HH.
- The thalassemia syndromes are globin chain synthetic defects.
- There are four clinical conditions of alpha thalassemia, each caused by gene deletions.
- Beta thalassemia major is the most severe of the beta thalassemic conditions.

- Individuals with beta thalassemia major have severe anemia, splenomegaly, and thalassemic facies.
- The majority hemoglobin in beta thalassemic major is Hgb F.
- Beta thalassemia minor is similar to IDA, with the exception of an elevated RBC and an elevated Hgb A_2.

CASE STUDY

A physician came into the clinical laboratory during the evening shift and asked to review the peripheral smear on one of his patients. This particular 40-year-old patient had been especially confusing for the physician because she came into the clinic with a CBC that indicated IDA, with MCV of 59 fL, Hgb of 11.3 g/dL, Hct of 34%, and RBC of 5.8×10^{12}/L. She complained of fatigue and lethargy. The physician had put her on a trial therapy with iron supplementation, but 3 weeks later her laboratory results were virtually the same. *What inherited hematologic condition shows a clinical picture similar to IDA?*

Insights to the Case Study

This case illustrates a frequent problem in the diagnosis and management of a patient with microcytic indices. The patient was diagnosed with IDA with no clear indication of her iron status and begun on a therapeutic trial of iron. She did not respond, as her CBC remained virtually the same. When Hgb A_2 was ordered, the results were found to be 8.5% (normal value 2% to 3%), and these results are indicative of beta thalassemia trait. This condition is an inherited disorder in which only one normal beta gene is present. An abnormal beta gene is inherited from one parent; consequently, a full complement of Hgb A is not formed, and Hgb A_2 is elevated. Patients have a lifelong moderate microcytic anemia, with an elevated RBC. Patients lead a normal life, but pregnancy or illness may cause the anemia to worsen, and transfusion may be warranted in such cases. If the information is available, individuals who carry the beta thalassemic trait should identify themselves to their supervising physician.

Review Questions

1. The morphologic classification of anemias is based on the
   a. RBC.
   b. Cause of the anemia.
   c. Red blood cell indices.
   d. Reticulocyte count.

2. Which of these symptoms is specific for IDA?
   a. Fatigue
   b. Koilonychia
   c. Palpitations
   d. Dizziness

3. Which of the following laboratory tests would be abnormal through each stage of iron deficiency?
   a. Serum iron
   b. Hemoglobin and hematocrit
   c. RBC
   d. Serum ferritin

4. A patient presents with a microcytic, hypochromic anemia with ragged-looking red blood cells in the peripheral smear and a high reticulocyte count. A brilliant cresyl blue preparation reveals inclusions that look like pitted golf balls. These inclusions are suggestive of
   a. Hgb H disease.
   b. Beta thalassemia major.
   c. Hereditary hemochromatosis.
   d. Beta thalassemic trait.

5. The most cost-effective therapy for a patient with hereditary hemochromatosis is
   a. Desferal chelation.
   b. Bone marrow transplant.
   c. Therapeutic phlebotomy.
   d. Stem cell transplant.

6. List two sets of laboratory data that can distinguish IDA from beta thalassemia trait.
   a. Serum iron and RBC
   b. Hemoglobin and hematocrit
   c. WBC and RDW
   d. Red blood cell indices and platelets

7. What is the majority hemoglobin in thalassemia major?
   a. Hgb A
   b. Hgb A_2
   c. Hgb F
   d. Hgb H

8. Of the four clinical states of alpha thalassemia, which is incompatible with life?
   a. Alpha thalassemia silent carrier
   b. Alpha thalassemia trait
   c. Hgb H disease
   d. Bart's hydrops fetalis

9. Which of the following hemoglobins has the chemical confirmation β_4?
   a. Hgb Bart's
   b. Hgb Gower
   c. Hgb H
   d. Hgb Portland

10. Although there are many complications in individuals with thalassemia major, which of the following is the leading cause of death?
    a. Splenomegaly
    b. Cardiac complications
    c. Hepatitis C infection
    d. Pathologic fractures

● TROUBLESHOOTING

What Do I Do When Red Blood Cell Inclusions Have Been Misidentified?

A 36-year-old woman with chronic alcoholism, liver disease, and pneumonia was admitted to the hospital. Her admission was for treatment of the pneumonia. Routine CBCs including differential were ordered daily to monitor her WBC during treatment. During evaluation of her peripheral smear, a shift to the left was observed. This is a term used to describe the presence of younger white blood cells from the bone marrow in response to infection and inflammation. On the second day after admission, the patient's smear was being examined on the evening shift by a new laboratory graduate. She noted red blood cell inclusions and identified them as Howell-Jolly bodies, but she felt insecure about the identity of the inclusion and no one was available to observe the inclusion. After consulting with the lead technologist, they reviewed the smear together to try to identify which inclusion was present. The student preliminarily identified the inclusions as Howell-Jolly bodies, which are single inclusion, DNA in origin, and usually located in the periphery of the red blood cell. Basophilic stippling was another possibility, but stippling is RNA in origin and seen throughout the red blood cells; the new employee noted that the inclusion was located toward the periphery of the cell. The next possibility was Pappenheimer bodies, small inclusions that look like grape clusters. Pappenheimer bodies are usually iron deposits either in the form of ferritin or hemosiderin. If they are suspected, an iron stain (Prussian blue) can confirm the presence of iron. A Prussian blue stain was performed, and the inclusions were confirmed to be siderocytes, iron-containing inclusions. These inclusions can be found in hemochromatosis, alcoholism, hemolytic anemia, and postsplenectomy.

WORD KEY

Chelation • Procedure to remove a heavy compound, such as a heavy metal

Collagen vascular disease • Disorder that affects primarily the joints and mobility

Dyspnea • Shortness of breath

Gastrectomy • Removal of a portion of the stomach

Jaundice • Yellow discoloration in the mucous membranes of the eyes and a yellow tone to the skin resulting from increase in bilirubin

Menorrhagia • Excessive menstrual bleeding

Vertigo • Dizziness

References

1. Ogedegbe HO, Csury L, Simmons BH. Anemias: A clinical laboratory perspective. Lab Med 35:177, 2004.
2. Hillman RS, Finch CA. Differential diagnosis of anemia. In: Hillman RS, Finch CA, eds. Red Cell Manual, 7th ed. Philadelphia: FA Davis, 1996; 71.
3. Hussong JW. Iron metabolism and hypochromic anemias. In: Harmening D, ed. Clinical Hematology and Fundamentals of Hemostasis. Philadelphia: FA Davis, 2002; 100.
4. Coleman M. Iron metabolism. In: Rodak B, ed. Hematology: Clinical Principles and Applications, 2nd ed. Philadelphia: WB Saunders, 2002; 118–119.
5. Annibale B, Caparso F, Delle Fave G. The stomach and iron deficiency anemia: A forgotten link. Liver Dis 35:288–295, 2003.
6. Gross S. Disorders of iron metabolism. In: Gross S, Roath S, eds. Routine Hematology: A Problem-Oriented Approach. Baltimore: Williams & Wilkins, 1996; 118.
7. Centers for Disease Control and Prevention. Recommendations to Prevent and Control Iron Deficiency in the United States. April 1998. Available at: http://www.cdc.gov/mmnr/preview/mmwrhtml/100051880.htm. Accessed September 24, 2006.
8. Doig K. Disorder of iron and heme metabolism. In: Rodak BF, Fritsma GA, Doig K, eds. Hematology: Clinical Principles and Applications, 3rd ed. St. Louis: Elsevier, 2007; 232–247.
9. Sullivan E. Identifying iron deficiency in pre-anemic infants. Lab Med 37:207, 2006.
10. Gross S. Disorders of iron metabolism. In: Gross S, Roath S, eds. Routine Hematology: A Problem-Oriented Approach. Baltimore: Williams & Wilkins, 1996; 125.
11. Spivak JL. Iron and the anemia of chronic disease. Oncology 9(Suppl 10):25–33, 2002.
12. Geffen D. Hepcidin, a key regulator of iron metabolism and mediator of anemia of inflammation. Blood 102:783–788, 2003.
13. Roy CN, Weinstein DA, Andrews NC. The molecular biology of the anemia of chronic disease: A hypothesis. Pediatr Res 53:507–512, 2003.
14. Kaplan LA, Pesce AJ. Iron, porphyrin and bilirubin metabolism. In: Kaplan LA, Pesce AJ, eds. Clinical Chemistry Theory, Analysis, Correlations, 3rd ed. St. Louis: Mosby, 1996; 700–701.
15. Weinberg ED. Laboratory contributions to the diagnosis of common iron loading disorders and anemias. Lab Med 32:507–508, 2002.
16. Galhenge SP, Viiala CH, Olynyk JK. Screening for hemochromatosis: Patients with liver disease, families and populations. Curr Gastroenterol Rep 6:44–51, 2004.
17. Cooley's Anemia Foundation. Leading the Fight Against Thalassemia. Available at: www.cooleysanemia.org, 2008.
18. Panich V, Pornpatku M, Sriroohgrueng W. The problem of the thalassemias in Thailand. Southeast Asian J Trop Med Public Health Suppl:23, 1992.
19. Teshima D, Hall J, Darniati E, et al. Microscopic erythrocyte morphologic changes associated with alpha thalassemia. Clin Lab Sci 6:236–240, 1993.
20. Hall RB, Haga JA, Guerra CG, et al. Optimizing the detection of hemoglobin H disease. Lab Med 26:736–741, 1995.
21. Vullo R, Moddel B, Georganda E. What Is Cooley's Anemia? 2nd ed. Nicosia, Cyprus/Geneva: Thalassaemia International Federation/World Health Organization, 1995; 17.
22. Eleftheriou A. Compliance to Iron Chelation Therapy with Desferrioxamine. Nicosia, Cyprus: Thalassaemia International Federation, 2000; 15.
23. Nuchprayoon I, Sukthawee B, Nuchprayoon T. Red cell indices and therapeutic trial of iron in diagnostic workup for anemic Thai females. J Med Assoc Thai 86(Suppl 2):S160–S169, 2003.

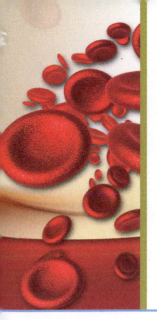

Chapter 6

The Macrocytic Anemias

Betty Ciesla

Objectives

After completing this chapter, the student will be able to:

1. Describe the criteria that define a macrocytic anemia as megaloblastic.

2. Compare and contrast the morphologic characteristics of megaloblasts and normoblasts in the bone marrow.

3. Differentiate red blood cell and white blood cell changes in the peripheral smear that are seen in the megaloblastic anemias.

4. Describe ineffective hematopoiesis as it relates to the megaloblastic process.

5. Describe the pathway of vitamin B_{12} and folic acid from ingestion through incorporation into the red blood cell.

6. Describe the clinical symptoms of a patient with megaloblastic anemia.

7. List the causes of vitamin B_{12} and folic acid deficiency.

8. Define pernicious anemia and its clinical and laboratory findings.

9. Describe the relevant laboratory tests used in the diagnosis of megaloblastic anemia.

10. Describe the treatments for the megaloblastic anemias.

11. Differentiate the anemias that are macrocytic but are not megaloblastic.

MACROCYTIC ANEMIAS AND THE MEGALOBLASTIC PROCESS

The macrocytic anemias are a morphologic classification of anemias having mean corpuscular volume (MCV) greater than 100 fL, elevated mean corpuscular hemoglobin (MCH), and mean corpuscular hemoglobin content (MCHC) within normal range. These anemias are termed macrocytic and normochromic. Broadly defined, the macrocytic anemias are divided into two categories: megaloblastic and nonmegaloblastic processes. If the source of the anemia is vitamin B_{12} or folic acid deficiency, the anemia is termed megaloblastic. If the source of the anemia is unrelated to a nutritional deficiency, the anemia is macrocytic but *not* megaloblastic. Vitamin B_{12} or folic acid deficiency leads to impaired DNA synthesis, a serious condition, and affects all readily dividing cells, skin cells, hematopoietic cells, and epithelial cells. The effects on the bone marrow, the peripheral smear, and the patient's quality of life are dramatic and substantive.

RED BLOOD CELL PRECURSORS IN MEGALOBLASTIC ANEMIA

Because megaloblastic processes damage DNA synthesis, nucleated cells are affected the most. There are multiple changes to white blood cells and red blood cells in the bone marrow structure that should be recognized and appreciated. The megaloblastic red blood cell precursors are larger, the nuclear structure is less condensed, and the cytoplasm is extremely basophilic or much bluer. There is asynchrony between the age of the nuclear material and the age of the cytoplasm, but this can best be appreciated by making a serious comparison of the nuclear and cytoplasmic material in megaloblastic precursor cells versus normoblastic precursor cells (Fig. 6.1). When a cell stage is asynchronous,

the nuclear age and the cytoplasmic age do not correspond. The normal red blood cell series is programmed for two specific functions: hemoglobin synthesis and nuclear expulsion. For the nucleus to be expelled, certain changes must occur in the size of the nucleus and the consistency of the nucleus structure. The chromatin that begins as fine, reticular, and smooth must take on a different texture and conformation before it is expelled from the orthochromic normoblast.

In megaloblastic erythropoiesis, the texture and condensation of the nuclear material are disrupted. Megaloblastic chromatin in the megaloblastic pronormoblast and megaloblastic basophilic normoblast is open-weaved, with a clockface arrangement of chromatin—easily imagined if you look closely at the chromatin pattern. The nuclear (or chromatin) material is fragile and lacks the composition and condensation of a nucleus ready to be delivered from the cell. Likewise, the cytoplasmic material in the early megaloblastic precursors is extremely basophilic, much bluer than normal precursors (Fig. 6.2). Students usually have a difficult time observing the difference between normal red blood cell precursors and megaloblastic precursors. A careful study of the nucleus:cytoplasm (N:C) ratio, cell size, nuclear material, and cytoplasm color in each stage of each cell can help differentiate one from the other.

INEFFECTIVE ERYTHROPOIESIS IN MEGALOBLASTIC ANEMIA

The bone marrow is hypercellular in megaloblastic conditions, and the white blood cell precursor cells are large, especially the metamyelocytes. The myeloid:erythroid (M:E) ratio is 1:1 or 1:3, reflecting erythroid

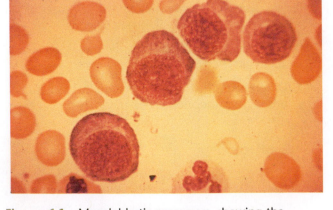

Figure 6.1 Megaloblastic precursors, showing the asynchrony between the nucleus and the chromatin; the cytoplasm of most cells is extremely basophilic.

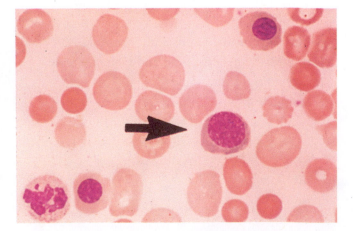

Figure 6.2 Normoblastic erythropoiesis with a polychromatophilic normoblast *(arrow).* From The College of American Pathologists, with permission.

hyperplasia that you would see in the bone marrow responding to anemia. Erythropoiesis in the megaloblastic processes is ineffective, however, meaning destruction in the bone marrow of red blood cell precursors before they reach the peripheral circulation (Table 6.1). Megaloblastic precursor cells, especially at the polychromatophilic and basophilic states, hemolyze before their maturation cycle is complete. Orthochromic normoblasts or reticulocytes or both do not have the opportunity to be delivered from the bone marrow as they *normally* would in response to anemic stress. Consequently, the reticulocyte count is inappropriately low. The peripheral smear does not show polychromasia or nucleated red blood cells, and bilirubin and lactate dehydrogenase (LDH) are elevated. The last two clinical developments signal **intramedullary hemolysis**. If erythropoiesis was *effective* and the bone marrow was responding to anemic stress, the peripheral smear would show evidence of a regenerative marrow process. Polychromasia and the presence of nucleated red blood cells would be self-evident (Table 6.2).

VITAMIN B$_{12}$ AND FOLIC ACID: THEIR ROLE IN DNA SYNTHESIS

DNA synthesis depends on a key structure, thymidine triphosphate (TTP). This structure cannot be formed unless it receives a methyl group from methyl tetrahydrofolate or folic acid. Vitamin B$_{12}$ is the cofactor responsible for transferring the methyl group to methyl tetrahydrofolate.[1] Sufficient quantities of vitamin B$_{12}$ and folic acid are key to the formation of TTP. If TTP cannot be synthesized, it is replaced by deoxyuridine triphosphate (DTP). The synthesis of this component leads to nuclear fragmentation and destruction of cells and impaired cell division. For this reason, vitamin B$_{12}$ and folic acid are essential elements in the DNA pathway.

Table 6.1 ◉ Consequences of Ineffective Erythropoiesis

- Bone marrow destruction of erythroid precursors
- Lack of regeneration of bone marrow elements during anemic stress
- Lack of nucleated red blood cells in peripheral smear
- Lack of polychromasia in peripheral smear
- Reticulocytopenia
- Intramedullary hemolysis
- Increased bilirubin and LDH
- Decreased haptoglobin

Table 6.2 ◉ Expected Bone Marrow Response to Anemic Stress

- Production of red blood cell precursor cells is accelerated
- M:E ratio is adjusted to reflect erythroid hyperplasia
- Precursor cells, orthochromic normoblasts, are prematurely released from the bone marrow
- Reticulocytes are prematurely released from the bone marrow
- Polychromasia is seen in the peripheral smear
- Nucleated red blood cells are present in the peripheral smear
- If the reticulocyte count is high, a slight macrocytosis might develop

NUTRITIONAL REQUIREMENTS, TRANSPORT, AND METABOLISM OF VITAMIN B$_{12}$ AND FOLIC ACID

Microorganisms and fungi are the main producers of vitamin B$_{12}$, a group of vitamins known as cobalamins. This vitamin may also be embedded in liver, meat, fish, eggs, and dairy products. The recommended daily allowance of vitamin B$_{12}$ is 2.0 µg, with the daily diet providing approximately 5 to 30 µg/day and storage of 1 to 2 mg in the liver. Dietary requirements increase during pregnancy and lactation. Depletion of vitamin B$_{12}$ stores takes years to develop because the storage rate is so high.

Folic acid is readily available in green leafy vegetables, fruit, broccoli, and dairy products. The minimum daily requirement is 200 µg, a much higher requirement than vitamin B$_{12}$, with body stores of 5 to 10 mg in the liver. Folic acid depletes quickly, within months, because the daily requirement is so much higher (Table 6.3). Pregnant women are encouraged to increase their folic acid intake because decreased folate may lead to neural tube defects.

INCORPORATING VITAMIN B$_{12}$ INTO THE BONE MARROW

The incorporation of vitamin B$_{12}$ into bone marrow and other tissues is a multistep process. Initially, the vitamin is taken in from the diet and separated from food by salivary enzymes. Next, vitamin B$_{12}$ is transported to the stomach, where it combines with intrinsic factor, a substance secreted by the parietal cells of the stomach. Intrinsic factor and vitamin B$_{12}$ form a complex that proceeds to the ileum. Vitamin B$_{12}$ is

Table 6.3 ● Sources of Vitamin B_{12} and Folic Acid

Vitamin B_{12}
- Meat, liver, kidney, oysters, clams, fish
- Eggs, cheese, and other dairy products

Folic acid
- Green leafy vegetables
- Broccoli
- Fruit
- Whole grains
- Dairy products

absorbed through the brush borders of the ileum, and intrinsic factor is degraded. When the vitamin leaves the ileum, it is carried into the plasma and forms a complex with transcobalamin II (TCII), which transports it to the circulation.[2] From the circulation, vitamin B_{12} is transferred to the liver, the bone marrow, and other tissues (Fig. 6.3).

The movement of folic acid into the circulation and tissues occurs with a little more ease. When folic acid is ingested and absorbed through the small intestine, it is

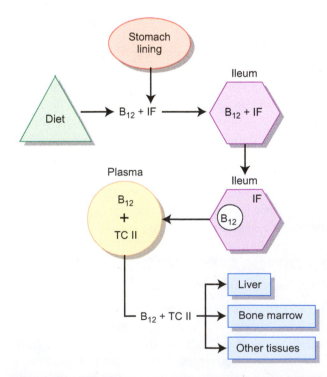

Figure 6.3 Vitamin B_{12} absorption and transport. Vitamin B_{12} must be combined with intrinsic factor (IF) before it enters the blood circulation: transcobalamin II (TC II) is the transport protein that carries vitamin B_{12} to the tissues.

reduced to methyl tetrahydrofolate through dihydrofolate reductase, an enzyme available in mucosal cells. The reduced form is delivered to the tissues. When inside the tissues, the methyl group is released to combine with homocysteine, an early precursor to DNA synthesis. Homocysteine is converted to methionine, an amino acid. If folate or vitamin B_{12} metabolism is flawed, homocysteine accumulates, potentially leading to thrombosis,[3] a potential consequence to the hemostatic system that is just being realized.

CLINICAL FEATURES OF PATIENTS WITH MEGALOBLASTIC ANEMIA

Megaloblastic anemia is usually a disease of middle age to older age, with a high predilection for women. More than 20% of elderly individuals may be vitamin B_{12} deficient, and these patients often go unrecognized. Expanding the definition of individuals who should be tested would potentially improve the diagnosis of megaloblastic anemia.[4] Severe anemia, in which the hemoglobin decreases to 7 to 8 g/dL, is accompanied by symptoms of anemia, such as shortness of breath, light-headedness, extreme weakness, and pallor. Patients may experience glossitis (sore or enlarged tongue), dyspepsia, or diarrhea. Evidence of neurologic involvement may be seen, with patients experiencing numbness, vibratory loss (**paresthesias**), and difficulties in balance and walking. Personality changes that may be observed include mania, disorientation, depression, and impaired memory. Vitamin B_{12} deficiency causes a **demyelinization** of the peripheral nerves, the spinal column, and the brain, which can cause many more severe neurologic symptoms, such as **spasticity** or **paranoia**. Jaundice may be seen because the average red blood cell life span in megaloblastic anemia is 75 days, a little more than one-half of the average red blood cell life span of 120 days. The bilirubin level is elevated, and LDH level is increased, signifying hemolysis.

HEMATOLOGIC FEATURES OF MEGALOBLASTIC ANEMIAS

The complete blood count (CBC) shows pancytopenia (low WBC, low RBC, and low platelet count), although the platelet count may be only borderline low (see normal values on the front cover of this textbook). Pancytopenia in the CBC combined with macrocytosis should raise the index of suspicion toward a megaloblastic process because few other conditions (i.e., aplastic anemia, hypersplenism) show this pattern.[5] Red blood cell inclusions such as basophilic stippling and Howell-Jolly bodies may be observed. Howell-Jolly bodies formed from megaloblastic erythropoiesis are larger and more fragmented than normal Howell-Jolly bodies. There is a low reticulocyte count (less than 1%), and the red blood cell distribution width (RDW) is increased, owing to schistocytes, targets, and teardrop cells. The blood smear in megaloblastic anemia is extremely relevant in the diagnosis and shows macrocytes, macro-ovalocytes, hypersegmented multi-lobed neutrophils, and little polychromasia with respect to the anemia (Fig. 6.4). The presence of hypersegmented neutrophils (lobe count of more than five lobes) in combination with macrocytic anemia is a morphologic marker for megaloblastic anemias. This qualitative white blood cell abnormality appears early in the disease and survives through treatment. It is usually the last morphology to disappear. MCV initially is extremely high and may be 100 to 140 fL. A bone marrow examination is not necessary for the diagnosis of megaloblastic anemia because the diagnosis of this disorder can be adequately made without this time-consuming, costly, and invasive procedure.

PERNICIOUS ANEMIA AS A SUBSET OF MEGALOBLASTIC ANEMIAS

Intrinsic factor is the most important ingredient to the absorption of vitamin B_{12} and subsequent delivery of vitamin B_{12} to the circulation. When problems with intrinsic factor develop, the condition is called pernicious anemia. Drs. George Minot and William Murphy of Boston were awarded the Nobel Prize in 1934 for their discovery that ingestion of liver successfully treated patients with pernicious anemia. Several factors may account for the lack of intrinsic factor in the

stomach, including physical factors such as partial or whole gastrectomy or genetic and immune factors. Whatever the cause, either intrinsic factor is not being secreted, or it is blocked or neutralized in some way. Atrophic gastritis may occur in which gastric secretions are diminished and intrinsic factor fails to be secreted. The reasons for this failure remain unclear, but age may play a role.[5]

Immune factors may arise that cause production of antibodies against intrinsic factor, thyroid tissue, and parietal cells, all of which decrease the production of intrinsic factor. Antibodies to intrinsic factor are present in 56% of patients with pernicious anemia, with 90% of patients showing parietal cell antibodies, suggesting a strong autoimmune component to this disorder. Additionally, pernicious anemia occurs more frequently in individuals with diabetes, thyroid conditions, and other autoimmune processes.[7] Pernicious anemia may occur genetically as an autosomal recessive trait in children before the age of 2 years. Cubilin, a receptor for vitamin B_{12} and intrinsic factor, has been identified since 1998, but its role in juvenile-onset pernicious anemia remains unclear.[8] Adult forms of congenital pernicious anemia occur and are associated with **achlorhydria** or malabsorption in relatives.

Pernicious anemia is more common in individuals with Irish and Scandinavian ethnicity. Patients with pernicious anemia experience all of the symptoms of megaloblastic anemia, but they have a higher tendency for neurologic involvement, including the neurologic manifestations already mentioned and degeneration of peripheral nerves and the spinal column. Neurologic manifestations may be slow to develop but include a vast array of symptoms. Patients may experience paresthesias in the limbs, an abnormal or clumsy walking pattern, or stiffness in the limbs. Treatment usually reverses these symptoms.

VITAMIN B_{12} AND FOLIC ACID DEFICIENCY

Dietary deficiencies are rarely the cause of vitamin B_{12} deficiency except in individuals who are strictly vegetarians or infants nursed by vegetarian mothers who do not supplement their diets. Other potential sources of vitamin B_{12} deficiency are the malabsorption syndromes, including cobalamin or intestinal malabsorption. *Helicobacter pylori* infections and long-term use of antacids may also contribute to severe food malabsorption.[9] Lack of intrinsic factor may occur after full or partial gastrectomy, and the parietal cells that secrete intrinsic factor would invariably be affected, thereby affecting vitamin B_{12} absorption. Added to this is a

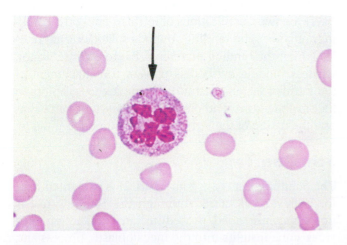

Figure 6.4 Peripheral smear from a patient with megaloblastic anemia. Note the hypersegmented neutrophils and the macro-ovalocytes. From The College of American Pathologists, with permission.

condition called blind loop syndrome, in which there is an overgrowth of bacteria in a small pocket of malformed intestine. Microorganisms take up vitamin B_{12}, making it unavailable for absorption. Although unusual, the fish tapeworm *Diphyllobothrium latum* may compete for vitamin B_{12} when it attaches to the intestine, and individuals who have this parasite exhibit signs of megaloblastic anemia, which can be corrected when the parasite is discovered and destroyed.

Dietary deficiency is a serious consideration in folic acid deficiency and may occur in pregnancy or infancy because of increased requirement or in elderly or alcoholic persons because of lack of availability. Folic acid is depleted from body stores within 3 to 6 months, and folic acid deficiency is one of the most common vitamin deficiencies in the United States in vulnerable populations. Tropical sprue is one of the most common malabsorption syndromes contributing to folic acid deficiency. This syndrome is usually seen in individuals from tropical or subtropical climates such as Haiti, Cuba, and Puerto Rico. Although rare, tropical sprue affects overall digestion and is thought to result from infection, overgrowth of bacteria, or poor nutrition. Normally, the villi that line the digestive tract are fingerlike projections whose job is to promote absorption from ingested food. The villi from individuals with tropical sprue are flattened, leading to poor absorption activity. Individuals with sprue present with diarrhea, indigestion, and weight loss. Finally, folic acid deficiency may be expected in individuals taking methotrexate or other chemotherapy drugs because many of these directly affect DNA synthesis of normal and abnormal dividing cells.

LABORATORY DIAGNOSIS OF MEGALOBLASTIC ANEMIAS

The megaloblastic anemias show striking similarities in clinical and hematologic presentations. Common features of the megaloblastic anemias include the following:

- Pancytopenia
- Increased MCV
- Hypersegmented neutrophils (five lobes or more in segmented neutrophils)
- Increased bilirubin
- Increased LDH
- Hyperplasia in the bone marrow
- Decreased M:E ratio
- Reticulocytopenia

The differential diagnosis of these disorders depends on a more sophisticated battery of laboratory tests that can help determine if the patient is lacking vitamin B_{12}, folic acid, or intrinsic factor.

Serum Vitamin B_{12} Levels and Folic Acid Levels

Presently, serum levels of vitamin B_{12} are determined by radioimmunoassay. Sample precautions must be taken because light degrades the vitamin. A value less than 200 ng/L indicates that additional testing may be necessary. Folate or folic acid deficiency is unusual in the 21st century because most foods are folate fortified. The serum test is available by the chemiluminescence technique and measures folate body stores.

Serum Methylmalonic Acid and Homocysteine

When vitamin B_{12} is deficient, the metabolites methylmalonic acid (MMA) and homocysteine are elevated and can be measured using reference laboratory techniques. MMA and serum homocysteine are valuable markers of even *mild* vitamin B_{12} deficiency and serve as important diagnostic indicators. When evaluated together, MMA and homocysteine can differentiate vitamin B_{12} from folate deficiency.[10]

Intrinsic Factor Antibodies

Parietal cell antibodies are seen in 90% of individuals at the time of initial diagnosis.[11] The presence of these antibodies is not specific for a diagnosis of pernicious anemia, however, because parietal cell antibodies are seen in some individuals with endocrine disorders. Intrinsic factor antibody evaluations are cost-effective, reliable, and highly specific for a diagnosis of pernicious anemia.[12] There are two classifications of intrinsic antibody: blocking antibodies and binding antibodies. Blocking antibodies inhibit the binding of vitamin B_{12} to intrinsic factor, whereas binding antibodies prevent the attachment of the intrinsic factor–vitamin B_{12} complex to receptors in the small intestine. Radioimmunoassay testing can delineate the nature of the intrinsic factor antibody.

Schilling Test

The Schilling test, part 1 and part 2, is presented here for its historical value. Although the Schilling test is not a recommended procedure, an explanation provides some insights into the megaloblastic process and pernicious anemia.

The procedure in part 1 is to give the patient an oral dose of vitamin B_{12} and then, within 2 hours, give a flushing dose of vitamin B_{12} via intramuscular injection. The flushing dose saturates all of the liver vitamin B_{12}–binding sites. The urine is collected in a 24-hour period, and the amount of vitamin B_{12} is measured. If intrinsic factor was present and vitamin B_{12} was absorbed, 5% to 30% of the initial radiolabeled vitamin B_{12} would be excreted. If less than this amount is excreted, some type of malabsorption has occurred. In part 2 of the test, intrinsic factor is added to the oral vitamin B_{12} dose, and the test proceeds as in part 1, including the flushing dose of vitamin B_{12}. If the excretion of vitamin B_{12} is in the proper amount, intrinsic factor is determined as the deficiency. If the excretion of vitamin B_{12} is less than expected, the patient is diagnosed with a malabsorption syndrome. Normal kidney function and conscientious urine collection are essential for the correct interpretation of this test (Fig. 6.5).

TREATMENT AND RESPONSE OF PATIENTS WITH MEGALOBLASTIC ANEMIA

Therapeutic vitamin B_{12} is available in the cyanocobalamin or hydroxycobalamin form. The vitamin can be administered orally, intramuscularly, or subcutaneously. If a patient is simply lacking in vitamin B_{12}, this vitamin can be taken orally at a daily dose of 1,000 μg.

Oral cyanocobalamin offers patients a substantial cost savings compared with intramuscular vitamin B_{12} injections, which must be administered by a healthcare professional.[13] Therapy is lifelong. For a patient with pernicious anemia, about 6,000 μg of vitamin B_{12} administered over a 6-day period is used as an initial dosage. At this dosage, all of the body stores are saturated. If therapy is successful, symptoms begin to diminish, and a rapid reticulocyte response begins in 2 to 3 days. Maintenance therapy of vitamin B_{12} needs to be given every 1 to 2 months for life, and the patient should be monitored by hematologic assays.

Folic acid deficiency is fairly easy to treat with oral folate at 1 to 5 mg/day for 2 to 3 weeks. Short-term therapy is usually all that is required, and patients are counseled to increase their dietary intake of folic acid. Changes in the peripheral circulation are noticed quickly as MCV returns to the reference range, the anemia is resolved, and some of the clinical symptoms abate. Dual therapy may be started in patients who have a combined deficiency; however, folic acid resolves the hematologic abnormalities long before the neurologic abnormalities are resolved.

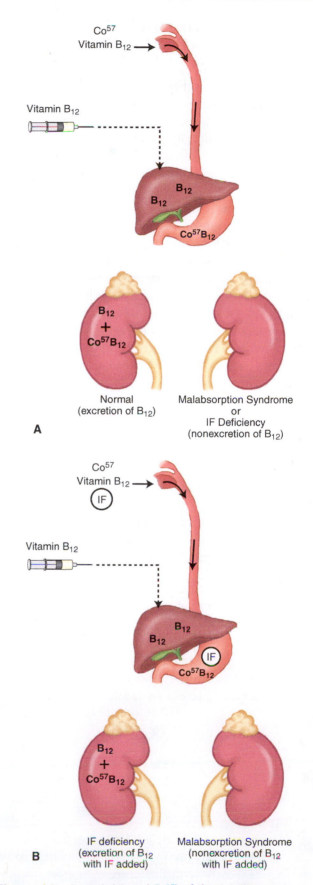

Figure 6.5 Parts 1 (*A*) and 2 (*B*) of the Schilling test. See text for explanation.

MACROCYTIC ANEMIAS THAT ARE NOT MEGALOBLASTIC

When macrocytes appear in the peripheral smear, it is important to observe them carefully for shape, color, or hypochromia because these morphologic clues can aid in determining if the macrocytosis is megaloblastic or nonmegaloblastic. Megaloblastic macrocytes are large and oval, with a thicker exterior membrane and lacking hypochromia. Macrocytes in the peripheral smear that lack any of these characteristics are usually not of megaloblastic origins.

Several conditions can contribute to a macrocytic blood picture without a deficiency in vitamin B_{12} and folic acid. The most frequently seen conditions are a compensatory bone marrow response to hemolytic anemia, in which case a reticulocytosis is seen. Because reticulocytes are polychromatophilic macrocytes and because reticulocytes are prematurely delivered from the bone marrow in response to hemolysis, it is easy to understand how a macrocytic blood picture would develop. In these cases, MCV is usually only slightly elevated, up to 105 fL. Macrocytosis may also be seen in conditions such as hypothyroidism, chronic liver disease, alcoholism, chemotherapy treatment, or a myelodysplastic disorder. In patients with chronic liver disease and alcoholism, the macrocytes are often targeted or hypochromic. Additionally, a macrocytic blood picture is noted in newborns because their bone marrow is immature and rapidly delivering nucleated cells and reticulocytes. For a differential diagnosis of macrocytes, see Figure 6.6.

Differential Diagnosis of Macrocyte

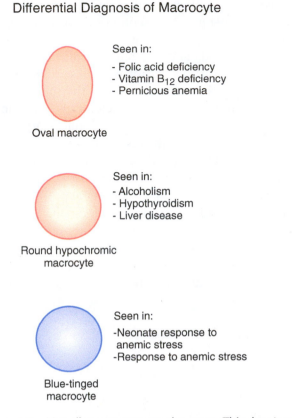

Seen in:
- Folic acid deficiency
- Vitamin B_{12} deficiency
- Pernicious anemia

Oval macrocyte

Seen in:
- Alcoholism
- Hypothyroidism
- Liver disease

Round hypochromic macrocyte

Seen in:
- Neonate response to anemic stress
- Response to anemic stress

Blue-tinged macrocyte

Figure 6.6   Not all macrocytes are the same. This drawing depicts three types of macrocytes, each differentiated by how they are produced with respect to the clinical condition.

CONDENSED CASE

The patient in this study is a 73-year-old woman who has long-standing anemia. She had always been a poor eater. Peripheral smears have consistently shown hypochromia with target and many Howell-Jolly bodies. She has no surgical history, and she shows no blood loss through either the gastrointestinal or the genitourinary tract. Her laboratory results are as follows:

WBC	2.7×10^9/L
RBC	2.25×10^{12}/L
Hgb	7.8 g/dL
Hct	25%
MCV	111 fL

Based on these findings, what is your initial clinical impression?

Answer

This patient most likely has a megaloblastic anemia. Her age, dietary habits, and CBC support that impression. With her dietary history, she may have initially had an iron deficiency condition, and her peripheral smear results seem to verify that. It seems as if her condition has shifted toward a vitamin B_{12} or folic acid deficiency, however. Serum vitamin B_{12} and folic acid assays should be ordered, and a Schilling test may be considered to rule in or rule out an intrinsic factor deficit.

Summary Points

- Macrocytic anemias have MCV of greater than 100 fL and normal MCHC.
- Megaloblastic anemias are macrocytic anemias in which vitamin B_{12} or folic acid or both are deficient.
- Not all macrocytic anemias are megaloblastic.
- Vitamin B_{12} and folic acid deficiencies lead to impaired DNA synthesis.
- The bone marrow in megaloblastic anemias is hypercellular with the red blood cell precursors showing distinct chromatin and cytoplasmic changes.
- Megaloblastic anemias show ineffective erythropoiesis in the bone marrow: premature destruction of red blood cell precursors before delivery into the circulation.
- The peripheral smear in megaloblastic anemia shows macrocytes, oval macrocytes, and hypersegmented neutrophils.
- Pancytopenia and reticulocytopenia are prominent features of the megaloblastic processes.
- Patients with megaloblastic anemia may exhibit symptoms of anemia and neurologic symptoms, gastrointestinal symptoms, and psychological symptoms.
- Many elderly individuals are not diagnosed with vitamin B_{12} deficiency because their symptoms are assumed to be related to other illnesses.
- Intrinsic factor, which is secreted by the parietal cells of the stomach, is necessary for vitamin B_{12} absorption.
- Intrinsic factor deficiency can lead to pernicious anemia, a subset of megaloblastic anemia.
- Intrinsic factor deficiency may develop because intrinsic factor is not being secreted or because it is being blocked or neutralized.
- Of individuals experiencing pernicious anemia, 90% have parietal cell antibodies.
- Folic acid deficiency is the most common vitamin deficiency in the United States.
- Serum vitamin B_{12}, folic acid, and red blood cell folate can be determined by radioimmunoassay.
- Individuals with vitamin B_{12} deficiency require lifelong therapy.
- Folic acid deficiency requires short-term therapy.
- Serum MMA and homocysteine are sensitive indicator tests of mild vitamin B_{12} deficiency.
- There are causes of a macrocytic anemia other than megaloblastic processes.
- Macrocytes may be seen in reticulocytosis, alcoholism, or liver disease.

CASE STUDY

Mrs. C., a 79-year-old woman, presented to the emergency department barely able to walk. She said that she had gotten progressively weaker in the past couple of weeks and that she had noticed that her appetite was failing. She had seen some yellow color to her eyes and skin, and that worried her. She had no desire to eat but she did crave ice. Mrs. C. was thin, emaciated, and pale; she had difficulty walking and seemed generally confused. CBC and peripheral smear were ordered, with more tests pending the initial results. The initial results were:

WBC	4.5×10^6/L
RBC	2.12×10^9/L
Hgb	7.5 g/dL
Hct	22%
MCV	103 fL
MCH	35.3 pg
MCHC	34.9
Platelets	105×10^6/L

The peripheral smear showed a mixture of microcytes and macrocytes, with target cells, schistocytes, few oval microcytes, rare hypersegmented neutrophils, and occasional hypochromic macrocytes. Because of the mixed blood picture, an iron profile was ordered as well as serum folate and serum vitamin B_{12}. *Which conditions show hypersegmented neutrophils?*

Insights to the Case Study

This case study presents a confusing morphologic picture because no *one red blood cell* morphology leads to any single clinical conclusion. The follow-up blood work showed serum iron of 25 µg/dL (reference range 40 to 150 µg/dL), TIBC

Continued

500 µg/dL (reference range 200 to 400 µg/dL), red blood cell folate 100 ng/mL (reference range 130 to 268 µg/dL), and serum vitamin B_{12} 200 pg/dL (reference range 100 to 700 µg/dL). Clearly, multiple nutritional deficiencies are present. Mrs. C. is in a vulnerable age range that is prone to poor dietary habits and noncompliance to health or food suggestions. As can be seen from her laboratory values, she is deficient in iron and folic acid. Folic acid deficiency is one of the most common vitamin deficiencies in the United States and easy to develop because folic acid stores are moderate, and the folic acid daily requirement is high. Add to this her iron deficiency, and you have a set of symptoms and a blood smear picture that represents a mixture of morphologies. She clearly showed a pancytopenia, but she did not show blatantly elevated MCV. Her elevated MCH could have been a clue to the megaloblastic process because MCV and MCH are usually elevated in the megaloblastic anemias. Her peripheral smear shows microcytes and macrocytes, with a few target cells and an occasional hypersegmented neutrophil. She was immediately started on oral iron and oral vitamin B_{12} supplementation, and her physical symptoms began to diminish. When her mental capacity was cleared, she began nutritional counseling, and she began to receive visits from Meals on Wheels to ensure that she had a balanced and varied diet.

Review Questions

1. Which bone marrow changes are most prominent in the megaloblastic anemias?
   a. M:E ratio of 10:1
   b. Hypocellular bone marrow
   c. Asynchrony in the red blood cell precursors
   d. Shaggy cytoplasm of the red blood cell precursors

2. Which morphologic changes in the peripheral smear are markers for megaloblastic anemias?
   a. Oval macrocytes and hypersegmented neutrophils
   b. Oval and hypochromic macrocytes
   c. Pappenheimer bodies and hypochromic microcytes
   d. Dimorphic red blood cells and Howell-Jolly bodies

3. Which is the most common vitamin deficiency in the United States?
   a. Vitamin A
   b. Folic acid
   c. Calcium
   d. Vitamin B_{12}

4. Which of the following group of symptoms is particular to patients with megaloblastic anemia?
   a. Pallor and dyspnea
   b. Jaundice and hemoglobinuria
   c. Difficulty in walking and mental confusion
   d. Pica and fatigue

5. Which one of the following substances is necessary for vitamin B_{12} to be absorbed?
   a. Transferrin
   b. Erythropoietin
   c. Intrinsic factor
   d. Cubilin

6. Which of the following clinical findings is indicative of intramedullary hemolysis in megaloblastic processes?
   a. Increased RBC
   b. Increased hemoglobin
   c. Decreased bilirubin
   d. Increased LDH

7. Which of the following adequately describes the pathophysiology of the megaloblastic anemias?
   a. Lack of DNA synthesis
   b. Defect in globin synthesis
   c. Defect in iron metabolism
   d. Excessive iron loading

8. Which of the following morphologic features is classic in the megaloblastic red cell precursors?
   a. Appropriate N:C ratio
   b. Asynchrony
   c. Basophilic cytoplasm
   d. Average size of cells

9. A macrocytosis that is not megaloblastic in origin can be seen in all of the following *except*:
   a. Chemotherapy
   b. Postsplenectomy
   c. Thyroid conditions
   d. Reticulocytosis

10. Ineffective erythropoieisis is defined as:
    a. An increase in M:E ratio
    b. A synthetic defect in hemoglobin
    c. Premature destruction of red blood cell precursors
    d. A DNA maturation defect

◉ TROUBLESHOOTING

What Clinical Possibilities Should I Consider in a Patient With an Increased MCV? What Preanalytic Variables May Increase MCV?

When a patient presents with a macrocytic blood picture, there are several clinical possibilities to consider. The most obvious reason for increased MCV is a patient with a megaloblastic process. Supporting laboratory data for this possibility would include a pancytopenia; a reticulocytopenia; increased LDH; and a peripheral smear with macro-ovalocytes, hypersegmented neutrophils, and other poikilocytes. Follow-up testing should initially include an assessment of the vitamin B_{12} and folic acid levels and testing for intrinsic factor antibodies.

A second patient population to consider when assessing a macrocytic anemia would be patients who have liver disease, alcoholic cirrhosis, hypothyroidism, or chemotherapy. These patients would *not* show a pancytopenia but would show moderate anemia with slightly increased MCV with round microcytes and perhaps siderocytes. A thorough review of the patient history should give insights into the nature of the macrocytic anemia. An often forgotten but fairly consistent reason for slightly increased MCV is regenerative bone marrow. Patients who have inherited blood disorders such as sickle cell anemia, thalassemia major, or other hemolytic processes are transfused on a regular basis as part of their disease management. Not only do the transfused cells lend some size variation to their clinical process, but also the chronic anemia in these patients leads to a premature release of reticulocytes, which are immature cells that are larger than normal red blood cells. When reticulocytes are stained with Wright's stain, polychromatophilic macrocytes appear in the peripheral smear. In a peripheral smear with increased polychromasia, a slightly macrocytic blood picture is often seen. A simple assessment for the reticulocytes would show an increased value, which is contributory to the source of increased MCV. Although MCV is a highly stable parameter, several preanalytic variables can alter MCV. If a sample fails a delta check as a result of an increase in MCV, several considerations are in order. Sample contamination may increase the red blood cell size, especially if the sample is drawn through an intravenous line or a line that has been flushed with anticoagulant. Another condition capable of increasing MCV is high glucose volume, either as a result of a diabetic episode or coma or as a result of blood drawn through the intravenous glucose infusion line. A quick check of the glucose level in the sample should reveal the source of the erratic MCV.

WORD KEY

Achlorhydria • Lack of hydrochloric acid in gastric contents

Intramedullary hemolysis • Premature hemolysis of red blood cell precursors in the bone marrow

Myelin • Fatty substance around a nerve

Paranoia • Mental condition characterized by systematic delusions

Paresthesias • Abnormal tingling or prickling sensation

Spasticity • Involuntary muscular contractions

References

1. Doig K. Anemias caused by defect of DNA metabolism. In: Rodak B, ed. Hematology: Clinical Principles and Applications, 2nd ed. Philadelphia: WB Saunders, 2002; 229.
2. Lotspeich-Steininger CA. Anemias of abnormal nuclear development. In: Steine-Martin EA, Lotspeich-Steininger CA, Koepke CA, eds. Clinical Hematology: Principles, Procedures and Correlations, 2nd ed. Philadelphia: Lippincott, 1998; 156.
3. Morrison HI, Schaubel D, Desmeules M, et al. Serum folate and the risk of fatal coronary heart disease. JAMA 275:1893–1896, 1996.
4. Andres E, Loukili NH, Noel E, et al. Vitamin B_{12} (cobalamin) deficiency in elderly patients. Can Med Assoc J 171:252–259, 2004.
5. Ishtiaq O, Baqai HZ, Anwer F. Patterns of pancytopenia in a general medical ward and a proposed diagnostic approach. J Ayub Med Coll Abbottabod 16:8–13, 2004.
6. Carmel R. Cobalamin, the stomach and aging. Am J Clin Nutr 66:750–759, 1997.
7. Taghizadeh M. Megaloblastic anemias. In: Harmening D, ed. Clinical Hematology and Fundamentals of Hemostasis, 4th ed. Philadelphia: FA Davis, 2002; 118.
8. Kozyraki R, Kristiansen M, Silahtaroglu A, et al. The human intrinsic factor, vitamin B_{12} receptor, cubilin: Molecular characterization and chromosomal mapping of the gene to 10 p within the autosomal recessive megaloblastic anemia (MCA 1) region. Blood 91:3593–3600, 1998.
9. Andres E, Voget T, Federici L, et al. Cobalamin deficiency in elderly patients: A personal view. Curr Gerontol Geriatr Res 848267, 2008.
10. Lindebaum J, Savage DG, Stables SP, et al. Diagnosis of cobalamin deficiency: II. Relative sensitivities of

serum cobalamin, methylmalonic acid, and total homocysteine concentrations. Am J Hematol 34:99–107, 1990.

11. Tejiani S. Pernicious anemia: Vitamin B_{12} to the rescue. ADVANCE for Medical Laboratory Professionals 10:16–18, 1998.

12. Ingram CF, Fleming AF, Patel M, et al. The value of intrinsic factor antibody test in diagnosing pernicious anemia. Cent Afr J Med 44:178–181, 1998.

13. Nyhols E, Turpin P, Swain D, et al. Oral vitamin B_{12} can change our practice. Postgrad Med J 79:218–220, 2003.

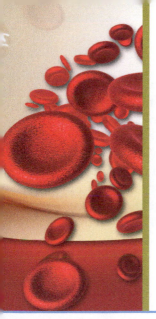

Chapter 7

Normochromic Anemias: Biochemical, Membrane, and Miscellaneous Red Blood Cell Disorders

Betty Ciesla

Objectives

After completing this chapter, the student will be able to:

1. Review the functions of the spleen as they relate to red blood cell membrane integrity.

2. Identify the red blood cell membrane defect in hereditary spherocytosis.

3. Describe the clinical findings and laboratory data in patients with hereditary spherocytosis.

4. Describe the relevant red blood cell morphology in patients with hereditary spherocytosis.

5. Describe the osmotic fragility test and its clinical usefulness.

6. Identify the red blood cell membrane defects in hereditary stomatocytosis, hereditary elliptocytosis, and hereditary pyropoikilocytosis.

7. Compare and contrast the clinical and peripheral smear findings from hereditary stomacytosis, hereditary elliptocytosis, and hereditary pyropoikilocytosis.

8. Define the pathophysiology of the red blood cell biochemical disorders.

9. Describe the mutations and ethnic distinctions in glucose-6-phosphate dehydrogenase deficiency.

10. Describe Heinz bodies with respect to their appearance in supravital and Wright's stain.

11. Define the defect in the rare membrane disorders of hereditary xerocytosis and Southeast Asian ovalocytosis.

12. Discuss the characteristics of aplastic anemia, paroxysmal nocturnal hemoglobinuria, paroxysmal cold hemoglobinuria, Fanconi's anemia, and Diamond-Blackfan syndrome.

ROLE OF THE SPLEEN IN RED BLOOD CELL MEMBRANE DISORDERS

The spleen plays a vital role in red blood cell health and longevity. Because 5% of cardiac output per minute is filtered through the spleen, this organ has ample opportunity to survey red blood cells for imperfections. Only red blood cells that are deemed "flawless" are conducted through the rest of the red blood cell journey. The four functions of the spleen have been explained in Chapter 2; when considering red blood cell membrane defects, the splenic filtration function is most relevant.

As each red blood cell passes through the spleen, the cell is inspected for imperfections. Imperfections may take many forms: inclusions, parasites, abnormal hemoglobin products, or an abnormal membrane. Inclusions may be removed from the cell, leaving the membrane intact and allowing the red blood cell to pass through the rest of circulation unharmed. If the red blood cell has abnormal hemoglobin (such as seen in thalassemia) or abnormal membrane components, red blood cell elasticity and deformability are harmed, and some degree of hemolysis usually results. In the case of spherocytes from hereditary spherocytosis (HS), the red blood cells are less elastic, and the exterior membrane of the cell is shaved off, leaving a smaller, more compact red blood cell structure, a spherocyte. A spherocyte represents abnormal red blood cell morphology with a shortened life span and a low surface area:volume ratio (Fig. 7.1).

HEREDITARY SPHEROCYTOSIS

Genetics and Pathophysiology of Hereditary Spherocytosis

Hereditary spherocytosis (HS) is a well-studied disorder that is common among individuals of northern European origin, with an incidence of 1:5,000.[1] In 75% of individuals, the mode of inheritance is autosomal dominant; 25% have an autosomal recessive presentation. The defect in HS is a deficiency of the key membrane protein, spectrin, and, to a lesser degree, a deficiency of membrane protein ankyrin (see Chapter 3) and the minor membrane proteins band 3 and protein 4.2. The red blood cell membrane disorders have been clearly defined genetically, with five gene mutations implicated in HS: *ANK1* (ankyrin), *SPTB* (spectrin, beta chain), *SLC4A1* (band 3), *EPB42* (protein 4.2), and *SPTA1* (spectrin, alpha chain).[2]

Spectrin and ankyrin are part of the cytoskeletal matrix proteins that support the lipid bilayer of the red blood cell. These proteins are responsible for elasticity and deformability, crucial properties of the red blood cell because the average red blood cell with a diameter of 6 to 8 μm must maneuver through circulatory spaces of much smaller diameter. A normal red blood cell is capable of stretching 117% of its surface volume (see Chapter 3) *only* if spectrin and ankyrin are in the proper amount and are fully functioning. The red blood cell membrane in patients with HS is stretchable, but it is less elastic and can expand only 3% before it ruptures.[3] With its low pH, low adenosine triphosphate (ATP), and low glucose, the spleen is a particularly caustic environment for spherocytes. Spherocytic red blood cells also exhibit problems with membrane diffusion. The active passive transport system of *normal* red blood cells allows ions and gases to pass across the red blood cell membrane in a balanced and harmonious fashion. As a result of the defective membrane proteins, the active passive transport system is disrupted, and spherocytes accumulate sodium at a higher rate than for normal red blood cells in the splenic microenvironment. They are less able to tolerate changes in their osmotic environment before they swell and lyse.[4] When an individual with HS has undergone splenectomy, red blood cell survival is longer, with fewer complications from chronic hemolysis. There is no evidence of spherocytes in the bone marrow environment, indicating that this phenomenon occurs within the level of the peripheral circulation.

Clinical Presentation in Hereditary Spherocytosis

Clinical presentations in HS are heterogeneous and range from disorders of lifelong anemia to disorders with subtle clinical and laboratory manifestations. Typically, a patient with HS presents with anemia, **jaundice**, and splenomegaly. Splenomegaly of varying degrees is the most common presentation, followed by a moderate anemia and recurrent jaundice, usually in younger children.[5] Older individuals have a

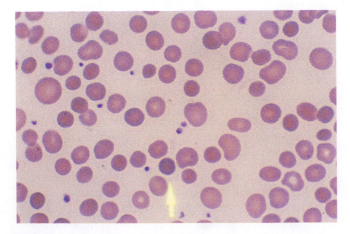

Figure 7.1 Spherocyte. Note the density of the cell with respect to the other red blood cells in the background.

From The College of American Pathologists, with permission.

well-compensated hemolytic process with little or no anemia. Compensated hemolytic processes indicate that the bone marrow production and destruction have reached equilibrium, and the peripheral indicators of hemolysis may not be present.

Reticulocytosis is a standard feature in individuals with HS, as evidenced by polychromatophilic macrocytes on the peripheral smear and reticulocyte counts ranging from 3% to 10%.[6] The peripheral smear also shows spherocytes in most patients with HS; however, the number of spherocytes varies considerably from field to field. Spherocytes have a *distinctive* morphology and are recognized as dense, small, round red blood cells lacking central pallor. With careful observation, the trained eye should be able to isolate and recognize spherocytes from the normal red blood cell population on the peripheral smear. Patients with HS show a moderate anemia, and 50% have elevated

mean corpuscular hemoglobin content (MCHC) of 36% or greater, a significant finding in the complete blood count (CBC). Mean corpuscular volume (MCV) is low normal, and red blood cell distribution width (RDW) is slightly elevated. Taken together, increased MCHC combined with elevated RDW adds strong predictive value in screening for HS.[7] Increased bilirubin is a frequent finding, owing to continued hemolysis, and younger patients tend to form gallstones. **Cholelithiasis**, or the presences of gallstones, is a common complication of patients with HS[8] and occurs most frequently in adolescents and young adults.

Documentation of spherocytes on a peripheral smear raises the index of suspicion of a hemolytic process. Spherocytes result from four mechanisms: HS (already discussed), autoimmune hemolytic anemia, thermal damage, or natural red blood cell death (Fig. 7.2). Spherocytes produced from an autoimmune

Spherocyte Formation

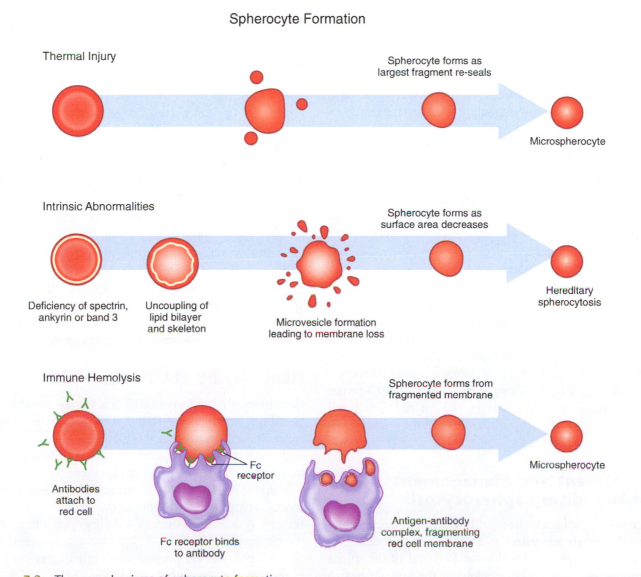

Figure 7.2   Three mechanisms of spherocyte formation.   Adapted from Glassy E. Color Atlas of Hematology: An Illustrated Guide Based on Proficiency Testing. Northfield, IL: College of American Pathologists, 1998, with permission.

process are the result of an antibody being attached to the red blood cell and then removed or sheared as the coated red blood cell passes through the spleen. As this occurs, the exterior membrane of the red blood cell is sheared, and a spherocyte is produced. A more moderated spherocyte-producing process is senescence, or natural red blood cell death. As the cell ages, it progressively loses membrane, leading to the production of spherocytes. In a normal peripheral smear, spherocytes are not seen, however, because they are removed by the spleen under normal circumstances of cell death.

Laboratory Diagnosis of Hereditary Spherocytosis

The laboratory diagnosis of HS is relatively easy in an individual with elevated MCHC, RDW, and the presence of spherocytes. Because most individuals with mild or moderate disease share a common clinical laboratory picture, additional laboratory testing is usually unnecessary. The confirmatory tests are labor-intensive and usually not offered as part of a regular laboratory menu of test items. The osmotic fragility test, incubated and unincubated, is the test of choice for confirming a diagnosis of HS. Red blood cells from patients suspected to have HS are subjected to varying saline solutions ranging from isotonic saline (0.85% NaCl) to distilled water (0.0% NaCl). Under isotonic conditions, normal red blood cells reach equilibrium and have little hemolysis. As the solutions become more hypotonic (less salt and more water), initial hemolysis occurs as red blood cells rupture.

The level of complete hemolysis is usually the only data reported on the patient sample. Normal red blood cells initially hemolyze at 0.45% NaCl. Red blood cells from patients with HS have a decreased surface:volume ratio and an increased osmotic fragility. They are less able to tolerate an influx of water and lyse at 0.65% (Fig. 7.3). An increased osmotic fragility curve is seen in conditions other than HS (e.g., some cases of autoimmune hemolytic anemia). Conditions such as thalassemia and iron deficiency anemia show a reduced osmotic fragility (hemolysis at 0.20%) owing to the high number of target cells, a red blood cell morphology with a capacity to take in a high influx of water before hemolysis.

Treatment and Management of Hereditary Spherocytosis

Because the spleen is the offending organ in HS, splenectomy is often suggested as a remedy for moderate to severe hemolysis in this disease. Removal of the spleen diminishes the anemia by allowing the spherocytes to

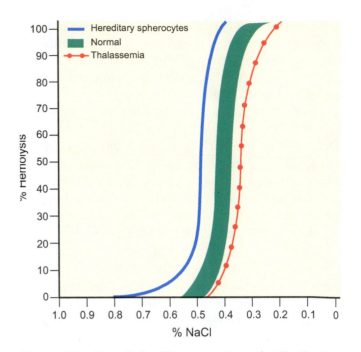

Figure 7.3 Osmotic fragility curves. Normal patient's plot is shown in the *shaded area*. The curve to the *right* shows a decreased fragility as seen in patients with sickle cell anemia. The curve to the *left* shows an increased fragility as seen in patients with hereditary spherocytosis.

remain in the circulation longer, reducing the need for blood transfusion and, in some cases, minimizing gallbladder disease. Splenectomy is a procedure that demands serious consideration before approval. Splenectomy in younger children poses serious risks by making them more vulnerable to infections with encapsulated organisms. **Prophylactic** penicillin should be offered after surgery to this age group, or a partial splenectomy surgical procedure should be considered. Partial splenectomy is known to reduce hemolysis, while preserving important immune splenic function.[9] If symptoms return as a result of remaining splenic tissue, a total splenectomy may be considered when the patient has the appropriate management and support.

HEREDITARY ELLIPTOCYTOSIS

Hereditary elliptocytosis (HE) is a highly variable red blood cell membrane disorder with many clinical subtypes. Its occurrence is 1:4,000, and it affects all racial and ethnic groups.[10] The inheritance is usually autosomal dominant. At the heart of this membrane defect is a defective or deficient spectrin and the proteins commonly associated with the alpha and beta spectrin regions. A decreased thermal stability occurs in each of the clinical subtypes.

Elliptocytes are present to varying degrees in each of the subtypes, and their red blood cell deformability is affected with degrees of hemolysis. Four clinical subtypes are discussed: common HE, Southeast Asian ovalocytosis, spherocytic HE, and hereditary pyropoikilocytosis.

Common Hereditary Elliptocytosis

The two clinical variants considered under common HE range from individuals who are silent carriers to transfusion-dependent individuals. Individuals with the silent carrier state of HE are hematologically normal, but family studies show that they are related to individuals with HE and hereditary pyropoikilocytosis. Common HE has two clinical presentations. In mild common HE, 30% to 100%[1] of the cells are elliptic, and most patients show no clinical symptoms (Fig. 7.4). Some patients may show slight hemolysis with elliptocytes and fragmented cells. The more severe variant of common HE, common HE with infantile pyropoikilocytosis, shows fragmented and bizarre red blood cell shapes from birth with a moderate hemolytic component and jaundice. As the patient ages, the disease converts to mild HE in presentation (Table 7.1).

Southeast Asian Ovalocytosis

Southeast Asian ovalocytosis is a common red blood cell condition in many Southeastern Asian populations in which the red blood cells are spoon-shaped and appear to have two bars across their center. Hemolysis may or may not be present, and this shape may give mild protection against all species of malaria.[11] Red blood cells with this disorder are strongly heat-resistant and rigid and are able to maintain their shape under temperatures that cause normal red blood cells to crenate or burst. This autosomal dominant disorder has a well-defined band 3 molecular defect (Fig. 7.5).

Table 7.1 ● Variants of Common Hereditary Elliptocytosis
• Silent carrier
• Mild common HE, either chronic hemolysis or moderate hemolysis
• Common HE with severe infant pyropoikilocytosis shows moderate hemolysis

Spherocytic Hereditary Elliptocytosis

Spherocytic HE is a cross between HE and HS. The red blood cells of affected individuals have more spherocytes and oval elliptocytes. This defect is common in individuals with northern European ancestry and shows a mild hemolysis and red blood cells of increased osmotic fragility. Gallbladder disease is a common feature, and splenectomy may be indicated if the hemoglobin decreases quickly because of increased hemolysis.

Hereditary Pyropoikilocytosis

Hereditary pyropoikilocytosis is a rare recessive disorder of the red blood cell membrane that primarily affects African American individuals. Two mechanisms are at work in the red blood cells of hereditary pyropoikilocytosis: a reduced assembly of alpha and beta spectrin on the membrane and increased susceptibility of mutant spectrin to degrade.[12] Hemoglobin values are extremely low (less than 6.5 g/dL), and the red blood cell morphology is extremely bizarre, with red blood cell budding, rare elliptocytes, and spherocytes. What makes these defective red blood cells unique is their heat sensitivity. Normal red blood cells show

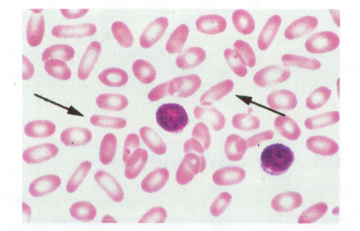

Figure 7.4 Elliptocytes. Note these cells are pencil-shaped.
From The College of American Pathologists, with permission.

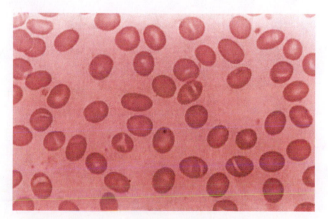

Figure 7.5 Photomicrograph of Southeastern Asian ovalocytosis.

crenation and hemolysis at 49°C, but red blood cells from patients with hereditary pyropoikilocytosis fragment at 46°C. Some may fragment at 37°C (body temperature) with prolonged heating. Individuals with this disorder have severe hemolysis, poor growth, and facial abnormalities as a result of the expanded bone marrow mass. MCV is extremely low (range 50 to75 fL).[13]

HEREDITARY STOMATOCYTOSIS AND HEREDITARY XEROCYTOSIS

Hereditary stomatocytosis is a rare hemolytic disorder in which red blood cells have an intrinsic defect related to sodium and potassium permeability. The defect, which is autosomal dominant, is identified as a deficiency in a membrane protein, stomatin, which is thought to regulate ions across the red blood cell channel.[14] Because of this transport lesion, the intracellular sodium content increases, leading to increased water content and a mild decrease in intracellular potassium. The red blood cells swell and take on a morphology that appears as if the cells have slits or bars in the center, as if the cell is "smiling." Peripheral smears show 10% to 30% stomatocytes (Fig. 7.6), with elevated MCV and decreased MCHC. Patients show a mild, moderate, or marked anemia that can be corrected by splenectomy; this is a dangerous procedure in this disorder, however, because many patients have thrombotic complications.[15] Stomatocytes may also be seen in individuals with Rh null disease—individuals who lack Rh antigens. These patients show a moderate anemia with a combination of spherocytes and stomatocytes.

Hereditary xerocytosis (Fig. 7.7) is a rare autosomal dominant condition in which red blood cells have an increased surface:volume ratio, leading to moderate to severe anemia, decreased osmotic fragility, and high

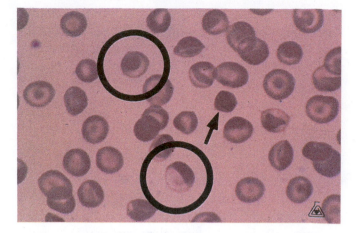

Figure 7.7   Hereditary xerocytosis.   From The College of American Pathologists, with permission.

MCHC.[16] Red blood cells are markedly dehydrated and show an irreversible potassium loss and formation of xerocytes, a peculiar red blood cell morphology in which the hemoglobin of red blood cells seems puddled at one end. The etiology of this disorder is unknown.

GLUCOSE-6-PHOSPHATE DEHYDROGENASE DEFICIENCY

A few inherited disorders of red blood cells are related to biochemical deficiencies. Glucose-6-phosphate dehydrogenase (G6PD) deficiency represents a fascinating and far-reaching disorder that has at its core a metabolic misstep. G6PD is the catalyst in the first stages of the oxidative portion of metabolism of the red blood cell and a key player in the phosphogluconate pathway, whose role it is to keep glutathione in the reduced state. Glutathione is the chief red blood cell antioxidant and serves to protect the red blood cell from oxidant stress caused by peroxide buildup and other compounds or drugs. The pathway to reduced glutathione is initiated when NADP is converted to NADPH by the action of G6PD, an essential enzyme in the phosphogluconate pathway. When this occurs, NADPH converts oxidized glutathione to reduced glutathione, and the red blood cell is protected.

Genetics of Glucose-6-Phosphate Dehydrogenase Deficiency

G6PD deficiency is the most common human enzyme deficiency in the world, present in more than 400 million people.[17] Despite this staggering number of affected individuals, G6PD deficiency has an extraordinarily low profile, which will be described later. G6PD was

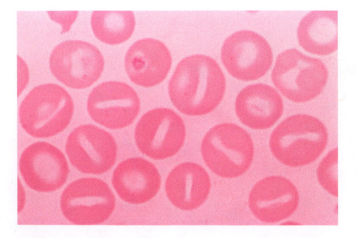

Figure 7.6   Stomatocytes.   From The College of American Pathologists, with permission.

discovered in America in 1950, when healthy African American soldiers developed hemolysis as a result of primaquine antimalarial drugs. The populations most affected are in West Africa, the Middle East, Southeast Asia, and the Mediterranean, and African Americans in the United States are affected. G6PD is inherited as an X-linked recessive disorder with mother-to-son transmission. Women are conductors of the aberrant genes; if they pass this gene to their sons, the sons inherit the disease. In heterozygous females, two populations of cells have been observed: a normal cell population and a G6PD cell population. The expression of G6PD deficiency is highly variable among heterozygotes and may sometimes cause disease. Homozygous females manifest the disease.

The human purified G6PD gene has 531 amino acids and is located near the genes for factor VIII and color blindness. More than 400 variants have been named, and many of the variants are caused by amino acid substitutions.[18] There are five known genotypes: two are normal and three are abnormal with varying amounts of hemolysis (Table 7.2). G6PD-deficient individuals are also afforded protection during malarial infections.[19] (For a Web-accessible database that details locus-specific mutations, see http://www.bioinf.org.uk/g6pd/.)

Clinical Manifestations of Glucose-6-Phosphate Dehydrogenase Deficiency

Acute Hemolytic Anemia

Four clinical conditions are associated with G6PD deficiency: drug-induced acute hemolytic anemia, favism, neonatal jaundice, and congenital nonspherocytic anemia. Classically, individuals with G6PD are hematologically normal and totally unaware that they possess a variant G6PD genotype. Proper red blood cell function requires only 20% of the enzyme. These individuals become exposed to a drug or have an infection and develop a self-limited but frightening hemolytic episode. Eventually, their G6PD status is investigated, and if a diagnosis is made, it becomes part of their medical record.

Affected individuals are made aware of a growing list of drugs that may cause hemolysis if injected or ingested. In a drug-induced process or an infection-induced hemolytic process, the patient experiences nausea, abdominal pain, and rapidly decreasing hematocrit within a 24- to 48-hour period. The level of hemolysis is alarming as the hemoglobin and hematocrit drop quickly and the intravascular lysis manifests as hemoglobinuria in which the urine has the color of Coca Cola, port wine, or strong tea.[20] LDH and reticulocytes are increased, whereas the anemia is normochromic and normocytic with the bone marrow showing erythroid hyperplasia. The peripheral smear shows marked polychromasia and a few bite cells. Bite cells (Fig. 7.8) are formed as Heinz bodies and are pitted from the red blood cells by the spleen. Heinz body inclusions (Fig. 7.9) are large inclusions (0.2 to 3 μm) that are rigid, distort the cell, and hang on the cell periphery (see Chapter 3). These inclusions form from denatured or precipitated hemoglobin that occurs in the G6PD-deficient individual on exposure to the oxidizing agent because the lack of the G6PD enzyme causes oxidative destruction of the red blood cell.

Heinz bodies are not visible on Wright's stain but may be seen when blood cells are stained with supravital stains such as crystal violet. The formation of Heinz bodies may be induced experimentally with phenylhydrazine. As the inclusion-laden red blood

Table 7.2 ● Genotypes of Glucose-6-Phosphate Dehydrogenase	
GdB+	Normal genotypes
GdA+	Normal genotype mutated gene in 20% of African Americans
GdA−	Abnormal genotype in 11% of African American males
Gd Med	Abnormal genotype seen in Caucasians, individuals of Mediterranean origin, Kurdish Jews
Gd Canton	Abnormal genotype seen in Thailand, Vietnam, Taiwan, other Asian populations

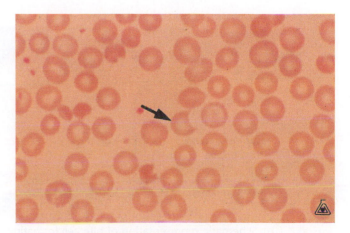

Figure 7.8 **Bite cells.** From The College of American Pathologists, with permission.

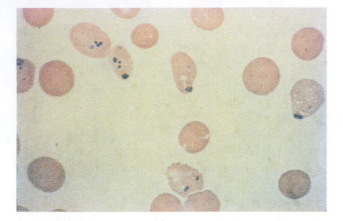

Figure 7.9   Heinz bodies.   From The College of American Pathologists, with permission.

Table 7.3 ●	Modified List of Compounds That May Cause Hemolysis in Glucose-6-Phosphate Dehydrogenase Deficient Individuals

- Aspirin
- Phenacetin
- Chloroquine
- Chloramphenicol
- Sulfacetamide
- Naphthalene
- Vitamin K
- Nitrofurantoin
- Nalidixic acid
- Sulfamethoxazole

cells pass through the spleen, the Heinz bodies are pitted from the cell surface, and bite or helmet cells (Fig. 7.10) remain. Heinz bodies and subsequently bite cells are a transient finding in G6PD-deficient individuals. The absence of this particular morphology cannot be used as a definitive argument against this diagnosis. For individuals who have a drug-induced hemolytic event, the hematologic consequences are self-limiting; however, individuals with G6PD variants must be cautioned about drug use or chemicals known to provoke a hemolytic episode in susceptible individuals (Table 7.3).

Favism

The second most severe clinical condition is favism. Favism is usually found in individuals of the G6PD Mediterranean or Canton type. Hours after ingesting young fava beans or broad beans, the individual usually becomes irritable and lethargic. Fever, nausea, and abdominal pain follow, and within 48 hours gross hemoglobinuria may be noted. Heinz bodies may or may not be observed. Patients present with a normochromic, normocytic process with polychromasia, decreased haptoglobin, and increased bilirubin. There have been incidents of favism from individuals inhaling fava beans pollen or from infants nursed by a mother who transmitted fava bean metabolites in breast milk. Fava beans trigger hemolytic episodes in only 25% of deficient individuals, however.

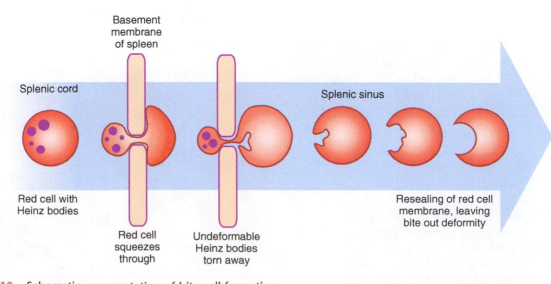

Basement membrane of spleen

Splenic cord   Splenic sinus

Red cell with Heinz bodies   Red cell squeezes through   Undeformable Heinz bodies torn away   Resealing of red cell membrane, leaving bite out deformity

Figure 7.10   Schematic representation of bite cell formation.   Adapted from Glassy E. Color Atlas of Hematology: An Illustrated Guide Based on Proficiency Testing. Northfield, IL: College of American Pathologists, 1998, with permission.

Neonatal Jaundice

Neonatal jaundice related to G6PD deficiency occurs within 2 to 3 days after birth. In contrast to patients with hemolytic disease of the newborn, patients with neonatal jaundice show more jaundice than anemia. Early recognition and management of the increasing bilirubin are essential to prevent neurologic complications (e.g., kernicterus) in these infants. Data on infants from Malaysia, the Mediterranean, Hong Kong, and Thailand have shown the incidence of neonatal jaundice to be quite frequent. Also notable is the increased sensitivity of these individuals to vitamin K substitutes, triple dye used to treat umbilical cords, and camphorated powder. These substances may cause a deterioration of the hematologic state. Phototherapy (intense light therapy) and transfusion support are used to treat affected infants.

Congenital Nonspherocytic Hemolytic Anemia

The final clinical condition is congenital nonspherocytic hemolytic anemia. Patients who have this condition have a history of neonatal jaundice complicated by gallstones, enlarged spleen, or both and may be investigated for jaundice or gallstones as adults. The anemia varies in severity from minimal to transfusion dependent. Splenectomy may be considered provided that the appropriate management (prophylactic therapy and management) is in place. The clinical picture suggests a chronic hemolysis that is mainly extravascular with hyperbilirubinemia, decreased haptoglobin, and increased reticulocytes.

Diagnosis of Glucose-6-Phosphate Dehydrogenase Deficiency

The detection of G6PD deficiency is complicated by the many genetic variants, the heterozygosity of the disorder, and the fact that young red blood cells show an increased enzyme level just by virtue of age. Several technical considerations must be kept in mind when determining a person's enzyme status. Appropriate timing of the test is critical for accurate results. If G6PD deficiency is tested for during an acute hemolytic episode, reticulocytes would be pouring from the bone marrow into the peripheral circulation. Testing should be performed after the hemolytic episode has resolved and the counts have returned to normal. G6PD enzyme assay of older red blood cells is recommended. Additionally, the fluorescent spot test that measures NADP to NADPH reduction may be used. The entire picture, including clinical presentation, CBC, peripheral smear, and enzyme status, must be analyzed before a diagnosis is made.

PYRUVATE KINASE DEFICIENCY

Pyruvate kinase deficiency is a rare enzyme disorder of the Embden-Meyerhof pathways. Red blood cells lacking this enzyme are unable to generate ATP from adenosine diphosphate (ADP) for red blood cell membrane function. Consequently, there is a buildup of 2,3-diphosphoglycerate. The result is rigid, inflexible cells that are sequestered by the spleen and hemolyzed. Both genders are affected in this autosomal recessive disorder. There is a high incidence in individuals of northern European origin and in the close-knit Amish population of Mifflin County, Pennsylvania.[21] Patients show a moderate hemolysis, with hematocrits between 18% and 36%,[22] and little abnormal morphology on the peripheral smear except for marked polychromasia and a few nucleated red blood cells. A fluorescent screening test is used followed by a specific assay for pyruvate kinase activity.

MISCELLANEOUS RED BLOOD CELL DISORDERS

Aplastic Anemia

Aplastic anemia is one of a group of hypoproliferative disorders in which there is cellular depletion and a reduced production of all blood cells, or pancytopenia. Discovered in 1888 by Ehrlich, this syndrome is usually idiopathic but is thought to result from two possible mechanisms: an antibody directed against an antigen on stem cells or an immune mechanism in which T lymphocytes suppress stem cell proliferation.[23] The following factors seem to predispose an individual to an aplastic episode:

- Radiation
- Chemotherapy or chemicals
- Benzene, either directly or indirectly
- Viruses, especially Epstein-Barr and hepatitis B and C

Clinical characteristics of aplastic anemia include decreased marrow cellularity, pancytopenia, and reticulocytopenia. This syndrome is an insidious process that progresses in a slow but orderly fashion with symptoms reflective of the depressed cellular elements. When red blood cells become significantly depleted, patients exhibit fatigue, heart palpitations, and dyspnea. As platelets become depleted, **ecchymosis** and mucosal bleeds develop, and WBC depletion leads to infections. In many cases, the peripheral smear shows lymphocytosis. Treatment for this normochromic, normocytic anemia includes transfusion support and steroids; a few patients recover spontaneously. Occasionally, stem cell transplantation is used to treat severe aplastic anemia.[24]

Fanconi's Anemia

Characterized by Fanconi in 1927, Fanconi's anemia is a rare autosomal recessive disorder that affects physical characteristics and bone marrow development. More than 400 cases have been reported worldwide, and a database, the International Fanconi Anemia Registry, provides current information concerning this disorder. Fanconi's anemia includes numerous chromosomal abnormalities, defective DNA repair, and many chromosomal breaks.[25] The bone marrow often shows a macrocytic morphology, with thrombocytopenia and leukopenia developing before red blood cell depletion. Hgb F values are increased. The physical characteristics of a patient with Fanconi's anemia include short stature, hyperpigmentation on the trunk and neck, microcephaly, broad nose, and structural abnormalities of the kidney.[26] Life span is shortened, with a mean survival of 16 years, and patients have a tendency to develop leukemia and other cancers. Treatment is supportive as complications from aplasia develop. The only curative therapy is a bone marrow transplant.

Diamond-Blackfan Anemia

Diamond-Blackfan anemia, discovered in 1938 by Diamond and Blackfan, shows dominant and recessive inheritance patterns. This congenital hypoplastic disorder is usually diagnosed in early infancy; 80% of individuals are severely anemic by age 6 months.[27] Several physical abnormalities have been observed, including short stature, low birth weight, head and facial abnormalities, and a tendency for children with Diamond-Blackfan anemia to look more like each other than family members. The bone marrow is usually lacking in red blood cell precursors with a slightly decreased number of leukocytes. The average hemoglobin is 7 g/dL, and Hgb F is increased. Treatment includes steroids and transfusional support with careful attention to the possibility of hemosiderosis. Spontaneous recovery occurs in 25% of patients.[28]

Paroxysmal Nocturnal Hemoglobinuria

The rare hemolytic anemia paroxysmal nocturnal hemoglobinuria (PNH) is notable because the increased susceptibility of the red blood cells to complement lysis is directly related to a clonal membrane defect. Classically in this disorder, red blood cells are destroyed while patients sleep because of their increased sensitivity to complement lysis; on arising, the patient notices bloody urine, or hemoglobinuria. PNH occurs because of a somatic mutation in the hematopoietic stem cells designated as phosphatidylinositol glycan A (PIGA). The X-linked mutation PIGA is essential for the synthesis of the glycosylphosphatidylinositol (GPI)-anchored proteins present in all cell lines. As a result of this mutation, nine cell surface proteins are missing from cells.[29] Two proteins in particular, CD55 decay accelerating factor and CD59 membrane inhibitor, offer protection to red blood cells against lysis by complement. The GPI mutation also affects white blood cells and platelets. There is a high variability of expression of these abnormal geneotypes in all of the affected cell lines; consequently, disease severity depends on the phenotypes involved. Intravascular lysis, however, is a primary manifestation of red blood cells missing these proteins. The intensity of lysis in the form of hemoglobinuria has been described by patients as having urine samples that range in color from strong tea to tar.

Patients with PNH have a variable presentation with an unexpected onset in 30% of cases. Marrow failure is part of the clinical picture, but its onset and its prevalence are not yet fully appreciated.[30] Patients may have a mild to severe anemia. Most are pancytopenic with reticulocyte levels that are elevated but not appropriate with respect to the level of anemia. Neutropenia is always present, but stainable iron is usually absent because of continued lysis. Many patients have a tendency toward thrombosis, especially in unusual sites, such as the dermal vessels, brain, liver, and abdomen.[31] In these patients, anticoagulant therapy may need to be considered because thrombosis can cause considerable mortality.

Treatment for patients with PNH includes transfusion support and, in selected younger patients, bone marrow transplant.[32] Iron therapy may also be included when the patient's iron status has been assessed. A new drug, eculizumab, blocks complement activity by binding to C5 and preventing hemolysis. This new monoclonal antibody treatment is well tolerated, and clinical trials have shown that it is effective in improving hemolysis and relieving symptoms.[33] Screening procedures usually employed in the diagnosis of PNH include the sugar water test and Ham's test. Flow cytometry is the most diagnostic and predictive procedure.

Sugar Water Test (for Historical Reference)

In the sugar water test, a 50% solution of the patient's washed ethylenediaminetetraacetic acid (EDTA) red blood cells are mixed with ABO/Rh-compatible serum, and sugar solution is added. The solutions are incubated for 30 minutes and then centrifuged. The percent hemolysis is determined by spectrophotometer. Normal cells show less than 5% hemolysis, and suspect cells show 10% to 80% hemolysis.

Ham's Test (Acidified Serum Test) (for Historical Reference)

Ham's test screens for PNH. The patient's serum is acidified using 0.2N HCl. A 50% solution of the patient's cells is added to tubes containing the patient's acidified serum, unacidified serum, and normal ABO-compatible serum. A normal red blood cell control is run. Normal red blood cells do not hemolyze, but cells from patients with PNH hemolyze with acidified serum from the patient and from normal ABO-compatible serum (Fig. 7.11). (*Note:* These tests are rarely performed in the laboratory because so few individuals have PNH, but they are simple and direct and yield some value.)

Flow Cytometry in the Diagnosis of Paroxysmal Nocturnal Hemoglobinuria

Currently available flow cytometry procedures can test white blood cells for the presence or absence of

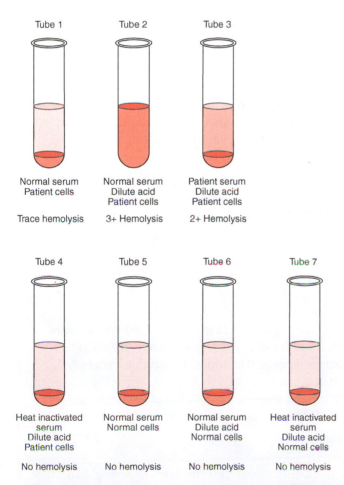

Figure 7.11 Ham's test. Note varying degrees of hemolysis in tubes 1, 2, and 3. Hemolysis occurs in tubes containing patient cells, patient serum, and acidified serum. Hemolysis does not occur in tubes with heat-inactivated serum and control cells because heat inactivates complement.

GPI-linked proteins. White blood cells can be examined for reactivity to anti-CD48, anti-CD55, and anti-CD59, all of which are anchored proteins.[34] A new diagnostic procedure, FLAER (fluorescent-labeled aerolysin), has proved effective in detecting smaller populations of abnormal leukocytes in PNH.[35] This technique may prove useful in determining PNH cell clones in individuals presenting with varying levels of bone marrow failure.

Cold Agglutinin Syndrome

Cold agglutinin syndrome (CAS) is another rare hemolytic disorder that primarily affects individuals older than 50 years. Also known as cold hemagglutinin disease (CHAD), the hemolysis in this disorder is caused by an IgM autoantibody of wide thermal range. Complement is fixed on the red blood cells during cold temperatures, 0°C to 5°C, and then red blood cells agglutinate and hemolyze as body temperature increases to 25°C to 30°C. Patients have acrocyanosis, or numbness and a bluish tone to the fingertips and toes; they also experience weakness, pallor, and weight loss. The lysis is intravascular with a positive direct **antiglobulin test** (with polyclonal antihuman globulin reagent or anti-C3d). Some hemoglobinuria may be present. If the antibody is strong, the CBC would need to be corrected because the antibody coats the red blood cells, causing agglutination and falsely elevated red blood cell indices and hematocrit. The sample should be warmed at 37°C for 15 to 30 minutes and then recycled through the instrument for accurate results. After warming, all parameters should be accurate. Treatment is circumstantial, depending on the level of hemolysis; many individuals move to warmer climates to avoid hemolytic episodes altogether. Additionally, transient cold agglutinin caused by *Mycoplasma pneumoniae* may be seen.

Paroxysmal Cold Hemoglobinuria

Paroxysmal cold hemoglobinuria (PCH) is a rare hemolytic anemia caused by anti-P, which attaches to the red blood cells at lower temperatures and then activates complement at warmer temperatures. Lysis occurs at body temperature. The lysis is intravascular and severe, with hemoglobinemia, hemoglobinuria, and increased bilirubin. The symptoms are similar to a hemolytic transfusion reaction, with back pain, fever, chills, and abdominal pain. Some patients may require transfusion.[33] The screening test for PCH is the Donath-Landsteiner test, which is rarely performed in the clinical laboratory.

Donath-Landsteiner Test

The patient's blood sample is split into two parts. The first aliquot is the control and should be incubated at 37°C for 1 hour. The second aliquot is placed at 4°C for 30 minutes and then incubated at 37°C for 30 minutes. Both aliquots are centrifuged and observed for hemolysis. The control should show no hemolysis. If the second aliquot shows hemolysis, that is evidence for PCH.

○ Summary Points

- The spleen plays a vital role in red blood cell health and longevity.

- HS is an autosomal dominant disorder of several membrane proteins, the key protein being spectrin.

- Spherocytes are less deformable and are more osmotically fragile.

- Patients with hereditary spherocytes have splenomegaly, jaundice, and an increased tendency for gallstone disease.

- The osmotic fragility test is a labor-intensive but valuable test to assess red blood cell response in different hypotonic salt solutions.

- HE is a membrane disorder of spectrin showing decreased thermal stability.

- There are several clinical variants of HE, including common HE, Southeast Asian ovalocytosis, and spherocytic HE.

- Hereditary pyropoikilocytosis is a recessive membrane disorder with a bizarre red blood cell morphology that shows hemoglobin budding.

- Hereditary stomatocytosis is a membrane disorder in which red blood cells have an intrinsic defect to sodium and potassium permeability.

- G6PD deficiency is the most common enzyme deficiency in the world.

- G6PD is an X-linked recessive disorder with more than 400 variants.

- Drug-induced or infection-induced hemolysis in G6PD is intravascular, brisk, and self-limiting.

- Most individuals with G6PD deficiency are totally unaware of their hematologic condition until they are challenged by a drug that produces oxidant stress.

- Pyruvate kinase deficiency is an enzyme deficiency of the Embden-Meyerhof pathway.

- Aplastic anemia is a hypoproliferative disorder in which there is cellular depletion and a reduced production of blood cells.

- Fanconi's anemia and Diamond-Blackfan anemia are rare hypoproliferative disorders with congenital malformations.

- PNH is a hemolytic anemia that is caused when nine red blood cell surface proteins are absent and red blood cells become increasingly sensitive to complement lysis.

- CAS is a disease affecting elderly individuals that is caused by an IgM autoantibody of wide thermal range.

- Paroxysmal cold hemoglobinuria is an extremely rare hemolytic disorder caused by anti-P of a wide thermal range.

CONDENSED CASE

A 2-year-old African American boy was seen in the sick baby clinic with vomiting, fever, and red-colored urine staining his diapers. His initial laboratory results showed hemoglobin of 5 g/dL and hematocrit of 15%. The most remarkable chemistry value was LDH of 500 IU/L (reference range 0 to 100 IU/L), which is extremely elevated. His peripheral smear revealed polychromasia and occasional bite cells.

When the mother was questioned about whether the boy had ingested anything out of the ordinary, she stated that he has been chewing on mothballs in her closet. The child was transported to the intensive care unit. *What is happening to this child?*

Answer

This child has severe intravascular lysis, as evidenced by the LDH value and the extremely low hemoglobin and hematocrit. Most likely, he has G6PD deficiency brought on by chewing on naphthalene, the active ingredient of mothballs. Naphthalene is an oxidizing chemical that in this case has put the child's red blood cells under oxidant stress. Occasional bite cells in the smear suggest the formation of Heinz bodies and their subsequent removal by the spleen.

CASE STUDY

A 28-year-old man presents to the emergency department with a complaint of abdominal pain. He appears quite ill with nausea, cold sweats, and tachycardia. He had taken aspirin when he started feeling sick. The patient appears slightly jaundiced and on further questioning admits that his urine had been dark and discolored that day. The preliminary impression was of acute appendicitis.

Pertinent Hematology Results (refer to inside cover for normal values)

WBC	6.3×10^9/L
RBC	1.00×10^{12}/L
Hgb	4.4 g/dL
Hct	12.6%
MCV	126 fL
MCH	43.9 pg
MCHC	34.8%

The white blood cell differential was essentially normal; however, the red blood cell morphology was abnormal, showing basophilic stippling, slight polychromasia, moderate teardrop cells, and occasional schistocytes and ovalocytes.

Pertinent Chemistry Results

Direct bilirubin	0.7 mg/dL (0.0 to 0.4 mg/dL)
Total bilirubin	7.9 mg/dL (0.1 to 1.4 mg/dL)
Indirect bilirubin	7.2 mg/dL (0.1 to 0.8 mg/dL)
SGOT	567 IU/L (0 to 100 IU/L)
LDH	2844 IU/L (0 to 100 IU/L)

Insights to the Case Study

This case is an example of a patient with G6PD deficiency. He has sustained a violent hemolytic episode as a result of drug exposure—in this case, aspirin. This previously healthy man has no idea that he has an abnormal G6PD variant. He is very ill, and his RBC, hemoglobin, and hematocrit are extremely depressed. His MCV is macrocytic and his MCH and RDW are also elevated. The indirect bilirubin, SGOT, and LDH all are increased, and these serum chemistry elevations are indicative of a hemolytic episode of monumental proportions.

MCV is increased because of increased reticulocytosis that manifests in the peripheral circulation as polychromasia and nucleated red blood cells, as seen in this patient's peripheral smear. A Heinz body preparation was performed by allowing equal volumes of EDTA blood to mix with crystal violet stain for 20 minutes. Several Heinz bodies were observed in this preparation. The hemolysis in G6PD deficiency is primarily intravascular as noted by the hemoglobinuria and hemoglobinemia. Most individuals who have G6PD deficiency remain in a steady state and are hematologically normal; they hemolyze only when exposed to an oxidative drug. These events are self-limiting, and, although troubling, their hematologic status returns to normal.

Review Questions

1. Which of the following inclusions cannot be visualized by the Wright-stained peripheral smear?
   a. Basophilic stippling
   b. Hgb H inclusion bodies
   c. Howell-Jolly bodies
   d. Heinz bodies

2. Which of the following functions most affect spherocytes as they travel through the circulation?
   a. They tend to form inclusion bodies.
   b. They are less deformable and more sensitive to the low glucose in the spleen.
   c. They tend to be sequestered in the spleen because of abnormal hemoglobin.
   d. They form siderotic granules and cannot navigate the circulation.

3. Many individuals with hereditary spherocytosis are prone to jaundice because of
   a. Epstein-Barr virus.
   b. Pathologic fractures.
   c. Gallstone disease.
   d. Skin pigmentation.

Continued

4. Which of the following are characteristics of hereditary pyropoikilocytosis?
   a. Elliptocytes with spherocytes intermixed in the peripheral smear
   b. Spherocytes with polychromasia and low MCV
   c. Elliptocytes, spherocytes, and budding red blood cells
   d. Mostly elliptocytes with a few other morphologies

5. Which red blood cell morphology is formed as a result of Heinz bodies being pitted from the red blood cell?
   a. Acanthocytes
   b. Bite cells
   c. Burr cells
   d. Stomatocytes

6. Which of the following hemolytic disorders has red blood cells that are especially sensitive to lysis by complement?
   a. Paroxysmal nocturnal hemoglobinuria
   b. Fanconi's anemia
   c. Aplastic anemia
   d. Hereditary spherocytosis

7. In the osmotic fragility test, normal red blood cells hemolyze at which level?
   a. 0.65%
   b. 0.45%
   c. 0.20%
   d. 0.30%

8. One of the least severe clinical manifestations of G6PD deficiency is
   a. Acute hemolytic anemia.
   b. Favism.
   c. Neonatal jaundice.
   d. Congenital nonspherocytic hemolytic anemia.

9. An anemia that manifests as decreased marrow cellularity, cytopenias in two cellular elements, and a reticulocytopenia is appropriately termed
   a. Megaloblastic anemia.
   b. Aplastic anemia.
   c. Sideroblastic anemia.
   d. Iron deficiency anemia.

10. Individuals with Fanconi's anemia characteristically show
    a. Intravascular hemolysis.
    b. Increased Hgb F.
    c. Ringed sideroblasts.
    d. Thrombocytosis.

○ TROUBLESHOOTING

What Kinds of Clinical Situations Come to Mind When the MCHC Is Greater Than 36.0%?

A 72-year-old man was seen in the emergency department for gastrointestinal bleeding and sepsis and was subsequently admitted. He had the usual emergency department tests ordered: chemistry panel, prothrombin time and activated partial thromboplastin time, urinalysis, and CBC. His CBC showed the following:

WBC	10.8×10^9/L
RBC	3.58×10^{12}/L
Hgb	10.7 g/dL
Hct	30.5%
MCV	85.3 fL
MCH	29.8 pg
MCHC	34.9%
Platelets	16×10^9/L
RDW	13.7%

During his 3-day stay, the patient's red blood cell indices began to fluctuate (MCH and MCHC), and his hemoglobin results showed variability. The CBC results on day 3 were as follows:

WBC	15.9×10^9/L
RBC	2.80×10^{12}/L
Hgb	9.3 g/dL
Hct	23.9%
MCV	85.5 fL
MCH	33.4 pg
MCHC	39.0%*
Platelets	79×10^9/L
RDW	15.1%

MCHC in the CBC was flagged (asterisk) and warranted further investigation. When the technologist first noticed these increases, several scenarios came to mind: (1) cold agglutinins, (2) lipemia, or (3) spherocytes. The technologist followed standard operating procedures (SOP) for elevated MCHC. First, the sample was warmed in a 37°C water bath for 30 minutes and then reanalyzed on the Coulter LH750. The results remained unchanged. Sometimes cold agglutinins require longer incubation in a water bath to correct. This was not the case with this particular specimen because it was incubated for 30 minutes longer. The MCHC refused to budge even after longer incubation. When a sample is incubated for 30 minutes or longer, cells settle away from the plasma, and the technologist can observe the plasma for the presence of lipemia. The observations revealed a slight increase (or cloudiness), but not true lipemia, which interferes with the MCHC. The final step was to look for spherocytes on the peripheral smear. The smear was negative for spherocytes. At this point, the technologist could not explain the MCHC and reported the results commenting under the MCHC: no hemolysis, no presence of cold agglutinins, and no spherocytes.

W O R D   K E Y

Antiglobulin test • Test used in immunohematology to determine if a patient has made an alloantibody present in the serum or an antibody that is coating the red blood cells

Cholelithiasis • Formation of gallstones

Crenation • Term used to describe the appearance of red blood cells that seem to have ridges around the edge

Ecchymosis • Bruising

Jaundice • Yellow color usually seen in the mucous membranes of the eyes and noticed as an overall skin color

Prophylactic • Preventive

References

1. Lux SE, Becker PS. Disorders of the red cell membrane skeleton: Hereditary spherocytosis and hereditary elliptocytosis. In: Scriver CR, Baudet AB, Sly US, et al, eds. The Metabolic Basis of Inherited Disease, 6th ed. New York: McGraw-Hill, 1989; 2367.
2. Iolascon A, Perrotta S, Stewart GW. Red blood cell membrane defects. Rev Clin Exp Haematol 7:22–56, 2003.
3. Evans EA, Waugh R, Melnik L. Elastic area compressibility modules of red cell membrane. Biophys J 16:585–595, 1976.
4. Vives Corrons JL, Besson I. Red cell membrane Na+ transport system in hereditary spherocytosis relevance to understanding the increased Na+ permeability. Ann Hematol 80:535–539, 2001.
5. Panigrahi I, Rhadke SR, Agarwal A, et al. Clinical profile of hereditary spherocytosis in North India. J Assoc Phys India 50:1360–1367, 2002.
6. Payne MS. Intracorpuscular defects leading to increased erythrocyte destruction. In: Rodak B, ed. Hematology: Clinical Principles and Applications, 2nd ed. Philadelphia: WB Saunders, 2002; 267.
7. Michaels LA, Cohen AR, Zhao H, et al. Screening for hereditary spherocytosis by use of automated erythrocytes indices. J Pediatr 13:957–960, 1997.
8. Tamary H, Aviner S, Freud E, et al. High incidences of early cholelithiasis detected by ultrasonography in children and young adults with hereditary spherocytosis. J Pediatr Hematol Oncol 25:952–954, 2003.
9. deBuys Roessingh AS, de Laguasie P, Rohrlich P, et al. Follow up of partial splenectomy in children with hereditary spherocytosis. J Pediatr Surg 37:1459–1463, 2002.
10. Gallagher PG, Forget BD, Lux SE. Disorders of the erythrocyte membrane. In: Nathan DG, Oski SH, eds. Nathan and Oski's Hematology of Infancy and Childhood, 5th ed. Philadelphia: WB Saunders, 1998; 544–664.
11. Cattani JA, Gibson FD, Alperes MP, et al. Hereditary ovalocytosis and reduced susceptibility to malaria in Papua New Guinea. Trans R Soc Trop Med Hyg 81:705–709, 1987.
12. Hanspal M, Hanspal JS, Sahr KE, et al. Molecular basis of spectrin deficiency in hereditary pyropoikilocytosis. Blood 82:1652–1660, 1993.
13. Palek J. Hereditary elliptocytosis and related disorders. Clin Hematol 14:45, 1985.
14. Fricke B, Argent AC, Chetley MC, et al. The "stomatin" gene and protein in overhydrated hereditary stomatocytosis. Blood 102:2268–2277, 2003.
15. Stewart GW, Amess JA, Eber SW, et al. Thromboembolic disease after splenectomy for hereditary stomatocytosis. Br J Hematol 93:303–310, 1996.
16. Glader BE, Fortier N, Abala MM, et al. Congenital hemolytic anemia associated with dehydrated erythrocytes and increased potassium ions. N Engl J Med 291:491–496, 1974.
17. Fiorelli G, Martinez di Montemuros F, Capellini MD. Chronic non-spherocytic hemolytic disorders associated with glucose 6 phosphate dehydrogenase variants. Baillieres Best Pract Res Clin Haematol 13:39–55, 2000.
18. Beutler E. Red cell enzyme defects. Hematol Pathol 4:103–114, 1990.
19. Mehta A, Mason PJ, Vulliam TJ. Glucose 6 phosphate dehydrogenase. Baillieres Best Pract Res Clin Haematol 13:21–38, 2000.
20. Lazzato L. G6PD deficiency and hemolytic anemias. In: Nathan DG, Oski FA, eds. Nathan and Oski's Hematology of Infancy and Childhood, 4th ed. Philadelphia: WB Saunders, 1993; 679.
21. Valentine WN, Koyichi RT, Paglia DE. Pyruvate kinase and other enzyme deficiency disorders of the erythrocyte. In: Scriver CR, Beaudet AL, Sly WS, Valle D, eds, The Metabolic Basis of Inherited Diseases, 6th ed. New York: McGraw-Hill, 1989; 1606–1628.
22. Brown BA. Hematology: Principles and Procedures, 6th ed. Philadelphia: Lea & Febiger; 1993; 298.

23. Gordon-Smith EC, Marsh JC, Gibson FM. Views on the pathophysiology of aplastic anemia. Int J Hematol 76(Suppl 12):163–166, 2002.

24. Trigg ME. Hematopoietic stem cells. Pediatrics 113(Suppl 4):1051–1057, 2004.

25. Bagby GC Jr. Genetic basis of Fanconi's anemia. Curr Opin Hematol 10:68–73, 2003.

26. Schroeder-Kurth TM, Auerbach AD, Obe G. Fanconi Anemia: Clinical, Cytogenetics and Experimental Aspects. Berlin: Springer-Verlag, 1989; 264.

27. Alter BP, Young NS. The bone marrow failure syndromes. In: Nathan DG, Oski FA, eds. Nathan and Oski's Hematology of Infancy and Childhood, 4th ed. Philadelphia: WB Saunders, 1992; 263.

28. Krijanovski OI, Seiff CA. Diamond-Blackfan anemia. Hematol Oncol Clin N Am 11:1061, 1997.

29. Lawrence LW, Harmening DM, Green R. Hemolytic anemia: Extracorpuscular defects and acquired intracorpuscular defects. In: Harmening D, ed. Clinical Hematology and Fundamentals of Thrombosis, 4th ed. Philadelphia: FA Davis, 2002; 202.

30. Young NS. Paroxysmal nocturnal hemoglobinuria: Current issues in pathophysiology and treatment. Curr Hematol Rep 4:103–109, 2005.

31. Hillmen P, Lewis SM, Bressler M, et al. Natural history of PNH. N Engl J Med 333:1253–1258, 1995.

32. Meyers G, Parker CJ. Management issues in paroxysmal nocturnal hemoglobinuria. Int J Haematol 77:125–132, 2003.

33. Hill A, Hillmen P, Richards SJ, et al. Sustained response and long-term safety of eculizumab in paroxysmal nocturnal hemoglobinuria. Blood 106:2559–2565, 2005.

34. Schubert J, Alvarado M, Uciechowski P, et al. Diagnosis of paroxysmal nocturnal haemoglobinuria using immunophenotyping of peripheral blood cells. Br J Haematol 79:487–492, 1991.

35. Brodsky RA, Mukhina GL, Li S, et al. Improved detection and characterization of paroxysmal nocturnal hemoglobinuria using fluorescent aerolysin. Am J Clin Pathol 114:459–466, 2000.

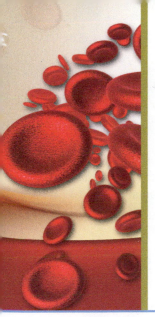

Chapter 8

The Normochromic Anemias Caused by Hemoglobinopathies

Betty Ciesla

Objectives

After completing this chapter, the student will be able to:

1. Recall the general characteristics of the hemoglobinopathies.

2. Describe the pathophysiology of the sickle disorders.

3. Identify the amino acid substitution in sickle cell disorders.

4. Identify the amino acid substitution in Hgb C disease.

5. Describe the inheritance patterns of the sickle disorders.

6. List the clinical and laboratory features of sickle cell anemia, sickle cell trait, Hgb C disease, Hgb C trait, and Hgb SC disease.

7. Review the physiologic conditions that most typically affect individuals with sickle cell anemia.

8. List conditions that may precipitate a sickle cell crisis.

9. Recognize normal hemoglobin patterns on hemoglobin electrophoresis at pH 8.6 and 6.2.

10. Recognize abnormal hemoglobin patterns on electrophoresis at pH 8.6 and 6.2.

11. Describe the treatment protocol for patients with sickle cell anemia.

12. Differentiate the clinical and laboratory features of other abnormal hemoglobins, such as Hgb E, Hgb O_{Arab}, Hgb D_{Punjab}, and Hgb G_{Phila}.

13. List the key features of sickle hemoglobin in combination with thalassemias.

14. Calculate the white blood cell correction formula when nucleated red blood cells are noted in the peripheral smear.

15. Summarize the general principles of acid and alkaline electrophoresis and isoelectric focusing.

GENERAL DESCRIPTION OF HEMOGLOBINOPATHIES

Disorders of the globin chain of the hemoglobin molecule have stirred the curiosity of scientists and hematologists for generations. Pauling discovered in 1949 that the altered hemoglobin migration pattern of sickle cell individuals was due to a change in globin and won the Nobel Prize for his discovery. Here was a description of the first molecular disease. Because proteins form the basis of the globin chain, there must be some abnormality *in* the chain to account for what was seen in the hemoglobin electrophoresis of individuals with sickle cell anemia. Ingram et al.[1] discovered the specific amino acid substitution located on the globin chain (valine substituted for glutamic acid), and the specific abnormal codon responsible for this substitution has been characterized. In molecular terms, the nucleotide triplet guanine-adenine-guanine codes for the amino acid glutamine in the sixth position of the normal beta chain. In sickle cell patients, adenine is replaced by thymine coding for the amino acid valine. When valine is substituted for glutamic acid, an abnormal hemoglobin, Hgb S, is produced.

Presently, more than 600 hemoglobin variants exist worldwide, and most are beta chain disorders.[2] To appreciate the magnitude of this statement, a brief review of the hemoglobin molecule is in order. All normal adult hemoglobins consist of two alpha chains, which have 141 amino acids in sequence, complemented by two nonalpha chains: beta, gamma, or delta. The nonalpha globin chains have 146 amino acids with amino acids linked together in sequence. Hemoglobinopathies occur as a result of one of four abnormal functions[3]:

1. A single amino acid substitution in one of the chains, usually the beta chain (i.e., sickle cell trait or disease)
2. Abnormal synthesis of one of the amino acid chains (i.e., thalassemia)

3. Fusion of hemoglobin chains (i.e., Hgb Lepore).
4. Extension of an amino acid chain (i.e., Hgb Constant Spring)

Single amino acid substitutions in the beta chain account for most of the hemoglobinopathies that manifest with hemolysis and clinical symptoms.

SICKLE CELL ANEMIA

Genetics and Incidence of Sickle Cell Anemia

The genetics of sickle cell anemia are not complicated. Sickle cell anemia is a beta chain variant, and inheritance of the beta chains is located on chromosome 11. Chromosome 11 has one location on each chromosome for the inheritance of a normal beta chain or an abnormal beta chain; sickle cell anemia is **autosomal** codominant, inherited in simple mendelian fashion (Fig. 8.1). At present, 80,000 Americans have sickle cell disorders: 65% with sickle cell disease, 24% with hemoglobin SC disease, and 10% with sickle cell beta thalassemia.[4] Individuals born with sickle cell trait were not included in the percentages. African American infants born with sickle cell disease occur with a frequency of 1:375. The sickle gene is especially prominent in African populations near areas endemic for malaria, including Central and West Africa, some parts of the Mediterranean, Asia, and India. The sickle gene is seen frequently in African American populations and with increasing frequency in nonblack populations.[5] The presentation of symptoms in individuals with sickle cell anemia is highly variable, a direct result of the different haplotypes of Hgb S that are inherited. Each haplotype differs from the other by possessing different sequences of some nucleotides in the DNA strands, but they all are located in the same gene cluster.

There are four primary haplotypes of the sickle beta gene: Asian, Senegal, Benin, and Bantu.[6] Haplotypes may be inherited homozygously or

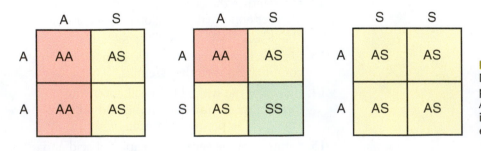

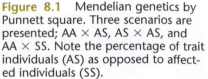

Figure 8.1 Mendelian genetics by Punnett square. Three scenarios are presented; AA × AS, AS × AS, and AA × SS. Note the percentage of trait individuals (AS) as opposed to affected individuals (SS).

heterozygously. Each of these haplotypes differs in the amount of Hgb F the red blood cell possesses. Higher Hgb F concentrations mean a less severe clinical presentation. The Asian haplotype is seen in Saudi Arabia and Asia; the Senegal haplotype, the west African coast; the Benin haplotype, West Africa; and the Mediterranean and Bantu haplotype, Central and South Africa (Table 8.1). Levels of Hgb F greater than 10% serve to lessen the clinical severity for sickle cell anemia patients.[7]

Pathophysiology of the Sickling Process

The beta chain has a carefully sequenced group of amino acids with glutamine or glutamic acid in the sixth position from the terminal end. If a person inherits the sickle gene, valine is substituted for glutamic acid in the sixth position of the beta chain, and the abnormal Hgb S is present in the person's red blood cells. Homozygous inheritance results in sickle cell disease, with most of the hemoglobin being Hgb S. Heterozygous inheritance results in sickle cell trait, in which Hgb S and Hgb A are present. The inheritance of one single abnormal amino acid means that the individual inherits Hgb S ($\alpha_2\beta_2^{6glu \rightarrow val}$) and sets in motion myriad events that alter the individual's quality of life and life span. Lives change when sickle cell disease is present, and the changes are dramatic and sometimes overwhelming.

It is essential for the hemoglobin in the red blood cells to remain soluble and pliable as the red blood cell passes through the oxygenated and deoxygenated rigors of circulation. Red blood cells possessing Hgb S as the majority hemoglobin are insoluble or rigid in areas of low oxygen concentration, such as the spleen, liver, kidneys, joints, and extremities. Instead of having a fluid hemoglobin content, Hgb S forms liquid tactoids or polymers of hemoglobin that appear as long, thin bundles of fibers under electron microscopy.[8] Consequently, affected red blood cells become rigid and inflexible and form an irreversibly sickled cell (ISC) with a pointed projection. These misshapen and inflexible red blood cells obstruct small vessels and adhere to vascular endothelium, increasing the viscosity of the blood as circulation is slowed. Less oxygen is available to the tissues, the pH of the blood decreases, and this combination of events quickly escalates the sickling process. Sickling is also induced by hypoxia, acidosis, dehydration, fever, and exposure to cold.

When red blood cells exit the spleen, they may return to the oxygenated environment of the lung, where they may be able to revert to the discoid shape or wheat shape (reversible sickle cell). For many Hgb S red blood cells, repeated sickling terminates their life span, and they are trapped in the splenic graveyard. The extent to which a red blood cell sickles depends on the amount of Hgb S, the amount of Hgb F, and the physiologic conditions present that may advance sickling.

Clinical Considerations for Sickle Cell Anemia

Sickle cell anemia is usually diagnosed through neonatal screening programs or between 6 months and 2 years of age. Before this time, red blood cells are protected from sickling with high levels of Hgb. Young children will manifest with symptoms of chronic hemolytic anemia, failure to thrive, infection, or dactylitis, which is painful swelling of hands and feet by sickled cells in the microcirculation. Basic clinical considerations for sickle cell patients fall under five categories as follows:

- Chronic hemolytic anemia
- Recurrent painful attacks
- Bacterial infections
- Deterioration of tissue and organ function
- Shortened life expectancy

Taken together, these conditions represent a complicated set of guideposts for medical management of a patient with sickle cell disease. Primary care physicians who treat sickle cell patients must be familiar with these particular complications (Table 8.2). Each patient has a unique presentation of the sickle state. Some have a lifetime of complications and hospitalizations, and others are not affected until later in life. Nevertheless, possessing Hgb S homozygously must not be ignored or trivialized.

Table 8.1 ⊙ Haplotypes of the Sickle Cell Gene		
Haplotype	Location	% Hgb F
Asian	Saudi Arabia, Asia	>20%
Senegal	West Africa Coast	5%–20%
Benin	West Africa, Mediterranean	<10%
Bantu	Central South Africa	5%–20%

Table 8.2 ● Clinical Considerations for Sickle Cell Anemia Individuals

Anemia
- Chronic hemolysis (20%–25% hematocrit)
- Reticulocytosis
- Shortened red blood cell life span
- Transfusion dependency (antibody development)

Spleen
- Loss of splenic filtration ability
- Functional asplenia
- Splenic sequestration

Lungs
- Pulmonary infarctions
- Pneumonia susceptibility in children
- Acute chest syndrome (leading cause of death)
- Pulmonary hypertension

Joints
- Painful tissue infarctions
- Painful swelling in joints
- Loss of mobility, partial paralysis for some

Genitals
- Priapism
- Erectile dysfunction

Eye
- Retinopathy
- Retinal lesions
- Possible blindness

Neurologic
- Stroke

Anemia

Most patients with sickle cell anemia have a chronic hemolytic process that is characterized by a hypercellular bone marrow, red blood cells that live only 10 to 20 days,[9] a marked reticulocytosis (8% to 12%), increased bilirubin, and cholelithiasis. The anemia is usually compensated with hematocrits in the range of 20% to 25%, and patients do well even with these low numbers. Complications occur in the form of aplastic anemia or splenic sequestration crisis. Acute aplastic anemia may develop as a result of infection, usually parvovirus, when the already overworked bone marrow simply fails to produce cells. The hematocrit may decrease by 10% to 15% per day.[10] Transfusion is essential because there is no backup therapy for bone marrow aplasia, and death may occur without transfusion intervention.

Spleen

The spleen bears the burden of the sickle process. Many patients have an initial splenomegaly, but by 5 to 6 years of age,[11] this organ drastically changes. Functional asplenia occurs within the first 2 years as the spleen loses its ability to clear abnormalities from red blood cells. Howell-Jolly bodies and other inclusions are evident in the peripheral smear, and there is increased incidence of severe infections, owing to the weakened immune function of the spleen. Repeated **infarctions** and congestion of the spleen lead to autosplenectomy, producing a fibrosed and shriveled organ. This scarred organ is dysfunctional, lacking the basic and most important splenic functions. Two consequences may develop: overwhelming sepsis and splenic sequestration. In an historical study performed in 1986, the incidence of infection decreased 85% with the use of oral penicillin compared with a **placebo** study in patients of the same age range.[12] *Streptococcus pneumoniae* infections are especially grave in this age group, but other encapsulated organisms such as *Haemophilus influenzae* and *Neisseria meningitidis* pose serious hazards. Acute splenic sequestration is most often a complication of young children. The onset is sudden, as large volumes of blood pool in the spleen. Distention of the abdomen and **hypovolemic** shock occur because of the rapid pooling. Recovery is not guaranteed because the condition often goes unrecognized, and treatment is delayed.

Lungs

Sickling can occur in any organ of the body, but the lungs are particularly susceptible to occlusions in the microenvironment of the pulmonary space. During the course of disease, patients may experience clinical lung conditions that are chronic or acute. Often, minute pulmonary infarctions may go undetected, but over time these may lead to impaired pulmonary function and pulmonary hypertension in 20% to 40% of patients, which carries a high risk of death.[13] Children with sickle cell anemia are 100 times more susceptible to pneumonia than other children.[14] Acute chest syndrome is characterized by fever, chest pain, hypoxia, and pulmonary infiltrates. These patients are critically ill, with an average hospitalization of 10 days. Older patients tend to have a more severe course of disease. Multiple causes are suggested, including pneumonia and other infectious agents and possibly fat **embolism**, although pulmonary infarction underlies each of these possibilities. Acute chest syndrome represents the leading cause of death and hospitalization in patients with sickle cell disease and should be considered in any sickle cell patient who is admitted for pain.[15]

Vaso-occlusive Episodes and Complications

Painful crisis is the trademark of patients with sickle cell disease. In African cultures, the descriptive words associated with this condition translate as "body biting" or "body chewing."[16] Tissue infarctions and sickling in small vessels produce several painful target points. Patients do not experience crisis episodes on a daily basis; for the most part, they are able to live reasonably normal lives. Certain events may trigger a sickling crisis, including fever, dehydration, cold, and stress. When a crisis occurs, the pain is described as gnawing, throbbing, and overwhelming, with few moments of relief. If the crisis is centered in the bones, patients experience tenderness, warmth, and swelling and some bone necrosis. Infarctions at the joint level lead to swelling, pain, and loss of mobility. Large, pitting ulcers that are slow to heal and difficult to treat may also result from joint infarction and poor circulation in the limbs. The pain of sickle cell crisis is intense and unrelenting and only temporarily relieved by analgesics. Clinicians may need to reevaluate the protocols and analgesics necessary for pain management in pediatric and adult sickle cell patients, with a goal of providing some relief and comfort.[17]

Priapism, Retinopathy, and Stroke

Priapism, a complication of vaso-occlusion, is the persistent painful erection of the penis that usually occurs around 15 years of age, the age of puberty. The condition may persist for hours, days, or weeks, with analgesics and sedation as the main course of treatment. Repeated episodes may resolutely alter sexual activity or the desire for sexual activity and lead to erectile dysfunction. There is a high incidence (35%) of priapism in males with sickle cell anemia, and this complication needs additional attention in the overall management of this disease.[18]

Retinopathy refers to the ophthalmologic complications that sickle cell patients experience resulting from sickling lesions and stasis of small blood vessels during the course of their disease. These complications may begin at 10 years of age and can include retinal detachment, retinal lesions, and possibly blindness.[19] Eye assessments must be conducted regularly for sickle cell patients so that appropriate treatment can be initiated and implemented.

Strokes are an infrequent complication of sickle cell anemia, affecting only 7% of children, but they may yield serious and unpredictable setbacks to this patient group. Young patients who experience a stroke may have some degree of paralysis, coma, or seizure.[20] Preventive measures include identifying children at risk through transcranial Doppler imaging, which may disclose the narrowing of arteries causing a blockage and hypoxia to the brain.[21] An additional strategy is to maintain Hgb S levels close to 30% through transfusion therapy. This method has been shown to reduce the recurrence of strokes or prevention of first-time events from 80% to 10%.[22]

Disease Management and Prognosis

Although sickle cell anemia was first described by Herrick in 1910, interest in sickle cell disease was sluggish, and progress for patients with sickle cell anemia was tentative at best. Two events signaled a significant advance in the disease profile: the passage of the national Sickle Cell Anemia Control Act of 1972 and the establishment of the Cooperative Study of Sickle Cell Disease (CSSCD) in 1979 under the auspices of the National Heart, Lung, and Blood Institute. The CSSCD aims to provide a central database to analyze treatment trends, social issues faced by patients, and disease data. Several key issues have been gleaned from 16 years of data, as follows[23]:

- Hospital visits are not the norm and are used only for crisis emergencies.
- In regard to hospital visits, 5% to 10% of patients account for 40% to 50% of visits.
- The average age of death is 42 years for men and 48 years for women.
- Patients who lived longer had a higher level of Hgb F.

Management of patients with sickle cell anemia revolves around prevention of complications and aggressive treatment if they occur. For children, prophylactic antibiotics and pneumococcal vaccines are encouraged as well as stroke prevention techniques mentioned earlier. Patients may need transfusions every 3 to 5 weeks to maintain a hemoglobin of 9 to 11 g/dL and a Hgb S concentration of less than 50%,[4] optimal standards to avoid complications. Although a worthy goal, this treatment may lead to iron overload and the development of alloantibodies that could make future transfusions difficult. Both of these occurrences need to be carefully monitored by laboratory screening. Serum ferritin levels and antibody screening should be done routinely in these patients. Perhaps one of the most auspicious developments for sickle cell patients was use of the drug hydroxyurea. Hydroxyurea increases the level of Hgb F in sickle cells, reducing vaso-occlusive episodes and dramatically improving clinical outlooks in these patients. First proposed by Charache et al.[24] in 1995, hydroxyurea was found to be successful in reducing crisis intervals and acute chest syndrome at a reasonable drug dose and with few reversible side effects. Hydroxyurea was a major breakthrough for this needy patient group, and the multicenter clinical study was halted earlier than usual to offer this promising drug to more patients. Sickle cell patients finally had a reason to be optimistic about their future. An additional, albeit more complex, treatment is bone marrow transplantation from a well sibling or allogeneic match. Limited studies have suggested bone marrow transplantation as a viable alternative, but the procedure itself has considerable risks.

Patients with sickle cell anemia have considerable needs on multiple levels. A thoughtful management plan should be developed and followed so that quality of life may be maximized in these patients. Table 8.3 presents a clinical management scheme for sickle cell

Table 8.3 ● Clinical Management Scheme for Sickle Cell Patients

Age 0–5 yr, monitor for

- Penicillin prophylaxis
- Splenic sequestration
- Fever or infection
- Stroke
- Pain
- Dental care
- Routine complete blood count
- Red blood cell antigen typing
- Pneumococcal vaccine administration

Age 5–10 yr, monitor for

- Pain
- Dental care
- Add urinalysis and liver function test to laboratory test panel
- Pulmonary function
- Chest radiograph
- Ultrasound
- Ophthalmologic examination

Age 10 yr and older

- Include all recommendations from age 5–10 yr
- Family planning and self-help groups
- Leg ulcers

patients. Additional help and advocacy can be obtained from the Sickle Cell Disease Association of America (www.sicklecelldisease.org) located in Baltimore, Maryland.

Laboratory Diagnosis

Patients with sickle cell anemia have a lifelong normochromic, normocytic anemia with decreased hemoglobin (6 to 8 g/dL), hematocrit, and RBC. The reticulocyte count is always elevated, leading to a slightly increased mean corpuscular volume (MCV) in many cases. Bilirubin and lactate dehydrogenase (LDH) are increased, and haptoglobin is decreased, indicating extravascular hemolysis. During crisis episodes, the peripheral smear shows marked polychromasia, many nucleated red blood cells, target cells, and the presence of irreversible and reversible sickle cells (Fig. 8.2). Peripheral smears from sickle cell patients not in crisis show minimal changes: a few oat-shaped reversible sickle cells and some polychromasia (Fig. 8.3). WBC may need to be corrected for nucleated red blood cells by applying the correction formula if automated instrumentation lacks this correction function (Fig. 8.4).

First-level screening procedures for adults include dithionite solubility, a solubility test based on the principle that Hgb S precipitates in high-molarity buffered phosphate solutions. The amount of Hgb S is insignificant in this screening procedure because the purpose of this procedure is to detect the presence of Hgb S in the test sample. The endpoint is easy to read as a turbid solution in the presence of Hgb S and a clear solution if Hgb S is not present (Fig. 8.5). Newborn screening for hemoglobinopathies occurs in most states and for all ethnic groups in the United States and provides the opportunity for early diagnosis and intervention for patients with sickle cell anemia, key ingredients for

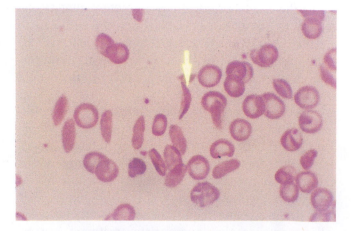

Figure 8.2   Irreversibly sickled cells. Note one pointed projection.   From The College of American Pathologists, with permission.

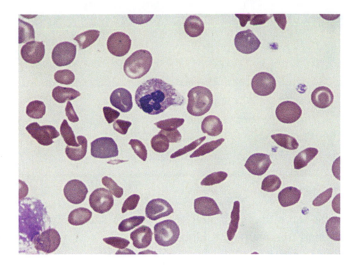

Figure 8.3   Reversible sickle cell. Note the blunted ends of the sickle cell.   Courtesy of Bernardino Madson, Casper College, Wyoming.

$$\frac{\text{Correct white count} = \text{original white count}}{100 + \text{nRBCs}} \times 100$$

Figure 8.4   White blood cell corrections based on number of nucleated red blood cells.

successful disease management. Most newborn blood samples are obtained by heel puncture, and the blood is collected onto filter paper and allowed to dry. The samples are analyzed by hemoglobin electrophoresis at alkaline or acid pH or both, isoelectric focusing, or high-performance liquid chromatography. If electrophoretic techniques are used, two bands, Hgb F and Hgb S, are seen in patients with sickle cell anemia because Hgb F is predominant in neonates. A healthy neonate shows two bands at Hgb A and Hgb F, whereas a neonate with sickle cell trait shows three bands: one at Hgb F, one at Hgb A, and one at Hgb S. (Table 8.4) shows the relative concentrations of Hgb A and Hgb F at different ages. Challenges in neonatal screening involve identifying unexpected bands and small amounts of Hgb A or Hgb S.[25]

Hemoglobin Electrophoresis

Hemoglobin electrophoresis is a time-honored quantitative procedure for isolating hemoglobin bands. This technique is based on the principle that hemoglobins migrate at different positions depending on pH, time of migration, and media used. Cellulose acetate and citrate agar are the media most often selected. Hemoglobin is isolated from a patient sample using various lysing agents, such as saponin or water. A small amount of sample is applied to the media and electrophoresed for the prescribed amount of time, and then each band is quantified using densitometry. Figure 8.6 is a comparison of cellulose acetate and citrate agar electrophoresis. What becomes immediately noticeable for both media is that several bands have the same migration point.

In analyzing each group of patterns, several features must be kept in mind to identify the abnormal hemoglobin properly (Table 8.5). On cellulose acetate in an alkaline electrophoresis, Hgb E, Hgb C, Hgb O_{Arab}, and Hgb A_2 migrate in the same position, and Hgb S, Hgb D_{Punjab}, and Hgb G_{Phila} travel together. On citrate agar in an acid pH, Hgb A, Hgb O, Hgb A_2, Hgb D_{Punjab}, Hgb G_{Phila}, and Hgb E migrate to the same point. This medium provides excellent separation, however, for Hgb S from Hgb D_{Punjab} and Hgb C from Hgb E. In practice, most laboratories use a screening technique followed by a known quantitative method that has been carefully developed for their hospital setting. Equipment costs, technologist time, and the number of samples to be evaluated factor into the decision as to whether the quantitative technique is performed on site or sent out to a reference laboratory.

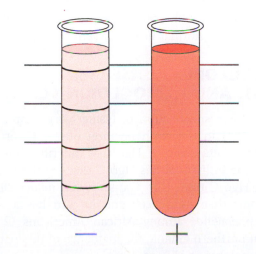

Figure 8.5   Sickle solubility test. An insoluble solution indicates the presence of Hgb S. Clear solution is from a normal patient.

Table 8.4 ○ Normal Hemoglobin A and Hemoglobin F Concentrations by Age		
Age	Hgb F (%)	Hgb A (%)
1 day	77.0 ± 7.3	23 ± 7.3
Up to 12 mo	1.6 ± 1.0	98.4 ± 1.0
Adult	<2.0	98

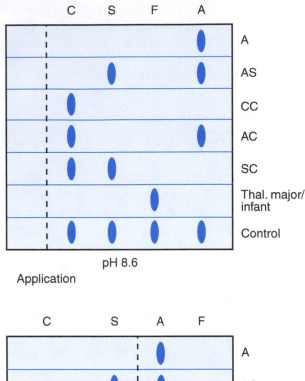

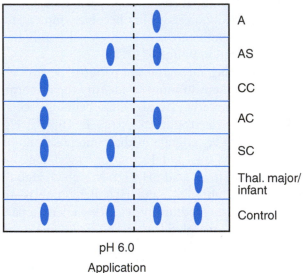

Figure 8.6   Hemoglobin electrophoresis at pH 8.6 and pH 6.0.

- What is the MCV of your patient?
- What is the strength of the band?
- What is the age of your patient?
- Does your patient have a transfusion history?

large-batch analysis, such as newborn screening performed in state health laboratories.

Sickle Cell Trait

Sickle cell trait is achieved through heterozygous inheritance of Hgb S, in which an individual possesses Hgb A at approximately 60% and Hgb S at approximately 40%. These individuals are hematologically normal. The prevalence of sickle cell trait is 8% to 10% among African Americans. Approximately 2.5 million people in the United States carry the sickle gene.[27] Population penetrance in parts of western Africa is 25% to 30%, and the protection against malaria is considered to be a large factor for the frequency of this gene in parts of Africa. Several circumstances may put an individual with sickle cell trait in jeopardy of having a crisis episode, such as air travel in an unpressurized cabin and high altitudes. Other than this, sickle trait individuals lead normal lives. In a perfect world, all African Americans would know their Hgb S status because a union with another individual carrying sickle cell trait could produce a child affected with sickle cell anemia (one in four chance). Generally, all health educators should encourage their African American students to be tested for the presence of sickle cell gene as part of their normal health screening.

HEMOGLOBIN C DISEASE, TRAIT, AND HEMOGLOBIN SC

Hgb C has a substitution of lysine for glutamic acid ($\alpha_2\beta_2^{glu \to lys}$) in the sixth position of the N-terminal end of the beta chain. If Hgb C is inherited homozygously, the individual has Hgb C disease; if heterozygously, Hgb C trait. Hgb C disease has *milder* clinical symptoms than sickle cell anemia and has a much lower prevalence among African Americans (2% to 3%). In northern Ghana, the incidence of this particular hemoglobin is 17% to 28%.[2]

The anemia is normochromic and normocytic, yet there is some increase in the mean corpuscular

Isoelectric Focusing

Isoelectric focusing (IEF) is the method of choice for most newborn screening in the United States. This refined electrophoretic procedure uses a pH range of 3 to 10 in polyacrylamide gel. Within this pH range, hemoglobins achieve their isoelectric point, their point of no net negative charge, and they focus into sharp distinct bands. Because each hemoglobin is a protein with a distinct amino acid composition, clearly defined points are achieved. This procedure is especially useful when small amounts of abnormal hemoglobin need to be detected.[26] The cost of equipment for IEF is prohibitive in most community hospital settings, but this technique has great value for hemoglobin content (MCHC) because red blood cells from homozygous individuals are denser. Most homozygous individuals show a moderate anemia with a hemoglobin value of 9 to 12 g/dL. There is a moderate reticulocytosis and splenomegaly. The red blood cell life span is 38 days, yet few patients exhibit any symptoms. Of particular interest is the possible presence of crystalline structures in the red blood cells that appear as blocks or "bars of gold" (Fig. 8.7). These peculiar crystals obstruct the microvasculature but melt in the splenic microenvironment. Consequently, splenic function is preserved, and little pitting occurs. Target cells (50% to 90%) are the predominant red blood cell morphology, and variations of targeting may include folded or "pocketbook"-shaped cells. Spherocytes may be present. Alkaline electrophoresis shows a single slow-moving band in the same position as Hgb A_2.

The heterozygous condition is termed Hgb A-C trait, with a ratio of 60% Hgb A and 40% Hgb C on alkaline electrophoresis. There are no clinical complications for individuals with this condition, and they may never be noticed except for the presence of 40% target cells on their peripheral smear, an extremely abnormal finding (see Fig. 3.16). Individuals who inherit Hgb C should be aware of their hemoglobin status and the hemoglobin status of prospective mates.

Hgb SC disease is a combination of two abnormal hemoglobins, Hgb S and Hgb C. Affected individuals have a moderate anemia, with an average hemoglobin of 8 to 10 g/dL, with a slight reticulocytosis. Red blood cell life span is reduced to approximately 29 days. Although the disease is less severe than sickle cell anemia, an individual may experience a painful crisis. Pregnant women may be severely affected. The peripheral smear shows high numbers of target cells; few reversible sickled cells; and folded cells, with a peculiar crystal shaped like the Washington Monument or a gloved hand showing in some cells (Fig. 8.8). The hemoglobin distribution on alkaline electrophoresis is 50% Hgb S and 50% Hgb C.

VARIANT HEMOGLOBINS

Hemoglobin S–Beta Thalassemia

The Hgb S–beta thalassemia combination hemoglobin may produce a clinical picture as severe as sickle cell anemia, with virtually no Hgb A present. The anemia is microcytic, hypochromic, showing the influence of the thalassemia gene, with nucleated red blood cells, target cells, polychromasia, and sickle cells. The red blood cell distribution width (RDW) and the reticulocyte count are increased. As opposed to the usual presentation of sickle cell anemia, splenomegaly is usually present. The severity of the condition overall depends on the beta thalassemia genotype inherited; patients inheriting B^0 have a more severe presentation. On alkaline electrophoresis, two bands are present—one at the location of Hgb S and one at the location of Hgb A_2.

Hemoglobin E

Hgb E has an extremely high occurrence in individuals from Southeast Asia. Individuals may inherit the hemoglobin either heterozygously or homozygously. The homozygous conditions of this abnormal hemoglobin present no clinical complications. Individuals show a marked microcytic, hypochromic picture, with some target cells and slight polychromasia, but are asymptomatic. On alkaline electrophoresis, there is a strong band located in the same position as Hgb C or

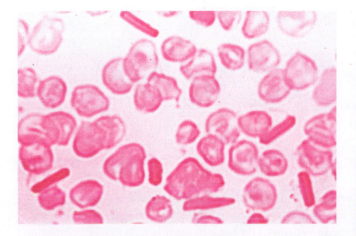

Figure 8.7 Hgb CC. Note the presence of crystals shaped like "bars of gold" and many target cells. © 1967 American Society of Clinical Pathologists. Reprinted with permission.

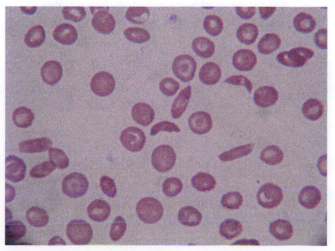

Figure 8.8 Hgb SC. Note the presence of crystals with pointed projections. Courtesy of Kathleen Finnegan, Stony Brook University, New York.

Hgb A₂. The heterozygous condition shows 70% Hgb A and 30% Hgb E. Hgb E is the second most common hemoglobin variant worldwide and is being seen with increasing frequency in the United States because of the large numbers of southeast Asians emigrating to North America (Fig. 8.9).

Hemoglobin D_{Punjab} and Hemoglobin G_{Phila}

Hgb D$_{Punjab}$ is a rare clinical variant in which both genetic states are asymptomatic. There is a higher incidence of Hgb D$_{Punjab}$ in Great Britain, and this is thought to reflect the large number of Indian wives brought to England during Great Britain's long occupation of the Punjab region of India and Pakistan. The prevalence of this variant in these regions is 3%.

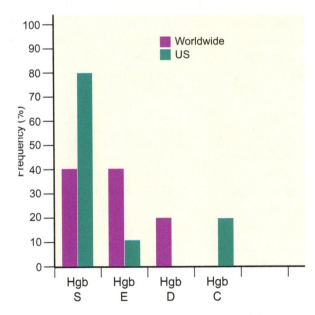

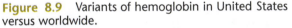

Figure 8.9 Variants of hemoglobin in United States versus worldwide.

Although rare, Hgb G$_{Phila}$ is seen in African Americans. It is an alpha chain variant that migrates in the same position as Hgb S at alkaline electrophoresis at pH 8.6. There are no hematologic abnormalities, but there is a high incidence of Hgb G$_{Phila}$ in Ghana.

Hemoglobin O_{Arab}

Hgb O$_{Arab}$ is an uncommon hemoglobin found in 0.4% of African Americans. Most individuals are asymptomatic, but this hemoglobin must be distinguished from Hgb C at alkaline electrophoresis because it migrates to the same location. Citrate electrophoresis at pH 6.4 isolates this band for positive identification.

○ *Summary Points*

- Most hemoglobinopathies are the result of single amino acid substitution in the beta chain.
- In sickle cell disorders, valine is substituted for glutamic acid in the sixth position of the beta chain.
- In Hgb C disorders, lysine is substituted for glutamic acid in the sixth position of the beta chain.
- The presence of Hgb S affords some protection against malarial infection of red blood cells.
- Cells containing Hgb S as the majority hemoglobin are insoluble in areas of the body with low oxygen tension.
- Sickle cells clog small vessels during sickling crisis, causing extensive organ damage and pain.
- Homozygous inheritance of Hgb S produces sickle cell anemia (Hgb SS); heterozygous inheritance produces sickle cell trait (Hgb AS).
- Hypoxia, acidosis, dehydration, cold, and fever predispose a patient to sickling episodes.

CONDENSED CASE

A 6-year-old Indian girl was brought to the emergency department with fever, malaise, and joint pain. Laboratory results were WBC = 13,000 × 10⁹/L, Hgb = 9.0 g/dL, Hct = 27%, and MCV = 85 fL. Her peripheral smear revealed a moderate number of target cells, with 2+ polychromasia and moderate oat-shaped cells. *Based on this sketch, what is the first diagnosis that comes to mind?*

Answer

Based on her peripheral smear and the fact that she is anemic with joint pain, sickle cell anemia is a strong possibility. She needs to have this condition confirmed with hemoglobin electrophoresis or IEF. Oat-shaped cells are reversible sickle cells seen in many patients with sickle cell anemia. Her bone marrow is responding because she is exhibiting polychromasia. Splenic function needs to be monitored carefully in pediatric patients.

- There is an 8% to 10% prevalence of the sickle cell gene among African Americans.
- Autosplenectomy is a consequence of repeated infarctions to the spleen in young children with sickle cell disease.
- Stroke and acute chest syndrome are serious complications in sickle cell patients.
- During sickle crisis episodes, patients show nucleated red blood cells, sickle cells, target cells, and polychromasia.
- WBC may need to be corrected due to nucleated red blood cells present during sickling episodes.
- Individuals with sickle cell trait are asymptomatic with rare abnormalities in the peripheral smear.
- Newborn screening for hemoglobinopathies is available in the United States through state health laboratories.
- Dithionite solubility is the usual screening procedure to determine if Hgb S is present.

- Acid or alkaline electrophoresis and IEF provide better methods to isolate hemoglobin bands.
- Hgb C disease occurs when Hgb C is inherited homozygously; Hgb C trait occurs when Hgb C is inherited heterozygously.
- Hgb C disease may produce Hgb C crystals on Wright's stain.
- Hgb SC is the result of inheriting two abnormal hemoglobins, Hgb S and Hgb C.
- Hgb SC may produce abnormal crystal formation resembling the Washington Monument or fingers in a glove.
- Hgb S–beta thalassemia may produce conditions as severe as sickle cell disease.
- Hgb E is the second most prevalent hemoglobin variant and is seen with great frequency in southeast Asia.
- Hgb D$_{Punjab}$ and Hgb G$_{Phila}$ migrate with Hgb S on alkaline electrophoresis.

Review Questions

1. What is the amino acid substitution in patients with sickle cell anemia?
   a. Adenine for thymine
   b. Lysine for valine
   c. Valine for glutamic acid
   d. Cytosine for guanine

2. Which of the following factors contributes to the pathophysiology of sickling?
   a. Increased iron concentration
   b. Hypochromia
   c. Fava beans
   d. Dehydration

3. Which of the following statements pertains to most clinically significant hemoglobin variants?
   a. Most are fusion hemoglobins
   b. Most are single amino acid substitutions
   c. Most are synthetic defects
   d. Most are extensions of the amino acid chain

4. Which of the following hemoglobins ranks second in variant hemoglobins worldwide?
   a. Hgb S
   b. Hbg E
   c. Hgb H
   d. Hgb C

5. Which of the following shows crystals appearing like bars of gold in the peripheral smear?
   a. Hgb CC disease
   b. Hgb DD disease
   c. Hgb EE disease
   d. Hgb SS disease

6. Which of the following conditions is the leading cause of hospitalization for sickle cell patients?
   a. Acute chest syndrome
   b. Priapism
   c. Painful crisis
   d. Splenic sequestration

7. Which of the following hemoglobin separation methods is used for most newborn hemoglobin screening?
   a. High-performance liquid chromatography
   b. Alkaline electrophoresis
   c. Isoelectric focusing
   d. Acid electrophoresis

8. Autosplenectomy is characteristic of
   a. Sickle cell trait.
   b. Hgb C disease.
   c. Thalassemia.
   d. Sickle cell anemia.

Continued

9. The Benin haplotype of sickle cell disease is prevalent in which country or countries?
   a. Saudi Arabia and Asia
   b. Senegal
   c. West Africa
   d. Central and South Africa

10. When the bone marrow temporarily ceases to produce cells in a sickle cell patient, a(n) _____ crisis has occurred.
   a. Aplastic
   b. Hemolytic
   c. Vaso-occlusive
   d. Painful

CASE STUDY

A 3-year-old boy of Ghanaian ethnicity came to the emergency department acutely ill, with fever, chest pain, and a heavy cough. He was accompanied by his parents, who said that he seemed to have a mild cold and slight fever. His condition, however, had become more serious in the last 24 hours. His temperature was 103°F. His parents informed the emergency department staff that he has a diagnosis of *sickle cell anemia,* but they thought that this episode was different from his previous crisis episodes. A complete blood count (CBC) was ordered, and he was helped to cough up a sputum sample for culture. He was given ibuprofen for pain and fever. Four hours from the time he was seen in the emergency department, he was admitted and put in the critical care unit, in grave condition. His breathing was compromised, and he was placed on mechanical ventilation and lapsed into a coma. He developed disseminated intravascular coagulation (DIC), using 10 U of fresh frozen plasma, 10 U of platelets, and 20 U of packed red blood cells to control the bleeding. He died from overwhelming sepsis 24 hours after admission. Initial results are listed (see cover for normal values). *What role does splenic function play in the management of sickle cell patients?*

WBC	20.0×10^9/L
RBC	3.50×10^{12}/L
Hgb	11.5 g/dL
Hct	34%
MCV	91 fL
MCH	32.9 pg
MCHC	35.9%
Platelets	160×10^9/L
RDW	18.0%

The differential showed a left shift with heavy toxic granulation and Döhle bodies. The initial coagulation results are as follows:

PT	12.0 seconds (normal value 11 to 13 seconds)
PTT	26.0 seconds (normal value less than 40 seconds)

Insights to the Case Study

This account represents the worst-case scenario for a young sickle patient. Patients in this age range who have sickle cell anemia are vulnerable to virulent infections by encapsulated organisms, acute chest syndrome, and dactylitis. When they are admitted to the hospital, coordinated care by a staff knowledgeable about sickle cell complications is crucial because time is usually the enemy, and the situation can rapidly escalate. In this case, even though the parent mentioned the child's sickle cell diagnosis, he was treated far too casually and not as a young child with special medical needs. *Streptococcus pneumoniae* grew from his sputum culture, and a gram-positive organism was seen on Gram stain, but he was not treated aggressively when one considers that his spleen was compromised. Functional asplenia is serious and life-threatening, especially if the patient becomes infected with an encapsulated organism. Patients such as this merit special attention. This patient died of overwhelming sepsis because of the streptococcal infection, which triggered DIC and uncontrollable bleeding. His platelet count plummeted to 40,000 within 2 hours of admission, and he began to bleed from the venipuncture site. He was too young to withstand the numerous assaults on his body system.

○ TROUBLE SHOOTING

What Is the Proper Procedure If the Automated WBC Does Not Correlate With a Slide Estimate?

A 14-year-old boy presented to the emergency department with a fever of unknown origin. CBC, blood cultures, and routine chemistries were ordered. The chemistries came back as normal, and the blood cultures would be read in 24 hours. CBC results were as follows:

WBC	35.0	H
RBC	4.19	L
Hgb	9.3	L
Hct	27.8	L
MCV	66.3	L
MCH	22.3	L
MCHC	33.5	
Platelets	598	H
RDW	21.0	H

The elevated WBC was flagged, and reflex testing indicated that a manual differential should be performed. The technologist performed the differential and noted several items:

- The WBC count of 35,000 did not correlate with the slide.
- 100 nucleated red blood cells were counted while completing the differential.
- The patient had anisocytosis, probably owing to younger polychromatic cells.
- The patient had poikilocytosis including moderate target and moderate sickle cells present.
- The patient had the presence of red blood cell inclusions: Pappenheimer and Howell-Jolly bodies.

It was obvious to the technologist that this was a sickle cell patient in a crisis with an elevated RDW and the peripheral smear indicative of sickle cell crisis. The presence of 100 nucleated red blood cells counted in the differential is a significant finding. Nucleated red blood cells were most likely being counted as white blood cells, falsely elevating the WBC. The Coulter LH750 usually corrects for the presence of nucleated red blood cells when the nucleated red blood cells are in the low range, but a nucleated RBC of 100 is fairly high, and the instrument calculation has not been reliable in the high range. The instrument reported WBC of 35,000, but the technologist thought that this count did not agree with the peripheral smear. The technologist needed to correct the WBC manually. To perform this function, the technologist referred to the raw data function available in the Coulter instrument to find what the WBC was before correction by the instrument. The number of the WBC was 49,800 and represents the raw number of white blood cells counted on the initial run of this sample. This number was used to correct for the nucleated red blood cells using the formula shown in Figure 8.4.

Uncorrected WBC × 100 ÷ 100 + 100 = 49,800 × 100 ÷ 200 = 49,800 ÷ 200 = 24,900, the corrected value

The corrected WBC was reported to the floor. This case illustrates the value of reflex testing, prompting the performance of a manual differential. A careful observation of the peripheral smear indicated that the instrument correction for nucleated red blood cells, 35,000, was not valid (WBC seemed lower) and that the technologist needed to intervene to provide a reliable WBC.

W O R D   K E Y

Autosomal • Referring to chromosome, a non–sex-linked chromosome

Embolism • Occlusion of a blood vessel

Infarction • Area of tissue that has been deprived of blood and has lost some of its function

Hypovolemic • Low blood pressure

Placebo • Substance having no medical effect when given to an individual as if a medicine

Viscosity • Thickness

References

1. Ingram VM. Gene mutations in human hemoglobins: The chemical differences between normal and sickle hemoglobins. Nature (Lond) 180:326, 1957.
2. Huisman TH, et al. A Syllabus of Human Hemoglobin Variants, 2nd ed. August, GA: The Sickle Cell Anemia Foundation, 1998.
3. McGhee DB. Structural defects in hemoglobin (hemoglobinopathies). In: Rodak B, ed. Hematology: Clinical Principles and Applications, 2nd ed. Philadelphia: WB Saunders, 2002; 321.
4. Smith-Whitley K. Sickle cell disease: Diagnosis and current management. Workshop material from the American

Society for Clinical Laboratory Sciences National Meeting, Philadelphia, July 2003.

5. Smith JA, Kinney TR (co-chairs). Sickle Cell Disease Guideline Panel: Sickle cell disease guideline and overview. Am J Hematol 47:152–154, 1994.

6. Pawars DR, Chan L, Schroeder WB. B^s-gene cluster haplotypes in sickle cell anemia: Clinical implications. Am J Pediatr Hematol Oncol 12:367–374, 1990.

7. Pawars DR, Weiss JN, Chan LS, et al. Is there a threshold level of fetal hemoglobin that ameliorates morbidity in sickle cell anemia? Blood 63:921–926, 1984.

8. Barnhart MI, Henry RL, Lusher JM. Sickle Cell. A Scope Publication. Kalamazoo, MI: The Upjohn Co., 1976; 12–14..

9. Armbruster DA. Neonatal hemoglobinopathy screening. Lab Med 21:816, 1990.

10. Singer K, Motulsky AG, et al. Aplastic crisis in sickle cell anemia. J Lab Clin Med 35:721, 1950.

11. Pearson HA, Cornelius EA, et al. Transfusion reversible functional asplenia in young children with sickle cell anemia. N Engl J Med 283:334, 1970.

12. Gaston MH, Vwerter JL, Woods G, et al. Prophylaxis with oral penicillin in children with sickle cell anemia: A randomized trial. N Engl J Med 314:1593–1599, 1986.

13. Gladwin MT, Sachdev V, Jison ML, et al. Pulmonary hypertension as a risk factor for death in patients with sickle cell disease. N Engl J Med 350:886–895, 2004.

14. Barnhart MI, Henry RL, Lusher JM. Sickle Cell. A Scope Publication. Kalamazoo, MI: The Upjohn Co., 1974; 45.

15. Vichinsky EP, Neumaur LD, Earles AN, et al. Causes and outcomes of acute chest syndrome in sickle cell disease. National Acute Chest Syndrome Study Group, 2000.

16. Konotey-Ahulu FI. Sickle cell disease. Arch Intern Med 133:616, 1974.

17. Dampier C, Ely E, Brodecki D, et al. Home management of pain in sickle cell disease: A daily diary study in children and adolescents. J Pediatr Hematol Oncol 24:643–647, 2002.

18. Adeyoju AB, Olujohungbe AB, Morris J, et al. Priapism in sickle cell disease: Incidence, risk factors and complications—an international multicenter study. BJU Int 90:898–902, 2002.

19. Babalola OE, Wambebe CO. When should children and young adults with sickle cell disease be referred for eye assessments? Afr J Med Sci 30:261–263, 2001.

20. Embury SH, et al. Sickle Cell Disease: Basic Principles and Clinical Practice. New York: Raven Press, 1994.

21. Adams RJ, et al. Prevention of a first stroke by transfusion in children with sickle cell anemia and abnormal results on transcranial Doppler ultrasonography N Engl J Med 317:781, 1987.

22. Pelehach L. Understanding sickle cell anemia. Lab Med 126:727, 1995.

23. Gaston M, Rosse WF; The Cooperative Group. The Cooperative Study of Sickle Cell Disease: Review of study designs and objectives. Am J Pediatr Hematol Oncol 4:197–201, 1982.

24. Charache S, Terrin ML, Moore RD, et al. Effect of hydroxyurea on the frequency of painful crisis in sickle cell anemia. N Engl J Med 332:1317–1322, 1995.

25. Pearson HA. Neonatal testing for sickle cell disease: A historical and personal view. Pediatrics 83(Suppl): 815–818, 1989.

26. Galacteros F, Kleman K, Caburi-Martin J, et al. Cord blood screening for hemoglobin abnormalities by thin layer isoelectric focusing. Blood 56:1068–1071, 1980.

27. Geist A. Hemoglobinopathies: Diagnosis and Care of Patients with Sickle Cell Disease. Indiana University Medical Center, personal correspondence.

Part III

White Blood Cell Disorders

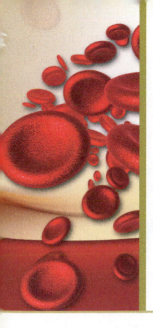

Chapter 9

Leukopoiesis and Leukopoietic Function

Betty Ciesla

Objectives

After completing this chapter, the student will be able to:

1. Describe leukopoiesis and the steps leading from immature forms to maturation.

2. List the maturation sequence of the granulocytic series.

3. Name four morphologic features that are helpful in differentiating the cells of the granulocytic series.

4. Describe the physiology and function of granulocytes.

5. Describe the features that differentiate the granules of the neutrophilic, eosinophilic, and basophilic cell lines.

6. Distinguish between the marginating and circulating pools of leukocytes.

7. Recognize the subtle morphologic clues that may distinguish one white blood cell from another.

8. Describe the lymphatic system and its relationship to lymphocyte production.

9. Describe the role of stimulated and unstimulated lymphocytes.

LEUKOPOIESIS

White blood cells are a remarkably versatile group of cells whose primary purpose is to defend against bacteria, viruses, fungi, and other foreign substances. To this end, most white blood cells are granulated. These granules contain enzymes that digest and destroy the invading organisms. In the bone marrow, the myeloid:erythroid (M:E) ratio is 3 to 4:1, indicating that four myeloid (white) cells are produced for one erythroid cell. Daily production of white blood cells is 1.5 billion. Transit from the bone marrow to the peripheral circulation occurs only after white blood cells have been held in the maturation storage pool of the bone marrow. Segmented neutrophils, the most mature of all of the white blood cells, are held for 7 to 10 days before their release into the peripheral circulation. Other white blood cell types remain in the maturation storage pool for a much shorter time.[1] After being released into the circulation, most white blood cells are short-lived before they migrate into tissues. White blood cells observed in the peripheral circulation are only a snapshot of white blood cells located in three distinct cell compartments: the bone marrow, the bloodstream, and the tissues.

White blood cells are referred to as leukocytes. For clarity, the word *leukocytic* applies to the white blood cells of all stages; *granulocytic* applies only to granulated white blood cells; and *myelocytic* describes a cell that originated from the myeloid stem cell. The term *myelocytic* may also be used interchangeably for *granulocytic* in conditions such as chronic granulocytic leukemia or chronic myelocytic leukemia. These three words—leukocytic, granulocytic, and myelocytic—all denote some stage of the white blood cell family. They are not meant to be confusing, but often are, despite good intentions.

White blood cells, or leukocytes, have a more complex maturation cycle than erythrocytes. There is only one mature red blood cell form as opposed to five mature white blood cell forms. Red blood cells journey through the circulation for 120 days, whereas white blood cells spend only *hours* in the circulating blood. Similar to red blood cells, white blood cells originate from the pluripotent stem cell. The pluripotent stem cell gives rise to the myeloid stem cell and the lymphoid stem cell. In response to stimulation from interleukins (chemical stimulators) and growth factors, a CFU-GEMM is structured to give rise to granulocytes, erythrocytes, monocytes, and macrophages. Megakaryocytes, eosinophils, and basophils have their own CFU: CGU-Meg and CFU-eosinophil and CFU-basophil. Lymphocytes originate not only from the bone marrow, but also from the

thymus, and they have a distinctive place on the hematopoietic maturation chart (see Fig. 2.3).

White blood cells perform most of their function in the tissues, and neutrophils reside here for 2 to 5 days. White blood cells that appear in the circulation are part of two distinctive cell pools: the marginating pool and the circulating pool. The marginating pool designates white blood cells located along the vessel endothelium, ready to migrate to a site of injury or infection. The circulating pool designates white blood cells actually in the bloodstream.[2] At any particular point in the peripheral circulation, the neutrophils divide evenly in either pool and transfer rapidly from pool to pool. The spleen, which harbors one-fourth of the white blood cell population, provides an additional site for granulocyte storage.

STAGES OF LEUKOCYTE MATURATION

The white blood cell series encompasses cells that are distinguished by their granules and cells that are agranular. In all, there are five morphologically distinct maturation stages for neutrophils, four for eosinophils and basophils, and three for monocytes and lymphocytes. Key features in distinguishing immature and mature stages of any of these cells are cell size, nucleus:cytoplasm ratio (N:C), chromatin pattern, presence or absence of nucleoli, cytoplasmic quality, and presence of granules. Nucleoli are a unique feature of immature cells and represent structures within the chromatin that appear lighter, more refractile, and more recognizable. Cell identification is an organized process. Each cell can be identified using the characteristics in the following list, and each student must survey the cell for each characteristic it presents. The stages of maturation for the neutrophilic series from least mature to most mature are as follows:

- Myeloblast
- Promyelocyte or progranulocyte
- Myelocyte
- Metamyelocyte
- Band
- Segmented neutrophil

FEATURES OF CELL IDENTIFICATION

Descriptions for this section represent composite criteria for each cell identification.[3–5] In addition to key distinguishing features, *differentiating characteristics* are presented for most cells. Cluster of differentiation (CD) markers, which represent surface antigen markers on the surface of circulating cells, are included when relevant.

Myeloblast

Size: 14 to 20 μm

N:C: 6:1; round, oval, or slightly indented central nucleus

Chromatin: Light red-purple with a fine meshlike and transparent structure and close-weaved texture; may see two to five nucleoli, which appear as lightened, refractile round structures

Cytoplasm: Moderate blue and usually without granules

Differentiating characteristic: Nucleus has thin chromatin strands that are distributed throughout the nucleus uniformly; chromatin appears smooth and velvety (Fig. 9.1)

CD45, CD38, CD34, CD33, CD13, human leukocyte antigen (HLA)-DR

Promyelocyte (Progranulocyte)

Size: 15 to 22 μm

N:C: 3:1; oval, round, or eccentric flattened nucleus

Chromatin: Light red-purple of medium density, may see single prominent nucleoli

Cytoplasm: Moderate blue color but difficult to observe because fine to large blue-red azurophilic granules are scattered throughout the chromatin pattern; granules are *nonspecific* or primary granules

Differentiating characteristic: Cell is usually larger than the blast, with large prominent

nucleoli; *nuclear chromatin is slightly coarse* (Fig. 9.2)

CD45, CD33, CD13, CD15

Myelocyte

Size: 10 to 18 μm

N:C: 2:1

Chromatin: Oval indented nucleus, denser, red-purple with slight granular appearance, coarser, clumped appearance

Cytoplasm: Specific or secondary granules present; neutrophilic granules are dusty, fine, and red-blue; eosinophilic granules, large red-orange and singular; basophil granules, large deep blue-purple

Last stage capable of dividing

Differentiating characteristic: Small pink-purple granules for neutrophilic myelocyte, nucleus stains deeper color, granular pattern to the chromatin, eccentric nucleus, with visible Golgi apparatus seen as a lighter area near nucleus (Fig. 9.3)

CD45, CD33, CD13, CD15, CD11b/11c

Metamyelocyte

Size: 10 to 15 μm

N:C: 1:1

Chromatin: Indented eccentric nucleus resembling kidney bean shape, patches of coarse chromatin in spots

Cytoplasm: Pale blue to pinkish tan with moderate specific granules

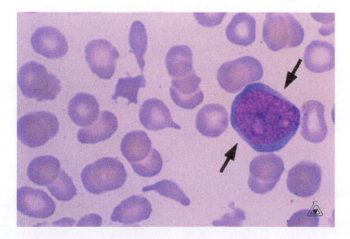

Figure 9.1 Myeloblast. Large cell with high N:C ratio and thin chromatin strands distributed evenly throughout the nucleus; no granules observed. From The College of American Pathologists, with permission.

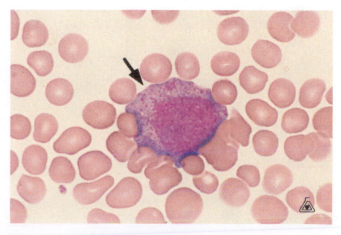

Figure 9.2 Promyelocyte. Prominent nuclei, prominent nonspecific granules, and slightly coarse nuclear chromatin. From The College of American Pathologists, with permission.

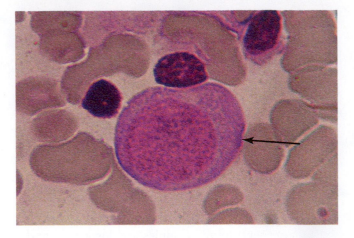

Figure 9.3 Myelocyte. Oval indented nucleus with small, specific granules and granular pattern to chromatin. Courtesy of Kathleen Finnegan, Stony Brook University, New York.

Differentiating characteristics: Nuclear indentation is less than half the diameter of the nucleus and condensed chromatin with no nuclei (Fig. 9.4)

CD markers are the same as for the myelocyte

Band

Size: 9 to 15 μm

Chromatin: Band-shaped similar to a cigar band, C- or S-shaped; filament not visible; coarsely clumped, almost like leopard-spot coarseness

Cytoplasm: Brown-pink, with many fine specific or secondary granules

Differentiating characteristics: Filament may resemble a metamyelocyte, but indentation

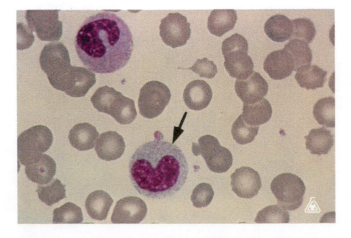

Figure 9.4 Metamyelocyte. Indented nucleus with condensed chromatin, small granules, and no nuclei. From The College of American Pathologists, with permission.

is more severe, and chromatin is more clumped (Fig. 9.5)

CD45, CD13, CD15, CD11b/11c

Segmented Neutrophil

Size: 9 to 15 μm

Chromatin: Two to five nuclear lobes connected by thin threadlike filaments, cannot observe chromatin pattern in filaments

Cytoplasm: Pale lilac with blue shading and many fine secondary dustlike granules

Distinguishing characteristics: Most filament-connecting lobes of nucleus are 0.5 μ. If filament cannot be observed, identification is based on the quality and age of chromatin (Fig. 9.6)

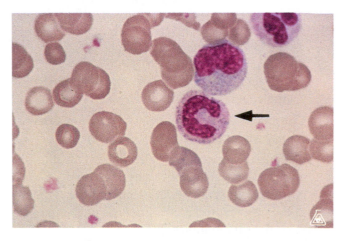

Figure 9.5 Band. No nuclear lobes, no filament, and clumped chromatin. From The College of American Pathologists, with permission.

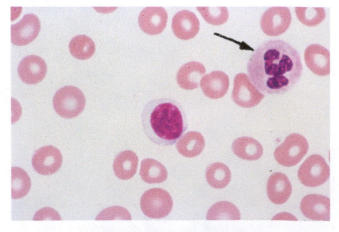

Figure 9.6 Segmented neutrophils. Note two to five lobes in the nucleus with well-distinguished filament and pale dustlike granules. From The College of American Pathologists, with permission.

Eosinophils and Basophils

Eosinophil (Mature)

Eosinophils can appear at the *myelocytic* stage and move through the maturation sequence

Size: 10 to 16 µm

N:C: Barely 1:2

Chromatin: Eccentric nucleus, usually bilobed

Cytoplasm: Large, distinctive red-orange *specific* granules with orange-pink cytoplasm, granules are highly metabolic and contain histamine and other substances

Distinguishing characteristics: Granules are uniformly round, large, and individualized; if stain is inadequate, observe granules carefully for their crystalloid nature (Fig. 9.7)

Basophil (Mature)

Basophils can appear at the *myelocytic* stage and move through the maturation sequence

Size: 10 to 14 µm

N:C: Difficult to determine

Chromatin: Coarse, clumped bilobed nucleus

Cytoplasm: Many large, *specific* secondary purple-black granules seem to obscure the large cloverleaf-form nucleus; may decolorize during staining leaving pale areas within cell; granules much larger than neutrophilic granules

Distinguishing characteristics: Size and color of granules obscure the nucleus (Fig. 9.8)

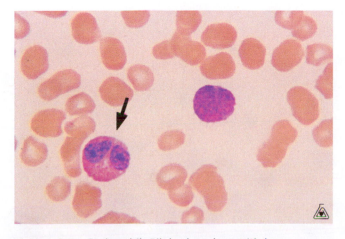

Figure 9.7 Eosinophil. Bilobed nucleus with large, uniformly round orange-red granules. From The College of American Pathologists, with permission.

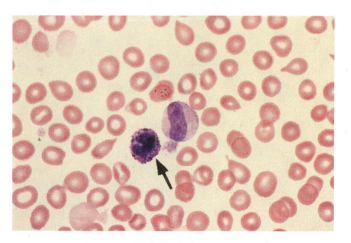

Figure 9.8 Basophil. Indistinguishable nucleus with large, purple-black granules. From The College of American Pathologists, with permission.

Monocytic Series

Monoblast

See description for myeloblast; however, nucleoli (one or two) are very prominent in monoblasts

Promonocyte

Size: 12 to 20 µm

N:C: 3:1

Chromatin: Irregular or indented, flattened nucleus; nucleoli may be present; folding, creasing, and crimping may be observed

Cytoplasm: Gray-blue, some blebbing may appear, rare granules, vacuoles may be present

Distinguishing characteristics: None noted

Monocyte

Size: 12 to 20 µm

N:C: 1:1

Chromatin: Nuclei take different shapes from brainy convolutions to lobulated and S-shaped; chromatin is loose-weaved, lacy, open, and thin

Cytoplasm: Abundant gray-blue with moderate nonspecific granules, may show area of protrusion or blebbing, may have numerous vacuoles

Distinguishing characteristic: Nuclear chromatin lacks density; open-weaved, soft, and velvetlike (Fig. 9.9)

CD33, CD13, CD14

Lymphocytic Series

Outlining CD markers for the lymphocyte cell population is a complex task and beyond the scope of this

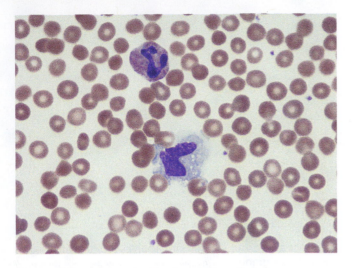

Figure 9.9 Monocyte. Nuclear chromatin is loose-weaved and open, with abundant gray-blue cytoplasm.
Courtesy of Bernardino Madsen, Casper College, Wyoming.

chapter. Lymphocytes develop subpopulations along the path to maturity, each with a unique CD subset. For this reason, this textbook includes only a modified CD list (Table 9.1).

Lymphoblast

Size: 10 to 20 μm

N:C: 4:1

Chromatin: One or two nucleoli with smudgy chromatin

Cytoplasm: Little, deep blue staining at edge

Table 9.1 ● Modified List of Antigen Markers of Lymphocytes*

First three entries are before 1980

LSC-HLA-DR

CD34, CD45

TdT

Pre-B (most mature)

CD19, CD24, CD45, CD10

TdT

Cyto μ

B cell (mature)

CD19, CD20, CD22, CD45

IgM, IgD

S Ig

T cell (most mature)

CD2, CD3, CD4, CD5, CD7, CD8

*List does not represent all possible CD cell designations. For a more extensive CD list, see flow cytometry (Chapter 20).

Distinguishing characteristics: Nucleoli are surrounded by dark rim of chromatin

Prolymphocyte

Size: 9 to 18 μm

N:C: 3:1

Chromatin: Nucleoli may be present, slightly coarse chromatin

Cytoplasm: Gray-blue, mostly blue at edges

Distinguishing characteristics: Moderate

Small Lymphocyte

Size: 7 to 12 μm

N:C: 4:1

Chromatin: Oval eccentric nucleus with coarse, lumpy chromatin with specific areas of clumping, a compact cell

Cytoplasm: Usually just a thin border, with few azurophilic, red granules

Distinguishing characteristics: Clumping of chromatin around nuclear membrane may help to distinguish this from a nucleated red blood cell (Fig. 9.10)

Large Lymphocyte

Size: 15 to 18 μm

N:C: 3:1

Chromatin: Looser chromatin pattern, more transparent

Cytoplasm: Larger amount of cytoplasm, lighter in color

Distinguishing characteristic: Cytoplasm is more abundant, with tendency for azurophilic granules (Fig. 9.11)

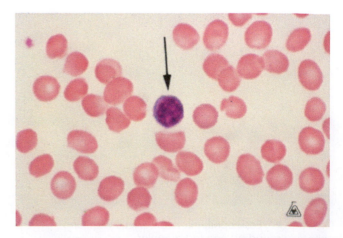

Figure 9.10 Small lymphocyte. Oval nucleus with coarse, lumpy chromatin. From The College of American Pathologists, with permission.

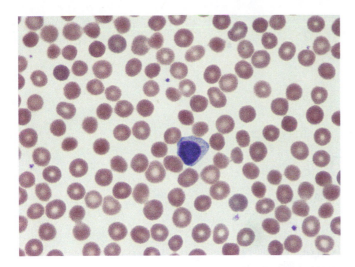

Figure 9.11 Large lymphocyte. Oval nucleus with looser, more transparent chromatin pattern. *Courtesy of Bernardino Madsen, Casper College, Wyoming.*

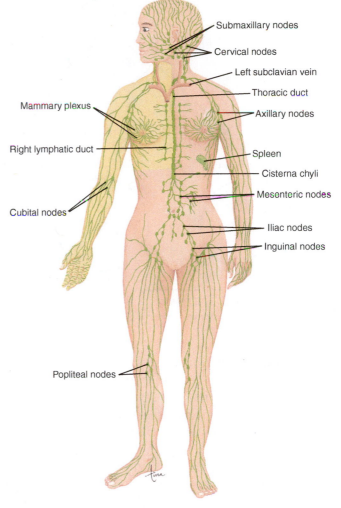

Figure 9.12 Lymphatic system.

LYMPHOCYTE ORIGIN AND FUNCTION

The lymphocytic series is distinctive in its presentation and function. In contrast to most other white blood cells, which derive solely from the bone marrow, lymphocytes derive from two locations. The primary lymphoid organs are the bone marrow and thymus. The secondary lymphoid organs are the spleen, lymph nodes, Peyer's patches of the gastrointestinal tract, and the tonsils. Additionally, the lymphatic system plays an essential role in lymphocyte development, differentiation, and function. More than 100 lymph nodes form a nexus known as the lymphatic system, which runs from the **cervical** lymph nodes of the neck to the inguinal lymph nodes in the groin area (Fig. 9.12). The lymphatic system plays an important role in blood filtration, fluid balance, antibody generation, and lymphopoiesis.[6] A major part of this system is lymph, a clear, thin fluid derived from plasma that bathes the soft tissues. After an injury, fluid accumulates through swelling, and the lymphatic system moves fluid from the affected area back to the circulation through the capillaries of the lymph nodes. Because the lymphatic system has no pumping mechanism such as the heart, it derives its circulatory ability from respiration, muscle movement, and pressure from nearby blood vessels. Excess fluid is transported to two large vessels: the thoracic duct near the left **subclavian** vein and the right thoracic duct near the right subclavian vein.

The primary function of lymphocytes is immunologic: recognizing what is foreign, nonself; forming antibodies; and securing immunity. Nonself or foreign substances may appear as bacteria, cell substances, proteins, or viruses.

Lymphocyte Populations

Two general subpopulations of lymphocytes—B lymphocytes and T lymphocytes—appear morphologically similar on peripheral smear. Their derivation and function, however, are quite different. B lymphocytes comprise,10% to 20% of the total lymphocyte population, whereas T lymphocytes **comprise** 60% to 80%. A third minor population, natural killer (NK) lymphocytes, constitutes less than 10% of the total lymphocyte population (Fig. 9.13).

B lymphocytes derive from bone marrow stem cells. Interleukin (IL)-1 and IL-6 activate the pluripotent stem cell, which differentiates into the lymphocyte stem cell (LSC). Generally, the LSC gives rise to the progression of the pre-B cell, the lymphoblast, the B cell, and the terminal cell, the plasma cell. The plasma

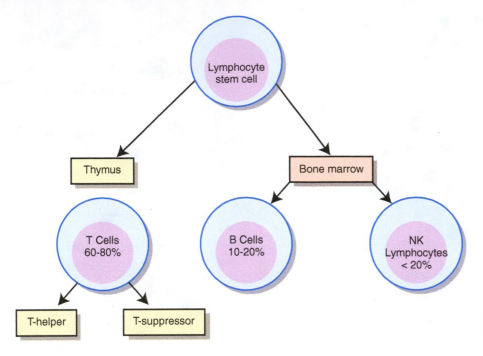

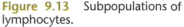

Figure 9.13   Subpopulations of lymphocytes.

cell is responsible for antibody production and **humoral** immunity. T cells arise from the LSC, which migrates to the thymus. The thymus, a gland located above the heart, gives rise to the prothymocyte, the T lymphoblast, and the T cell responsible for cell-mediated immunity. This gland, although highly active in infants and children, is not functional in adults. Determining lymphocyte life span is difficult. Long-lived lymphocytes produce cytokines, whereas short-lived lymphocytes produce antibodies. Plasma and tissue environmental influences either promote or delay longevity. There has been speculation that some lymphocytes may live 4 years.[7]

T cells and B cells are dependent on their interaction with their microenvironment: bone marrow versus thymus versus lymph nodes versus peripheral blood. The surface membrane markers they possess and their stimulation toward a particular immune response define their specific derivation. Classification of stages of T cells and B cells is complex and dominated by which CD markers or surface antigens they possess.

Travel Path of Lymphocytes

Lymphocytes may originate in the bone marrow, the thymus, and the lymphatic system. Because the lymphatic system is a network of tissues, the travel path of lymphocytes from blood to thymus to lymphatics is not straightforward. Most white blood cells proliferate and mature in the bone marrow and are released into the peripheral circulation. From the circulation, they

may either migrate to tissues or wind their way through the circulation until they degenerate. Lymphocytes travel two paths, either between areas of inflammation or moving from the bone marrow to the thymus and then into secondary lymphoid tissue, the lymphatic system. Mature lymphocytes primarily move back and forth between the lymphatic system, whereas immature lymphocytes move from the bone marrow to the thymus and then into the lymphatic system. Because the lymphocyte is a highly mobile cell, it interacts with the endothelial cells of blood vessels as it migrates to tissues. This migration is carefully orchestrated through a series of receptors and cytokines from the endothelial network. Lymphocytes spend far more time traveling through tissues than through the marrow or circulation.[8] Extensive transit is meant to increase their opportunities to become exposed to foreign antigenic stimuli and mount an appropriate response.

Lymphocytes and Development of Immunocompetence

Initially, lymphocytes developing and maturing in the bone marrow and thymus do not respond to provocative antigens. It is only when they reach the lymphatic system that they begin to develop a response to antigenic stimulation and become immunocompetent. Migration through the lymphatic system is carefully orchestrated through a series of receptors and chemokines on the endothelial network of blood vessels surrounding lymphatic tissue.[8] Immunoblasts are large activated lymphocytes capable of mustering an immune response. Antigenic presentation to lymphocytes may take many forms—from altered cells to the body or foreign antigens or proteins. When a foreign antigen is presented to the body, it is usually phagocytized and destroyed by the macrophages of the lymph nodes or tissues. If this mechanism is incomplete and some part of the invading mechanism is left behind, an immune response begins to occur. Lymphocytes become activated and proceed to "battle" foreign antigens with many immune capabilities. Activated lymphocytes take on many roles and proliferate in the first few days after recognizing a foreign antigen or antigenic products. B cells begin to synthesize antibodies to the particular antigen as a primary response. When the antigen is presented to T cells by macrophages or B cells, T cells respond by participating in cell-mediated immunity activities, including the following:

- Delayed hypersensitivity
- Tumor suppression
- Resistance to intracellular organisms

In addition to each of these responses, T cells release lymphokines, which activate B lymphocytes and assist in humoral immunity and the production of plasma cells. T cells play a vital role in cell-mediated and humoral response and are essential to immune development.

Response of Lymphocytes to Antigenic Stimulation

When resting lymphocytes respond to antigenic stimulation, they begin to synthesize receptors, signals, or antigenic markers. T cells, which represent 60% to 85% of total lymphocytes, can be subdivided into two populations: T helper (CD4) or T cytotoxic/suppressor (CD8). T helper cells interact with monocytes and macrophages, secrete cytokines, and promote humoral immunity. T cytotoxic cells promote memory cells and help to eliminate nonself by promoting enzyme activity, which can significantly alter the cell membrane. B cells, which represent 10% to 20% of total lymphocytes, differentiate into plasma cells. This transformation occurs as T cells recognize antigens and release lymphokines. Lymphokines help B lymphocytes transform into plasma cells, detect antigens, and produce antibodies. NK cells represent a small subpopulation of lymphocytes with a highly specific function. These cells are non-T or non-B in origin and do not need antigenic stimulation to function. Originating in the bone marrow, their primary role is resisting bacteria, viruses, and fungi.

Lymphocyte Cell Markers and Cluster of Differentiation

Before 1980, lymphocytes were demarcated by surface and cytoplasmic immunoglobulins, HLA markers, and terminal deoxynucleotidyl transferase (TdT) antigens. See Table 9.1 for a listing of CD markers in unstimulated B cells and T cells. At the present time, most lymphocyte subpopulations are recognized by their CD (cluster of differentiation) markers or antigens. These antigens are determined through a series of monoclonal antibodies manufactured by public and private companies to identify surface antigens on the many lymphocyte (and other cell) subsets. Lymphocytes can be identified at successive stages in their maturation by their pattern of reaction to monoclonal antibodies. Most lymphocytes have several CD designations that they may initially possess and then lose throughout their maturation sequence; this often occurs during a disease process. Flow cytometry is presently the primary method used to determine CD markers.

LEUKOCYTE COUNT FROM COMPLETE BLOOD CELL COUNT TO DIFFERENTIAL

WBCs reported on the complete blood count (CBC) are counted either directly from an automated instrument or manually. The age of the patient directly influences whether this number is within or outside of the reference range (Table 9.2). Pediatric reference ranges vary more than adult ranges. Some of the peculiarities of newborns include highest WBCs at 3 months.

The WBC differential is an evaluation of the types of mature white blood cells in the peripheral circulation. Although the differential provides only a snapshot of the white blood cell population at a particular moment in time, it offers valuable information about an individual's hematologic status and the individual's response to any circumstances that may alter that status. Generally, the differential is performed on a well-stained, well-distributed peripheral smear.

Table 9.2 ● Leukocyte Counts at Different Ages	
Age	**Leukocyte Count***
Birth	4–40
4 Years	5–15
Adult	4–11

*All values × 10^9/L.

The peripheral smear is evaluated for distribution at 10× and then a white blood cell estimate is performed at 40× (see Chapter 20 for procedures). Next, a differential count is performed; 100 white blood cells are counted, and the percentage and identification of each type of white blood cell are recorded. These percentages are compared with the reference ranges for an individual according to age (Table 9.3). White blood cell estimates provide important quality control data for the technologist performing the differential. A white blood cell estimate that fails to agree with the automated count may indicate that the wrong smear was pulled, warranting an investigation to correct this error.

In most cases, 100 white blood cells are carefully counted and identified, but there are circumstances that may warrant counting 200 white blood cells. Students need to refer to the standard operating procedure at each clinical site for recommendations for counting a 200-cell differential. If a 200-cell differential is done, the physician should be aware of this. Table 9.4 lists general conditions when a 200-cell differential may be desirable. Critical values outside of the reference range have been established for each clinical facility regarding the CBC and the differential. These values are usually flagged by the automated instrument and must be reported to the physician or the pathologist, or both, in a timely fashion. Laboratory personnel keep careful records concerning notification of a patient with a critical value. Date, time, and person giving and receiving the information are usually recorded. Table 9.5 provides a list of sample critical values.

Manual Differential Versus Differential Scan

Most automated hematology instruments have the capacity to perform a differential count. This advance in instrumentation has dramatically shifted work patterns because less time is spent in reviewing peripheral smears. When a differential is ordered and reported from instrumentation, there are some conditions in which the automated differential count may be questionable. If certain parameters in the differential have been flagged or if a peripheral smear requires review because of a delta check or reflex testing, the peripheral smear is reviewed by a laboratory professional. In these circumstances, there are two levels of technologist review: a manual leukocyte differential count or a differential scan (diff scan). A manual leukocyte differential count implies counting 100 white blood cells along with red blood cell morphology and platelets estimate. A differential scan implies that approximately 50 cells are reviewed to verify the automated result. The criteria for performing either a full differential count or a differential scan are usually well outlined in the standard operating procedure for each clinical facility. Generally, these criteria include items such as total leukocyte count, lymphocytes, and monocytes above a certain level; an abnormal scatter plot; or thrombocytopenia. Patients whose peripheral smears need review usually are seriously ill or their conditions

Table 9.3 ● Manual Differential Reference Ranges for Different Ages		
	Adults	**Up to 4 Years**
Segmented neutrophils	50%–70%	20%–44%
Bands	2%–6%	0%–5%
Lymphocytes	20%–44%	48%–78%
Monocytes	2%–9%	2%–11%
Eosinophils	0%–4%	1%–4%
Basophils	0%–2%	0%–2%

Table 9.4 ● When to Consider Counting More Than 100 Cells on Differential*
• WBC >35.0 × 10⁹/L
• Lymphocytes >40% or <17%
• Monocytes >12%
• Blasts (first-time patient)

*These values vary with every clinical site.

Table 9.5 ● Sample Critical Values	
WBC	Low 3.0 × 10⁹/L
	High 25.0 × 10⁹/L
Hemoglobin	Low 7.0 g/dL
	High 17.0 g/dL
Platelet	Low 50.0 × 10⁹/L
	High 1.0 × 10¹²/L
Differential	For criteria for performing a manual differential, refer to the standard operating procedure for each facility. *Blasts*, which are reported on a new patient, are always a critical result

are deteriorating or changing. Reviewing peripheral smears on these patients requires a high level of morphologic skill from the laboratory professional.

Relative Versus Absolute Values

Relative and absolute counts refer to the WBC differential. The absolute count refers to the count derived from the total WBC multiplied by the percentage of any particular white blood cell. The relative count refers to the percentage of a particular cell counted from the 100 WBC differential. Absolute reference ranges have been compiled for each cell in the WBC differential (Table 9.6). An example of how to calculate and interpret the relative and absolute count follows:

If the WBC is
5.0 × 10⁹/L

And the differential reads:

Segmented neutrophils: 40%
(Ref. range = 50% to 70%)

Bands: 3%
(Ref. range = 2% to 6%)

Lymphocytes: 55%
(Ref. range = 20% to 44%)

Monocytes: 2%
(Ref. range = 2% to 9%)

Then the absolute count of lymphocytes would be 5000 × 0.55 = 2500.

Reference range for absolute lymphocyte count = 1700 to 3500

In this patient, there is a relative lymphocytosis but not an absolute lymphocytosis.

Table 9.6 • Absolute Reference Range for Adult Differential*

• Neutrophils	2.0–7.5
• Lymphocytes	1.2–3.4
• Monocytes	0.0–0.9
• Eosinophils	0.0–0.6

*All values × 10⁹/L.

Summary Points

- The myeloid:erythroid ratio (M:E) in the bone marrow is 3 to 4:1.
- Segmented neutrophils are held in the marginating pool for 7 to 10 days before release to circulation.
- The maturation sequence for neutrophils, from least mature to most mature, is myeloblast, promyelocyte, myelocyte, metamyelocyte, band, and segmented neutrophil.
- Cell identification is based on cell size, N:C ratio, presence or absence of granules, presence or absence of nucleoli, chromatin pattern, and texture of cytoplasm.
- The marginating pool designates white blood cells located along the vessel endothelium.
- The circulating pool designates white blood cells present in the bloodstream.
- Lymphocytes originate not only from the bone marrow, but also from the thymus gland and the lymphatic system.

CONDENSED CASE

A routine CBC was received in the clinical laboratory on a patient who had been receiving daily blood work. On this particular day, the computer flagged various parameters pertaining to the CBC, and a delta check was performed. The flagged parameters were WBC, hemoglobin, hematocrit, and MCV. *What are the steps needed to investigate the discrepancy in this patient's results?*

Answer

- Realize that the delta check is the historical reference on the patient. If the results are flagged, there is a discrepancy in patient results.
- Visually inspect the CBC tubes, and peel back the label, looking for identification.
- Check the sample for a clot.
- Rerun the sample to ensure there is the proper amount of sample and proper mixing.
- Check whether there is a transfusion history on the patient.
- Call the floor and ask how the sample was drawn.

After performing these steps, decide on a course of action.

- The bone marrow and the thymus are the primary lymphoid organs.
- Spleen, lymph nodes, Peyer's patches, and tonsils are the secondary lymphoid organs.
- The lymphatic system plays an important role in blood filtration, fluid balance, antibody generation, and lymphopoiesis.
- T cells represent 60% to 80% of the total lymphocyte count.

- B cells represent 10% to 20% of the total lymphocyte count.
- T helper and T cytotoxic/suppressor cells are essential in cell-mediated immunity.
- B cells are responsible for humoral immunity, which is antibody production by plasma cells.
- Absolute counts are derived from the total WBCs multiplied by the relative percentage of a particular white blood cell in the differential.

CASE STUDY

A 45-year-old woman presented to the emergency department with vague complaints of dizziness, right-sided abdominal pain, and intermittent blurred vision. A baseline CBC was drawn with the following results:

WBC	6.5×10^9/L
RBC	4.02×10^{12}/L
Hgb	13.2 g/dL
Hct	37.3%
MCV	92.8 fL
MCH	31.4 pg
MCHC	35.4%
Platelets	30.3×10^9/L

Is this a critical platelet count?

Insights to the Case Study

The patient was admitted to the hospital as a result of the extremely low platelet count. The risk of spontaneous bleeding was a consideration. No further testing was ordered because it was the weekend, and a hematology consultation could not be arranged before Monday. The patient had two subsequent CBCs during this time, and eventually a peripheral smear was pulled. When the peripheral smear was stained and reviewed, the technologist noted that most of the platelets were spreading around the neutrophils, a condition known as *platelet satellitism* (see Fig. 10.18). This condition is a reaction by some patients to the EDTA in the lavender top tubes. When this reaction was observed, the patient's blood was redrawn in a sodium citrate tube and cycled for a platelet count. The platelet count on this sample was recorded at 230,000. Ordinarily, a flag on the platelet count probably would not warrant a peripheral smear review. This situation may serve as a catalyst, however, for reviewing the flagging policy.

Review Questions

1. The primary lymphoid organs are the
   a. Liver and spleen.
   b. Gallbladder and liver.
   c. Bone marrow and thymus.
   d. Spleen and tonsils.

2. Which one of the following features distinguishes a monocyte from a lymphocyte?
   a. Nucleoli
   b. Abundant gray-blue cytoplasm
   c. Irregularly shaped flattened nucleus
   d. Large blue-black granules

3. In which stage of neutrophilic maturation are specific secondary granules first seen?
   a. Myeloblast
   b. Metamyelocyte
   c. Myelocyte
   d. Band

4. Which CD marker is specific for monocytes?
   a. CD45
   b. CD19
   c. CD20
   d. CD14

5. Which subpopulation of T cells alters the cell membrane?
   a. T cytotoxic
   b. T helper
   c. NK cells
   d. None of the above

6. Lymphocyte concentrations in peripheral blood are greatest during what age interval?
   a. Immediately after birth
   b. Older adult (40 to 70 years)
   c. Young adult (16 to 40 years)
   d. Young child (1 to 4 years)

7. The marginating pool of neutrophils is located
   a. In the kidneys.
   b. In the tissue.
   c. Next to marrow sinuses.
   d. On the blood vessel walls.

8. The CBC results for a 3-month-old infant are as follows:
   WBC 9.5×10^9/L differential
   RBC 3.4×10^{12}/L
   Hgb 6.7g/dL
   Hct 25%
   Segmented neutrophils 25%
   Hgb 6.7 g/dL
   Lymphocytes 75%
   The absolute lymphocyte count in this patient would be
   a. 1.2×10^9/L.
   b. 2.4×10^9/L.
   c. 7.1×10^9/L.
   d. 7.5×10^9/L.

9. Which of the following CD markers is more appropriately associated with the myelocyte?
   a. CD4, CD8
   b. CD33, CD13, CD14
   c. CD45, CD33, CD13
   d. CD19, CD22

10. One of the primary glands in an infant responsible for lymphocyte origination is the
    a. Thymus gland.
    b. Adrenal gland.
    c. Thyroid gland.
    d. Pituitary gland.

○ TROUBLESHOOTING

What Do I Do When Samples Are Sent to the Laboratory Within Minutes on the Same Patient and the Results Do Not Match?

A 74-year-old patient in the critical care unit was having daily hematology blood work performed. The first sample was sent to the laboratory at 2:23 p.m. Hemoglobin and hematocrit were the only analyses requested. The results were verified without delta flags. The second sample was sent 20 minutes later with a request for hemoglobin and hematocrit. Both samples were cycled through the automated instrument, and a full CBC was obtained. Only the hemoglobin and hematocrit were reported. The results were as follows:

	First Sample at 2:23 p.m.	Second Sample at 2:43 p.m.
WBC	16.9×10^9/L	12.5×10^9/L
Hgb	9.3 g/dL	8.4 g/dL
Hct	26.5%	24.2%
Platelets	104×10^9/L	97×10^9/L

Hemoglobin and hematocrit were the only two tests ordered, and both results seem totally verifiable.

Because the technologist had access to the complete CBC on the computer screen, she noticed the disparity in WBCs. The change in WBC was troubling and alerted the technologist to possible problems with the sample. She considered the following possibilities:

1. Is the specimen clotted or contaminated?
2. Was the blood in specimen 1 and specimen 2 drawn from the same patient?
3. How was the specimen obtained?

Both samples were checked for clots. After contacting the floor nurse, the following information was obtained. Both samples were drawn through an arterial line, an "A line." Arterial lines are inserted in critically ill patients who have frequent blood draws and receive frequent medications. The procedure when drawing through an A line is to draw off and discard the first 10 mL of blood and then proceed with the blood draw, usually filling tubes directly from the line. In this case, the blood draw for the first sample was difficult, and the blood from the A line was not free flowing. The second sample was obtained without difficulty. Proper

Continued

blood drawing procedure with the A line was followed with both samples. After consultation with the lead technologist and the nurse, it was decided to release the second set of results and remove the first set from the computer. The patient had a blood bank history and had received units of packed red blood cells and fresh frozen plasma. Because the parameter in question was the WBC, this information was not relevant in this case.

WORD KEY

Cervical • Relating to the neck

Humoral • When referring to immunity, antibody formation

Inguinal • Relating to the groin area

Subclavian • Situated beneath the clavicle or collar bone

Thoracic • Relating to the chest

Thymus • Ductless gland located above the heart that plays a role in immunity

References

1. Turgeon ML. Clinical Hematology: Theory and Procedures. Philadelphia: Lippincott Williams & Wilkins, 1999; 160.
2. Parsons D, Marty J, Strauss R. Cell biology, disorders of neutrophils, infectious mononucleosis and reactive lymphocytes. In: Harmoning DM, ed. Clinical Hematology and Fundamentals of Hemostasis, 4th ed. Philadelphia: FA Davis, 2002; 252.
3. Heckner F, Lehman P, Kao Y. Practical Microscopic Hematology, 4th ed. Philadelphia: Lea & Febiger, 1994; 14–16.
4. Carr JH, Rodak BF. Clinical Hematology Atlas. Philadelphia: WB Saunders, 1999.
5. O'Connor BH. A Color Atlas and Instructional Manual of Peripheral Blood Cell Morphology. Baltimore: Williams & Wilkins, 1984.
6. Brown B. Hematology: Principles and Procedures, 6th ed. Philadelphia: Lippincott Williams & Wilkins, 2000; 74–79.
7. Rossi MI, Yokota T, Medin KL, et al. B lymphopoiesis is active throughout human life, but there are developmental age related changes. Blood 101:576–584, 2003.
8. Steine-Martin EA, Lotspeich-Steininger CA, Koepke JA. Clinical Hematology: Principles, Procedures, and Correlations, 2nd ed. Philadelphia: Lippincott, 1998; 326–327.

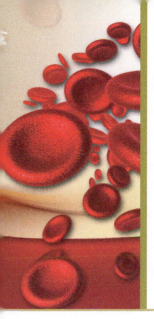

Chapter 10

Abnormalities of White Blood Cells: Quantitative, Qualitative, and the Lipid Storage Diseases

Betty Ciesla

Objectives

After completing this chapter, the student will be able to:

1. Identify the physiology and function of granulocytes.

2. Explain the steps involved in phagocytosis.

3. Identify conditions that cause a quantitative increase or decrease in a particular white blood cell line.

4. Describe the changes observed when white blood cells respond to infection.

5. Compare and contrast the acquired and inherited qualitative changes in the white blood cell.

6. Identify conditions that lead to hyposegmentation or hypersegmentation of segmented neutrophils.

7. Define the probable causes for an increased lymphocyte count.

8. Define the differences seen in the lymphocyte count of an adult versus a child.

9. Describe the effects of HIV on the CBC and the peripheral smear.

10. Describe the process of reactive lymphocytosis in infections with Epstein-Barr virus and cytomegalovirus.

11. Define white blood cell–related terms such as leukocytosis, left shift, leukemoid reaction, and leukoerythroblastic reaction.

12. Describe briefly lipid storage diseases, such as Gaucher's disease, Niemann-Pick disease, and Tay-Sachs disease.

INTRODUCTION TO WHITE BLOOD CELL DISORDERS

Because white blood cells have such a short time span in the peripheral circulation, alterations either in the quantity or in the quality of a particular white blood cell can be quite dramatic. With the normal differential reference ranges for adults and children as a benchmark, any increase or decrease in a particular type of cell signals the body's unique response to "assaults" of any kind. Infection, inflammation, chronic disease, and parasitic infestations all are examples of an unexpected occurrence and an opportunity for white blood cells to mobilize. As white blood cells respond to infection or other stimuli, changes are seen in the number and types of a particular cell line. When a cell line is increased, the suffix used to designate an increase is "osis" or "philia" (e.g., "eosinophilia" and "leukocytosis"). When a cell line is decreased, the suffix used to designate a decrease is "penia" (e.g., "neutropenia"). Changes are observed in the complete blood count (CBC) and in the peripheral blood smear.

An interesting situation is the role that granules from a particular cell line play in producing symptoms. For example, eosinophilic granules contain histamine. In patients with allergy, eosinophils are usually seen in excess. When histamine is released from eosinophils, this chemical stimulates allergy-related symptoms such as watery, itching eyes and **rhinorrhea**. Most allergy medications contain antihistamines that are formulated to block allergy symptoms.

In most cases, patients who have newly acquired infections show an increase in white blood cells from the reference range. Care must be taken, however, when assessing a patient with an increased WBC. Ethnic differences have been suggested in the normal white blood cell reference range, with blacks having a lower normal WBC than whites. Symptoms that reflect an infection combined with an elevated WBC strongly suggest an infectious process.[1]

QUANTITATIVE CHANGES IN WHITE BLOOD CELLS

Various conditions give rise to increases or decreases in a particular cell line. These conditions are usually transient, and when the underlying condition has resolved itself, for the most part the counts return to normal. A partial list of disorders that increase or decrease leukocytes follows.* Table 10.1 lists disorders that affect lymphocytes quantitatively.

Conditions With Increased Neutrophils

- Infections
- Inflammatory response
- Stress response
- Malignancies
- Surgery
- Physical conditions (heat, cold, shock)
- Drugs

Conditions With Increased Eosinophils

- Skin disease
- Parasitic disease
- Transplant rejection[2]
- Myeloproliferative disorders
- Asthma

Conditions With Increased Basophils

- Myeloproliferative disorders
- Hypersensitivity reactions
- Ulcerative colitis
- Chronic inflammatory conditions

Conditions With Increased Monocytes

- Chronic infections (e.g., tuberculosis)
- Malignancies
- Leukemias with a strong monocytic component
- Bone marrow failure

Conditions That Decrease Neutrophils

- Drugs (e.g., chloramphenicol)
- Chemotherapy
- Infectious disease
- Autoimmune disease

Conditions That Decrease Eosinophils

- Acute infections
- Adrenocorticotropic hormone (ACTH)
- Bone marrow aplasia

---

*The information is taken in part from Wu A, Teitz HB. Clinical Guide to Laboratory Tests, 4th ed. St. Louis: WB Saunders.

Conditions That Decrease Basophils

- Steroid treatment
- Inflammation

Conditions That Decrease Monocytes

- Autoimmune processes
- Hairy cell leukemia

Perhaps the most significant finding regarding decreased cell lines is neutropenia, in which the absolute neutrophil count is lower than $2.0 \times 10^9/L$. This occurs as a result of medications, bone marrow assaults secondary to chemicals, viral infections, or splenic sequestration.[3] Table 10.2 provides specific terminology relating to quantitative changes to white blood cells.

Table 10.1 ● Nonmalignant Quantitative Changes in Lymphocytes	
Increase in	**Decrease in**
EBV	HIV
CMV	Malnutrition
Hepatitis viruses	Chemotherapy
HIV	Radiation
Chronic bacterial infections	Renal failure
Autoimmune disorders	
Drugs	

Taken in part from Wu A, Teitz HB. Teitz Clinical Guide to Laboratory Tests, 4th ed. St. Louis: WB Saunders, 2006; 1194.

Table 10.2 ● White Blood Cell Terminology

- **Neutrophilia** Increase in segmented neutrophils
- **Leukocytosis** Increase in white blood cells
- **Left shift** Increase in bands and metamyelocytes in the peripheral smear; seen in response to infection
- **Leukemoid reaction** Exaggerated response to infection; resulting in high WBC and increased numbers of metamyelocytes, bands, and possibly younger cells
- **Leukoerythroblastic picture** Immature white blood cells, immature red blood cells, and platelet abnormalities seen in peripheral smear

STAGES OF WHITE BLOOD CELL PHAGOCYTOSIS

The phagocytic process by which bacteria and other infectious agents are recognized and destroyed is a critical function of neutrophils and monocytes. The role of the neutrophil in phagocytosis is localized and immediate; the role of the monocyte is related to immune response and is more tissue-oriented. The process by which bacteria are digested and immobilized can be broken down into several simplified steps (Fig. 10.1).

- *Stage 1—chemotaxis*: Foreign body invades tissues; neutrophils, which usually move in random motion through the tissue, are attracted directly to site of invasion through chemical signals stimulated by foreign body (bacteria). The release of interleukin-8 and complement helps neutrophils mobilize to site of infection.
- *Stage 2—opsonization*: Neutrophilic attachment of the invading foreign body can take place only after the foreign body has been opsonized or prepared to be ingested through

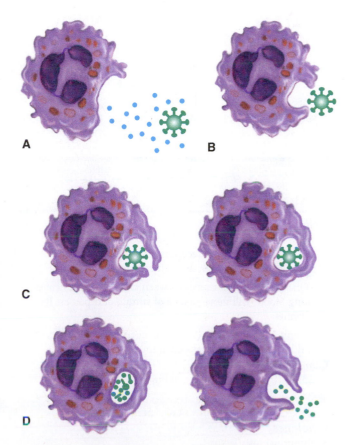

Figure 10.1 Mechanism of phagocytosis. Stages depicted are (*A*) chemotaxis and directed motility, (*B*) opsonization, (*C*) ingestion, (*D*) degranulation and digestion.

interaction with the complement system and other immunoglobulins.

- *Stage 3—ingestion*: The opsonized foreign body is ingested by the neutrophil. The foreign body is engulfed by the neutrophilic pseudopod membranes.
- *Stage 4—killing*: The neutrophilic granules release their contents, which contain various lytic elements. The pH of the cell is reduced, and hydrogen peroxide is produced by the neutrophil as a result of respiratory burst and released to accelerate the destruction process. The neutrophil is also destroyed in this process.

Bacteremia or sepsis may occur if invading organisms or foreign bodies are not destroyed when they enter the body. The organisms may locate in secondary sites such as the lymph nodes, where they rapidly multiply and release toxins.

Phagocytic activity is a complex process involving phagocytic cells, the complement system, cytotoxins, and acute-phase reactants. Each of these systems must have coordinated activities to ensure that pathogens are destroyed (Table 10.3).[4]

QUALITATIVE DEFECTS OF WHITE BLOOD CELLS

Qualitative changes of the white blood cell occur either in the cytoplasm or in the nucleus. These changes are classified as inherited or acquired. Acquired defects are seen with much greater frequency than inherited

---

Table 10.3 ◯ Essential Elements Leading to Phagocytosis

Cells
- Neutrophils: Attracted to pathogen, are activated by endothelial cell surface receptors, will recruit more neutrophils to infection site through cell surface receptors
- Monocytes: Cells in transit between marrow, tissues circulating blood, will move to area of stimuli and possess lytic enzymes
- Basophils, eosinophils: React in concert with complement and hormones to suppress inflammation

Complement
- C5a: Coats the pathogen, making it "tasty" to phagocytic cells
- C3b: Causes increase in vascular permeability

Cytokines
- Tumor necrosis factor
- Interleukins 1, 8, and 10

---

defects. When a patient has developed an increased WBC, toxic changes of the white blood cells usually occur as a result of stress during maturation and as a result of activity in the circulation or tissue. A careful and patient review of the peripheral smear of these individuals reveals many of the changes discussed (Fig. 10.2).

Toxic Changes in White Blood Cells

The visible response of white blood cells to infection or inflammation occurs along two paths. As white blood cells increase, the peripheral smear usually shows either increased numbers of segmented neutrophils, giving rise to a neutrophilia, or a shift to the left, where younger cells are noted. In either of these cases, toxic changes, such as toxic granulation, toxic vacuolization, or the presence of Döhle bodies, may be observed. Careful examination of the neutrophils for these toxic changes is extremely important.

Toxic Granulation

Normal granulation in the segmented neutrophils has a dustlike appearance, with the red and blue granules

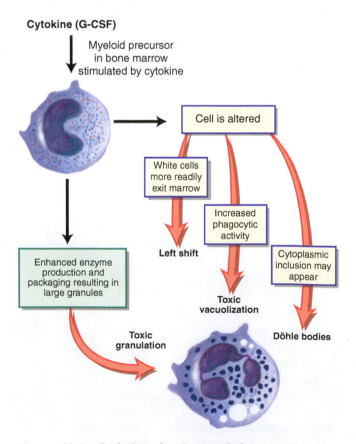

Figure 10.2   Evolution of toxic granulation.   Adapted from Glassy

E. Color Atlas of Hematology: An Illustrated Guide Based on Proficiency Testing. Northfield, IL: College of American Pathologists, 1998, with permission.

being difficult to observe. Toxic granulation is excessive in amount and intensity, with more prominent granules in segmented neutrophils and bands in direct response to enhanced lysosome enzyme production. These granules are more frequent and have much more vivid blue-black coloration (Fig. 10.3). Clusters of toxic granules usually appear in neutrophils. Sometimes the granulation is so heavy as to resemble basophilic granules.

Toxic Vacuolization

Toxic vacuolization occurs in the segmented neutrophil. Vacuoles appear in the cytoplasm of this cell and may be small or large (Fig. 10.4). Prolonged exposure of blood to drugs such as sulfonamides or chloroquine or prolonged storage may lead to phagocytosis of granules or cytoplasmic contents.[5] Additionally,

small, uniformly placed vacuoles may be seen in a peripheral smear made from blood that has been held for an extended period. In cases where the creation of peripheral smears has been delayed, pseudovacuolization can be recognized. This phenomenon must be distinguished from pathogenic toxic vacuolization. Larger vacuoles unevenly distributed throughout the cytoplasm usually signal serious infections and possible **sepsis**. Studies have shown that when 10% of neutrophils are affected by vacuoles in a fresh sample, this ranks as a serious and significant **prognostic indicator** (Table 10.4).[6]

Döhle Bodies

Döhle bodies are cytoplasmic inclusions that consist of ribosomal RNA. They range from 1 to 5 μm in size, are located near the cytoplasmic membrane, and appear as a rod-shaped, pale bluish gray structure (Fig. 10.5).

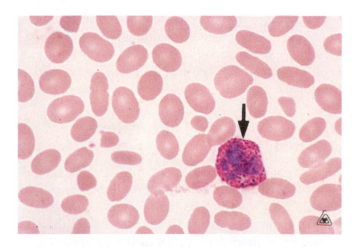

Figure 10.3 Toxic granulation. Note heavier granulation throughout the cytoplasm. From The College of American Pathologists, with permission.

Table 10.4 ⊙ Significant Alterations in Neutrophils in Peripheral Smears

- Döhle bodies
- Toxic granulation
- Toxic vacuolization
- Hyposegmentation
- Hypersegmentation
- Bacteria (intracellular or extracellular)
- Platelet satellitism
- Chédiak-Higashi granules

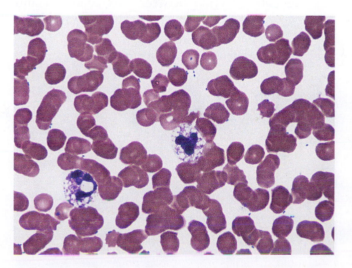

Figure 10.4 Toxic vacuolization. Note large vacuoles located in the cytoplasm. Courtesy of Bernardino Madsen, Casper College, Wyoming.

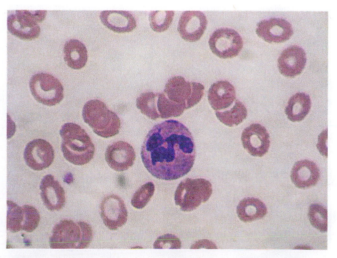

Figure 10.5 Döhle bodies are inclusions that are pale, peripherally located in the cytoplasm, and rodlike. Courtesy of Bernardino Madsen, Casper College, Wyoming.

These transient inclusions are frequently observed in neutrophils but may be seen in monocytes and bands. Döhle bodies are difficult to observe under light microscopy, and peripheral smears must be carefully scrutinized for their presence. Döhle bodies may also be seen in nonpathologic conditions such as pregnancy.

Human Ehrlichiosis

Named for the noted microbiologist Ehrlich, human ehrlichiosis and anaplasmosis infections are a relatively new group of tick-borne diseases that show a notable white blood cell inclusion in some cases. There are two varieties: human monocytic ehrlichiosis (HME), caused by the *Rickettsia*-like bacteria *Ehrlichia chaffeensis,* and human granulocytic anaplasmosis (HGA), which is caused by the *Rickettsia*-like bacteria *Anaplasma phagocytophilum.* These diseases are difficult to diagnose because patients present with vague symptoms that are often mistaken for other infectious diseases. HME cases are usually located in the southeastern and mid-Atlantic United States,[9] and patients initially present with flu-like symptoms. Patients with HGA, who are usually located in the Midwestern United States, present with an acute onset of high fever, chills, and headache.[10] Common to both illnesses are low WBC, extremely elevated liver enzymes, and thrombocytopenia. Inclusions, known as morulae, may be seen in the granulocytes or monocytes from the bone marrow or peripheral smear; these inclusions are large (1 to 3 μm) and resemble berries in appearance (Fig. 10.6). If identified, morulae are specific for HME and HGA, but they are difficult to observe and are not seen in every case. Peripheral smears and bone marrow

smears should be carefully reviewed for identification of these inclusion bodies.

Nuclear Abnormalities: Hypersegmentation

Normal segmented neutrophils have between three and five lobes in the nucleus. Hypersegmentation is defined as a segmented neutrophilic nucleus having more than five lobes (Fig. 10.7). This condition is usually seen in megaloblastic processes, such as folic acid deficiency, pernicious anemia, or vitamin B_{12} deficiency, and is usually accompanied by oval macrocytes.

HEREDITARY WHITE BLOOD CELL DISORDERS

May-Hegglin Anomaly

May-Hegglin anomaly is an inherited disorder that is associated with thrombocytopenia and giant platelets. Abnormal bleeding may be seen in a few affected individuals. Döhle-like bodies are seen in the cytoplasm of neutrophils and are larger than the Döhle bodies seen in neutrophils responding to infections or inflammation.

Alder's Anomaly (Alder-Reilly Anomaly)

Alder's anomaly is a rare genetic disorder that is associated with the presence of coarse, dark granules in neutrophils, lymphocytes, monocytes, eosinophils, and basophils (Fig. 10.8). This granulation is thought to consist of lipid depositions in the cytoplasm as a result of decreased mucopolysaccharide production.[7] Prominent deposition of granules in *every* cell line is a differentiating feature between this condition and

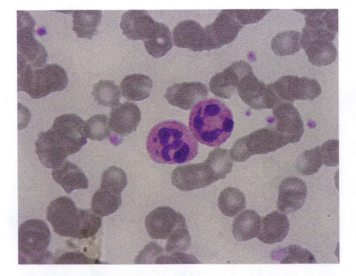

Figure 10.6 Human ehrlichiosis. Courtesy of Ms. Kathy Finnegan, MS, MT (ASCP)SH, Stony Brook Medical Center, Stony Brook, NY.

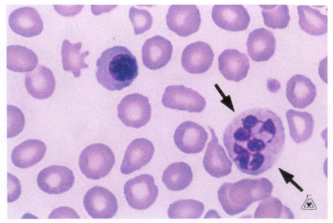

Figure 10.7 Hypersegmented neutrophil. From The College of American Pathologists, with permission.

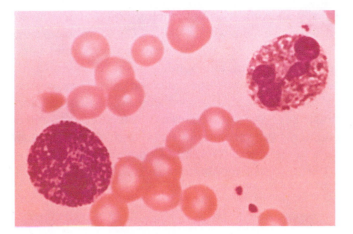

Figure 10.8 Alder's anomaly. Note deep granulation.
© 1967 American Society of Clinical Pathologists. Reprinted with permission.

toxic granulation, which appears in clusters only in neutrophils and monocytes.

Pelger-Huët Anomaly

Pelger-Huët anomaly is a fairly common inherited disorder that shows hyposegmentation of the nucleus of segmented neutrophils. In heterozygotes, the nucleus is seen as peanut-shaped, dumbbell-shaped, or pince-nez–shaped (Fig. 10.9). In homozygotes, the nucleus is spherical with no lobes and prominent nuclear clumping. When initially observing cells with Pelger-Huët anomaly, they may appear as bands or metamyelocytes. When considering these cells in a peripheral smear, it is important to make two judgments: Is the hyposegmentation seen in most neutrophils? Is the nuclear content mature? Even experienced morphologists have misidentified these cells as bands or

metamyelocytes, greatly skewing the peripheral smear results. In a true Pelger-Huët anomaly, almost 70% to 95% of the neutrophils show hyposegmentation. The cells are functional neutrophils, however. There are numerous conditions in which the neutrophils may have a pseudo–Pelger-Huët appearance, such as leukemias, myeloproliferative disorders, and severe infections.

Chédiak-Higashi Syndrome

Chédiak-Higashi syndrome is a rare autosomal disorder of neutrophilic granules. Neutrophils in these individuals show giant purple-gray cytoplasmic granules (Fig. 10.10). Lymphocytes and monocytes may show a single red granule in the cytoplasm. Current studies suggest that these individuals have a defective fusion protein, which is crucial to lysosomal secretion.[8] White blood cells in patients with Chédiak-Higashi syndrome are not fully functioning and show reduced chemotaxis and bactericidal killing function. Affected children show neutropenia, **albinism**, and photophobia and develop recurrent infections with *Staphylococcus aureus*. Hepatosplenomegaly and liver failure may develop. Platelet function is affected with abnormal bleeding times and small vessel bleeding. The prognosis is poor in most children, who usually die young because of complications of infections.

REACTIVE LYMPHOCYTOSIS IN COMMON DISEASE STATES

It is normal for young children 1 to 4 years old to have a relative lymphocytosis. The white blood cell differential in this age group shows a reversal in the number of lymphocytes to segmented neutrophils from the adult

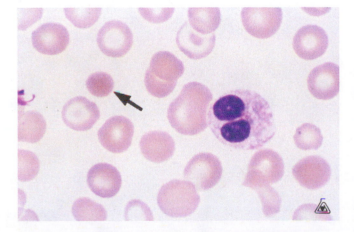

Figure 10.9 Pelger-Huët anomaly. Note spherocyte (at *arrow*) and the typical bilobed appearance of Pelger-Huët cells. From The College of American Pathologists, with permission. American Pathologists, with permission.

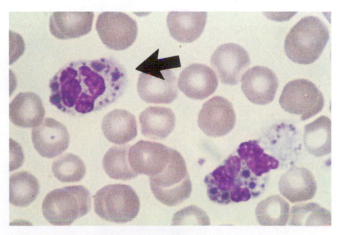

Figure 10.10 Chédiak-Higashi syndrome. Note large gray-green granules in the cytoplasm. From The College of American Pathologists, with permission.

reference range. The lymphocytes, however, have normal morphology (Fig. 10.11).

The most common disease entity displaying variation in lymphocytes is infectious mononucleosis. This viral illness is caused by Epstein-Barr virus (EBV), a member of the human herpesvirus family, type 4. Although young children may become infected with EBV, the virus has a peak incidence at around 20 years of age. Most adults have been exposed to EBV by midlife, and this is recognized by demonstrable antibody titer whether or not they have had an active case of infectious mononucleosis. The virus is found in body fluids, especially saliva, and is frequently passed through exchanges such as kissing, sharing food utensils, or sharing drinking cups. The virus, which incubates for 3 to 4 weeks, enters through the oral passages and infects B lymphocytes. Normal lymphocytes become infected and are transformed into "reactive" (old terminology, "atypical") lymphocytes. Symptoms include sore throat, fatigue, anorexia, fever, and headache. The lymph nodes are usually enlarged, and there may be hepatosplenomegaly. Most individuals have a self-limited course of disease, which is uncomfortable but uncomplicated. Autoimmune hemolytic anemia and elevated liver enzymes may be a complication in less than 1% of patients. Rarely, patients with infectious mononucleosis may experience a cold autoimmune hemolytic anemia, and occasionally thrombocytopenia related to hypersplenism is noted.

Differential diagnosis includes careful examination of the peripheral smear, the results of rapid agglutination tests, and more sophisticated procedures such as enzyme-linked immunosorbent assay (ELISA) or indirect immunofluorescence, which track EBV antigen positivity and measure IgG titers in **convalescence**. The peripheral smear is particularly impressive and

usually shows a reactive lymphocytosis, with 10% to 60% reactive lymphocytes (Fig. 10.12). Morphologically, these lymphocytes are larger than the normal large lymphocytes, with an abundant royal blue cytoplasm, sometimes scalloping the red blood cells. They are easily identified with clumped chromatin material and must be recorded separately (on the differential counter) from other nonreactive normal lymphocytes seen in the smear (Table 10.5). Sometimes the diagnosis of infectious mononucleosis is difficult to make if

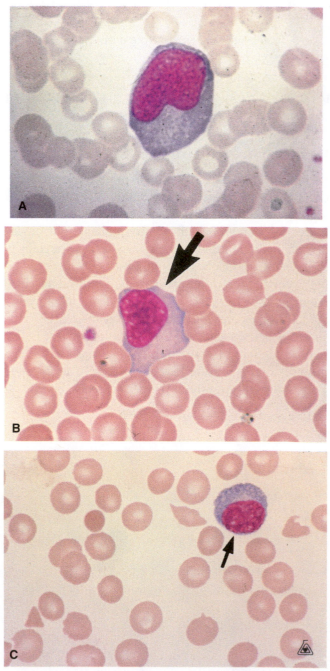

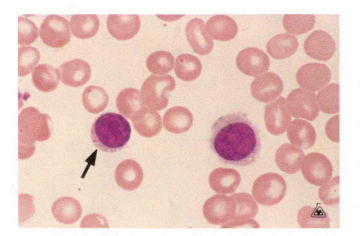

Figure 10.11 **Normal lymphocyte.** From The College of American Pathologists, with permission.

Figure 10.12 Reactive lymphocytes. Note large cells with abundant basophilic cytoplasm. From The College of American Pathologists, with permission.

Table 10.5 ● Lymphocyte Morphologies

	Reactive Lymphocyte	Resting Small Lymphocyte
Size	Large (9–30 μm)	Small (8–12 μm)
N:C ratio	Low to moderate	High to moderate
Cytoplasm	Abundant, colorless to dark blue	Scant, colorless to light blue
Nucleus	Round to irregular	Round
Chromatin	Coarse to moderately fine	Coarse
Nucleoli	Absent to distinct	Absent
Typing	Polyclonal	Polyclonal

the rapid agglutination test is negative, which it is in 10% of cases.[11] The clinician should rely on symptoms, peripheral smear, and professional experience in diagnosing the disease. Although highly accurate, molecular diagnostics are expensive and specialized procedures. There is no treatment for infectious mononucleosis except bed rest and treatment of additional symptoms or possible subsequent infections.

Other Sources of Reactive Lymphocytosis

In most cases, viral disorders affect the CBC in a similar pattern. Most viral disorders have an increased WBC with a depressed number of segmented neutrophils and an increased lymphocyte count. Cytomegalovirus (CMV) and hepatitis A, B, and C viruses may show reactive lymphocytes of a morphology similar to infectious mononucleosis. CMV is a virus that is endemic worldwide. A member of the herpesvirus family, CMV was discovered in 1957 and is similar to EBV. CMV has been isolated from respiratory secretions, urine, semen, and cervical secretions, but it is also found in transplanted organs and donor blood. Anti-CMV titers are present in 40% to 90% of all blood donors, indicating that they have been exposed and have mounted an antibody response.

Most individuals have a subclinical infection and do not even realize that they have had a viral infection. Some individuals have a mononucleosis-like syndrome with low-grade fever and flu-like symptoms. CMV disease can be severe and potentially fatal, however, to immunocompromised individuals, pregnant women, and other vulnerable individuals. Congenital CMV occurs when the mother develops an active CMV infection or when latent CMV becomes reactivated

because of pregnancy. CMV is the leading congenital viral disease. Affected infants may have low birth weight, jaundice, and an enlarged spleen, and the disease may predispose to psychomotor defects or deafness. Affected mothers often are not even aware that they are infected. Donor blood administered to premature infants, patients with multiple transfusions, or immunocompromised patients must be CMV negative.

EFFECT OF HIV/AIDS ON HEMATOLOGY PARAMETERS

HIV is the causative agent of AIDS. In this disease, immune function is eventually obliterated, and patients frequently die of opportunistic infections, such as *Pneumocystis carinii* (now known as *P. Jiroveci*) and *Mycobacterium avium,* or neoplasms, such as Kaposi's sarcoma. Lymphocytes are primarily involved in this disease process, particularly CD4 helper, inducer cells and CD8 suppressor, cytotoxic cells. The normal CD4:CD8 ratio is 2:1. In HIV infection, the level of CD4 cells is drastically reduced, and the CD4:CD8 ratio is reversed, leading to a decline in immune capabilities. Patients have the anemia of inflammation with decreased WBC, decreased platelet count, impaired iron studies, and reticulocytopenia.[12] The lymphocytes show reactive changes, such as extremely basophilic cytoplasm or possibly clefting and vacuolization.

LIPID STORAGE DISEASES

Briefly, the lipid storage diseases are a group of diseases in which a strategic metabolic enzyme is missing or inactive, usually as a result of a single gene deletion (Table 10.6). Because of this missing enzyme, undigested metabolic products accumulate in cells, and cell integrity is affected. Cells of the reticuloendothelial system (RES) are most often affected. The RES is a network of cells seen throughout the circulation and tissues that provide the phagocytic defense system. This network comprises histiocytes; monocytes; macrophages; and the cells of the bone marrow, liver, spleen, and lymph nodes. Consequently, large, easily identifiable cells specific to each disease are located in the bone marrow and are part of the diagnostic picture of many of these disorders. For this reason, these disorders are not frequently observed in the clinical laboratory.

Common Features of a Few Lipid Storage Diseases

Gaucher's disease, Tay-Sachs disease, and Niemann-Pick disease are the three most common lipid storage

Table 10.6 ○	Enzyme Deficiencies in Specific Lipid Storage Diseases
Disease	**Missing Enzyme**
Gaucher's disease	β-Glucocerebrosidase
Niemann-Pick disease	Sphingomyelinase
Tay-Sachs disease	Hexosaminidase A

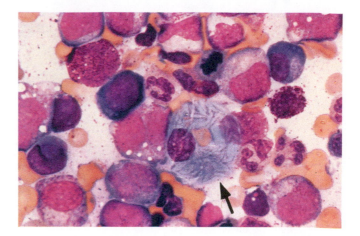

Figure 10.13 Gaucher's cells (bone marrow). Note crinkled tissue paper appearance of cytoplasm. From The College of American Pathologists, with permission.

diseases, and they have many common features. All are autosomal recessive disorders resulting from a single-gene mutation. Abnormal facial features and liver enlargement are seen in Gaucher's disease and Niemann-Pick disease but not Tay-Sachs disease. Although there is a wide range of clinical presentation, from infant onset to adult onset, patients with infant onset have a more severe clinical presentation and a shorter life span. Many of these diseases have a high incidence in the northeast European Jewish population (the Ashkenazi), and for this reason prenatal counseling and genetic screening are highly recommended in affected or extended families. Central nervous system involvement is often a feature of infantile forms of disease, especially Tay-Sachs disease, and short life spans usually prevail.[13] There is no cure for lipid storage diseases, and only supportive therapy can be offered for the most severe manifestations. Enzyme replacement therapy using biosynthetic enzyme material is available in limited quantities.[14] Bone marrow transplantation is also available, but the risks and benefits of this procedure in young children must be carefully considered.

Bone Marrow Cells in Lipid Storage Disorders

Gaucher's disease and Niemann-Pick disease have specific bone marrow cells that are representative of the particular disorder. For Gaucher's disease, the cell is large (20 to 100 μm) with rod-shaped inclusions that appear like crinkled tissue paper in the bone marrow (Fig. 10.13). For Niemann-Pick disease, the cell is equally large but appears round, with evenly sized lipid accumulations (Fig. 10.14). In their own right, each of these cells is striking on bone marrow examination because they are infrequently observed. In Tay-Sachs disease, there is no large identifiable bone marrow cell, but most of these individuals have a deficiency of hexosaminidase A, which can be tested for prenatally.[15] The lymphocytes in each of these disorders may show vacuolization, and although it is a common finding, it is not specific for lipid storage disorders.

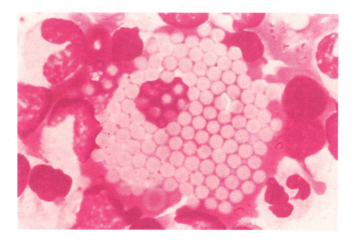

Figure 10.14 Niemann-Pick cell (bone marrow). Cytoplasm shows lipid accumulation. ©1967 American Society of Clinical Pathologists. Reprinted with permission.

BACTERIA AND OTHER UNEXPECTED WHITE BLOOD CELL CHANGES

The presence of bacteria in a peripheral smear indicates bacteremia or sepsis, a condition that may have severe consequences to the patient. Blood is a sterile environment, and the presence of gram-positive or gram-negative bacteria or fungi is unwanted. Bacteria may be seen intracellularly or extracellularly as either cocci or rods. In either case, bacteria must be recognized, and the appropriate health-care providers must be alerted (Figs. 10.15 and 10.16). Precipitated stain may sometimes resemble bacteria; it is important to be positive in identification of bacteria because artifacts may be confusing (Fig. 10.17).

Platelet satellitism has been discussed in a case study in a previous chapter. It is a phenomenon that must be recognized as an unexpected event in a peripheral smear. The blood of some patients reacts

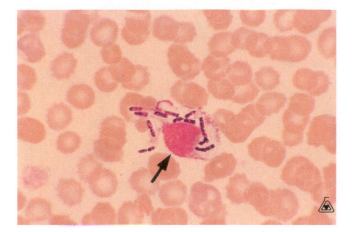

Figure 10.15   Intracellular bacteria in a segmented neutrophil.   From The College of American Pathologists, with permission.

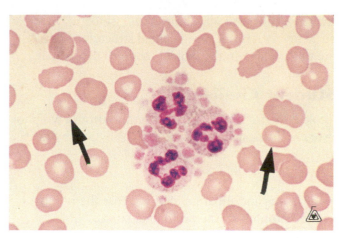

Figure 10.18   Platelet satellitism.   From The College of American Pathologists, with permission.

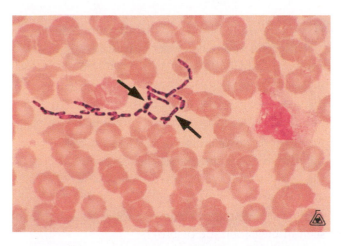

Figure 10.16   Extracellular bacteria in peripheral blood.
From The College of American Pathologists, with permission.

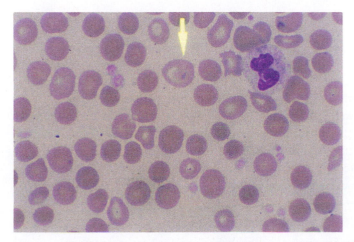

Figure 10.17   Precipitated stain, not bacteria.

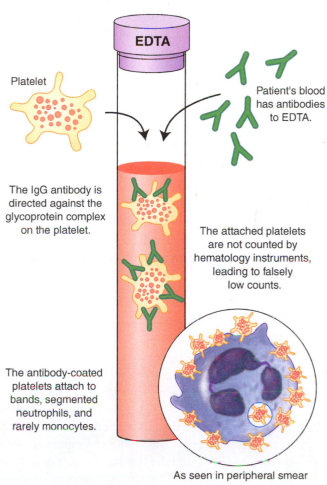

EDTA

Platelet

Patient's blood has antibodies to EDTA.

The IgG antibody is directed against the glycoprotein complex on the platelet.

The attached platelets are not counted by hematology instruments, leading to falsely low counts.

The antibody-coated platelets attach to bands, segmented neutrophils, and rarely monocytes.

As seen in peripheral smear

Figure 10.19   Platelet satellitism formation. An unexpected reaction of the patient to EDTA causes platelets to ring around segmented neutrophils.   Adapted from Glassy E. Color Atlas of Hematology: An Illustrated Guide Based on Proficiency Testing. Northfield, IL: College of American Pathologists, 1998, with permission.

with EDTA, causing platelets to form a ring around neutrophils. This is described as platelet satellitism (Fig. 10.18). This event produces a falsely low platelet count and can be corrected only when the patient sample is collected in a sodium citrate tube for an accurate platelet count (Fig. 10.19). An additional peripheral cell change that may occur in segmented neutrophils is **pyknosis**, or pyknotic changes. Pyknosis is seen in degenerated neutrophils as the segmented nucleus becomes an amorphous, smooth, bloblike structure with no clear segmented structure. These cells are not counted in the white blood cell differential.

Student Challenge

Look at Figure 10.20. Is the cell at the arrow a lymphocyte or a nucleated red blood cell? Why or why not?

○ *Summary Points*

• Infections and inflammation increase the number of neutrophils in the peripheral smear.

• Leukocytosis means an increase in WBC.

• Eosinophils are increased in skin diseases, parasitic infections, allergic response, and transplant rejection.

• A left shift signifies that younger white blood cells appear in the peripheral smear, such as occasional metamyelocytes, many bands, and segmented neutrophils.

• Leukemoid reaction is an exaggerated response to infection or inflammation.

• In the leukoerythroblastic picture, young white blood cells, young red blood cells, and abnormal platelets are seen.

• Phagocytosis is a process by which bacteria and other infectious agents are recognized and destroyed by neutrophils and monocytes.

• Toxic changes in white blood cells are observed as toxic granulation, toxic vacuolization, and Döhle bodies.

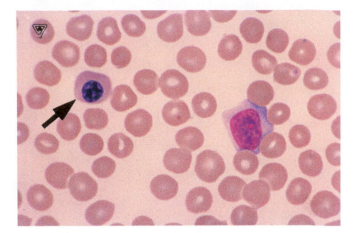

Figure 10.20   Is this a lymphocyte or a nucleated red blood cell? From The College of American Pathologists, with permission.

• Hereditary white blood cell disorders include May-Hegglin anomaly, Pelger-Huët anomaly, Alder's anomaly, and Chédiak-Higashi syndrome.

• Pelger-Huët anomaly is a hyposegmentation disorder in which the lobes of the segmented neutrophils are peanut-shaped or bilobed.

• Alder's anomaly is a disorder in which lipid deposition produces coarse, dark granules in the cytoplasm of granulocytes and occasionally agranulocytes.

• A hypersegmented nucleus, five lobes or more, is seen in megaloblastic disorders.

• Chédiak-Higashi syndrome is a rare autosomal disorder of neutrophilic granules.

CONDENSED CASE

A hemoglobin and hematocrit were ordered on a patient for a surgical floor. The test was performed on the Coulter LH 750, and the hemoglobin and hematocrit were compatible with previous results. The instrument routinely reports the complete CBC, and while observing the entire nine parameters, the operator noticed that the platelet count was only 23,000, a critical value. The delta check on the patient from the previous day showed that the platelet count was 257,000, a significant difference. Corrective action needed to be taken. The operator decided to check the tube that she had just cycled through the instrument for clots, and a small clot was found. *How many times should a purple top tube be inverted when drawn to prevent clotting?*

Answer

The specimen that was sent from the floor was an improper sample that probably had not been properly collected. When drawing blood into a purple top tube, the tube must be inverted five to seven times for proper mixing of the anticoagulant and blood. When the technologist noticed a small clot, corrective action needed to be taken. The technologist now had the responsibility of notifying the nurse of the erroneous results and asking for a redraw. Additionally, the erroneous results needed to be removed from the computer, and documentation of the situation and corrective action needed to be recorded. The sharp eye of the technologist/technician in this case made it possible for reliable results eventually to be obtained.

- Human ehrlichiosis and human granulocytic anaplasmosis represent a group of tick-borne diseases caused by the rickettsia-like bacteria *Ehrlichia chaffeensis* and *Anaplasma phagocytophilum*. Inclusions, known as morulae, may be observed in the granulocytes and monocytes in the bone marrow.

- Reactive lymphocytes are lymphocytes transformed by viral infections or other disorders.

- Reactive lymphocytes are characterized by abundant basophilic cytoplasm, lower N:C ratio, and clumped chromatin material. Marginal erythrocyte molding is seen.

- Infectious mononucleosis is caused by Epstein-Barr virus; patients have low-grade fever, sore throat, swollen glands, anorexia, and headache.

- Individuals with AIDS show pancytopenia and a reversal in CD4 and CD8 lymphocyte ratios.

- Bacteria may appear intracellularly in neutrophils or may appear within the peripheral smear.

- Lipid storage diseases are a group of inherited disorders in which a key metabolic enzyme is missing or inactive.

- Gaucher's disease and Niemann-Pick disease are lipid storage disorders that show large histiocytic-like cells in the bone marrow.

CASE STUDY

A 60-year-old woman was sent for preoperative blood testing before elective gallbladder surgery. Her surgeon ordered a CBC, chemistry panel, and coagulation profile. Her chemistry panel and coagulation profile were normal. Her CBC showed numerous band forms, however, which were flagged on the automated differential. This was an unexpected result, and the surgeon called for a repeat sample. Because her differential was flagged, a slide was pulled and observed for a slide review. *Which conditions may show a high number of bands?*

Insights to the Case Study
The CBC on this patient showed all normal parameters except for the band count in the automated differential. The automated differential in this patient reported 50% bands, clearly unexpected results. Reflex testing was ordered, and a peripheral smear was reviewed. The smear showed large numbers of segmented neutrophils with bilobed or peanut-shaped nuclear material, suggestive of Pelger-Huët anomaly. Pelger-Huët anomaly, discovered in 1928, is an inherited abnormality of the segmented neutrophils in which there is hyposegmentation of the nuclear material. In most cases, it is a heterozygous disorder, and the white blood cells still function normally showing active phagocytic ability and normal leukocyte function. When the disorder occurs homozygously, a single round nucleus is seen. It is essential to differentiate Pelger-Huët anomaly from true band cells because the reporting of 50% bands could lead the physician to suspect septicemia or other serious infectious conditions, which would warrant a left shift. In this case, the surgeon was notified, and the surgery was completed as scheduled.

Review Questions

1. Which of the following inclusions are more likely seen only in the bone marrow?
   a. Toxic granulation
   b. Chédiak-Higashi granules
   c. Morulae from *Ehrlichia* infections
   d. Bacteria

2. In which of the following conditions are monocytes increased?
   a. Tuberculosis
   b. Parasitic infections
   c. Ulcerative colitis
   d. Skin diseases

3. Which of the following is the causative agent in infectious mononucleosis?
   a. HIV
   b. EBV
   c. CMV
   d. CBC

4. The process of ingesting, digesting, and killing bacteria is termed
   a. Opsonization.
   b. Phagocytosis.
   c. Neutrophilia.
   d. Mobilization.

Continued

5. Qualitative changes in the white blood cell include all of the following *except*
   a. Toxic granulation.
   b. Toxic vacuolization.
   c. Gaucher's cells.
   d. Döhle bodies.

6. A 17-year-old boy is admitted to the hospital for a fever of unknown origin. His WBC is $20.0 \times 10^9/L$. All of the following can be seen on his peripheral smear *except*
   a. Toxic granulation.
   b. Reactive monocytes.
   c. Increased band neutrophils.
   d. Döhle bodies.

7. A typical blood picture in infectious mononucleosis is an absolute
   a. Lymphocytosis and anemia with many reactive lymphocytes.
   b. Lymphocytosis without anemia and with many reactive lymphocytes.
   c. Monocytosis and anemia with many atypical monocytes.
   d. Monocytosis without anemia and with many atypical monocytes.

8. Opsonization of neutrophils is defined as
   a. Preparing neutrophils to be ingested.
   b. Degranulation.
   c. Fusion of cytoplasmic granules.
   d. Bactericidal activity.

9. A white blood cell disorder that manifests with a low WBC, thrombocytopenia, and a mulberry-like inclusion in the monocytes is
   a. May-Hegglin anomaly.
   b. Chédiak-Higashi anomaly.
   c. Human ehrlichiosis.
   d. Alder's anomaly.

10. All of the following are mechanisms by which neutropenia is usually produced *except*
   a. Decreased production by the bone marrow.
   b. Impaired release from the bone marrow to the blood.
   c. Increased destruction.
   d. Bacterial infection.

● TROUBLESHOOTING

Is It Precipitated Stain or Is It Bacteria?

A 24-year-old man presented to the emergency department with a fever of unknown origin. CBC, blood cultures, and routine chemistries were ordered. The chemistries came back as normal, and the blood cultures would be read in 24 hours. The CBC results were as follows:

WBC	$35.0 \times 10^9/L$	H
RBC	$3.23 \times 10^{12}/L$	L
Hgb	9.3 g/dL	L
Hct	27.8%	L
MCV	86.0 fL	N
MCH	28.7 pg	N
MCHC	33.5%	N
Platelets	$598 \times 10^9/L$	H
RDW	21.0	H

The elevated WBC was flagged, and reflex testing required that a manual differential be completed. The technologist, on reviewing the peripheral smear, noted several items:

The $35.0 \times 10^9/L$ WBC count correlated with the slide.

Many band forms were seen.

Toxic granulation was noted.

The patient's peripheral smear seemed to show the presence of bacteria intracellularly and extracellularly; however, the technologist was new to the hospital facility, and because this was such an important finding, he needed assistance in making a definite identification.

Differentiating precipitated stain from bacteria is often difficult, but there are some distinct characteristics that can make the identification easier. Microorganisms or bacteria are uniform in size and shape and are usually dispersed throughout the slide. They may be found randomly throughout the peripheral smear, and in most cases, it is lucky that they are visualized at all. Precipitated stain tends to appear in aggregates, which are localized and plentiful. Additionally, precipitated stain tends to lack an organized morphology and looks smudgy or clumpy. In the case of our patient, the technologist consulted several of his peers. Through consensus, it was agreed the inclusions were bacteria. The pathologist was notified, and the floor was contacted. The blood cultures were positive, and the patient was started on high-dose antibiotics and made a complete recovery.

WORD KEY

Albinism • Partial or total absence of pigment in the hair, skin, and eyes

Convalescence • Period of recovery after a disease or surgery

Photophobia • Unusual intolerance of light

Prognostic • Prediction of the chance for recovery

Pyknosis • Shrinkage of nucleus or nuclear material through degeneration

Rhinorrhea • Excessive watery discharge from nose

Sepsis • Systemic inflammatory response to infection that includes symptoms such as fever, hypothermia, tachycardia, and others

References

1. Van Assendelft OW. Reference values for the total and differential leukocyte count. Blood Cells 11:77–96, 1985.
2. Barnes EJ, Abdel-Rehim MM, Goulis Y, et al. Application and limitation of blood eosinophilia for the diagnosis of acute cellular rejection in liver transplantation. Am J Transplant 3:432–438, 2003.
3. Wiseman BK. A newly recognized granulopenic syndrome caused by excessive splenic leukolysis and successfully treated by splenectomy. J Clin Invest 18:473, 1939.
4. Turgeon ML. Clinical Hematology: Theory and Procedures, 4th ed. Baltimore: Lippincott Williams & Wilkins, 2005; 196–200.
5. Ponder E, Ponder RV. The cytology of the polymorphonuclear leukocyte in toxic conditions. J Lab Clin Med 28:316, 1942.
6. Malcolm ID, Flegel KM, Katz M. Vacuolation of the neutrophil in bacteremia. Arch Intern Med 139:675, 1979.
7. Foley A. Nonmalignant hereditary disorders of leukocyte. In: Steine-Martin EA, Lotspeich-Steininger CA, Koepke JA. Clinical Hematology: Principles, Procedures, Correlations, 2nd ed. Philadelphia: Lippincott, 1998; 365.
8. Baetz K, Isaaz S, Griffith SG. Loss of cytotoxic T lymphocyte function in Chediak-Higashi syndrome arises from a secretory defect that prevents granule exocytosis. J Immunol 154:6122, 1995.
9. Eng TR, Harkess JR, Fishbein DB, et al. Epidemiological clinical and laboratory findings of human ehrlichiosis in the U.S. in 1988. JAMA 264:2252–2258, 1990.
10. Bakken JS. Ask the experts: Differentiating human ehrlichiosis from other tick borne illnesses. Infect Dis News September:14–15, 1995.
11. James E. Unmasking infectious mononucleosis. ADVANCE for Medical Laboratory Professionals. March 22, 2004.
12. Cosby C, Holzemer WL, Henry SB, et al. Hematologic complications and quality of life in hospitalized AIDS patients. AIDS Patient Care STDS 14:269, 2000.
13. Kolodney EH, Tenembaum AL. Storage diseases of the reticuloendothelial system. In: D. Nathan and F. Oski, eds., Nathan and Oski's Hematology of Infancy and Childhood, 4th ed. Philadelphia: WB Saunders, 1992; 1453–1464.
14. Graubowski GA, Pastores GM. Enzyme replacement therapy in type I Gaucher disease. Gaucher Clin Perspect 1:8, 1993.
15. Harmening DM, Spier CM. Lipid (lysosomal) storage disease and histiocytosis. In: Harmening DM, ed. Clinical Hematology and Fundamentals of Hemostasis, 4th ed. Philadelphia: FA Davis, 2002; 633.

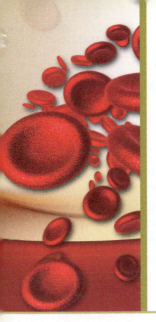

Chapter 11

Acute Leukemias

Barbara Caldwell

Objectives

After completing this chapter, the student will be able to:

1. Compare and contrast acute versus chronic leukemia with respect to age of onset, presenting symptoms, and organ involvement.

2. Describe acute leukemia with emphasis on symptoms and peripheral blood and bone marrow findings.

3. Classify acute leukemias according to the French-American-British (FAB) classification system.

4. Briefly describe the World Health Organization (WHO) classification for acute myeloid leukemias and related myeloid proliferations.

5. Describe how cytochemical staining can aid in the diagnosis of acute leukemias.

6. Identify the most consistent cytogenetic abnormalities in acute leukemias.

7. List the most pertinent CD markers for various acute leukemias.

8. Briefly explain the WHO classification of acute lymphoblastic leukemia/lymphoma.

9. Describe acute lymphoblastic leukemia with emphasis on age of onset, symptoms at presentation, prognosis, and laboratory findings.

10. State the factors that may influence the prognosis in acute lymphoblastic leukemias/lymphomas.

DEFINITION OF LEUKEMIA

Leukemia is caused by the mutation of the bone marrow pluripotent or most primitive stem cells. This neoplastic expansion results in abnormal, leukemic cells and impaired production of normal red blood cells, leukocytes, and platelets. As the mutant cell line takes hold and normal hematopoiesis is inhibited, the leukemic cells spill into the peripheral blood and invade the reticuloendothelial tissue, specifically the spleen, liver, lymph nodes, and sometimes the central nervous system (CNS). The leukemic stem cells have abnormal growth and maturation capability. The mutant clone may show unique morphologic, cytogenetic, and immunophenotypic features that can be used to aid in the classification of the particular type of leukemia. Many leukemias have similar clinical features, but regardless of the subtype, the disease is fatal if left untreated.

COMPARING ACUTE AND CHRONIC LEUKEMIA

The initial evaluation of leukemia includes the following:

1. Noting the onset of symptoms
2. Analyzing the complete blood count (CBC) results
3. Observing the *type* of cells that predominate (cell **lineage**)
4. Assessing the *maturity* of cells that predominate

Because leukemia is a disease of the bone marrow that causes normal bone marrow cell production to be crowded out as the abnormal, neoplastic cells take over, the CBC results commonly show a decreased RBC or anemia and a decrease in platelets or thrombocytopenia. The level of anemia and thrombocytopenia tends to be more severe in acute leukemia. Leukocytosis is a hallmark feature of chronic leukemia, and because the spleen also becomes a site of extramedullary (outside of the bone marrow) hematopoiesis, prominent hepatosplenomegaly is also most often associated with chronic leukemia.

The type of cell that predominates in the peripheral blood and the bone marrow is defined according to *cell lineage* as either myeloid or lymphoid. The myeloid stem cell gives birth to granulocytes, monocytes, megakaryocytes, and erythrocytes (see Fig. 2.3). As described in subsequent sections of this chapter, myeloid leukemias can involve proliferation of any stage of these four cell lines. By contrast, the lymphoid stem cell gives rise solely to lymphocytic lineage cells.

Cell maturity can be used to separate the initial diagnosis between acute and chronic leukemias. When blasts or other immature cells predominate, the leukemia is classified as *acute*; when more mature cell types predominate, the leukemia is classified as *chronic*. The onset of acute versus chronic leukemia is distinctly different. Acute leukemia has a quick onset, whereas chronic leukemia has a slow, insidious course and may be discovered on routine physical examination. Age is another factor that is often consistent in the different leukemic variants. Although acute leukemia may occur at any age, chronic leukemia is usually seen in adults (Table 11.1).

Using the cell lineage and the maturity of cells that predominate, leukemias can be categorized into the following four broad groups:

1. Acute myelogenous leukemias (AMLs)
2. Acute lymphoblastic leukemias (ALLs)
3. Chronic myelocytic leukemias (CMLs) (see Chapter 12)
4. Chronic lymphocytic leukemias (CLLs) (see Chapter 13)

LEUKEMIA HISTORY

It is important to give credit to early scientists who were able to recognize and define leukemia through astute clinical observations and postmortem analysis in

Table 11.1 ● Comparison of Characteristics of Acute and Chronic Leukemia

Characteristic	Acute Leukemia	Chronic Leukemia
Onset	Abrupt	Subtle
Morbidity	Months	Years
Age	All	Adults
WBC	Variable	Elevated
Predominant cells	Blasts and other immature white blood cells	Mature
Anemia, thrombocytopenia	Present	Variable
Neutropenia	Present	Variable
Organomegaly	Mild	Marked

an age when little technology existed save a crude microscope. A brief discussion of the pertinent discoveries that occurred more than 100 years ago gives one a great appreciation of just how far the science of hematology has progressed in such a short time.

In 1845, two scientists in separate countries made early descriptions of leukemia. Virchow[1] in Germany and Bennett[2] in Scotland both studied a series of autopsy findings from individuals who died with very enlarged spleens and livers (hepatosplenomegaly). Virchow is credited with assigning the term *weisses blut* ("white blood"), which is translated into Greek as *leukemia.* Both Bennett and Virchow came to believe that leukemia is caused by a cancerous overgrowth of the white blood cells. Virchow showed by further studies that one could classify the cases into two groups—cases with mostly large spleens and cases with predominantly lymph nodes enlarged.[3] We now know that these groups represent a distinction between CML and CLL.

The next conceptual proposal came in 1878 from Neumann,[4] who suggested that the origin of blood cells was the bone marrow, and leukemia was a disease of the bone marrow. He used the term *myelogene,* which is the origin of the later term *myelogenous leukemia.* In 1889, Epstein[5] was the first to use the term *acute leukemia,* designating cases wherein the patients died within months from manifestation of first symptoms. He noted that these patients had very purulent blood and surmised by this gross observation of "white blood" that there was an incredible increase in white blood cells. He was eventually able to lead the hematology forefathers of his day to recognize a separation between what we now call AML and a more chronic, slow onset that we now recognize as CML.

Proof of these early scientists' ingenuity is the fact that until 1877, when Ehrlich developed a polychromatic stain that allowed blood cells to be distinguished, scientists were able to observe only colorless cells under the microscope.[6] When the use of Ehrlich's stains became widespread, scientists around the turn of the 20th century were able to show that acute leukemia was associated with early blast cells, and chronic leukemia was associated with more mature cells. The description of a myeloblast and a myelocyte were documented by Naegeli in 1900.[7] Several years later, Schilling first described the existence of monoblastic leukemia. Hirschfield[8] made the important connection that red blood cells and white blood cells share a common cell of origin.

The combined discoveries of these scientists laid the foundation for current understanding of leukemia.

As new research and application of new techniques continue to refine the classification of leukemia, changes in treatment protocols lead to improved survival statistics.

ACUTE MYELOID LEUKEMIA

AML is a malignant, clonal disease that involves proliferation of blasts in bone marrow, blood, or other tissue. The blasts most often show myeloid or monocytic differentiation. Almost 80% of patients with AML have chromosome abnormalities, usually a mutation resulting from a chromosomal translocation (the transfer of one portion of chromosome to another).[9] The translocation causes abnormal **oncogene** or tumor suppressor gene expression, and this results in uncontrolled cellular proliferation. Genetic syndromes and toxic exposure contribute to the pathogenesis in some patients.

Although the diseases grouped into the AML categories have similar clinical manifestations, the morphology, immunophenotyping, and cytogenetic features are distinct. Cytochemical stains are used along with morphology to help identify the lineage of the blast population. Electron microscopy may also be used to subclassify the various leukemias. Flow cytometry is increasingly used specifically to tag the myeloid or lymphoid antigens and classify the acute leukemias. Molecular studies are employed to establish clonality and identify translocations and gene mutations (Table 11.2).

Epidemiology

The incidence of AML increases with age, accounting for 80% of acute leukemias in adults and 15% to 20% of acute leukemias in children. When congenital leukemia (occurring during the neonatal period) does rarely occur, however, it is paradoxically AML rather than ALL, and it is often monocytic. The rate of occurrence of AML is greater in males than females, and there is an increased incidence in developed, more industrialized countries. Eastern European Jews have an increased risk of developing AML, whereas Asians have a decreased risk.[10]

Table 11.3 lists the conditions that have been documented as predisposing to development of AML. The high incidence of individuals with congenital defects (e.g., Down syndrome [DS]) and bone marrow failure syndromes (e.g., Fanconi's anemia) has shown that these factors are often implicated in the pathogenesis of AML. It is also well documented that leukemia is associated with exposure to ionizing radiation, as

Table 11.2 ◉ Methods Useful in the Diagnosis of Acute Leukemia

Morphology	• Provides initial diagnostic information
	• Can often distinguish acute leukemia from a reactive process
	• Helps to distinguish AML, ALL, and myelodysplastic syndrome
Cytochemistry	• Rapid, readily accessible type of testing
	• Provides quick diagnostic information
Immunophenotyping	• Differentiates ALL from AML
	• Classifies subtypes of AML
	• Separates precursor B-ALL from precursor T-ALL
	• Provides vital information for treatment decisions
	• Provides prognostic information
	• Detects minimal residual disease
Cytogenetics	• Classifies subtypes of AML and ALL
	• Provides prognostic information
Molecular studies	• Identifies translocation and gene mutations
	• Establishes clonality
	• Detects minimal residual disease

Table 11.3 ◉ Conditions and Disorders with Increased Risk for Development of Acute Leukemia

Congenital Defects	Acquired Diseases	Environmental Factors
Down syndrome	Aplastic anemia	Ionizing radiation
Klinefelter syndrome	Myeloma	Alkylating agents
Turner syndrome	Sideroblastic anemia	Cytotoxic drugs
Monosomy 7 syndrome	Acquired genetic changes	Pesticide exposure
Fanconi's anemia	Translocations	Solvents
Wiskott-Aldrich syndrome	Inversions	
Neurofibromatosis	Deletions	
Familial aplastic anemia	Point mutations	
Fraternal twins and nonidentical siblings	Paroxysmal nocturnal hemoglobinuria	
Combined immunodeficiency syndrome	Transition from other hematopoietic diseases (myeloproliferative disorders)	
Blackfan-Diamond syndrome		

this was most notably reported with the increase in leukemia that occurred after the release of atomic bombs over Hiroshima and Nagasaki in 1945. The fallout from atomic bombs and exposure to nuclear reactor plants have caused much well-founded public apprehension, fear, and concern over the past 50 years.[11,12] A wide variety of chemicals and drugs have been linked to AML. In a study involving factories in China, the risk of developing leukemia was five to six times higher in workers with recurrent exposure to benzene than in the general population.[13] Many drugs, particularly therapy-related alkylating drugs, are associated with post-treatment AML. All of the chronic myeloproliferative disorders—CML, idiopathic myelofibrosis (IMF), polycythemia vera, and essential thrombocythemia—have an increased propensity for terminating in AML, with 60% to 70% of CML cases undergoing a transition to AML.

Clinical Features

All of the signs and symptoms that occur so abruptly in patients with AML are caused by the infiltration of the bone marrow with leukemic cells and the resulting failure of normal hematopoiesis. These leukemic cells that invade the bone marrow are dysfunctional, and without the normal hematopoietic elements the patient is at risk for developing life-threatening complications of anemia, infection secondary to functional neutropenia, and hemorrhage from thrombocytopenia (Table 11.4).

Fatigue and weakness are the most common complaints that reflect the development of anemia. Pallor, **dyspnea** on exertion, heart palpitations, and a general loss of well-being have been described.[14] Fever is present is about 15% to 20% of patients and may be the result of bacterial, fungal, and, less frequently, viral infections, or may result from the leukemic burden of cells on tissues and organs. Easy bruising, petechiae, and mucosal bleeding may be found secondary to thrombocytopenia. Other, more severe symptoms related to decreased platelet counts that occur less commonly are gastrointestinal or genitourinary tract symptoms and CNS bleeding. CNS infiltration with high numbers of leukemic cells has been reported in 5% to 20% of children and approximately 15% of adults with AML.[15,16] Headache, blindness, and other neurologic complications are indications of meningeal involvement. Leukemic blast cells circulate through the peripheral blood and may invade any tissue. Extramedullary hematopoiesis is common in monocytic or myelomonocytic leukemias. Organs that were active in fetal hematopoiesis may be reactivated to produce cells when stressed by the poor performance of the overladen leukemic bone marrow. Hepatosplenomegaly and lymphadenopathy may occur but are not as prominent as in the chronic leukemias. Skin infiltration is very characteristic in monocytic leukemia, particularly gum infiltration that is termed **gingival hyperplasia**. When leukemic cells crowd the bone marrow of the long bones, joint pain may be produced.

Laboratory Features

Peripheral Blood and Bone Marrow Findings

CBC and examination of peripheral blood smear are the first steps in the laboratory diagnosis of leukemia. Blood cell counts are variable in patients with AML. WBC may be normal, increased, or decreased. It is markedly elevated (greater than 100×10^9/L cells) in less than 20% of cases. Conversely, WBC is less than 5.0×10^9/L, with an absolute neutrophil count of less than 1.0×10^9/L, in about half of patients at the time of diagnosis.[17] Blasts are usually seen on the peripheral smear, but in leukopenic patients, the numbers may be few and require diligent search to uncover. Cytoplasmic inclusions known as **Auer rods** are often present in a small percentage of the myeloblasts, monoblasts, or promyelocytes that occur in the various subtypes of AML. Auer rods are elliptical, spindlelike inclusions composed of azurophilic granules. Nucleated red blood cells may be present, as well as myelodysplastic features, including pseudohyposegmentation (pseudo–Pelger-Huët cells) or hypersegmentation of the neutrophils and hypogranulation.

Anemia is a very common feature resulting from inadequate production of normal red blood cells. The reticulocyte count is usually normal or decreased. Red blood cell anisopoikilocytosis is mildly abnormal, with few poikilocytes present. Thrombocytopenia, which can be severe, is almost always a feature at diagnosis. Giant platelets and agranular platelets may be seen. Disseminated intravascular coagulation (DIC) is most commonly associated with the type of AML known as acute promyelocytic leukemia (APL). DIC is caused by the release of tissue factor–like procoagulants from the azurophilic granules of the neoplastic promyelocytes,

Table 11.4 ⊙ Clinical Findings in Acute Leukemia	
Pathogenesis	**Signs and Symptoms**
Bone marrow infiltration	
Neutropenia	Fever, infection
Anemia	Pallor, dyspnea, lethargy
Thrombocytopenia	Bleeding, petechiae, ecchymosis, intracranial hematoma, and gastrointestinal or conjunctival hemorrhage (rare)
Medullary infiltration	
Marrow	Bone pain and tenderness, limp, arthralgia
Extramedullary infiltration	
Liver, spleen, lymph nodes, thymus	Organomegaly
CNS	Neurologic complications including dizziness, headache, vomiting, alteration of mental function
Gums, mouth	Gingival bleeding and hypertrophy
Skin	Lesions or granulocytic sarcoma

which activate coagulation and further consume platelets, leading to dangerous bleeding diathesis.

Before treatment, serum uric acid and lactate dehydrogenase levels often are mildly or moderately increased.

The hallmark feature of acute leukemia is always a hypercellular bone marrow, with 20% to 90% leukemic blasts at diagnosis or during relapse. The blast population grows indiscriminately because these cells have only limited differentiation capability and are frozen in the earliest stage of development. The lineage of blasts that predominate depends on the specific type of acute leukemia. The most current classification for hematologic and lymphoid tumors published by the World Health Organization (WHO) recommends that the requisite blast percentage for a diagnosis of AML be greater than or equal to 20% myeloblasts in the blood or marrow.[18] When performing a peripheral blood smear on a patient with a suspected diagnosis of leukemia, at least 200 white blood cells should be classified. It is recommended that the blast percentage in the bone marrow be derived from a 500-cell differential count. If the WBC is less than 2.0×10^9/L, buffy coat smears should be prepared for differential count.

Myeloblasts may be distinguished from lymphoblasts in three ways: presence of Auer rods, reactivity with cytochemical stains, or reactivity with cell surface markers (e.g., cluster of differentiation [CD] groups CD13 and CD33) on blasts with specific monoclonal antibodies. An experienced morphologist can often determine the morphology of blasts; however, other supporting tests are always needed to confirm the initial designation. Figure 11.1 shows the features that can be used to differentiate a myeloblast from a lymphoblast. The chromatin material of a myeloblast is usually much finer than that of a lymphoblast. A myeloblast often has more cytoplasm than a lymphoblast. Size of the blast and number of nucleoli may not be helpful characteristics. Although a myeloblast is usually larger than a lymphoblast, sufficient variations are seen that this is not the best factor to consider. Along the same lines, the number of nucleoli that can be seen in a myeloblast is one to four, and the number of lymphoblasts is one to two, so when deciding lineage on a blast with two obvious nucleoli, either choice would be acceptable. Of the characteristic features listed in Figure 11.1, the chromatin staining pattern is usually the most helpful. As mentioned previously, other methods besides morphologic examination must be used to confirm the type of blasts present and often to quantify the number of blasts, particularly when two blast populations coexist in the significant amounts in the leukemic bone marrow.

Five percent to 10% of AMLs have a preleukemic presentation termed "myelodysplastic syndrome." These patients are usually older than 50 years and have anemia, thrombocytopenia, and monocytosis but with bone marrow blast percentages of less than 20% (see Chapter 14). Other studies that can be used to aid in the diagnosis of acute leukemias include cytochemical

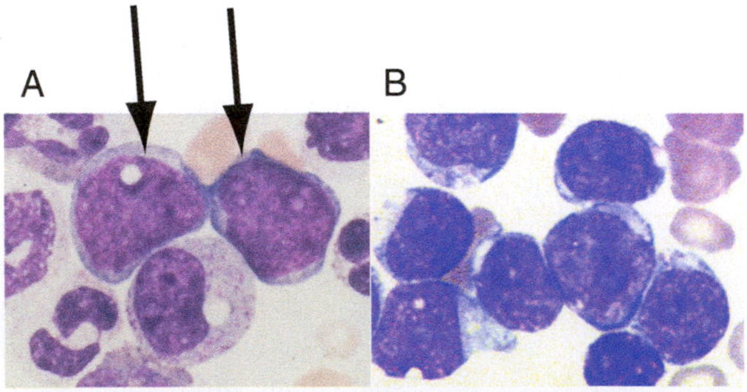

	Myeloblast	*Lymphoblast*
Size	15-20 μm	10-15 μm
Chromatin	Fine	Moderately condensed
Nucleoli	1-4, prominent	1-2, often inconspicuous
Cytoplasm	Moderate, basophilic	Scant
Auer rods	May be present	Absent

Figure 11.1 Comparison of myeloblast (A) and lymphoblast (B) morphology.

stains, chromosome analysis, molecular genetic studies, DNA flow cytometry, and electron microscopy.

Cytochemical Stains

Cytochemical stains are very helpful in the diagnosis and classification of acute leukemias (Table 11.5). These stains are usually performed on bone marrow smears but may also be done on peripheral smears or bone marrow touch preparations. Because the special stains are used to identify enzymes or lipids within the *blast* population of cells, the reaction in mature cells is not important. Positive reactions are associated with a particular lineage. With some stains (e.g., myeloperoxidase [MPO] and Sudan black B [SBB]), the fine or coarse staining intensity indicates the lineage of blast cells. All of the cytochemical stains described subsequently yield negative results in lymphoid cells (with rare exceptions), so a positive result with any of these most often rules out ALL (Table 11.6). Many institutions have replaced cytochemical stains with immunologic testing that uses flow cytometry or immunohistochemistry or both.

Myeloperoxidase

Primary granules of myeloid cells contain peroxidase. The granules are found in the late myeloblast and exist throughout all the myeloid maturation stages. Because primary granules are absent in myeloblasts, there is limited MPO activity in early myeloblasts; however, the blasts that are closer to maturing to the promyelocyte stage stain positive. Promyelocytes, myelocytes, metamyelocytes, and band and segmented neutrophils stain strongly positive, indicated by the presence of blue-black granules. Monocytic granules stain faintly positive. Because lymphoid cells, nucleated red blood cells, and megakaryoblasts lack this enzyme, they stain negative. This negative reaction is useful in initially differentiating ALL from AML. Eosinophils also stain positive for MPO. Auer rods are strongly positive for peroxidase. The enzymatic activity in blood smears fades over time, so slides should not be held for staining for more than 3 weeks. MPO stain is positive in AML (greater than 3% positive), APL (90% to 100% positive), acute myelomonocytic leukemia, acute monoblastic and monocytic leukemia (variable), and the myeloblasts present in acute erythroid leukemia (myeloblasts greater than 3% positive).

Sudan Black B

Phospholipids and other intracellular lipids are stained by SBB. Phospholipids are found in the primary (nonspecific) and secondary (specific) granules

Table 11.5 ● Acute Leukemia Cytochemistry

Cytochemical Stain	Cellular Element Stained	Blasts Identified
MPO	Neutrophil primary granules	Myeloblasts strong positive; monoblasts faint positive
SBB	Phospholipids	Myeloblasts strong positive; monoblasts faint positive
Specific esterase (CAE)	Cellular enzyme	Myeloblasts strong positive
NSE	Cellular enzyme	Monoblasts strong positive
TdT	Intranuclear enzyme	Lymphoblasts positive
PAS	Glycogen	Variable, coarse or blocklike positivity often seen in lymphoblasts and pronormoblasts, myeloblasts usually negative, although faint diffuse reaction may occasionally be seen

Table 11.6 ● Cytochemical Reactions in Acute Leukemia

Acute Leukemia	MPO/SBB	CAE	NSE	PAS
AML	++	+ (myeloblasts)	+ (monoblasts, diffuse ++)	+/−
ALL	Negative	Negative	Negative (majority) (rare +)	++ (block +)

CAE, chloroacetate esterase; MPO, myeloperoxidase; NSE, non-specific esterase; PAS, periodic acid–Schiff; SBB, Sudan Black B.

of neutrophilic cells and eosinophils and in smaller quantities in monocytes and macrophages. The stain is negative in lymphocytes, although rarely azurophilic granules of lymphoblasts may show positivity. SBB pattern of staining mimics MPO stain in that it is very sensitive for granulocyte precursors, increases in staining intensity with the later stages of granulocytic maturation, and stains weakly positive with monocytic cells. This stain can also be used to differentiate AML from ALL. A distinct advantage of SBB over MPO stain is that the SBB-stained slides are stable for a longer period.

Specific Esterase (Naphthol AS-D Chloroacetate Esterase)

The specific esterase enzyme is present in the primary granules of myeloid cells. Myeloblasts and other neutrophilic cells in AML stain positive. Naphthol AS-D chloroacetate esterase (CAE) also is positive in basophils and mast cells but negative in eosinophils, monocytes, and lymphocytes. The specific esterase enzymatic reaction is stable in paraffin-embedded tissue sections, making this an extremely useful stain for identifying cells of myeloid lineage in extramedullary myeloid tumors.[19]

Nonspecific Esterase (Alpha-Naphthyl Butyrate or Alpha-Naphthyl Acetate Esterase)

Nonspecific esterase (NSE) stains are used to identify monocytic cells and stain negative with granulocytes. Different substrates are available, with alpha-naphthyl butyrate stain considered more specific and alpha-naphthyl acetate stain considered more sensitive. Many cells in addition to monocytes stain positive (macrophages, histiocytes, megakaryoblasts, and some carcinomas), so the sodium fluoride inhibition step is used to differentiate the positivity. With this step, after initial staining, NSE activity of monocytes and macrophages is inhibited (reaction was positive, then reaction is negative), whereas the activity of the other cells remains positive. Mature T lymphocytes stain a coarse dotlike pattern. NSE stain is used to identify the monoblast and promonocyte populations in acute monoblastic leukemia and acute myelomonocytic leukemia. In 10% to 20% of cases of acute monoblastic leukemia, NSE stain is weakly positive or negative, however. In these cases, immunophenotyping can be used to confirm monocytic differentiation.[18]

Terminal Deoxynucleotidyl Transferase

Terminal deoxynucleotidyl transferase (TdT) is an intranuclear enzyme found in stem cells and immature lymphoid cells within the bone marrow but not in mature B lymphocytes. It is present in 90% of ALLs

but only 5% to 10% of acute myeloblastic leukemias.[20] TdT has also been shown in one-third of cases of the blast crisis stage of CML and is a good prognostic indicator in these patients.[21,22]

Immunophenotype

Immunophenotyping is routinely used to help to classify the clone of leukemic blasts by employing monoclonal antibodies that are directed against cell surface markers. The specific lineage and stage of maturation can be tagged, and this information is used to recommend appropriate therapy and can be correlated to prognosis. The blasts in many subtypes of acute leukemias have characteristic immunophenotyping reactions. Clinicians would have difficulty making a diagnosis without this information, whereas in other cases the immunophenotype is just one additional piece of diagnostic information. Immunophenotyping can help differentiate ALL from acute myeloblastic leukemia, distinguish precursor B and precursor T ALL, and identify subtypes of AML.

Immunophenotyping is performed by flow cytometry or by immunohistochemistry methods. Multiple antigens can be detected simultaneously on a single cell using flow cytometry. Table 11.7 shows a selected panel of monoclonal antibodies.

Molecular Analysis

Molecular analysis can be used to identify clonality, such as immunoglobulin gene rearrangements. It can also be performed to establish translocations such as

Table 11.7 ⊙ Immunophenotypic Classification	
Lineage	**Marker**
Hematopoietic precursor	CD117 (HLA-DR), CD34
Myeloid	CD11b, CD13, CD33, CD15
T lineage	CD1, CD2, CD3, CD4, CD5, CD7, CD8, TdT
B lineage	CD10, CD19, CD20, CD21A, CD22, CD23, CD24, CD79a, TdT
Erythroid	Glycophorin A
Monocytic	CD14, CD4, CD11b, CD11c, CD36, CD64
Megakaryocytic	CD41, CD42, CD61

PML/RARA fusion resulting from 15:17 translocation in APL and to identify gene mutations (e.g., *FLT3*, *KIT* mutations). As with immunophenotyping, molecular analysis is helpful for detecting minimal residual disease and establishing prognostic indicators.

Genetic Studies

The 2008 WHO classification of AMLs defines numerous diseases that can be identified by specific genetic markers.[23] Particular gene mutations and gene rearrangements secondary to chromosomal translocations are also included. Many of the most important mutations that may be seen in AML are described subsequently.

The assignment of the particular nomenclature for the type of leukemia is based on the combined morphologic, immunophenotypic, cytochemical, cytogenetic, and sometimes molecular information and any unique clinical presentation. The array of cytologic and clinical information is used to suggest the best approximation of the subtype of leukemia, recognizing that knowledge is sometimes imperfect and that changes in these classifications will undoubtedly occur again in the future as understanding of the science of leukemia evolves.

Classifications

The morphologic variants of AML may occur as a primary presentation or may be the result of a clonal evolution from other disorders such as the myeloproliferative disorders of CML, IMF, or essential thrombocythemia. Acute leukemias are categorized according to the cell line and stage of maturation that predominate. To classify acute leukemias consistently, in 1976 the French-American-British (FAB) group developed a system of nomenclature that separated AMLs from ALLs. As it evolved over the years, the FAB classification scheme designated multiple subtypes for the various AMLs (M0 to M7), and three subtypes (L1 to L3) for the ALLs (Table 11.8). The classification was initially based solely on morphology of the cells present; however, later results of cytochemistry staining reactions were incorporated into the classification. The requisite blast percentage derived from bone marrow examination using the FAB classification is greater than 30%.

The FAB classification has been problematic for several reasons. Immunophenotyping, cytogenic analyses, and molecular analyses are not well defined for the individual subtypes. Also, the FAB classification does not clearly separate out the groups of patients with positive clinical outcomes. Because of these limitations, and because of the discovery of numerous genetic lesions that can predict clinical outcomes much better than just a morphology-based delineation, hematopathologists convened by WHO in 1997 proposed a new classification for AMLs. The resulting scheme proposed by the WHO group incorporated specific genetic data into the classification of hematopoietic and lymphopoietic tumors.[24] The use of these genetic data provides objective definitions for acute leukemia disease recognition and helps to identify antigens, genes, or pathways that are targeted for therapy.

The fourth edition of the *World Health Organization Classification of Tumours of Haematopoietic and Lymphoid Tissues*[23] incorporates changes into the first four original categories as defined in the third WHO edition (AML with recurrent genetic abnormalities, AML with myelodysplasia-related changes, therapy-related myeloid neoplasms, and AML not otherwise specified [NOS]) and added three new categories (myeloid sarcoma, myeloid proliferations related to DS, and blastic

Table 11.8 ● FAB Classification of Acute Leukemia*	
Designation	**Descriptive Name**
M0	Acute myeloblastic leukemia, minimally differentiated
M1	Acute myeloblastic leukemia without maturation
M2	Acute myeloblastic leukemia with maturation
M3	Acute promyelocytic leukemia, hypergranular
M3v	Acute promyelocytic leukemia, microgranular
M4	Acute myelomonocytic leukemia
M4Eo	Acute myelomonocytic leukemia with eosinophilia
M5a	Acute monoblastic leukemia, poorly differentiated
M5b	Acute monoblastic leukemia, with differentiation
M6	Erythroleukemia
M7	Acute megakaryoblastic leukemia
L1†	Acute lymphoblastic leukemia
L2†	Acute lymphoblastic leukemia
L3†	Acute lymphoblastic leukemia, leukemic phase of Burkitt's lymphoma

*For historic review only.
†Based on blast morphology

plasmacytoid dendritic cell neoplasms) (Table 11.9). In addition, leukemias with no single lineage differentiation are described as "*acute leukemias of ambiguous lineage.*" Notably, the most significant change from the FAB classification is that the required blast percentage for a diagnosis of AML using the WHO criteria is greater than or equal to *20%* myeloblasts in the blood or marrow compared with the FAB blast percentage criteria of *30%* that has been used for many years.[18]

Because the WHO classification is the most current classification, each of the subtypes of AMLs and related myeloid proliferations is briefly discussed (Table 11.10). Because technology of genetic and molecular analysis is moving so rapidly, however, it is

---

Table 11.9 ● 2008 World Health Organization (WHO) Categories of Acute Myeloid Leukemia and Related Myeloid Proliferations

Descriptive Name

Acute myeloid leukemia with recurrent genetic abnormalities	Myeloid sarcoma
Acute myeloid leukemia with myelodysplasia-related changes	Myeloid proliferations related to Down syndrome
Therapy-related myeloid neoplasms	Blastic plasmacytoid dendritic cell neoplasm
Acute myeloid leukemia, not otherwise specified	

Table 11.10 ● 2008 WHO Classification of Acute Myeloid Leukemias and Related Myeloid Proliferations

Acute myeloid leukemia with recurrent genetic abnormalities (chromosome abnormality and fusion genes listed)
- AML with t(8;21)(q22;q22); *RUNX1-RUNX1T1*
- AML with inv(16)(p13.1q22) or t(16;16)(p13.1;q22); *CBFB-MYH11*
- APL with t(15;17)(q22;q12); *PML-RARA*
- AML with t(9;11)(p22;q23); *MLLT3-MLL*
- AML with t(6;9)(p23;q34); *DEK-NUP214*
- AML with inv(3)(q21q26.s) or t(3;3)(q21;q26.2); *PRN1-EVl1*
- AML (megakaryoblastic) with t(1;22)(p13;q13); *RBM15-MKL1*

Acute myeloid leukemia with myelodysplasia-related changes
Therapy-related myeloid neoplasms
Acute myeloid leukemia not otherwise specified
- AML with minimal differentiation
- AML without maturation
- AML with maturation
- Acute myelomonocytic leukemia
- Acute monoblastic and monocytic leukemia
- Acute erythroid leukemia
- Acute megakaryoblastic leukemia
- Acute basophilic leukemia
- Acute panmyelosis with myelofibrosis

Myeloid sarcoma
Myeloid proliferations related to Down syndrome
Blastic plasmacytoid dendritic cell neoplasm

likely that modifications to this classification scheme will be necessary on a periodic basis.

I. Acute Myeloid Leukemia With Recurrent Genetic Abnormalities

The most important features of AMLs with recurrent genetic abnormalities are the recurrent genetic abnormality and favorable prognosis. The abnormalities that are commonly identified involve reciprocal translocations. Four subtypes are described. The reader is referred to other hematology reference texts for an in-depth discussion of immunophenotypes and genetics that are characteristic for each disorder.

Acute Myeloid Leukemia With t(8;21)(q22;q22); *RUNX1-RUNX1T1*

AML with t(8;21) occurs most often in children or young adults and represents 5% to 12% of AML cases.[25] The translocation t(8;21)(q22;q22) and, more recently, the *RUNX1-RUNX1T1* fusion gene are the hallmark features of this subtype. The morphology associated with this AML includes the presence of myeloblasts with abundant cytoplasm, often containing azurophilic granules and sometimes containing large, pseudo–Chédiak-Higashi granules. Auer rods are common, and maturation in the neutrophil lineage (promyelocytes, myelocytes, neutrophils) is seen. **Dysplastic** neutrophilic features that may be seen include pseudo–Pelger-Huët hyposegmentation and hypogranulation. Eosinophils are often increased, and monocytes are usually decreased (Fig. 11.2). AML with t(8;21) is associated with good response to chemotherapy and long-term survival rates.

Acute Myeloid Leukemia With inv(16)(p13q22) or t(16;16)(p13;q22); *CBFB-MYH11*

AML with inv16 and t(16;16) occurs in all age groups but most often in younger patients. The translocation inv(16)(p13q22) is found in approximately 5% to 8% of all AML cases.[23] Various stages of myelocytic, monocytic, and eosinophilic maturation are present and abnormally large granulation in the immature eosinophils (Fig. 11.3). Rarely, cases of AML with inv(16)(p13q22) lack eosinophilia.[26] Myeloblasts and monoblasts show greater than 3% positivity, and monoblasts and promonocytes stain positive for NSE stain. In most cases, the translocation inv(16)(p13q22) results in the fusion of the core binding factor beta (*CBFB*) subunit gene at 16q22 to the *MYH11* gene at 16p13.1, an abnormality that is detectable by fluorescence in situ hybridization or reverse transcriptase polymerase chain reaction analysis.[23] AML with inv16 and t(16;16) has high complete remission rates.

Acute Promyelocytic Leukemia (Acute Myeloid Leukemia) With t(15;17)(q22;q12); *PML-RARA*

APL accounts for 5% to 8% of AMLs and can occur at any age but occurs most often in middle-aged patients.[27] Abnormal, hypergranular promyelocytes predominate in the bone marrow in APL with t(15;17)(q22;q12). Numerous Auer rods (fused azurophilic granules) are present in the myeloblasts and promyelocytes, and bundles of Auer rods ("faggot cells") may be seen (Fig. 11.4, *C*). The azurophilic granules from leukemic promyelocytes have procoagulant activity and predispose the patient to a bleeding

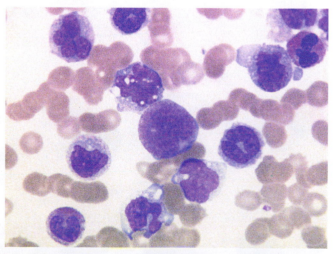

Figure 11.3 AML with inv(16)(p13;q22). Monoblasts, promonocytes, and abnormal monocytes are present. Also note few eosinophils that are often characteristically increased in AML with this cytogenetic abnormality. *Courtesy of Dr. Sidonie Morrison and Kathleen Finnegan, Stony Brook University, New York.*

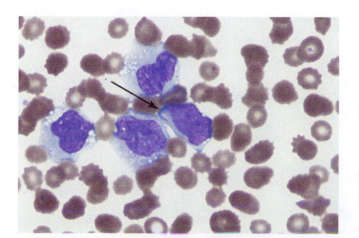

Figure 11.2 AML with t(8;21)(q22;q22). Note Auer rod in myeloblast. *Courtesy of Bernardino Madsen, Casper College, Wyoming.*

diathesis resulting from DIC. MPO reaction is strongly positive in promyelocytes. In about 20% of APL cases, a variant type of APL, referred to as microgranular APL, is found. These cases are characterized by cells with convoluted or lobulated nuclei that mimic promonocytes (Fig. 11.4, *D*). These leukemic promyelocytes contain such small azurophilic granules that they are not visible by light microscopy. These cells can be confused with acute monocytic leukemia, but the strong positive MPO reaction (weak in acute monocytic leukemia) and the bundles of Auer rods are clear clues pointing to a diagnosis of microgranular APL. In addition, WBC is often markedly elevated in the microgranular variety of APL with a rapid doubling time.

APL is characterized by the presence of the retinoic acid receptor alpha (*RARA*) gene on 17q12, which fuses with a nuclear regulatory factor gene on 15q22 (*PML* gene) yielding the *PML-RARA* fusion gene product. Cytogenetic abnormalities are seen in approximately 40% of cases, and the *FLT3* mutation is noted in 34% to 45% of cases of APL.[23] The prognosis in APL

patients with t(15;17)(q22;q12) treated with the drug all trans retinoic acid (ATRA) is very good, better than any other AML subtype.

Acute Myeloid Leukemia With t(9;11)(p22;q23); *MLLT3-MLL*

The t(9;11)(p22;q23) translocation cytogenetic abnormality is found in approximately 10% of pediatric and 2% of adult AML cases.[23] It occurs more often in children but can occur at any age. Monoblasts and promonocytes predominate in the bone marrow and peripheral blood, and patients may present with DIC. Monoblasts have abundant cytoplasm (often showing pseudopodia) and fine nuclear chromatin with one or more nuclei. Azurophilic granules are often seen in monoblasts, and cytoplasmic vacuoles may be present in monoblasts and promonocytes (Fig. 11.5). NSE reaction is strongly positive in monoblasts and promonocytes, and MPO reaction is often negative. Molecular genetic studies in patients with AML with t(9;11)(p22;q23) show a fusion gene designated as

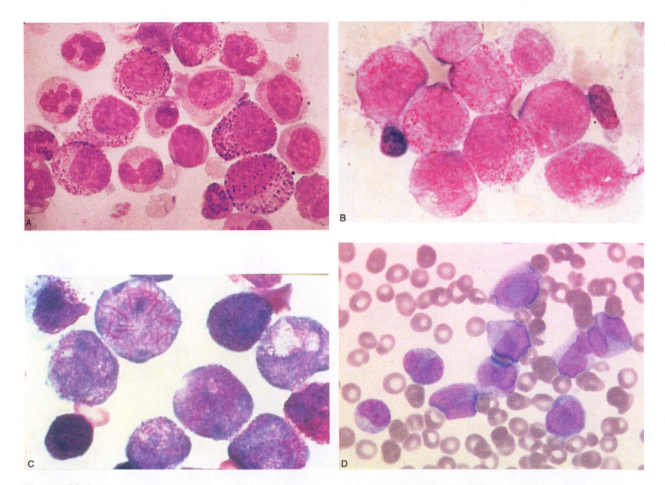

Figure 11.4 (*A, B*) Hypergranular APL with t(15;17)(q22;q12), promyelocytes with prominent azurophilic granules. (*C*) Hypergranular APL with multiple Auer rods. (*D*) Microgranular APL variant; these abnormal promyelocytes have lobulated nuclei and absent or fine azurophilic granules.

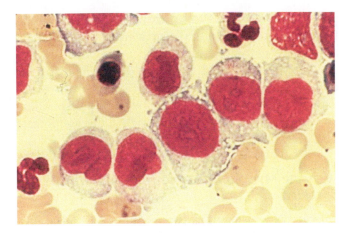

Figure 11.5 AML with t(9;11)(p22;q23). Note monoblastic leukemia features: monoblasts have abundant cytoplasm, often showing pseudopodia, and fine nuclear chromatin, with one or more nucleoli.

MLLT3. The prognosis in AML with 11q23 abnormalities is intermediate.

Acute Myeloid Leukemia With t(6;9)(p23;q34); *DEK-NUP214*

The t(6;9)(p23;q34) translocation cytogenetic abnormality is found in 0.7% to 1.8% of AMLs and occurs in children and adults. The morphology seen in AML with maturation and acute myelomonocytic leukemia is the most common. Auer rods may be seen in about one-third of cases. The blasts stain MPO-positive but may be positive or negative for NSE. An unusual morphologic finding is the presence of peripheral blood and bone marrow basophilia, which may be seen in 44% to 62% of cases.[23] Myelocytic and erythroid dysplasia may also be present. Molecular genetic studies in patients with AML with t(6;9)(p23;q34) show a fusion of *DEK* on chromosome 6 with *NUP214* on chromosome 9. *FLT3-ITD* mutations are also very common in this translocation abnormality. Patients with AML with t(6;9)(p23;q34) have a poor prognosis.

Acute Myeloid Leukemia With inv(3)(q21q26.2) or t(3;3)(q21;q26.2); *RPN1-EVI1*

AML with inv(3)(q21q26.2) is rare, occurs predominately in adults, and represents 1% to 2% of all AMLs. As with other leukemias, patients present with anemia; however, an elevated platelet count (marked thrombocythemia, not thrombocytopenia) is found in 7% to 22% of patients. Hypogranular neutrophils and platelets may be seen in the peripheral blood, along with giant platelets and dwarf megakaryocytes (uninuclear, "bare" megakaryocytes with no cytoplasm). The morphologic and cytochemical features are not distinctive, but multilineage dysplasia of nonblast bone marrow cells is common. Megakaryocytic hyperplasia is usually noted in the bone marrow; however, the atypical megakaryocytes are small and hypolobulated. Increased levels of marrow eosinophils, basophils, or mast cells may be seen in this AML. Common cytogenic abnormalities that are responsible for leukemic transformation and increased cell proliferation include the chromosome 3 abnormalities involving the inversion (3)(q21q26.2) and the translocation t(3;3)(q21;q26.2). The oncogenes *EVl1* and *PRN1* are implicated cytogenetic aberrations. This AML is associated with a poor prognosis and a short survival.

Acute Myeloid Leukemia (Megakaryoblastic) With t(1;22)(p13;q13); *RBM15-MKL1*

AML with t(1;22)(p13;q13) is rare (less than 1% cases) and usually occurs in infants or young children with marked organomegaly. The blasts have the morphology of acute megakaryoblastic leukemia not otherwise specified (NOS) with medium to large blasts that may be mixed with lymphoblastic-appearing cells. The basophilic cytoplasm may show cytoplasmic pseudopod formation.

Immunophenotype markers are consistent with typical reactions that are positive for glycoprotein, CD41 (glycoprotein IIb/IIIa), or CD61 (glycoprotein IIIa). The genetic abnormality is the translocation t(1;22)(p13;q13), and molecular marker is a fusion of RNA-binding motif protein 15 (*RBM15*) and megakaryocyte leukemia-1 (*MKL1*) yielding the *RBM15-MKL1* gene product. Prognosis is currently considered to be promising after AML chemotherapy.

Acute Myeloid Leukemia With Gene Mutations

Gene mutations other than inversions and translocations are also found in AMLs. The most common are fms-related tyrosine kinase 3 (*FLT3*) and nucleophosmin (*NPM1*). Less common mutations include *KIT*, *MLL*, and *CEBPA* gene mutations. *MPM1* mutation and *CEBPA* mutation are associated with a favorable prognosis, whereas the other gene mutations are poor prognostic markers. The reader is referred to other texts for a more in-depth discussion of these AMLs with gene mutations.

II. Acute Myeloid Leukemia With Myelodysplasia-Related Changes

AML with myelodysplasia is seen primarily in adults.[28] The blast percentage in blood or bone marrow is 20% or greater, with abnormal characteristics, called **dysplasia**, observed in at least two cell lines. Dysplastic features that can be observed in neutrophils include hypogranulation, hyposegmentation, pseudo-Pelger neutrophils, and bizarre segmented nuclei. In the erythroid cell line, dyserythropoiesis may manifest as nucleated red blood cells with nuclear fragments or multinucleated cells, megaloblastic features, cytoplasmic vacuoles, or karyorrhexis. Ringed sideroblasts may also be seen. The platelet cell line may also be dysplastic, as micromegakaryocytes having one lobe instead of being multilobed are often present. The ability to recognize these dwarf megakaryocytes is important because they may be seen by a technologist performing a peripheral smear examination and can be confused with other cells having a round nucleus (e.g., mimicking the appearance of a myelocyte). Dysplasia must be present in at least two cell lines to fit the criteria for this category of AML. AML with myelodysplasia may follow a myelodysplastic syndrome (see Chapter 14). Patients with this disorder often present with decreased WBC, RBC, and platelet count, termed pancytopenia. The prognosis of patients with AML with myelodysplasia is poor.[29]

III. Therapy-Related Myeloid Neoplasms

Treatment with cytotoxic chemotherapy or radiation therapy or both has been associated with the development of AML and myelodysplastic syndrome. These disorders have been designated therapy-related AML, therapy-related myelodysplastic syndrome, and therapy-related myelodysplastic/myeloproliferative neoplasms.[23] The two major agents implicated are alkylating agents/radiation and topoisomerase II inhibitors.[30] These therapy-related leukemias have different epidemiologies because the alkylating agent/radiation–induced disorders usually occur 5 to 6 years after exposure, whereas the topoisomerase II inhibitor disorders occur after an of 2 to 3 years after exposure.[31] Alkylating agent–related AMLs usually start with a myelodysplastic presentation, including a blast percentage less than 5% and typical myelodysplastic features. Nuclear hypolobulation, cytoplasmic hypogranulation, dyserythropoiesis, and an increase in ringed sideroblasts are characteristic features. This condition may develop into an AML or a more pronounced myelodysplastic syndrome. A generally poor prognosis is associated with alkylating agent/radiation therapy–related AML.

Topoisomerase II inhibitor–related AML does not usually have a preleukemic or myelodysplastic phase. This type of therapy-related AML often has a morphology consistent with that seen in acute monoblastic or myelomonocytic leukemia, although cases showing involvement of other cell lineages have been described. Cytogenetic abnormalities occur in almost 100% of

patients. Most cases of therapy-related AML and therapy-related myelodysplastic syndrome are characterized by chromosomal translocations that involve 11q23 (*MLL*) or 21q22 (*RUNX1*). There is no specific corresponding immunophenotype. The prognosis is usually poor but is influenced by the corresponding karyotype abnormality and the original disease process that necessitated cytotoxic therapy.

IV. Acute Myeloid Leukemia Not Otherwise Specified

Leukemias with features that do not fit into the previously described categories fall into the group AML NOS. Although leukemias encompass a diverse morphologic and cytochemical spectrum, cytogenetic studies and gene mutation analysis may provide more prognostic information than the actual morphologic and cytochemistry subtypes. As with other AMLs, the presence of at least 20% blasts in the peripheral blood or bone marrow is a hallmark characteristic; the promonocytes in AML are now considered to be "blast equivalents." WHO recommends determining the blast percentage by examining a 500-cell differential count in the bone marrow and evaluating at least 200 cells in the peripheral blood.[23] If leukopenia is present, a buffy coat preparation may be evaluated. Many cases previously designated into the AML NOS group may now be classified into other, more defined categories by use of cytogenetic and gene mutation studies.

Acute Myeloid Leukemia With Minimal Differentiation

There is little evidence of maturation beyond the blast stage in AML with minimal differentiation, and the marrow is replaced by a homogeneous population of blasts (Fig. 11.6). The myeloid lineage of blasts is defined by immunophenotyping with a positive expression of CD13, CD33, CD34, and CD117. MPO and SBB cytochemical stains are usually negative (less than 3% blasts reacting), and Auer rods are absent. *RUNX1* (*ANL-1*) mutation occurs in 27% of cases, and *FLT3* mutation occurs in 16% to 22% of cases. There are no characteristic chromosome abnormalities in the AML with minimal differentiation category. This phenotype accounts for approximately 5% of AML cases and is associated with a poor prognosis.

Acute Myeloid Leukemia Without Maturation

Similar to AML with minimal differentiation, the category of AML without maturation also involves cases in which at least 90% of the nonerythroid cells in the

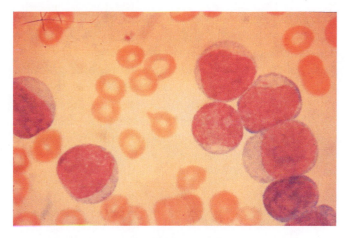

Figure 11.6 AML with minimal differentiation.

bone marrow are myeloblasts (Fig. 11.7). Approximately 5% of the blasts—usually a much higher percentage—have a positive reaction with MPO or SBB, however, and Auer rods may be present. AML without maturation constitutes about 5% to 10% of AML cases; most patients are adults. The blasts in this AML variant express CD13, CD33, CD34, and CD117. No specific chromosomal abnormalities are associated with this subtype. AML without maturation seems to have a poor prognosis, especially in patients with a markedly increased WBC.[18]

Acute Myeloid Leukemia With Maturation

AML with maturation is a common leukemia, accounting for approximately 10% of all AML cases. In accordance with the definition for acute leukemia, blasts constitute at least 20% of all nucleated cells in the bone marrow; however, in this variant, greater than 10% of neutrophils with maturation beyond the promyelocyte stage are observed. Additionally, the

monocytic component constitutes less than 20% of bone marrow cells. Blasts are seen with and without granules, frequently showing Auer rods (Fig. 11.8). Variable degrees of dysplasia may be seen. More than 50% of the blasts and maturing cells are MPO-positive and SBB-positive. The morphology of the previously described AML with t(8;21)(q22;q22) is usually the morphology of AML with maturation. The blasts in this AML variant express CD13, CD33, CD34, CD11b, and CD15. No specific chromosomal abnormalities are associated with this subtype. This phenotype responds variably to chemotherapy, with t(8;21) cases having a favorable prognosis.

Acute Myelomonocytic Leukemia

A mixture of malignant cells with myelocytic and monocytic features is found in the blood and bone marrow of patients with acute myelomonocytic leukemia. This subtype accounts for approximately 5% to 10% cases of AML. The bone marrow has greater than 20% blasts, with myeloid cells and monocytic cells each constituting greater than 20% of all marrow cells. The monoblasts are large cells with abundant, basophilic cytoplasm having fine azurophilic granules and often showing pseudopod cytoplasmic extensions; the nucleus has a lacy chromatin and one to four nucleoli. Promonocytes have a more convoluted nucleus with a more condensed, mature chromatin pattern and may have cytoplasmic vacuoles (Fig. 11.9). The monocytic component may be more prominent in the peripheral blood than in the bone marrow. NSE reaction is usually strongly positive in acute myelomonocytic leukemia, and at least 3% of the blasts are MPO-positive. Naphthol ASD chloroacetate esterase (specific esterase) reaction is also positive. The leukemic cells variably express myeloid antigens of

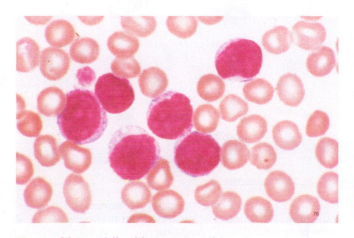

Figure 11.7 **AML without maturation.** Courtesy of Dr. Sidonie
Morrison and Kathleen Finnegan, Stony Brook University, New York

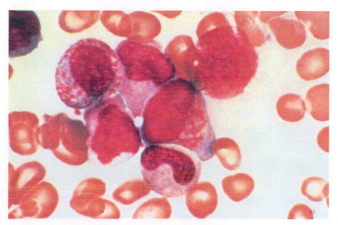

Figure 11.8 Acute myeloid leukemia with maturation. Note myeloblast with multiple Auer rods.

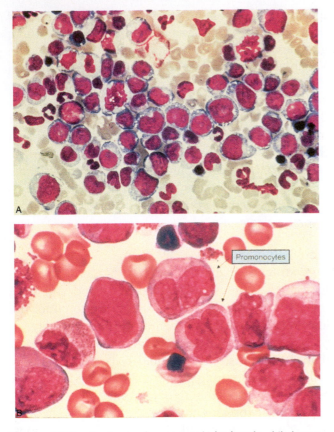

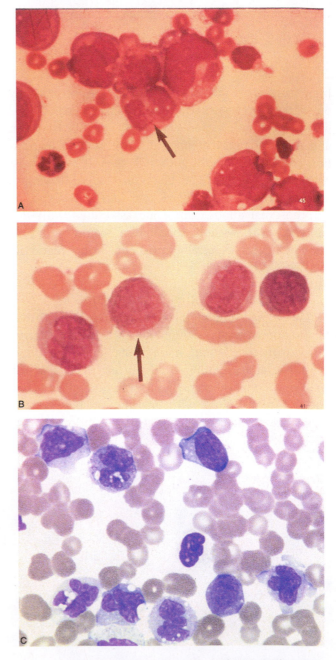

Figure 11.9 Acute myelomonocytic leukemia. (*A*) Acute myelomonocytic leukemia with prominent monoblasts, promonocytes, and spectrum of myeloid/monocytic cells. (*B*) Acute myelomonocytic leukemia with promonoblast, promonocytes, and eosinophil on edge of frame at arrow.

CD13, CD33, CD15, and CD65 and usually show one or more monocytic-associated antigens, such as CD14, CD4, CD11c, CD11c, CD64, CD36, CD68, CD163, and lysozyme.[18,23] This particular variant is associated with a favorable prognosis.

Acute Monoblastic and Acute Monocytic Leukemia

Acute monoblastic leukemia and acute monocytic leukemia each account for approximately 5% of AMLs.[23,27] The bone marrow in each of these leukemias shows greater than 20% blasts, with greater than 80% of the cells having monocytic origin, including monoblasts, promonocytes, and monocytes. The distinction between monoblastic and monocytic leukemia subtypes depends on the proportions of monoblasts and promonocytes present in the bone marrow. Acute monoblastic leukemia has a predominance of monoblasts, which are large cells with moderate to intensely basophilic, abundant cytoplasm and prominent round nuclei with fine chromatin. A spectrum of monocytic cells is seen in acute monocytic leukemia, with most cells being promonocytes

(Fig. 11.10). The nuclear chromatin of promonocytes is more condensed, and these cells often have a convoluted or cerebriform configuration. The cytoplasm of promonocytes contains azurophilic granules and may be vacuolated. Less than 20% of the cells are of granulocytic origin. Auer rods are usually absent in acute monoblastic leukemia. In most cases, monoblasts and promonocytes stain intensely positive with NSE. Monoblasts are typically MPO-negative or

Figure 11.10 (*A*) Acute monocytic leukemia with Auer rods. (*B*) Acute monocytic leukemia with monoblast and three promonocytes. (*C*) Acute monocytic leukemia with monoblast, several promonocytes, and monocytes. C, Courtesy of Dr. Sidonie Morrison and Kathleen Finnegan, Stony Brook University, New York.

SBB-negative; promonocytes may be very weakly positive with these staining reactions. Characteristic positive immunoreactivity of monocytic leukemic cells for lysozyme is also a common finding.

Acute monoblastic leukemia may occur at any age, but most patients tend to be younger, with increased blast percentages in the peripheral blood, and with a poor prognosis.[32] Acute monocytic leukemia is more common in adults (median age 49 years). A hallmark clinical feature of monocytic leukemias is extramedullary disease, and the most predominant finding is the cutaneous and gum infiltration, which results in gingival hypertrophy. Other clinical features include bleeding disorders secondary to DIC and a high incidence of CNS or meningeal disease either at the time of diagnosis or as a manifestation of relapse during remission.[33] High WBC is another common finding reported in 10% to 30% of patients.

Characteristic immunophenotypic markers for cells of monocytic differentiation include CD14, CD4, CD11b, CD11c, CD36, CD64, and CD68. There is a strong association between acute monocytic leukemia and the translocation t(8;16)(p11.2;p13.3) in most

cases. Generally, acute monoblastic leukemia and acute monocytic leukemia have an unfavorable prognosis because of shorter duration of treatment response and poor prognostic factors.

Acute Erythroid Leukemia

Acute erythroid leukemias are predominantly characterized by abnormal proliferation of erythroid precursors. The additional presence or absence of a myeloid element defines the two subtypes, erythroleukemia or pure erythroid leukemia. More than 50% of bone marrow cells are erythroid precursors, and at least 20% are myeloblasts in erythroleukemia (erythroid/myeloid) (Fig. 11.11). Pure erythroid leukemia is defined by most marrow cells (greater than 80%) comprising erythroid precursors, without a myeloid proliferation.[18]

Erythroleukemia (erythroid/myeloid) is usually found in patients 50 years old or older and accounts for less than 5% of AML cases. Pure erythroid leukemia is extremely rare. Characteristics that are commonly seen in the abundant erythroid precursors include dysplastic features, such as bizarre multinucleation,

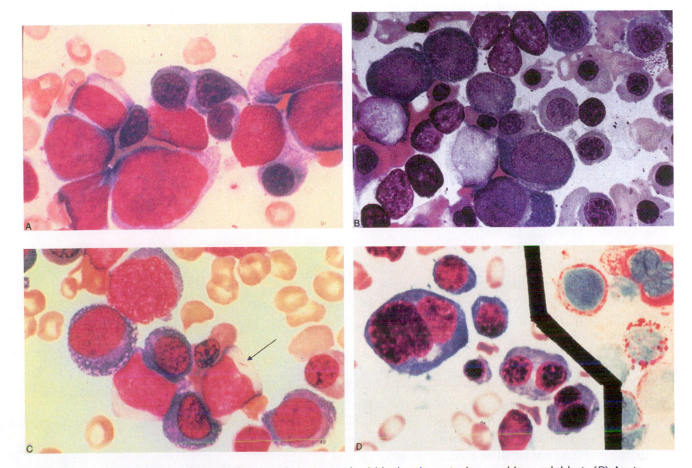

Figure 11.11   (A, B) Acute erythroid leukemia. (C) Acute erythroid leukemia; note Auer rod in myeloblast. (D) Acute erythroid leukemia; left frame shows binucleated pronormoblasts and dysplastic features, and right frame shows PAS block positivity in a ring around the nucleus.

cytoplasmic vacuolization, and megaloblastic nuclear changes. The differential diagnosis includes megaloblastic anemia; however, patients with vitamin B_{12} or folic acid deficiency respond to treatment with these vitamins, and the dysplastic features are not as pronounced as those dysplastic features seen in cases of erythroleukemia (erythroid/myeloid).

Myeloblasts containing Auer rods may be observed in up to two-thirds of patients with erythroleukemia (erythroid/myeloid).[34] Abnormal megakaryocytes may also be noted. Anemia is often markedly severe in patients with erythroid leukemias; it may be more profound than the degree seen in other AML subtypes. The peripheral blood may contain a striking amount of nucleated red blood cells. It is interesting to note, however, that the crowding of the normal elements of the bone marrow by the leukemic cell population results in ineffective erythropoiesis, which leads to reticulocytopenia. The bone marrow iron stain often shows ringed sideroblasts, and the periodic acid–Schiff (PAS) stain may be positive in the classic "block" or show coarse positivity in the pronormoblasts. The myeloblasts are MPO-positive and SBB-positive.

Pure erythroid leukemia is the rarer subtype of the two acute erythroid leukemias and may be seen in patients of any age. The stem cells in this leukemia give rise predominantly to erythroid lineage; any myeloid cell markers are negative. The pronormoblasts can be identified by immunohistochemical reactivity with antibody to Hgb A and expression of glycophorin A, a red blood cell membrane protein.[18]

Erythromyeloleukemia may evolve to an acute myeloblastic leukemia, with similar prognostic results as other subtypes in patients of similar ages.[35] Pure erythroid leukemia is usually associated with an aggressive clinical course.

Acute Megakaryoblastic Leukemia

Acute megakaryoblastic leukemia is a rare form of AML that accounts for approximately less than 5% of cases. This diagnosis is made if at least 20% blasts in the bone marrow are observed and if at least 50% of these are megakaryoblasts. This leukemia occurs in children and adults. Although adult patients usually present with the typical acute leukemia symptoms related to cytopenias of pallor, weakness, and excessive bleeding, in contrast to other leukemias, organomegaly is uncommon at diagnosis. Thrombocytosis may rarely occur, and dysplastic features of platelets, immature myeloid, and erythroid cells may be seen.

Megakaryoblasts are small or medium-to-large in size and are often found as a heterogeneous mix in the same patient in regard to size, with some blasts being small or medium with scant basophilic cytoplasm and others being much larger with more abundant cytoplasm and distinct blebbing pseudopod formation. The nucleus is round or slightly indented with delicate chromatin and one to three prominent nucleoli. Although megakaryoblasts may be difficult, if not impossible, to identify by light microscopy, the presence of blasts with cytoplasmic blebbing may provide a hallmark clue regarding the lineage of the blasts. Megakaryoblastic fragments or micromegakaryocytes and giant, hypogranular platelets are sometimes present (Fig. 11.12).

The diagnosis of acute megakaryoblastic leukemia is usually made based on immunophenotyping results because megakaryoblasts express one or more of the platelet glycoproteins: CD41 (glycoprotein IIb/IIIa), CD61 (glycoprotein IIIa), and, less frequently, CD42 (glycoprotein Ib). Cytochemical stains are not as useful because MPO, SBB, and TdT are negative, and the alpha-naphthyl acetate esterase reaction is usually positive with a negative alpha-naphthyl butyrate esterase reaction. Both types of nonspecific esterase would be positive in acute monocytic leukemia. Megakaryoblasts manifest platelet peroxidase activity that can be identified by electron microscopy cytochemistry.

There are no specific chromosomal abnormalities associated with this subtype. A poor prognosis is typical of most cases of acute megakaryoblastic leukemia.

Acute Basophilic Leukemia

Accounting for less than 1% of all AMLs, acute basophilic leukemia is a very rare leukemia that may occur de novo or more commonly may arise as a blastic transformation in patients with a preceding CML.

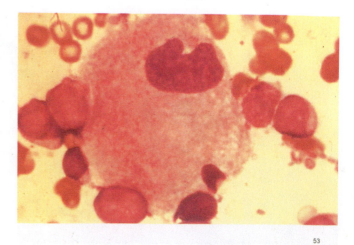

Figure 11.12 Acute megakaryoblastic leukemia.

The predominant circulating cell appears blastlike with one to three nucleoli and a prominent but variable number of coarse, basophilic granules. The cells stain positive with the metachromatic stain toluidine blue. Additionally, the blasts stain positive with acid phosphatase and show block positivity with PAS but are negative with MPO, SBB, and NSE stains. The blasts usually are positive for myeloid markers CD13, CD33, and CD34 and show reactivity with CD11b, CD123, and CD203c.[23]

Because of hyperhistaminemia, cutaneous lesions are often seen in these patients, in addition to the typical leukemic symptoms of hepatosplenomegaly and bone marrow failure. The clinical symptoms, special stains, immunophenotyping, and cytogenetic features distinguish acute basophilic leukemia from APL because the early basophilic myelocytes may be confused with promyelocytes. Acute basophilic leukemia should also be distinguished from other AML categories with basophilia, such as AML with t(6;9) (p23;q34).

Acute Panmyelosis with Myelofibrosis

Acute panmyelofibrosis with myelofibrosis (APMF), a rare leukemia of adults, is characterized by marked peripheral blood pancytopenia and panmyeloid marrow hyperplasia of the erythroid, granulocytic, and megakaryocytic components, combined with a variable degree of reticulin fibrosis. Dysplastic myeloid precursors and dysplastic megakaryocytes (small, hypolobulated with eosinophilic granules) may be observed. Differential diagnosis from chronic IMF can be made because more immature cells are seen in the acute process, and the splenomegaly that is a hallmark feature of IMF is absent in APMF. The heterogeneous blasts in APMF are positive for CD34. This subtype of acute leukemia is usually associated with a poor prognosis.

V. Myeloid Sarcoma

Myeloid sarcoma is defined as a tumor that consists of myeloblasts with or without any significant myeloid maturation that is found in the lymph nodes, bone, gastrointestinal tract, skin, or any soft tissue. It may precede or occur at the same time with AML, or it may arise as a result of a blast transformation of a myelodysplastic syndrome. A myeloid sarcoma tumor mass displaces the normal architecture of the tissue. The cytochemistry reactions of the tissue imprints are usually positive for MPO, chloroacetate esterase, and NSE stains. Positive CD markers include CD30, CD34, CD56, CD68, CD99, and CD117. Chromosome aberrations are seen in approximately one-half of cases.

VI. Myeloid Proliferations Related to Down Syndrome

An estimated 10-fold to 100-fold increased risk of developing leukemia is present in individuals with Down syndrome (DS), particularly in children younger than 5 years. Children with DS are at risk to develop all forms of leukemia, including AML and ALL. Of AMLs in children with DS younger than 4 years, 70% are of the acute megakaryoblastic leukemia variety.[23] This subtype has a unique marker, *GATA1* mutation, which is helpful in distinguishing it from other leukemias.

About 10% of children with DS have a *transient abnormal myelopoiesis*, which resolves spontaneously over weeks to several months. In 20% to 30% of cases, acute megakaryoblastic leukemia may develop in subsequent years.

VII. Blastic Plasmacytoid Dendritic Cell Neoplasm

Blastic plasmacytoid dendritic cell neoplasm is a very rare but aggressive tumor that can develop at any age but usually is seen in adults. The plasmacytic dendritic cells are medium-sized blasts with irregular nuclei, one to two small nucleoli, and fine chromatin. These cells are unique because they produce a large amount of alpha-interferon. Patients present with one or more skin lesions that may appear as nodules or plaques and bone marrow involvement. Cytopenias may be minimal early on, but as the disease progresses and bone marrow failure is evident, the cytopenias intensify. Some of these cases involve a transition to acute leukemia, either AML or acute myelomonocytic leukemia. The tumor cells express many CD markers, and the reader is referred to other texts for a more in-depth discussion of the immunophenotyping and genetic studies. The prognosis is poor for patients with this neoplasm.

ACUTE LEUKEMIAS OF AMBIGUOUS LINEAGE

The WHO group has combined several types of acute leukemias into the acute leukemia of ambiguous lineage classification. These include leukemias in which the morphologic, immunophenotypic, or cytochemical findings are not helpful in the classification of a particular type of myeloid or lymphoid process or, conversely, in which the features indicate a combination of both processes.[39–41] *Undifferentiated acute leukemias* lack markers consistent with a specific lineage. *Mixed phenotype acute leukemias with t(9;22)(q34;q11.1); BCR-ABL1* manifest with dimorphic blast populations that contain different populations of cells that express myeloid and lymphoid markers (myeloblasts and lymphoblasts). *Mixed phenotype acute leukemias with t(v;11q23); MLL rearranged* are typified by a dimorphic blast population, one morphologically appearing as monoblasts and the other appearing as lymphoblasts, and having the translocation involving the *MLL* gene. *Mixed phenotype acute leukemias, T/myeloid NOS* involve a proliferation of cells that have myeloid and T lineage specific antigens on the same blast population[18] but without the cytogenetic abnormality listed earlier.

ACUTE LYMPHOBLASTIC LEUKEMIA

ALL is a malignant disease that evolves as a result of a mutation of lymphoid precursor cells originating in the marrow or thymus at a particular stage of maturation. The immunophenotype reflects the antigen expression of the stage of differentiation of the dominant clone. The leukemic cells persistently accumulate in intramedullary and extramedullary sites, constantly competing with normal hematopoietic cell production and function. This situation results in anemia, thrombocytopenia, neutropenia, and an overpopulation of lymphoblasts in tissues such as liver, spleen, lymph nodes, meninges, and gonads.

Epidemiology

ALL is predominantly a disease of children, with the highest incidence occurring in children 2 to 6 years old. It accounts for 76% of all leukemias diagnosed in children younger than 15 years.[42] According to National Cancer Institute statistics, an increased incidence of ALL occurs in all age groups in males compared with females of European or African descent.[43] The exception is a slight female predominance in infancy.[44] Although more uncommon in adults, ALL occurs in all age groups, and incidence rates increase with increasing age, with a second peak incidence in elderly adults.

The etiology of ALL is unknown in most cases. Environmental agents such as ionizing radiation and chemical mutagens have been implicated, and evidence suggests a genetic factor in some patients. Children with DS have an increased risk of leukemia, particularly precursor B lymphoblastic leukemia. Childhood ALL occurs more frequently in industrialized countries compared with developing countries. It has also been postulated that some cases of childhood leukemia stem from adverse cellular response to common infections that occur at a later age than was typically experienced in past centuries.[45,46] These "delayed" exposures are believed to increase the risk of genetic mutations in the lymphoid precursors leading to development of leukemia.

Clinical Features

Clinical presentation is variable; symptoms may be subtle and develop over months, or they may be acute and quite severe. The presenting symptoms are directly related to the degree of bone marrow failure or extramedullary involvement (see Table 11.4). In about half of patients, symptoms include fever that stems from the leukemic process itself (tumor burden) and from neutropenia, pallor, and fatigue that are caused by anemia. Bleeding, purpura, and bone and joint pain are other common presenting complaints. Children often present with a limp or the inability to walk because of pain caused by leukemic infiltration of the periosteum (bone covering) or bone itself, causing osteoporosis or bone erosion. Hepatosplenomegaly and lymphadenopathy may be prominent symptoms. Uncommon symptoms include cough, dyspnea, cyanosis, and syncope related to a bulky mediastinal mass that can compress blood vessels or the trachea.[47]

Classifications

The FAB classification developed in 1976 defined three morphologic subtypes (L1, L2, and L3) based on the appearance of the blasts that predominate. L1 lymphoblasts are small with scant cytoplasm, are uniform in size, and have indistinct nucleoli. L2 blasts are larger, are more pleomorphic, and often contain abundant cytoplasm and prominent nucleoli (Table 11.11). L1 and L2 blasts cannot be determined from morphology alone because they are easily confused with myeloblasts seen in AML. L3 lymphoblasts are characterized by intensely basophilic cytoplasm that has many vacuoles.

Because of the differences in prognosis based on immunophenotype and cytogenetics, the 2008 WHO classification has recognized three major immunophenotypic categories: B lymphoblastic leukemia (B-ALL)/lymphoblastic lymphoma (B-LBL) NOS, B-ALL/B-LBL with recurrent genetic abnormalities, and T lymphoblastic leukemia (T-ALL)/T lymphoblastic lymphoma (T-LBL). There are seven subtypes of precursor B-ALL in the B-ALL/B-LBL category with recurrent genetic abnormalities (Table 11.12).

B Lymphoblastic Leukemia/B Lymphoblastic Lymphoma Not Otherwise Specified

B-ALL/B-LBL is a malignancy in which B-lineage lymphoblasts predominate in the bone marrow (B-ALL),

Table 11.11 ⦿ FAB Morphologic Classification of Acute Lymphoblastic Leukemia*			
Feature	**L1**	**L2**	**L3**
Cell size	Small, regular	Large, mixed sizes	Large
Nuclear chromatin	Fine or condensed	Fine or condensed	Fine
Nuclear shape	Regular, cleft or indentation possible	Irregular, cleft or indentation more common	Regular, round or oval
Nucleoli	Indistinct	1–2, prominent	1–2, prominent
Cytoplasm	Scant	Variable, often moderately abundant	Deeply basophilic, vacuolated

*For historic review only.

Table 11.12 ⦿ 2008 WHO Classification of Acute Lymphoblastic Leukemia/Lymphoblastic Lymphoma

B lymphoblastic leukemia/B lymphoblastic lymphoma not otherwise specified

B lymphoblastic leukemia/B lymphoblastic lymphoma with recurrent genetic abnormalities

Cytogenetic subtypes

B lymphoblastic leukemia/B lymphoblastic lymphoma with:

- t(9;22)(q34;q11.1); *BCR-ABL1*
- t(v;11q23); *MLL* rearranged
- t(12;21)(p13;q22); *TEL-AML1(ETV6-RUNX1)*
- Hyperdiploidy
- Hypodiploidy (hypodiploid ALL)
- t(5;14)(q31;q32); *IL3-IGH*
- t(1;19)(q23;p13.3); *E2A-PBX1 (TCF3-PBX1)*

T lymphoblastic leukemia/T lymphoblastic lymphoma

and sometimes there is primary involvement of lymph nodes or extranodal sites (B-LBL). More than 25% of bone marrow cells must be identified as lymphoblasts to meet the WHO definition of ALL; however, the bone marrow aspirate typically consists almost entirely of lymphoblasts at diagnosis. When the leukemic process is limited to a mass lesion and 25% or less lymphoblasts are seen in the marrow, the designation **lymphoma** is used.[18] B-ALL accounts for approximately 85% of all childhood ALL, whereas B-LBL is a rare type of lymphoma and constitutes approximately 10% of lymphoblastic lymphoma cases.[48] B-ALL may also develop in adults, and the prognosis is generally much poorer in adults.

Bone marrow and blood manifest blasts in all cases of B-ALL. Extramedullary sites of hematopoiesis cause hepatosplenomegaly, and there is a predilection for CNS (**meningeal leukemia**), lymph node, and gonadal involvement. Bone pain from marrow hyperplasia is also a frequent clinical symptom. Asymptomatic head and neck lymphadenopathy is particularly common in B-LBL.

Laboratory Features

WBC is variable in B-ALL—markedly elevated, normal, or decreased. As with all other acute leukemias, anemia and thrombocytopenia are apparent at diagnosis. The blood and bone marrow contain lymphoblasts with small, scanty cytoplasm and condensed nuclear chromatin approximately twice the size of normal small lymphocytes or larger blasts with a moderate amount of basophilic cytoplasm, prominent nucleoli, and homogeneous, more dispersed nuclear chromatin (Fig. 11.13). Coarse azurophilic granules may be present in lymphoblasts of 10% of cases. Vacuoles may be present but not to the degree seen in Burkitt cells. Lymphoblasts with pseudopod projections, termed "hand-mirror cells," may be found occasionally. Although not as important as the immunophenotypic characterization, cytochemistries may be helpful until further studies can be performed to help separate the preliminary diagnosis of lymphoid from myeloid leukemia. Myeloid stains SBB and MPO are negative or very weakly positive compared with the intensely positive stain seen in myeloblasts. NSE reaction is generally negative. By contrast, PAS stain is positive in greater than 70% of ALL cases, with the nuclei often giving the appearance of being rimmed with a punctate PAS-positive string of beads.

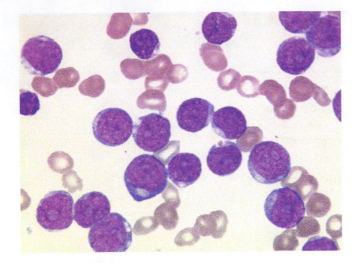

Figure 11.13 Precursor B lymphoblastic leukemia. Courtesy of Dr. Sidonie Morrison and Kathleen Finnegan, Stony Brook University, New York.

Immunophenotype

As previously noted, immunologic classification should be performed in all cases because it allows for more precise diagnosis and important prognostic correlations. To define a particular population of lymphoblasts in leukemia, evaluation of the results of a panel of antibodies used to distinguish the CD groups is done. Because no one surface marker is 100% specific, a panel is needed to establish the diagnosis and sort the leukemia into the appropriate subtype. To be able to interpret CD information, it is important to have a basic understanding of lymphocyte ontogeny.

Each of the two lineages of lymphocytes (B cells and T cells) can be subclassified into several maturational stages by the expression of their surface antigens. ALLs are divided by immunophenotype, first into B-cell or T-cell lineages. In leukemia, the lymphoblasts are "frozen" at a specific stage of maturation; using CD markers, these blasts can be categorized further into the particular stage of differentiation (i.e., precursor B cells or T cells and mature B cells or T cells).

The lymphoblasts in B-ALL/B-LBL are uniformly TdT-positive, HLA-DR-positive, and *PAX5*-positive. The flow cytometric immunophenotype in most cases is positive for CD10, CD19, CD20, CD24, cytoplasmic CD22, and CD79a (Fig. 11.14).

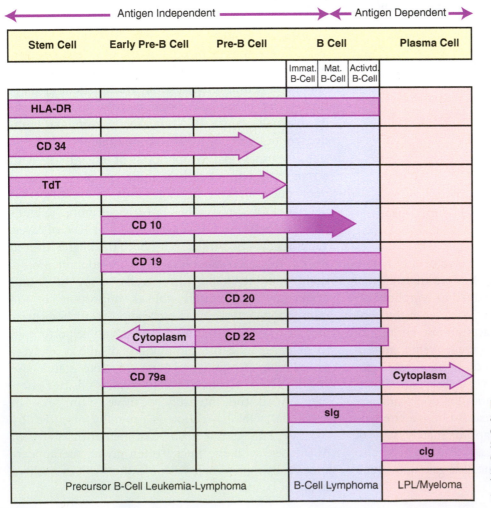

Figure 11.14 B-lineage antigen expression. Stages of B-cell differentiation can be shown by antigen expression. cIg, cytoplasmic immunoglobulin; sIg, surface immunoglobulin; TdT, terminal deoxynucleotidyl transferase.

Cytogenetic Findings

In addition to immunophenotype, chromosomal alterations that are considered prognostically important have been identified in most cases of B-ALL/B-LBL. These abnormalities are used to define the specific subtype and are discussed subsequently. B-ALL has a good prognosis in children but is not associated with such a positive outcome in adults.

B Lymphoblastic Leukemia/B Lymphoblastic Lymphoma With Recurrent Genetic Abnormalities

The seven subtypes of B-ALL/B-LBL are linked because each represents a balanced translocation or other chromosomal abnormality, and each has distinctive clinical or phenotypic markers that carry important prognostic correlations (see Table 11.12).

B Lymphoblastic Leukemia/B Lymphoblastic Lymphoma With t(9;22)(q34;q11.2); *BCR-ABL1*

The translocation between the *BCR* gene on chromosome 22 and the *ABL1* gene on chromosome 9 is the hallmark of the t(9;22) B-ALL subtype, which affects adults more often than children, representing 25% of adult ALL but only 2% to 4% of ALL in children.[23] Typically, there is an associated hyperleukocytosis, frequent CNS disease, and resistance to chemotherapy treatment. The t(9;22) B-ALL has the worst prognosis of all of the ALLs.

B Lymphoblastic Leukemia/B Lymphoblastic Lymphoma With t(v;11q23); *MLL* Rearranged

The translocation between the *MLL* gene at band 11q23 and other fusion partners causes the rearranged product that is the characteristic finding of the t(v;11q23) B-ALL subtype. Although it is the most common ALL in infants younger than 1 year, it is uncommon in older children; however, this ALL increases in frequency as age increases in adulthood. Markedly elevated WBC and CNS involvement produce two distinctly negative prognostic indicators.

B Lymphoblastic Leukemia/B Lymphoblastic Lymphoma With t(12;21)(p13;q22); *TEL-AML1(ETV6-RUNX1)*

The translocation between the *TEL (ETV6)* gene on chromosome 12 with the *AML1 (RUNX1)* gene on chromosome 12 accounts for the t(12;21) B-ALL subtype. It accounts for approximately 25% of B-ALL in children and is associated with a very favorable outcome (i.e., cures of greater than 90% in children treated).[23]

B Lymphoblastic Leukemia/B Lymphoblastic Lymphoma With Hyperdiploidy

Hyperdiploidy with blasts containing 50 to 66 chromosomes is found in approximately 25% of cases of childhood B-ALL and about 5% of adult B-ALL. Hyperdiploidy can be detected by routine karyotyping, flow cytometry, or fluorescence in situ hybridization analysis. This subtype of B-ALL has a very favorable outcome, with cures obtained in greater than 90% of children.

B Lymphoblastic Leukemia/B Lymphoblastic Lymphoma With Hypodiploidy (Hypodiploid Acute Lymphoblastic Leukemia)

The blasts in hypodiploid ALL contain less than 45 chromosomes. This subtype is present in 2% to 9% of ALL cases and occurs in children and adults.[23] Overall, hypodiploidy is considered to have a poor prognosis. The prognosis depends, however, on the number of chromosomes; ALLs with 44 to 45 chromosomes have the best prognosis, and ALLs with a near-haploid number of chromosomes, found in only about 1% of cases, have a very poor prognosis.

B Lymphoblastic Leukemia/B Lymphoblastic Lymphoma With t(5;14)(q31;q32); *IL3-IGH*

The rare t(5;14) subtype of B-ALL is reported in less than 1% of cases of ALL and occurs in children and adults. The translocation between the *IL3* gene on chromosome 5 and the *IGH* gene on chromosome 14 is responsible for this neoplasm of B lymphoblasts. Besides the finding of CD19-positive and CD10-positive lymphoblasts, the unusual finding with this subtype is the presence of peripheral blood eosinophilia.

B Lymphoblastic Leukemia/B Lymphoma With t(1;19)(q23;p13.3); *E2A-PBX1 (TCF3-PBX1)*

The t(1:19) subtype of ALL is usually found in children and is responsible for approximately 6% of B-ALL cases. The t(1:19) translocation is the most frequent translocation identified in precursor ALL. The translocation may be balanced or unbalanced and occurs between the *E2A(TCF3)* gene on chromosome 19 and the *PBX1* gene on chromosome 1.[23] These pre–B-ALL blasts are CD19-positive and CD10-positive and are also cytoplasmic μ heavy chain–positive. Previously, this genetic subtype was associated with a poor prognosis; however, current therapy has produced a more promising prognosis.

T Lymphoblastic Leukemia/T Lymphoblastic Lymphoma

T-ALL/T-LBL is a malignancy of lymphoblasts having T-lineage markers. The small to medium-sized lymphoblasts may involve the bone marrow and peripheral blood (T-ALL). When the lymphoblasts primarily involve lymph nodes or extranodal sites, the neoplasm is termed T-LBL. As in B-ALL, more than 25% of bone marrow cells must be identified as lymphoblasts to meet the WHO definition of ALL; however, the bone marrow aspirate typically consists almost entirely of lymphoblasts at diagnosis. When the leukemic process is limited to a mass lesion, and 2% or less of lymphoblasts are seen in the marrow, the designation *lymphoma* is used.[18]

T-ALL represents approximately 15% to 20% of all childhood ALL. It is more prevalent in adolescents than young children and is seen more frequently in males than females. T-ALL accounts for 25% of adult cases. T-LBL is the subtype of 85% to 90% of lymphoblastic lymphomas[18] and is seen more frequently in males.

Bone marrow and blood manifest blasts in all cases of T-ALL. T-ALL and T-LBL patients often present with large mediastinal or other tissue mass; other sites of involvement include lymph nodes, liver, spleen, thymus, skin, CNS, and gonads. Precursor T-ALL manifests more commonly as a lymphoma, with minimal or no bone marrow involvement compared with B-ALL.

Laboratory Features

The leukocyte count may be quite high in T-ALL (greater than $100 \times 10^9/L$). Lymphoblast morphology shows medium-sized blasts with a moderate amount of cytoplasm and prominent nucleoli; occasional nuclear clefting (previously L2 FAB morphology classification); or, less frequently, smaller blasts, a high nuclear:cytoplasmic ratio, scant cytoplasm, and indistinct cytoplasm (previously L1 FAB morphology). Sometimes, a patient has a mixture of small and medium-sized blasts (Fig. 11.15; see Table 11.11). The number of mitotic blast cells is usually greater in T-ALL than in B-ALL.

Immunophenotype

Most precursor T-ALL malignancies have an immunophenotype that corresponds to an immature thymocyte (prothymocyte) stage, originating in the bone marrow.[49] The lymphoblasts in T-ALL are TdT-positive, cytoplasmic CD3-positive, and CD7-positive, and variably express CD1 CD2, CD4, CD5, CD8, or CD10. The myeloid-associated antigens CD13 and CD34 are often present; this may still be consistent with the diagnosis of T-ALL/T-LBL (Fig. 11.16).

Cytogenetic Findings

Reciprocal translocations of the T-cell receptor loci have been detected in about one-third of patients

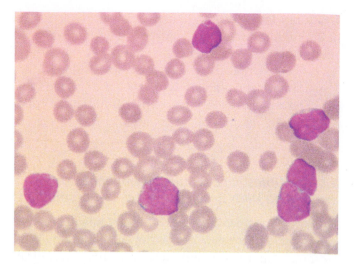

Figure 11.15   Precursor T lymphoblastic leukemia.
Courtesy of Dr. Sidonie Morrison and Kathleen Finnegan, Stony Brook University, New York.

with T-ALL/T-LBL.[18] These translocations arise from mistakes in the normal recombination mechanisms that generate antigen receptor genes. The cellular rearrangements that occur in T-ALL cases affect the proteins that have vital functions in cell proliferation, differentiation, or survival.[50] The association of clinical findings, specific lymphoblast phenotype, and particular chromosomal abnormalities has been shown to have prognostic significance. The reader is referred to other texts for a more detailed discussion of the genes affected by chromosomal translocations in B-ALL and T-ALL.

Prognosis in Acute Lymphoblastic Leukemia

Although children with ALL have an overall complete remission rate of almost 95%, the disease-free, long-term response rate is about 70% to 80%.[51,52] The cure rate in adults is more variable at 60% to 85%.[18] (Table 11.13) lists the prognostic indicators for ALL. Although the prognosis of T-ALL is found to be poorer in children compared with the prognosis of B-ALL, the opposite is true in adults, in whom prognosis of T-ALL is better than prognosis of B-ALL.

Age and WBC are used for risk assessment in all pediatric clinical trials, with WBC less than $50 \times 10^9/L$ as the minimal criteria for low-risk ALL.[53] Other prognostic factors used to determine outcome are gender, immunophenotypic and cytogenetic profiles, and response to treatment. The two most important tests having the greatest prognostic prediction power when the sample of hematopoietic material is limited are flow cytometry and cytogenetics.

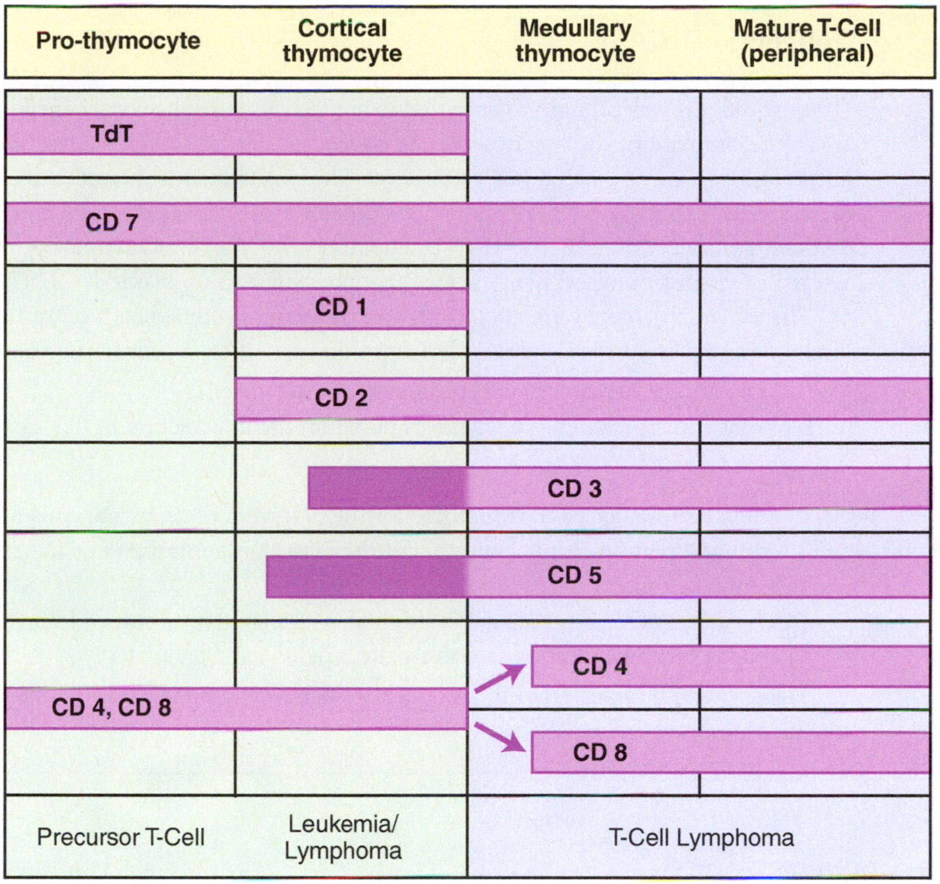

Pro-thymocyte	Cortical thymocyte	Medullary thymocyte	Mature T-Cell (peripheral)
TdT			
CD 7			
	CD 1		
	CD 2		
	CD 3		
	CD 5		
		CD 4	
CD 4, CD 8		CD 8	
Precursor T-Cell	Leukemia/Lymphoma	T-Cell Lymphoma	

Figure 11.16 T-lineage antigen expression. T-cell development originates with prothymocytes in the bone marrow. Further development takes place after these cells migrate to the thymus, where the maturation of the thymocyte can be classified, using specific CD markers, according to the various membrane antigens that are expressed.

Table 11.13 ○ Prognostic Factors in Acute Lymphoblastic Leukemia

Risk Factors	Favorable	Unfavorable
WBC	Less than 10×10^9/L	Greater than 50×10^9/L
Hemoglobin	Greater than 10 g/dL	Less than 7 g/dL
Age	2–9 years	Less than 2 and greater than 10 years
Race	White	Black
Gender	Female	Male
Response to treatment	Less than 14 days	Greater than 28 days
CNS leukemia	Absent	Present
Immunophenotype	CD10 positive	CD10 negative
Cytogenetic	Hyperploidy greater than 50	Hypoploidy
	Translocations	Translocations
	• t(12;21)(p13;q22); *TEL-AML1*	• t(9;22)(q34;q11.2); *BCR-ABL1*
		• t(v;11q23); *MLL-AF4*

The combination of conventional clinical and morphologic findings with now standard immunophenotypic, cytogenetic, and molecular testing affords the pathologist and oncologist the most valuable and comprehensive information to "get to know" each disease entity and its characteristics. Good communication between the clinician, the laboratory staff, and the pathologist is now even more imperative in gathering the important prognostic data to apply the most specific diagnosis and treatment.

CONDENSED CASE

A 10-year-old girl was brought to an outpatient clinic because she complained of sore throat and a lump in her neck. On examination, she was observed to have a tonsillar abscess, swollen glands, and widespread bruising in the extremities. She also had a low-grade fever. She was treated with antibiotics and released, but she failed to progress over the next 2 days. Hematology laboratory tests revealed a WBC of 8.0×10^9/L, a hematocrit of 28%, and a platelet count of 10×10^9/L. The peripheral blood differential count revealed 3 band neutrophils, 25 segmented neutrophils, 8 lymphocytes, 1 monocyte, and 63 blasts.

The patient's parents were contacted, and the girl was immediately admitted to the hospital. A bone marrow examination was performed and revealed an infiltration of blast cells in the marrow.

1. Why are the hematocrit and platelet count decreased?
2. What is the presumptive diagnosis based on the information in this case?

Answers

1. Many typical signs and symptoms for the diagnosis of acute leukemia are present. The depressed hematocrit and platelet count indicate that the blast burden in the bone marrow is crowding out all the normal elements, causing low counts.
2. The differential count results indicate an acute leukemia; however, further immunophenotype and genetic testing is needed to classify the type of acute leukemia.

This girl will be transferred to an oncology facility and most likely will be treated aggressively after her leukemia is appropriately classified.

○ *Summary Points*

- Leukemia is caused by the mutation of bone marrow pluripotent stem cells.
- Individuals with acute leukemia present with variable WBCs, anemia, and platelet counts.
- When blast cells accumulate in the bone marrow and peripheral smear, leukemia is classified as acute.
- Hepatosplenomegaly or lymphadenopathy is more prominent in chronic leukemias than acute leukemias.
- According to WHO, the peripheral smear must contain greater than or equal to 20% myeloblasts for a diagnosis of acute leukemia.
- Skin infiltration is characteristic of monocytic leukemias; extramedullary hematopoiesis is common in monocytic or myelomonocytic leukemias.
- Headache, blindness, and other neurologic complications are indicative of blast cells crossing the blood-brain barrier.
- Cytochemical staining can assist in the diagnosis of acute leukemias based on staining patterns, particularly AMLs.
- Auer rods are composed of fused primary granules and may be present in myeloblasts, monoblasts, and promyelocytes.

- Immunophenotyping can help to classify the clone of leukemic cells by using monoclonal antibodies in flow cytometry or immunohistochemistry procedures.
- Cytogenetic abnormalities such as translocations and deletions are an important prognostic feature of many acute leukemias.
- APL is associated with DIC.
- Treatment with cytotoxic chemotherapy or radiation therapy is associated with the development of acute leukemia and myelodysplastic syndrome.
- AML with maturation is the most common type of AML.
- ALL is the leukemia of childhood, predominately occurring between the ages of 2 and 6 years.
- ALLs account for 76% of all leukemias diagnosed in children younger than 13 years.
- Children with DS have an increased risk of leukemia.
- Lymphoblasts frequently cross the blood-brain barrier causing neurologic involvement.
- In the pediatric age group, children with ALL have an overall complete remission rate of almost 95%.

Review Questions

1. Which of the following is most often associated with acute leukemia?
   a. Erythrocytosis and thrombocytosis
   b. Neutropenia and thrombosis
   c. Anemia and thrombocytopenia
   d. Lymphocytosis and thrombocythemia

2. What is the requisite blast percentage for the diagnosis of acute myeloid leukemia recommended by the World Health Organization (WHO)?
   a. 10%
   b. 20%
   c. 30%
   d. 40%

3. Auer rods may be seen in which of the following cells?
   a. Myeloblasts
   d. Myelocytes
   c. Lymphoblasts
   d. Megakaryoblasts

4. Myeloperoxidase stain is strongly positive in
   a. Acute lymphoblastic leukemia.
   b. Acute monocytic leukemia.
   c. Acute megakaryoblastic leukemia.
   d. Acute myeloblastic leukemia.

5. Acute promyelocytic leukemia has a high incidence of which of the following cytogenetic abnormalities?
   a. t(8;21)(q22;q22)
   b. inv(16)(p13;q22)
   c. t(15;17)(q22;q12)
   d. t(9;11)(p22;q23)

6. Which cytochemical reaction is most helpful in identifying the blasts in acute monoblastic leukemia?
   a. NSE
   b. TdT
   c. PAS
   d. SBB

7. The monoclonal marker that is often positive in B lymphoblastic leukemia/B lymphoblastic lymphoma is
   a. CD1.
   b. CD7.
   c. CD10.
   d. CD41.

8. The basic pathophysiology mechanism responsible for producing signs and symptoms in leukemia includes all of the following *except*
   a. Replacement of normal marrow precursors by leukemic cells.
   b. Decrease in functional leukocytes causing infection.
   c. Hemorrhage secondary to thrombocytopenia.
   d. Decreased erythropoietin production.

9. Migration to extramedullary sites is a feature of which of the following leukemias?
   a. Acute progranulocytic leukemia
   b. Acute myelocytic leukemia
   c. Acute monocytic leukemia
   d. Acute lymphocytic leukemia

10. A patient presents with generalized lymphadenopathy and WBC of 100×10^9/L. This blood picture would most likely be seen in
    a. Chronic lymphocytic leukemia.
    b. Acute lymphocytic leukemia.
    c. Burkitt's lymphoma.
    d. Hairy cell leukemia.

⦿ TROUBLE SHOOTING

What Does the Laboratory Technologist Do When the WBC Is Beyond the Reportable Range?

CBC Results

WBC	194.1×10^9/L	
RBC	3.89×10^{12}/L	
Hgb	11.3 g/dL	
Hct	34.0%	
MCV	87.4 fL	
MCH	29.1 pg	
MCHC	33.2 g/dL	
RDW	17.2%	
Platelets	41×10^9/L	
WBC differential	NE, LY, MO, EO, BA all have R* flags	

Flags

+++ WBC beyond reportable range, upper linearity limit is 99.9×10^9/L

The entire CBC and differential was "flagged" and considered nonreportable.

1. Which of these CBC results are unacceptable to report to the clinician without further workup?
   ALL: WBC out-of-range, inaccurate RBC/Hct/RBC indices, questionable inaccurate platelets

2. What are the next steps that should be taken to provide accurate results?
   Resolution steps

   - Dilute blood 1:10 with diluent, rerun
   - Calculate to get accurate WBC
   - Subtract RBC from WBC (i.e., RBC − WBC = accurate RBC)
   - Perform microhematocrit (spun Hct)
   - Report only WBC, RBC, platelets
   - Perform manual WBC differential, verify platelet count (or perform manually)

Example:

1. 1:10 dilution of blood—WBC result was 24.9×10^9/L

   - Calculate to get **accurate WBC**
     WBC 24.9×10^9/L
     24.9×10 (dilution factor) = 249×10^9/L = *accurate WBC*

2. Subtract WBC from original RBC, as white blood cells are included in original count, to obtain **accurate RBC**
   3.89 (original RBC) − 0.249 (WBC expressed in millions unit of measure) = 3.64×10^{12}/L = *accurate RBC count*

3. Microhematocrit = 33.5%
   - Be careful to exclude the buffy coat when reading the microhematocrit

4. Perform manual WBC differential and platelet estimate

*R, review flags on all CBC parameters.

W O R D   K E Y

Auer rods • Elliptical, spindlelike inclusions composed of fused azurophilic granules that may be present in myeloblasts, monoblasts, or promyelocytes in the various acute myelocytic leukemias

Cytochemical stains • Special stains usually performed on bone marrow samples that are examined microscopically to identify enzymes, lipids, or other chemical constituents within the blast population of cells in acute leukemia

Dypsnea • Shortness of breath

Dysplasia • Abnormal maturation of cells in the bone marrow

Gingival hyperplasia • Swelling of the gingival tissues (gums); in leukemia, this is due to infiltration of the gum tissues with leukemic cells

Immunophenotyping • Process of using monoclonal antibodies directed against cell surface markers to identify antigens unique to the specific lineage and stage of maturation

Lineage • Referring to one specific cell line

Lymphoma • Neoplasm involving abnormal proliferation of cells arising in the lymph nodes; these tumor cells may also metastasize to involve extranodal sites

Meningeal leukemia • Leukemic cells proliferating in the central nervous system

Myelodysplasia • Abnormal maturation or differentiation, or both, of granulocytes, erythrocytes, monocytes, and platelets

Oncogene • Gene that is responsible for the development of cancer

References

1. Virchow R. Weisses Blut. Froiep's Notizen 36:151, 1845.
2. Bennett JH. Two cases of disease and enlargement of the spleen in which death took place from the presence of purulent matter in the blood. Edinburgh Med Surg J 64:413, 1845.
3. Virchow R. Die farblosen Blutkorperchen. In: Gesammelte Abhandlungen sur Wissen schaftlichen Medizin. Frankfurt: Meidinger, 1856.
4. Neumann E. Ueber myelogene leukäemie. Berl Klin Wochenschr 15:69, 1878.
5. Ebstein W. Ueber die acute Leukämie und Pseudo-leukämie. Dtsch Arch Klin Med 44:343, 1889.
6. Erlich P. Farbenanolytische Untersuchungen zur Histologie und Klinik des Blutes. Berlin: Hirschwald, 1891.
7. Naegeli O. Ueber rothes Knochenmark und Myeloblasten. Dtsch Med Wochenschr 26:287, 1900.
8. Hirschfield H. Zur Kenntnis der Histogenese der granulirten Knochenmarkzellen. Arch Pathol Anat 153:335, 1898.
9. Look AT. Oncogene transcription factors in human acute leukemias. Science 278:1059, 1997.
10. Sandler DP, Ross JA. Epidemiology of acute leukemia in children and adults. Semin Oncol 24:3–16, 1997.
11. Caldwell GG, Kelley D, Zack M, et al. Mortality and cancer frequency among military nuclear test (SMOKY) participants 1957 through 1979. JAMA 250:620–624, 1983.
12. United Nations Scientific Committee on the Effects of Atomic Radiation. Sources and effects of ionizing radiation. Publ E.94.IX.2. New York: United Nations, 1972.
13. Sullivan AK. Classification, pathogenesis, and etiology of neoplastic diseases of the hematopoietic system. In: Lee GR, Bithell TC, Foerster J, et al, eds. Wintrobe's Clinical Hematology, 9th ed. Philadelphia: Lea & Febiger, 1993; 1725–1791.
14. Chang JC. How to differentiate neoplastic fever from infectious fever in patients with cancer: Usefulness of naproxen test. Heart Lung 16:122, 1987.
15. Golub TR, Weinstein HJ, Grier, HE, Acute myelogeneous leukemia. In: Pizzo P, Poplack D, eds. Principles and Practice of Pediatric Oncology, 3rd ed. Philadelphia: Lippincott, 1997; 463–482.
16. Rohatiner A, Lister TA. The general management of the patient with leukemia. In: Henderson ES, Lister TA, Greaves MF, eds. Leukemia, 6th ed. Philadelphia: WB Saunders, 1996; 247–255.
17. Burns CP, Armitage JO, Frey AL, et al. Analysis of presenting features of adult leukemia. Dancer 47:2460, 1981.
18. Jaffe ES, Harris NL, Stein H, et al. World Health Organization Classification of Tumours: Pathology and Genetics of Tumours of Haematopoietic and Lymphoid Tissues, 3rd ed. Lyon: IARC Press, 2001.
19. Traweek ST, Arber DA, Rappoport H, et al. Extramedullary myeloid tumors: An immunohistochemical and morphologic study of 28 cases. Am J Surg Pathol 17:1011–1019, 1993.
20. Chilosi M, Pizzolo G. Review of terminal deoxynucleotidyl transferase: Biologic aspects, methods of detection, and selected diagnostic application. Appl Immunohistochem 3:209–221, 1995.
21. Kung PC, Long JC, McCaffrey RP, et al. Tdt in the diagnosis of leukemia and malignant lymphoma. Am J Med 64:788, 1978.
22. Marks SM, Baltimore D, McCaffrey R. Terminal transferase as a predictor of initial responsiveness to vincristine and prednisone in blastic chronic myelogenous leukemia: A cooperative study. N Engl J Med 298:812, 1978.
23. Swerdlow SH, Campo E, Harris NL, et a., World Health Organization Classification of Tumours of Hematopoietic and Lymphoid Tissues, 4th ed. Lyon: IARC Press, 2008.
24. Harris NL, Jaffe ES, Diebold J, et al. World Health Organization classification of neoplastic diseases of the hematopoietic and lymphoid tissues: Report of the Clinical Advisory Committee meeting—Airlie House, Virginia, November, 1997. J Clin Oncol 17:3835–3849, 1999.
25. Caligiuri MA, Strout MP, Gilliland DG. Molecular biology of acute myeloid leukemia. Semin Oncol 24:32–34, 1997.
26. Stark B, Resnitzky P, Jeison M, et al. A distinct subtype of M4/M5 acute myeloblastic leukemia (AML) associated with t(8;16)(p11;13), in a patient with the variant t(8;19)(p11;q13)—case report and review of the literature. Leuk Res 19:367–379, 1995.
27. Stanley M, McKenna RW, Ellinger G, et al. Classification of 358 Cases of Acute Myeloid Leukemia by FAB Criteria: Analysis of Clinical and Morphologic Findings in Chronic and Acute Leukemias in Adults. Boston: Martin Nijhoff Publishers, 1985.
28. Head DR. Revised classification of acute myeloid leukemia. Leukemia 10:1826–1831, 1996.
29. Leith CP, Kopecky KJ, Godwin J, et al. Acute myeloid leukemia in the elderly: Assessment of multidrug resistance (MDR1) and cytogenetics distinguishes biologic subgroups with remarkably distinct responses to standard chemotherapy. A Southwest Oncology Group study. Blood 89:3323–3329, 1997.
30. Pui CH, Relling MV, Rivera GK, et al. Epipodophyllotoxin-related acute myeloid leukemia: A study of 35 cases. Leukemia 9:1990–1996, 1995.
31. Ellis M, Ravid M, Lishner M. A comparative analysis of alkylating agent and epipodophyllotoxin-related leukemias. Leuk Lymphoma 11:9–13, 1993.

32. Scott CS, Stark AN, Limbert HJ, et al. Diagnostic and prognostic factors in acute monocytic leukemia: An analysis of 51 cases. Br J Haematol 69:247–252, 1988.

33. Finaux P, Vanhaesbroucke C, Estienne MH, et al. Acute monocytic leukaemia in adults: Treatment and prognosis in 99 cases. Br J Haematol 75:41, 1990.

34. Brunning RD, McKenna RW. Acute leukemias. In: Atlas of Tumor Pathology. Tumors of the Bone Marrow. Washington, DC: Armed Forces Institute of Pathology, 1994; 19–142.

35. Davey FR, Abraham N Jr, Bronetto VL, et al. Morphologic characteristics of erythroleukemia (acute myeloid leukemia; FAB-M6): A CALGB study. Am J Hematol 49:29, 1995.

36. Bernstein J, Dastugue N, Haas OA, et al. Nineteen cases of the t(1;22)(p13;q13) acute megakaryoblastic leukaemia of infants/children and a review of 39 cases: Report from a t(1;22) study group. Leukemia 14:216–218, 2000.

37. Nichols CR, Roth BJ, Heerema N, et al. Hematologic neoplasms associated with primary mediastinal germ-cell tumors. N Engl J Med 322:1425–1429, 1990.

38. Bowman WP, Melvin SL, Aur RJ, et al. A clinical perspective on cell markers in acute lymphocytic leukemia. Cancer Res 41:4752–4766, 1981.

39. Hanson CA, Abaza M, Sheldon S, et al. Acute biphe-notypic leukaemia: Immunophenotypic and cytoge-netic analysis. Br J Haematol 84:49–60, 1993.

40. Legrand O, Perrot JY, Simonin G, et al. Adult biphenotypic acute leukaemia: An entity with poor prognosis which is related to unfavorable cytogenet-ics and P-glycoprotein over-expression. Br J Haematol 100:147–155, 1998.

41. Matutes E, Morilla R, Farahat N, et al. Definition of acute biphenotypic leukemia. Haematologica 82:64–66, 1997.

42. Gurney JG, Davis S, Serverson RK, et al. Trends in cancer incidence among children in the U.S. Cancer 78:532, 1996.

43. SEER Cancer Statistics Review, 1973–1995. Bethesda, MD: National Cancer Institute, 1998.

44. Reaman GH, Sposto R, Sensel MG, et al. Treatment outcome and prognostic factors for infants with acute lymphoblastic leukemia treated on two consecutive trials of the Children's Cancer Group. J Clin Oncol 17:445, 1999.

45. Greaves MF. Aetiology of acute leukaemia. Lancet 349:344, 1997.

46. Kinlen LJ. High-contact paternal occupation, infection and childhood leukaemia: Five studies of unusual population mixing of adults. Br J Cancer 76:1539, 1997.

47. Ingram L, Rivera GK, Shapiro DN. Superior vena cava syndrome associated with childhood malignancy: Analysis of 24 cases. Med Pediatr Oncol 18:476, 1990.

48. Borowitz MJ, Croker BP, Metzgar RS. Lymphoblastic lymphoma with the phenotype of common acute lymphoblastic leukemia. Am J Clin Pathol 79: 387–391, 1983.

49. Weiss LM, Bindl JM, Picozzi VJ, et al. Lymphoblastic lymphoma: An immunophenotype study of 26 cases with comparison to T cell acute lymphoblastic leukemia. Blood 67:474–478, 1986.

50. Look AT. Oncogenic transcription factors in the human acute leukemias. Science 278:1059, 1997.

51. Reiter A, Schrappe M, Tiemann M, et al. Improved treatment results in childhood B-cell neoplasms with tailored intensification of therapy: A report of the Berlin-Frankfurt-Münster group trial NHL-BFM90. Blood 94:3294, 1999.

52. Bowman W, Shuster JJ, Cook B, et al. Improved sur-vival for children with B-cell acute lymphoblastic leukemia and stage IV small noncleaved-cell lym-phoma: A Pediatric Oncology Group study. J Clin Oncol 14:1252, 1996.

53. Smith M, Arthur D, Camita B, et al. Uniform approach to risk classification and treatment assignment for chil-dren with acute lymphoblastic leukemia. J Clin Oncol 14:18, 1996.

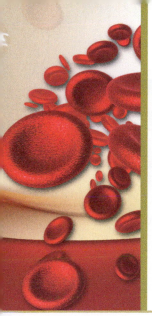

Chapter 12

Chronic Myeloproliferative Disorders

Kathleen Finnegan

Objectives

After completing this chapter, the student will be able to:

1. Define the term myeloproliferative disorders.

2. List and discuss classification of myeloproliferative disorders.

3. Identify the major cell lines involved with myeloproliferative disorders.

4. Discuss the pathogenesis of myeloproliferative disorders.

5. Identify and differentiate clinical features and signs associated with chronic myeloproliferative disorders.

6. Identify and describe the peripheral and bone marrow abnormalities associated with chronic myeloproliferative disorders.

7. Compare and contrast the clinical and laboratory features of chronic myeloproliferative disorders.

8. Identify the diagnostic criteria for chronic myeloproliferative disorders.

9. Discuss the treatment of and prognosis for chronic myeloproliferative disorders.

10. Discuss the cytogenetic abnormalities associated with chronic myeloproliferative disorders.

INTRODUCTION TO CHRONIC MYELOPROLIFERATIVE DISORDERS

Chronic **myeloproliferative** disorders (CMPDs) are a group of disorders that are considered **clonal** malignancies of the hematopoietic stem cell.[1] CMPDs include chronic myelogenous leukemia (CML), idiopathic myelofibrosis (IMF), polycythemia vera (PV), and essential thrombocythemia (ET). Significant changes have evolved in the last decade with regard to terminology of leukemias and associated disorders. In conjunction with the Society for Hematopathology and the European Association of Hematopathology, the World Health Organization (WHO) published a new classification for myeloid and lymphoid neoplasms.[1,2] The WHO classification is based on morphologic, genetic, immunophenotypic, biologic, and clinical features. For lymphoid disorders, the WHO classification uses the Revised European-American Lymphoma (REAL) Classification. The myeloid disorders include the criteria of the French-American-British (FAB) classification and the guidelines of the Polycythemia Vera Study Group (PVSG).[3,4]

The WHO classification of CMPDs recognizes seven entities (Table 12.1).[1–3] These disorders are unified but independent. Each disease has overlapping clinical features but different etiologies. CMPDs are characterized by proliferation of one or more cell lines and are predominantly mature in cell morphology. Bone marrow shows varying degrees of abnormal proliferation of myeloid, erythroid, and megakaryocytic elements. In the peripheral blood, the RBC, WBC, and platelet count vary, and each disorder is identified by the predominant cell that is present. Table 12.2 summarizes the characteristics of CMPDs. Other common features shared by these disorders are splenomegaly, hepatomegaly, increased leukocytosis, thrombocytosis,

and erythrocytosis. There may be various degrees of bone marrow fibrosis. Interrelationships between the disorders are present in all CMPDs. Transitions are common between disorders, and many disorders finally terminate in acute myelogenous leukemia (AML).[1] Figure 12.1 illustrates these interrelationships. A very small percentage of CMPDs terminate in acute lymphoblastic leukemia (ALL). An increase in the percentage of blasts in the peripheral blood and bone marrow indicates the onset of an accelerated stage or transformation to an acute process.

CMPDs are primarily diseases of adults. The peak onset is in the fifth to seventh decades.[1] The major clinical and pathologic findings are unregulated proliferation of cells in the bone marrow, which result in increased numbers of mature cells in the peripheral blood. The increase is found in the granulocytes,

---

Table 12.1 ● 2001 WHO Classification of Chronic Myeloproliferative Diseases

Chronic myelogenous leukemia (CML)

Chronic neutrophilic leukemia (CNL)

Chronic eosinophilic leukemia (CEL) (synonym: hypereosinophilic syndrome)

Polycythemia vera (PV)

Chronic idiopathic myelofibrosis (IMF)

Essential thrombocythemia (ET)

Chronic myeloproliferative disease, unclassifiable

Adapted from Jaffe ES, Harris NL, Stein H, Vardiman JW, eds. World Health Organization Classification of Tumors: Pathology and Genetics of Tumors of Haematopoietic Lymphoic Tissues. Lyon: IARC Press; 2001.

Table 12.2 ● Characteristics of Chronic Myeloproliferative Disorders

CMPD	Cell Line	WBC	Bone Marrow Fibrosis	Philadelphia Chromosome (Ph1)	Organ Involvement
CML	Myeloid	Increased	Variable	Present	Splenomegaly Hepatomegaly
PV	Erythroid, myeloid megakaryocyte	Increased	None	Absent	Splenomegaly Hepatomegaly
IMF	Teardrop erythrocytes Fibroblasts	Variable	Increased	Absent	Splenomegaly Hepatomegaly
ET	Megakaryocyte	Normal	None	Absent	Splenomegaly

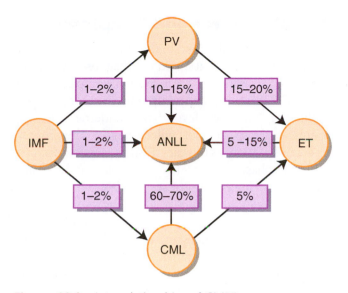

Figure 12.1 Interrelationships of CMPDs.

usually the neutrophils, platelets, or red blood cells. These disorders typically manifest a normocytic, normochromic anemia involving all three cell lines. The dysfunction in CMPDs is a loss of regulatory signals that control the production of the mature cells. An important bone marrow finding that overlaps the various CMPDs is marrow fibrosis. *Fibrosis* is defined as the replacement of normal bone marrow elements with connective tissue. Classification of these diseases is based on the lineage of the predominant cell present, marrow fibrosis, and clinical and pathologic findings.

New World Health Organization Classification

CMPDs are a group of disorders that result in the overproduction of one or more blood cells (red blood cells, white blood cells, and platelets) in the peripheral blood. In 2001, the WHO classification incorporated clinical, morphologic, and genetic features to diagnose the hematopathologic process. Diagnosis was based primarily on clinical and morphologic features. The classification had four major diagnostic entities and three less common entities (see Table 12.1). Since 2001, more has been learned about the pathophysiology of CMPDs and tyrosine kinase activation as a common mechanism. This defect involves signal transduction in the proliferative pathways and involves the *BCR-ABL* gene in CML and *JAK-2* mutation. Other molecular associations have begun to emerge.

In 2008, the WHO classification changed its terminology. CMPDs are now called *myeloproliferative*

neoplasms (MPNs), and primary idiopathic myeloproliferative disorders are now called *primary myelofibrosis*. The refurbished classification also contains new entities and shifts (Table 12.3). The new entities are clonal eosinophilic disorders and mast cell disorders. Shifted entities include hypereosinophilic syndromes with abnormalities in *PDGFRA*, *PDGFBB*, or *FGRII*.

Molecular testing is now essential for diagnosis of MPNs, and the identification of molecular markers *BCR-ABL* and *JAK-2* is incorporated into the diagnosis. The clinical criteria for diagnosis of MPNs have been modified because of these markers. The bone marrow morphology is not a major criterion when a molecular marker is present. Molecular testing is becoming the cornerstone of diagnosis, prognosis, and monitoring response to therapy. For learning purposes, we continue to focus on the major myeloproliferative entities (CML, PV, IMF, ET) for understanding of pathophysiology, morphology, and symptoms.

CHRONIC MYELOGENOUS LEUKEMIA
Disease Overview

CML is a hematopoietic proliferative disorder associated with a specific gene defect and a very characteristic blood picture.[5] Synonyms for this disorder include chronic granulocytic leukemia and chronic myelocytic leukemia. A marked neutrophil leukocytosis is present with some circulation of immature neutrophils and an increase in basophils. The gene defect is the translocation of genetic

Table 12.3 ● 2008 WHO Classification of Myeloproliferative Neoplasms (MNPs)
Chronic myelogenous leukemia *BCR-ABL1* positive
Chronic neutrophilic leukemia
Polycythemia vera (PV)
Primary myelofibrosis
Essential thrombocypenia (ET)
Chronic eosinophilic leukemia (NOS)
Mastocytosis
Cutaneous mastocytosis
Systemic mastocytosis
Mast cell leukemia
Mast cell sarcoma
Extracutaneous mastocytoma
Myeloproliferative neoplasm, unclassifiable

material between chromosome 9 and chromosome 22 t(9:22), which is positive in 90% to 95% of cases.[6,7] This gene mutation is called the Philadelphia chromosome (Ph). This translocation leads to a formation of a hybrid gene called *BCR-ABL*. This fusion gene mutation affects maturation and differentiation of the hematopoietic cells.

CML is usually diagnosed in the chronic phase of the disorder. The peripheral blood picture shows an extremely high WBC showing the whole spectrum of neutrophilic cell development. As the disease evolves, the chronic phase deteriorates to an aggressive or accelerated phase and terminates in an acute phase or blast crisis. CML is one of the most common forms of chronic leukemia.[1] Table 12.4 summarizes key facts for CML.

Pathophysiology

CML is a clonal proliferative disorder. The hallmark of the initial phase is the excess of mature neutrophils in the peripheral blood. The expansion of the myeloid cell results in an alteration of self-renewal and differentiation. There now is an increase in cells. The formation of Ph plays a significant role in the understanding of the pathogenesis of CML. The main portion of the long arm of chromosome 22 is deleted and translocated to the distal end of the long arm of chromosome 9, resulting in an elongated chromosome 9 or 9q+. A small part of chromosome 9 is reciprocally translocated to the broken end of chromosome 22, forming the *BCR-ABL* hybrid gene, which codes for a 210-kDa protein, or p210, which has increased tyrosine kinase activity.[5,8] Tyrosine kinase activity provides an important mediator to regulate metabolic pathways causing abnormal cell cycling. The activation of tyrosine kinase activity may suppress apoptosis (natural cell death) in hematopoietic cells and provide the mechanism for excess cell production.[6,9]

Clinical Features and Symptoms

Most patients are diagnosed in the chronic phase. Many patients are asymptomatic and are diagnosed when an elevated WBC is found on a routine complete blood count (CBC). Common symptoms include fatigue, weight loss, low-grade fever, bone tenderness, loss of appetite, night sweats, and splenomegaly. The chronic phase can last months to years. CML is characterized by a chronic phase, an accelerated phase, and a blast phase. As the disease progresses, the features worsen.

The accelerated phase of CML shows an increasing peripheral blood count, the appearance of peripheral blasts and promyelocytes, increased splenomegaly, bone pain, thrombocytopenia, and worsening anemia. The acute phase or blast crisis is similar to acute leukemia. Bone marrow and peripheral blood blast counts are greater than 20%.[1] Excessive bleeding, infection, petechiae, ecchymosis, and bruising are seen more in the later stage secondary to bone marrow failure.

Peripheral Blood and Bone Marrow

The peripheral blood smear shows the presence of a severe leukocytosis with the entire spectrum of myeloid cell development. A mild normocytic, normochromic anemia with nucleated red blood cells is a common finding. Eosinophils, basophils, and myelocytes increase in number. Thrombocytosis is present in the chronic phase. Figure 12.2 illustrates the spectrum of neutrophilic maturation seen in CML. As the disease progresses, the anemia worsens, and thrombocytopenia and younger cells are seen. In the acute phase, the blast count increases and may be greater than 20%.

Table 12.4 ⊙ Chronic Myelogenous Leukemia: Key Facts

- Clonal stem cell disorder
- Marked leukocytosis with all stages of granulocyte maturation
- Hepatosplenomegaly
- Thrombocytosis is common in chronic phase
- Three phases—chronic, accelerated, blast
- Philadelphia chromosome
- *BCR-ABL* fusion gene
- LAP score <10

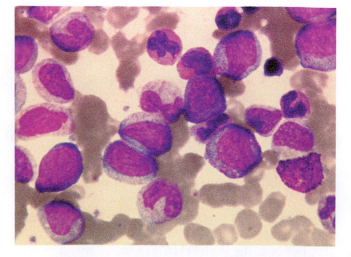

Figure 12.2 Spectrum of neutrophil maturation seen in CML. Courtesy of Dr. Sidonie Morrison and Kathleen Finnegan, Stony Brook University, New York.

Examination of the bone marrow reveals a hypercellular marrow with marked myeloid **hyperplasia**. The myeloid:erythroid (M:E) ratio is 10:1 and can reach 25:1. A normal M:E ratio is 3–4:1. The bone marrow may become fibrotic as the disease progresses. Table 12.5 summarizes the peripheral blood and bone marrow findings in the three phases of CML.

Diagnosis

CML must be distinguished from other myeloproliferative disorders. The presence of the Ph chromosome or *BCR-ABL* fusion gene and a low or absent leukocyte alkaline phosphatase (LAP) score is diagnostic for CML. The LAP score is a cytochemical stain that is used to differentiate CML from a leukemoid reaction. LAP enzyme is located in the granules of the neutrophil and bands. LAP activity increases with the maturity of the neutrophil. To determine the LAP score, 100 mature neutrophils and bands are stained, counted, and scored for stain intensity and granulation. In a leukemoid reaction, the LAP score is high, and in CML, it is low. A leukemoid reaction is caused by a severe infection or inflammation. This reaction can resemble a leukemic process. Table 12.6 summarizes the differentiation of a neutrophilic leukemoid reaction and CML.

Treatment

The goal of treatment for CML is to achieve hematologic remission, which consists of a normal CBC, no **organomegaly**, and a negative Ph1 chromosome or negative *BCR-ABL* fusion gene. The chronic phase can be controlled with hydroxyurea, interferon-alfa, or busulfan therapy.[10] This type of therapy is called myelosuppressive therapy, with the goal of controlling the hyperproliferation of the myeloid elements. The drug tries to decrease the WBC by interfering with cell division. Cytotoxic drug therapy cannot prevent the blast crisis. Another treatment is leukapheresis, which uses a cell separator to decrease the WBC rapidly (red blood cells are reinfused) and a cytotoxic drug to keep the patient in a longer remission.[5,7]

A new treatment approach involves the direct inhibition of the abnormal molecule using a tyrosine kinase inhibitor. This inhibitor reacts to the *BCL-ABL* tyrosine kinase associated with the Ph chromosome. The drug is called imatinib mesylate (Gleevec), and it inhibits proliferation, slows cell growth, and induces cell death.[11–13] An additional treatment for CML is allogeneic bone marrow or stem cell transplantation. Bone marrow transplantation, however, has a high mortality rate due to graft-versus-host disease (GVHD).[14] Allogeneic bone

Table 12.5 ○ Peripheral Blood and Bone Marrow Findings in the Three Phases of Chronic Myelogenous Leukemia			
	Chronic Phase	**Accelerated Phase**	**Blast Phase**
Peripheral blood	Leukocytosis with the presence of neutrophils in all stages of maturation	Increase in promyelocytes	Blasts greater than 20%
	Blasts greater than 2%	Blasts increased	Increase in promyelocytes
	Increased basophils	Basophils greater than 20%	Increase in basophils and eosinophils
	Increased eosinophils	Increase in circulation nucleated red blood cells	Thrombocytopenia
	Thrombocytosis	Erythrocytes	
	Mild anemia	Persistent thrombocytopenia	
	Nucleated red blood cells	Anemia	
Bone marrow	Hyperplasia myeloid	Dysplasia	Blasts greater than 20%
	Blasts less than 5%	Blasts greater than 5% and less than 20%	Large clusters of blasts
	M:E ratio 10:1	Left shift of mature neutrophils	Increased fibrosis
	Increased immature forms of basophils	Increased basophils	Marked dysplasia of all three cell lines
	Reduced erythrocytes	Megakaryocytic proliferation in sheets and clusters	
	Increased megakaryocytes	Fibrosis	

Table 12.6 ○ Differentiating a Neutrophilic Leukemoid Reaction and CML

Criterion	CML	Leukemoid Reaction
Neutrophil	Whole spectrum of cells mature to the blast	Shift to the left, more bands, metamyelocytes, blast very rare
Eosinophil	Increased	Normal
Basophil	Increased	Normal
Platelet	Increased with abnormal forms	Normal
Anemia	Usually present	Not typical
LAP score	Decreased	Increased
Ph1 chromosome	Present	Absent
Toxic granulation	Absent	Increased
Döhle bodies	Absent	Increased

marrow transplantation is currently the only curative therapy.[1] Many clinical trials are in progress searching for better prognosis.

Prognosis

The chronic phase of CML is highly responsive to treatment. The median survival is 4 to 6 years, with a range of 1 year to longer than 10 years. Survival after developing an accelerated phase is usually less than 1 year, and after blast crisis, survival is only a few months.[15] Poor prognosis in patients with CML is associated with the following factors:

- Age
- Phase of CML
- Amount of blasts in the peripheral blood and bone marrow
- Size of the spleen at diagnosis
- Marrow fibrosis
- General health

For patients lacking the Ph1 chromosome, median survival is about 1 year.[16]

CHRONIC NEUTROPHILIC LEUKEMIA

Chronic neutrophilic leukemia (CNL) is a rare CMPD characterized by an elevated neutrophil count. The bone marrow is hypercellular with an increase in the granulocytic proliferation. An enlarged spleen and liver are also present. There is no significant dysplasia in any cell line, and bone marrow fibrosis is uncommon.[1] The Ph1 chromosome or *BCR-ABL* fusion gene is absent.[17]

CHRONIC EOSINOPHILIC LEUKEMIA

Chronic eosinophilic leukemia (CEL) is a CMPD characterized by an elevation and proliferation of eosinophils.[1] Eosinophils increase in the peripheral blood, bone marrow, and peripheral tissue, resulting in tissue and organ damage. CEL is diagnosed when the blood eosinophil count is greater than 1,500/µL, there are no other causes for increased eosinophils, and clinical signs and symptoms indicate organ damage. No Ph1 chromosome or *BCL-ABL* fusion gene is found. Synonyms for CEL include hypereosinophilic syndrome.

POLYCYTHEMIA VERA

Disease Overview

PV (polycythemia rubra vera) is a clonal disorder characterized by overproduction of mature red blood cells, white blood cells, and platelets.[19,20] Increased production of red blood cells results in increased hemoglobin, hematocrit, and *red blood cell mass* (RCM). Erythrocytosis is the most prominent clinical manifestation of PV. The bone marrow is usually hypercellular with hyperplasia of all three bone marrow elements. This disorder usually occurs in the sixth or seventh decade of life. All causes of secondary erythrocytosis must be excluded before a diagnosis of PV can be made. Table 12.7 summarizes the key facts for PV.

Pathophysiology

The etiology of PV has become clearer recently. The primary defect involves the pluripotential stem cell

Table 12.7 ○ Polycythemia Vera: Key Facts

- Increase in all three cell lines
- Absolute increase in RCM
- Normal oxygen saturation
- Splenomegaly
- Recommended treatment is phlebotomy
- Thrombosis and hemorrhage
- *JAK2* mutation present in most

that has the capability of differentiating into red blood cells, white blood cells, and platelets. The *JAK2 V617F* mutation has been discovered in most patients with PV.[18] This mutation, which is a phenylalanine-to-valine mutation at position 617, activates JAK2 kinase, leading to red blood cell production that is **independent** of erythropoietin. Erythroid precursors in PV are very sensitive to erythropoietin, leading to an increased red blood cell production. The increased red blood cell production leads to an increase in RCM and increased blood viscosity. For this reason, patients are predisposed to arterial and venous thrombosis or increased bleeding, or both. The elevated hematocrit and platelet counts are directly proportional to the number of thrombotic events.[18]

Clinical Features and Symptoms

Patients tend to be asymptomatic at the time of diagnosis. Symptoms are often insidious in onset. As the red blood cells and platelets increase, more symptoms become evident. The major symptoms are related to hypertension, hyperviscosity, and vascular abnormalities caused by the increased RCM. Symptoms of hyperviscosity and increased hematocrit include headache, light-headedness, blurred vision or visual disturbances, fatigue, and plethora. **Plethora** is a condition of a red or ruddy complexion caused by the expanded blood volume. Plethora manifests in the nail beds, hands, feet, face, and conjunctivae. Thrombosis in the small blood vessels leads to painful dilation of the vessels in the extremities. Sometimes ulceration or gangrene can occur in the fingers and toes. Thrombosis in the larger vessels can lead to myocardial infarction, **transient ischemic attacks**, stroke, and **deep vein thrombosis** (DVT).

Abnormalities in platelet function can lead to bleeding from the nose (epistaxis), easy bruising, and gingival bleeding. The increased blood cell turnover can cause hyperuricemia, **gout**, and stomach ulcers. As the disease progresses, patients develop abdominal pain because of hepatomegaly and splenomegaly. Splenomegaly is present in 75% of patients at the time of diagnosis, and hepatomegaly is present in about 30%.[20,21] **Pruritus**, which results from increased histamine levels released from the basophil, is a common extenuating symptom.

Peripheral Blood and Bone Marrow Findings

PV is characterized by pancytosis, an increased cell count in all three cell lines. The major characteristics of PV are normoblastic erythroid proliferation in the

bone marrow and an increased number of normocytic, normochromic red blood cells in the peripheral blood. Figure 12.3 illustrates the increase in red blood cells. The reticulocyte count tends to be normal or slightly increased. Neutrophilia with a shift to the left and basophilia are common in the blood smear.[1] At disease onset, RBC, hemoglobin, and hematocrit are increased. The red blood cell distribution width (RDW) tends to be higher than normal. The granulocyte and platelet counts are found to be increased. The LAP score is usually elevated. Platelet counts are increased and have abnormal morphology and function.

Characteristically, the bone marrow biopsy specimen is hypercellular, and peripheral pancytosis is seen as the result of the increased cellularity. The increased number of erythroid and megakaryocytic precursors is more significant. The bone marrow biopsy specimen shows increased reticulin or fibrosis. The amount of reticulin is directly proportional to the amount of cellularity. The iron stores of the bone marrow are usually depleted.

As the disease progresses, the erythroid activity in the marrow decreases. The classic leukoerythroblastic picture emerges when immature white blood cell and red blood cell precursors are found in the peripheral blood with marked morphology. Microcytes, elliptocytes, and dacryocytes (teardrop cells) develop. Granulocytes and platelet morphology are abnormal with increases in younger and younger cells.

Diagnosis

The major diagnostic issue related to PV is distinguishing it from secondary and relative erythrocytosis. Secondary erythrocytosis is an increase in the RCM

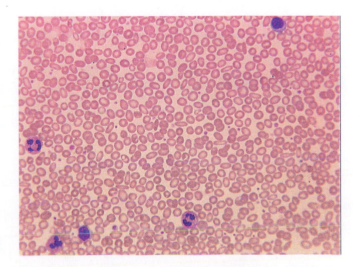

Figure 12.3 Increased red blood cells in PV. Courtesy of Dr. Sidonie Morrison and Kathleen Finnegan, Stony Brook University, New York.

without evidence of changes in the other cell lines. Table 12.8 summarizes the causes of secondary erythrocytosis. Relative erythrocytosis is due to dehydration and hemoconcentration. Elevated hematocrit and hemoglobin counts are a result of an elevated RBC and a low plasma volume.

Table 12.9 summarizes the diagnostic criteria of the national Polycythemia Vera Study Group (PVSG).[1,22] PV is present when a patient shows all of the major or primary criteria (elevated hematocrit or RCM, normal arterial oxygen saturation, and splenomegaly) or some major criteria together with secondary or minor criteria (thrombocytosis, leukocytosis, elevated LAP score, and increased serum vitamin B_{12}). The most significant finding in PV is increased RCM, splenomegaly, and the *JAK2* mutation with increase in leukocytes and platelets. Other tests that are helpful in the diagnosis of PV are a bone marrow aspirate and biopsy. Although these invasive procedures are unnecessary to establish a diagnosis, a hypercellular marrow with hyperplasia of erythroid, granulocytic, and megakaryocytic elements supports the diagnosis. Serum erythropoietin levels in patients with PV are often found to be low compared with patients with secondary and relative erythrocytosis.[20,23]

There is no consistent or unique cytogenetic abnormality associated with PV. Cytogenetic abnormalities are found in 8% to 20% of patients at the time of diagnosis.[24] The most frequent cytogenetic abnormality are **trisomy** of 1q, 8, 9 or 9p, del 3q, del 20q or interstitial deletions of chromosome 13 or 20.[24]

Treatment

Initial treatment decreases hematocrit and hemoglobin, reducing plasma viscosity. Therapy recommendations

Table 12.8 ⊙ **Causes of Secondary Erythrocytosis**
• Hypertension
• Arterial hypoxemia
• Impaired tissue oxygen delivery
• Smoking
• Renal lesions
• Renal disease
• Endocrine lesions
• Drugs
• Alcohol
• Hepatic lesions

Table 12.9 ⊙ **Diagnostic Criteria for Polycythemia Vera**	
A1	Elevated RCM greater than 25% above mean normal predicted
	Hemoglobin greater than 18.5 g/dL in men or greater than 16.5 g/dL in women
A2	No cause or absence of secondary erythrocytosis
A3	Splenomegaly
A4	Presence of *JAK2 V617F* mutation or other cytogenetic abnormalities in hematopoietic cells
A5	Endogenous erythroid colony formation in vitro
B1	Thrombocytosis greater than 400×10^9/L
B2	WBC greater than 12×10^9/L
B3	Bone marrow biopsy specimen with panmyelosis with prominent and megakaryocytic proliferation
B4	Low serum erythropoietin levels
A1 + A2 + any other category of A present = PV diagnosis.	
A1 + A2 + any two of category B present = PV diagnosis.	

Adapted from Jaffe ES, Harris NL, Stein H, Vardiman JW, eds. Organization Classification of Tumors: Pathology and Genetics of Tumors of Haematopoietic Lymphoid Tissues. Lyon: IARC Press, 2001; and Pearson TC, Messinezy M, Westwood N, et al. A polycythemia vera update: Diagnosis, pathobiology and treatment. Hematology Am Soc Hematol Educ Program 51–68, 2000.

are based on age, sex, clinical manifestations, and hematologic findings. Treatment recommendations for patients with PV include phlebotomy, radioactive phosphorus (^{32}P), myelosuppressive agents, and interferon-alfa.[25] The target goal for therapy is to decrease the hematocrit. For men, the hematocrit target value is less than 45%, and for women, it is less than 40%.[26] **Therapeutic phlebotomy** is an immediately effective therapy and is usually the first choice of the recommended treatments. An aggressive therapeutic phlebotomy regimen results in iron deficiency in some patients.

Prognosis

PV is a chronic disease. The median survival is more than 10 years with treatment.[1] The major causes of death in untreated patients are hemorrhage and thrombosis. Other causes of death are complications of myeloid metaplasia or the development of leukemia.[1] The incidence of transformation into an acute leukemia is greater in patients treated with radioactive phosphorus or alkylating agents.[26]

During the later stages of PV, a post–polycythemic myelofibrosis phase occurs, characterized by a leukoerythroblastic peripheral blood picture with an increase in immature white blood cells and red blood cells. The red blood cells appear in a teardrop shape, with an increase in shape changes. The spleen increases in size secondary to extramedullary hematopoiesis. The main characteristics of this stage are the increase in reticulin and fibrosis in the bone marrow.[27]

IDIOPATHIC MYELOFIBROSIS

Disease Overview

IMF is a CMPD characterized by bone marrow fibrosis, proliferation of megakaryocytic and granulocytic cells, and extramedullary hematopoiesis. IMF manifests with an elevated WBC, teardrop red blood cells, normocellular or hypercellular bone marrow, leukoerythroblastic anemia, splenomegaly, and the absence of the Ph chromosome.[28,29] IMF is a clonal hematopoietic stem cell expansion in the bone marrow with the production of reticulin and bone marrow fibrosis.[30,31] Table 12.10 summarizes key facts for IMF. There are many synonyms for IMF, including agnogenic myeloid metaplasia, chronic idiopathic myelofibrosis, myelofibrosis with myeloid metaplasia, primary myelofibrosis, leukoerythroblastic anemia, and myelosclerosis with myeloid metaplasia.

Pathophysiology

The etiology of IMF is unknown, and the mechanism of myelofibrosis is poorly understood. The clonal proliferation of hematopoietic stem cells is thought to produce growth factors and an abnormal cytokine release that mediates a bone marrow reaction that leads to fibrosis of the bone marrow.[32,33] Platelets, megakaryocytes, and monocytes are thought to secrete cytokines, transforming growth factor-beta (TGF-beta), platelet-derived growth factor (PDGF), interleukin (IL)-1, and fibroblast growth factor, which may result in formation of the bone marrow matrix.[32,33]

Table 12.10 ● Idiopathic Myelofibrosis: Key Facts

- Leukoerythroblastosis
- Extramedullary hematopoiesis
- Fibrosis of bone marrow/reticulin silver stain
- Teardrop red blood cells
- Absence of Ph chromosome
- Hepatosplenomegaly
- *JAK2* mutation may be present

IMF has an evolutionary disease process. The initial phase is the prefibrotic stage, which is characterized by a hypercellular bone marrow with minimal reticulin. The second phase is the fibrotic stage, which is characterized by bone marrow with marked reticulin or collagen fibrosis. Normal hematopoiesis is blocked as the bone marrow becomes more fibrotic. This stage is characterized by a leukoerythroblastic blood smear: immature white blood cells and nucleated red blood cells combined with teardrop red blood cells. Patients become pancytopenic (decrease in all three cell lines). Extramedullary hematopoiesis contributes to the leukoerythroblastic blood picture, splenomegaly, and hepatomegaly. Myelofibrosis is a complicating reactive feature of the primary disease process.

Clinical Features and Symptoms

In the early stages of IMF, the patient may be asymptomatic. Patients with myelofibrosis exhibit splenomegaly, anemia, and marrow fibrosis. Many of the signs and symptoms are attributed to the pancytopenia associated with the presence of a fibrotic bone marrow. Pancytopenia occurs as a result of decreased cell production because of the marrow fibrosis or ineffective hematopoiesis with increased spleen sequestration. Most patients exhibit symptoms of anemia. Patients who are thrombocytopenic and neutropenic are prone to bleeding tendencies and infection. Other symptoms include night sweats, low-grade fever, weight loss, and anorexia. Patients often complain of left upper quadrant discomfort because of enlarged spleen and liver. Patients with myelofibrosis develop **osteosclerosis**, which can cause severe joint pain.

Peripheral Blood and Bone Marrow Findings

The peripheral blood and bone marrow biopsy provide information for diagnosis. The WBC and platelet count may increase initially but decrease as the disease progresses. The typical picture is a blood smear that shows leukoerythroblastosis and teardrop red blood cells (Fig. 12.4). Large platelets, megakaryocyte fragments, and immature blood cells may be found because of the crowding out of normal cell development by fibrosis in the bone marrow. A normocytic, normochromic anemia is present with hemoglobin of less than 10 g/dL.

The bone marrow is hypercellular with increased and abnormal megakaryocytes and megakaryocyte clusters. Bone marrow aspirates result in dry taps in about 50% of patients. A "dry tap" refers to the inability of the physician to obtain a sample because the

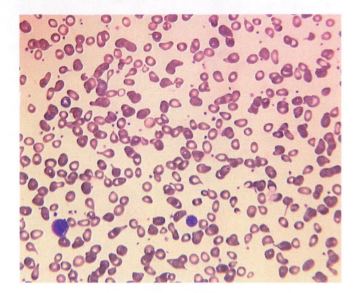

Figure 12.4 Teardrop red blood cells in IMF. Courtesy of Dr. Sidonie Morrison and Kathleen Finnegan, Stony Brook University, New York.

Table 12.11 ○ Diagnostic Criteria for Idiopathic Myelofibrosis

Clinical criteria

A1	No preceding or allied subtype of CMPDs
A2	Early clinical stages
	Normal hemoglobin
	Slight or moderate splenomegaly
	Thrombocythemia platelets greater than $400 \times 10^9/L$
A3	Intermediate clinical stage
	Anemia
	Definitive leukoerythroblastic blood picture/teardrop red blood cells
	Splenomegaly
	No advance signs
A4	Advanced clinical stage
	Anemia
	One or more adverse signs

Pathologic criteria

B1	Megakaryocytic and granulocytic proliferation
	Reduction in red blood cell precursors
	Abnormal giant-sized megakaryocytes

Adapted from Spivak JL, Barosi G, Tognoni G, et al. Chronic myeloproliferative disorders. Hematology 1:200–224, 2003.

normal architecture of the bone marrow is disrupted by fibrotic tissue, also known as reticulin.

Diagnosis

Diagnosis is made on the basis of detecting splenomegaly and the results of the CBC. Splenomegaly is the most common finding, followed by hepatomegaly.[34] The PVSG has criteria for myelofibrosis as follows: splenomegaly, fibrosis of the bone marrow, a leukoerythroblastic blood picture, absence of increased RCM, absence of the Ph chromosome, and exclusion of any other systemic disease. Table 12.11 summarizes the diagnostic criteria for IMF.[35]

There are no specific genetic defects. Cytogenetic abnormalities occur in about 60% of patients.[36] Cytogenetics rule out CML, myelodysplastic syndrome, and other chronic myeloid disorders. Various chromosomal abnormalities may occur, most commonly del(13q), del(20q) and partial trisomy 1q.[36]

Treatment

No treatments are available to reverse the process of IMF. Asymptomatic patients are observed and require no treatment. Therapy for IMF is mainly supportive for anemia and thrombocythemia. Hydroxyurea is used as a cytoreductive therapy to control leukocytosis, thrombocytosis, and organomegaly.[28] Interferon-alfa is used in patients younger than 45 years. Splenectomy may be considered for treating patients with symptomatic splenomegaly that is refractory to hydroxyurea.[37] Radiation may be used to treat symptomatic

extramedullary hematopoiesis. A more aggressive approach is allogeneic peripheral stem cell or bone marrow transplantation.[38]

Prognosis

IMF has the worst prognosis of all the myeloproliferative disorders. The median survival is approximately 3 to 5 years from diagnosis.[29] Major causes of death are infection, cardiovascular disease, hemorrhage, thrombosis, progressive marrow failure, and transformation into an acute leukemia.[29,31] Prognostic factors that affect survival include age, anemia, leukopenia, leukocytosis, circulating blasts, and karyotype abnormalities. There is a shorter survival with poor prognostic values.[28,39]

ESSENTIAL THROMBOCYTHEMIA
Disease Overview

Primary ET is a CMPD characterized by a clonal proliferation of megakaryocytes in the bone marrow. The peripheral blood platelet counts exceed $600 \times 10^9/L$

and can be greater than $1,000 \times 10^9/L$. This disease is characterized by an increased platelet count, a megakaryocytic hyperplasia, and an absence of increased RCM. The clinical course is complicated by hemorrhage or thrombotic episodes. The etiology is unknown; the disorder usually occurs between age 50 and 70 years.[1] Table 12.12 summarizes key facts for ET.

Pathophysiology

ET is considered a clonal disorder of the multipotential stem cell.[35] ET has many biologic characteristics in common with PV and other myeloproliferative disorders. This disorder can affect all three cell lines, but its main characteristic is the increase in the megakaryocyte. Bone marrow and peripheral blood are the principal sites of involvement in this disorder. Megakaryocytes are hypersensitive to several cytokines, including IL-3, IL-6, and thrombopoietin, leading to increased platelet production.[40] Platelet survival and platelet aggregation studies are normal.

The increased platelet count can cause increased thrombotic and hemorrhagic episodes. Qualitative abnormalities in the platelet contribute to the increased risk of thrombotic and hemorrhagic complications. Age, previous thrombotic event, increased or greater than $600 \times 10^9/L$ platelet counts, duration of disease, and prior symptoms are considered high-risk factors. The increased thrombotic risk that accompanies aging has been attributed to vascular disease or hypercoagulable platelets.

Clinical Features and Symptoms

Most often, patients are asymptomatic at the time of diagnosis. The elevated platelet count is discovered on a routine CBC. The clinical signs and symptoms are similar to those of PV. The most frequent symptoms are weight loss, low-grade fever, weakness, pruritus, hemorrhage, headache, and dizziness. Bleeding is usually mild and may manifest as epistaxis and the tendency to bruise easily. The gastrointestinal tract is the primary site for bleeding complications. Patients who present with microvascular occlusion may have transient ischemic attacks with symptoms of unsteadiness, syncope, and seizures. Thrombosis of the large veins and main arteries is common. Occlusion of the leg arteries and renal arteries may be involved. When ET is diagnosed, approximately 50% of patients present with an enlarged spleen, and approximately 20% of patients present with an enlarged liver.[1]

Peripheral Blood and Bone Marrow Findings

The hallmark for ET is an unexplained elevated platelet count. The blood platelet count is usually greater than $1,000 \times 10^9/L$, and the platelets have anisocytosis ranging from small to large forms. Figure 12.5 illustrates the increased platelet count. The peripheral blood may reveal a leukocytosis with an occasional immature cell (myelocytes and metamyelocytes); erythrocytosis; and a mild normocytic, normochromic anemia. A mild basophilia and eosinophilia may be seen. Leukoerythroblastosis and teardrop cells are not features of ET.

The bone marrow shows increased cellularity. Megakaryocytic hyperplasia is the most striking feature. Giant megakaryocytes and clusters of megakaryocytes are frequently seen. The megakaryocytes have

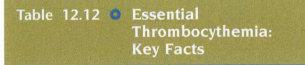

Table 12.12 ●	Essential Thrombocythemia: Key Facts

- Marked thrombocytosis (platelet count greater than $600 \times 10^9/L$)
- Usually no fibrosis
- Neurologic manifestations
- Abnormal platelet function
- Megakaryocyte fragments in peripheral blood and bone marrow
- Absent Ph chromosome
- *JAK2* mutation may be present

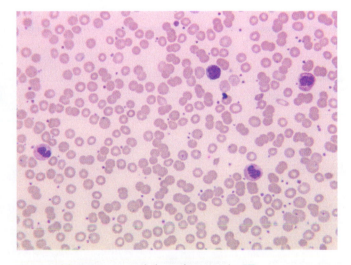

Figure 12.5 • Increased thrombocytes in ET. Courtesy of Dr. Sidonie Morrison and Kathleen Finnegan, Stony Brook University, New York.

abundant, mature cytoplasm and hyperlobulated nuclei. Proliferation of erythroid precursors may be found in some cases. The network of reticulin fibers is normal or slightly increased.[1] Increased reticulin or collagen fibrosis points more toward IMF than ET. Stainable iron is present.

Diagnosis

Distinguishing ET from reactive thrombocytosis and the other myeloproliferative disorders is a diagnostic challenge. For the diagnosis of ET, reactive thrombocytosis needs to be excluded. Secondary or reactive thrombocytosis is associated with many acute and chronic infections. Table 12.13 summarizes the causes of relative thrombocytosis. In reactive thrombocytosis, the platelet count is less than 1 million/µL and is transient. Leukocytes and erythrocytes are normal. Platelet function is normal, and the spleen and liver are not enlarged.

Diagnostic requirements for ET include a normal RCM (increased with PV), a hemoglobin of less than 13 g/dL (elevated in PV), the absence of the Ph1 chromosome (associated with CML), and the absence of teardrop red blood cells or significant increase in bone marrow fibrosis (seen in IMF). Diagnosis for ET follows the gold standard criteria of the PVSG.[3] Table 12.14 summarizes the diagnostic criteria for ET.[3,41] There are no characteristic cytogenetic or molecular abnormalities that are associated with ET or establish diagnosis for patients with ET.[41,42]

Treatment

The treatment goal for ET is to prevent or reduce the risk of complications from vaso-occlusion or

Table 12.13 • Causes of Relative Thrombocytosis

- Inflammatory states
- Infection
- Trauma
- Blood loss
- Postsplenectomy
- Acute hemorrhage
- Malignancy
- Postoperative
- Hemolytic anemia

Table 12.14 • Diagnostic Criteria for Essential Thrombocythemia

	Platelet count greater than 600×10^9/L
II.	Hematocrit less than 40 or normal RCM (men less than 36 mL/kg, women less than 32 mL/kg)
III.	Stainable iron in marrow or normal serum ferritin or normal red blood cell mean corpuscular volume
IV.	Absent Ph1 chromosome or *BCR-ABL* gene rearrangement
V.	Collagen fibrosis of marrow
	A. Absent, *or*
	B. Less than one-third of biopsy specimen involved and neither marked splenomegaly nor a leukoerythroblastic reaction
VI.	No cytogenetic or morphologic evidence for myelodysplastic syndrome
VII.	No cause for reactive thrombocytosis

Adapted from Murphy S, Peterson P, Iland H, Laszio J. Experience of the Polycythemia Vera Study Group with essential thrombocythemia: A final report on diagnostic criteria, survival and leukemic transition by treatment. Semin Hematol 34:29, 1997; and Nimer S. Essential thrombocythemia: Another "heterogeneous disease" better understood? Blood 93:415–416, 1999.

hemorrhage. The treatment of ET can vary from no treatment, if patients are asymptomatic; to low-dose aspirin for low-risk patients; to treatment with hydroxyurea, anagrelide, or alfa-interferon to reduce the platelet count.[43,44] Patients with life-threatening hemorrhagic or thrombotic events should be treated with platelet pheresis in combination with myelosuppressive therapy to reduce the platelet count to less than $1,000 \times 10^9$/L.[40] Maintaining a platelet count of less than 400×10^9/L is necessary to reduce the risk of a thrombotic event.

Prognosis

Prognosis depends on the age of the patient and the history of thrombotic events (Table 12.15). The survival rate is 10 years for 64% to 80% of the patients, particularly younger patients.[4,46] Less than 10% of patients with ET convert to AML and less than 5% convert to IMF.[47] Most patients die as a result of thrombotic complications.

Table 12.15 ● Differentiation of Myeloproliferative Disorders

Laboratory Findings	CML	IMF	PV	ET
Hematocrit	Normal/decreased	Decreased	Marked increased	Normal/decreased
WBC	Marked neutrophilia with shift to the left Basophilia and eosinophilia	Increased Left shift with myeloblasts (occ) Basophilia and eosinophilia	Normal/increased Leukocytosis with neutrophilia and basophilia	Normal/increased Leukocytosis usually mild
RBC	Normal Few nucleated red blood cells	Teardrop reticulocytosis Nucleated red blood cells	Normal morphology as disease progresses; iron-deficient morphology	Normal morphology and maturation
Platelets	Normal/increased Enlarged and fragments	Normal/decreased/increased Giant and abnormal megakaryocytes present	Increased	Increased Platelet count greater than 600,000/μL Giant size Bizarre shapes Micromegakaryocytes and megakaryocytic fragments
Immature granulocytes	Increased	Increased	Absent or shift	Rare
LAP	Decreased	Normal/increased	Increased	Normal
Ph chromosome	Present	Absent	Absent	Absent
Spleen	Normal/enlarged	Enlarged	Enlarged	Normal/enlarged
Bone marrow	Hypercellular predominantly granulocytic Decreased iron stores	Increased fibrosis Megakaryocytic hyperplasia RBCs and WBCs usually normal Bone marrow aspirate dry tap	Hypercellular moderate to severe All three lines increased with normal maturation Deceased iron stores	Hypercellular mild to moderate Megakaryocytic hyperplasia Clusters and sheets of megakaryocytes Some marrow fibrosis
Diagnostic criteria	Complete spectrum of all stages of neutrophil maturation Less than 5% blasts in peripheral blood Ph chromosome present in 90%–95% of cases Three clinical phases: Chronic Accelerated Blast	Leukoerythroblastic picture with teardrop red blood cells Fibrotic marrow as disease progresses Enlarged spleen	Excessive red blood cell production Increased red blood cell volume, normal O_2 saturation, all three lines increased Enlarged spleen	Platelet count greater than 600×10^9/L with no known cause for reactive thrombocytosis Complications of thrombosis and hemorrhage

Adapted from Finnegan K. Leukocyte disorders. In: Lehmann C, ed. Saunders Manual of Clinical Laboratory Science. Philadelphia: WB Saunders, 1998: 903–944.

CONDENSED CASE

A 44-year-old woman went to her physician as part of a physical examination for life insurance. Her medical history was unremarkable, but she complained of loss of appetite with a full feeling in her upper abdomen. She appeared to be in good physical condition, but her spleen was palpable. Her physician ordered a complete CBC. **What condition could cause an enlarged spleen?**

Answer

An enlarged spleen can occur primarily as a result of hemolysis and sequestered cells or as a result of extramedullary hematopoiesis. In this case, the CBC revealed a 50,000 WBC and a differential that showed the entire family of white blood cells. LAP was ordered, and it was negative. This patient was diagnosed with early-stage chronic myelocytic leukemia. She was in no acute distress, but she was cautioned that since her spleen was enlarged, her movements should be restricted so as not to cause a rupture.

○ Summary Points

- CMPDs are caused by abnormal stem cells that lead to unchecked autonomous proliferation of one or more cell lines.

- The most common CMPDs are chronic granulocytic leukemia, PV, IMF, and ET.

- The bone marrow in CMPDs may show hyperplasia or elements of fibrosis.

- Most CMPDs are seen in older adults and show a normochromic, normocytic anemic process.

- Individuals with CML show an extremely high WBC, moderate anemia, and the entire spectrum of white blood cells in the peripheral smear.

- Of patients with CML, 90% have the Ph chromosome, a cytogenetic abnormality in which a small part of chromosome 9 is translocated to the broken arm of chromosome 22.

- A hybrid gene, *BCR-ABL*, is also manifested with the Ph chromosome, and this gene prevents natural cell death or apoptosis.

- In the accelerated phase of CML, a higher blast count may be present and eventually ends in blast crisis, all blasts in the bone marrow.

- PV is a clonal disorder of red blood cells in which the patient shows a pancytosis: high RBC, high WBC, and high platelet count.

- The *JAK2 V617F* mutation has been shown in large numbers of patients with PV and in fewer patients with ET and IMF.

- Patients with PV have symptoms related to hyperviscosity, including hypertension and vascular abnormalities.

- The LAP score is usually elevated in PV and low in CML.

- Patients with PV must be distinguished from patients with secondary or relative erythrocytosis.

- The major causes of death in patients with PV are hemorrhage and thrombosis.

- IMF is characterized by marrow fibrosis, extramedullary hematopoiesis, and the leukoerythroblastic blood smear.

- In patients with IMF, the accelerating fibrosis may contribute to leukopenia and thrombocytopenia.

- In 50% of patients with IMF, bone marrow aspirates are impossible because of increased fibrosis (the dry tap).

- IMF has the worst prognosis of all of the myeloproliferative disorders.

- ET is a clonal proliferation of megakaryocytes in the bone marrow.

- The peripheral platelet count of patients with ET is extremely elevated, sometimes up to $1,000 \times 10^9/L$.

- The increased platelet count in ET can cause hemorrhagic and thrombotic episodes, including gastrointestinal bleeding, epistaxis, and transient ischemic attacks.

- Diagnosis for ET involves ruling out any causes for reactive thrombocytosis other than the clonal proliferation of megakaryocytes.

CASE STUDY

A 45-year-old male police officer sustained a fall from his motorcycle while driving at low speed while on patrol. He started to experience light-headedness, headache, and left upper quadrant abdominal pain. He was brought to a local hospital emergency department. On the basis of a physical examination, he was scheduled for surgery because of a ruptured spleen. A STAT CBC was performed before surgery, with the following results:

Laboratory Data		Differential	
WBC	199×10^9/L	Basophils	5%
Hgb	10.6 g/dL	Eosinophils	5%
Hct	32%	Metamyelocytes	15%
Platelets	850×10^9/L	Myelocytes	8%
Bands	17%	Promyelocytes	7%
Neutrophils	32%	Blasts	7%
Lymphocytes	3%		
Monocytes	1%		

Which conditions show a differential with these abnormalities?

Insights to the Case Study

This case study contains many pieces of abnormal laboratory data. Chief among these is the exorbitant WBC and platelet count. When you combine these unexpected data with the patient's enlarged spleen and the peripheral smear findings, a likely diagnosis is chronic myelocytic leukemia. The patient seems to be in the chronic phase of the disease because his blast count is low. This phase can last months to years. Cytogenetic studies need to be run to determine if he is positive for Ph chromosome. Myelosuppressive therapy will probably be instituted to reduce his WBC, and he will be followed closely to monitor his progress and the progression of the disease.

Review Questions

1. A hallmark in the diagnosis of a patient with CML is
   a. Splenomegaly.
   b. Presence of teardrop cells.
   c. Thrombocytosis.
   d. M:E ratio of 10:1 or greater.

2. The *BCR:ABL* fusion gene leads to
   a. Increased LAP activity.
   b. Increased tyrosine kinase activity.
   c. Organomegaly.
   d. Increased platelet count.

3. Blast crisis in CML means that there are more than _____ blasts in the peripheral smear.
   a. 10%
   b. 20%
   c. 5%
   d. 15%

4. The origin of the dry tap in IMF occurs as a result of
   a. Extramedullary hematopoiesis.
   b. The presence of teardrop cells in IMF.
   c. The infiltration of fibrotic tissue in IMF.
   d. The increase of megakaryocytes in IMF.

5. Thrombotic symptoms in PV are generally related to
   a. Hyperviscosity syndrome.
   b. Increased M:E ratio.
   c. Increased LAP.
   d. Splenomegaly.

6. Pancytopenia in IMF may be caused by
   a. An aplastic origin.
   b. Increase in reticulin fiber in the bone marrow.
   c. Extramedullary hematopoiesis.
   d. The Ph chromosome.

7. The diagnostic criteria for essential thrombocythemia includes all of the following criteria *except*
   a. Increased platelet count.
   b. Absence of collagen fibers.
   c. Increased hematocrit.
   d. No cytogenic abnormalities.

Continued

8. Myocardial infarctions, transient ischemic attacks, and deep vein thrombosis are more likely to be complications of
   a. Chronic myelocytic leukemia.
   b. Acute myelocytic leukemia.
   c. Polycythemia vera.
   d. Idiopathic myelofibrosis.

9. A dry tap is a characteristic of idiopathic myelofibrosis secondary to
   a. Increased infiltration of blast cells.
   b. Increased infiltration of abnormal platelets.
   c. Increased infiltration of abnormal red blood cells.
   d. Increased infiltration of fibrotic elements.

10. What effect does the Ph chromosome have on the prognosis of patients with chronic myelocytic leukemia?
    a. It is not predictive.
    b. The prognosis is better if the Ph chromosome is present.
    c. The prognosis is worse if the Ph chromosome is present.
    d. The disease usually transforms into AML when the Ph1 chromosome is present.

○ TROUBLESHOOTING

How Do I Obtain a Valid WBC When My Patient's WBC Is Outside of the Linearity Range?

Consider the case study presented earlier in this chapter. The WBC is 199×10^9/L, which is out of the linearity range. The technologist must use special techniques to obtain a valid WBC on this sample. The technologist will notice that the WBC is seen as a vote out ++++ on the automated screen; this is the first alert that the WBC may be too high (out of the linearity range) to be recorded by the instrument. The first step is to dilute a small amount of the patient's sample, usually 1:2 dilution, and rerun it to see if a number can be obtained. If this dilution is still out of range, several more dilutions are tried until a reading can be obtained. When a reading is obtained, the technologist must remember to multiply it by the dilution factor to obtain an accurate WBC. The WBC is a critical value and must be called and reported to a responsible party. Additionally, each of the other parameters of the CBC must be examined to evaluate whether they are credible. The troubleshooting case in Chapter 11 outlines each of the steps necessary to resolve the total CBC on a troublesome patient such as this, examining each CBC parameter and the resolution steps. Although each of these procedures seems exhaustive, they are necessary to give the physician an accurate account of this patient's CBC.

WORD KEY

Clonal • Disease arising from a single cell

Deep vein thrombosis • Formation of a blood clot in the deep veins of the legs, arms, or pelvis

Gout • Arthritic disorder marked by crystal formation (usually uric acid) in the joints or tissues

Hyperplasia • Increase in the number of cells in the bone marrow

Myelofibrosis • Increase in the reticulin or fibrotic tissue in the bone marrow

Myeloproliferative • Disease that results in the uncontrolled overproduction of normal-appearing cells in the absence of an appropriate stimulus

Organomegaly • Enlargement of the organs

Osteosclerosis • Abnormal increase in the thickening or density of bone

Plethora • Excess blood volume

Pruritus • Itching

Therapeutic phlebotomy • Withdrawing blood for a medical purpose

Transient ischemic attack • Neurologic defect, having a vascular cause, producing stroke symptoms that resolve in 24 hours

Trisomy • In genetics, having three homologous chromosomes instead of two

References

1. Jaffee ES, Harris NL, Stein H, Vardiman JW, eds. World Health Organization Classification of Tumors: Pathology and Genetics of Tumors of Haematopoietic Lymphoid Tissues. Lyon: IARC Press, 2001.

2. Vardiman JW, Harris NL, Brunning RD. The World Health Organization (WHO) classification of the myeloid neoplasms. Blood 100:2292–2302, 2002.

3. Murphy S, Peterson P, Iland H, Laszio J. Experience of the Polycythemia Vera Study Group with essential thrombocythemia: A final report on diagnostic criteria, survival and leukemic transition by treatment. Semin Hematol 34:29, 1997.

4. Berlin NI. Diagnosis and classification of the polycythemias. Semin Hematol 12:339–351, 1975.

5. Melo JV, Hughes TP, Apperley JF. Chronic myeloid leukemia. Hematology 1:132–152, 2003.

6. Drucker BJ, Sawyers CL, Kantarjian H, et al. Activity of a specific inhibitor of the BCR-ABL tyrosine kinase in the blast crisis of chronic myeloid leukemia and acute lymphoblastic leukemia with Philadelphia chromosome. N Engl J Med 344:1038–1042, 2001.

7. Goldman JM, Melo JV. Chronic myeloid leukemia—advances in biology and new approach in treatment. N Engl J Med 349:1451–1464, 2003.

8. Deininger MW, Goldman JM, Melo JV. The molecular biology of chronic myeloid leukemia. Blood 96:3342–3356, 2000.

9. Calabretta B, Perrotti D. The biology of CML blast crisis. Blood 103:4020–4022, 2004.

10. Faderl S, Talpaz M, Estrov Z, Kantarjian HM. Chronic myelogenous leukemia: Biology and therapy. Ann Intern Med 131:207–219, 1999.

11. O'Brien SG, Guilhot F, Larson RA, et al. Imatinib compared with interferon and low-dose cytarabine for newly diagnosed chronic-phase chronic myeloid leukemia. N Engl J Med 348:994–1004, 2003.

12. Obrien SG, Tefferi A, Valent P. Chronic myelogenous leukemia and myeloproliferative disease. Hematology 1:146–162, 2004.

13. Sawyers CL, Hochhaus A, Feldman E, et al. Imatinib induces hematologic and cytogenetic responses in patients with chronic myelogenous leukemia in myeloid blast crisis: Results of a phase II study. Blood 99:3530–3539, 2002.

14. Reiffers J, Trouette R, Marit G, et al. Autologous blood stem cell transplantation for chronic granulocytic leukemia in transformation: A report of 47 cases. Br J Haematol 77:339–345, 1991.

15. Sawyers CL. Chronic myeloid leukemia. N Engl J Med 340:1330–1340, 1999.

16. Onida F, Ball G, Kantarjian HM, et al. Characteristics and outcome of patients with Philadelphia chromosome negative, BCR/ABL negative chronic myelogenous leukemia. Cancer 95:1673–1684, 2002.

17. Bohm J, Schaefer HE. Chronic neutrophilic leukemia: 14 new cases of an uncommon myeloproliferative disease. J Clin Pathol 55:862–864, 2002.

18. Campbell PJ, Green AR. Management of polycythemia vera and essential thrombocythemia. Hematology Am Soc Hematol Educ Program 201–205, 2005.

19. Bilrami S, Greenburg BR. Polycythemia rubra vera. Semin Oncol 22:307–326, 1995.

20. Spivak JL. Polycythemia vera: myths, mechanisms, and management. Blood 100:4272–4290, 2002.

21. Streiff MB, Smith B, Spivak JL. The diagnosis and management of polycythemia vera since the Polycythemia Vera Study Group: A survey of American Society of Hematology practice patterns. Blood 99:114–119, 2002.

22. Pearson TC, Messinezy M, Westwood N, Green AR, et al. A polycythemia vera update: Diagnosis, pathobiology and treatment. Hematology Am Soc Hematol Educ Program 51–68, 2000.

23. Cazzola M, Guarnone R, Cerani P, et al. Red blood cell precursor mass as an independent determinant of serum erythropoietin level. Blood 91:2139–2145, 1998.

24. Swolin B, Weinfeld A, Westin J. A prospective long term cytogenetic study in polycythemia vera in relation to treatment and clinical course. Blood 72:386–395, 1998.

25. Lengfelder E, Berger U, Hehlman R. Interferon alpha in the treatment of polycythemia. Hematology 79:103–109, 2000.

26. Berk PD, Goldberg JD, Donovan PB, et al. Therapeutic recommendations in polycythemia based on Polycythemia Vera Study Group protocols. Trans Assoc Am Physicians 99:132–143, 1986.

27. Georgii A, Buesche G, Kreft A. The histopathology of chronic myeloproliferative diseases. Baillieres Clin Haematol 11:721–749, 1998.

28. Barosi G. Myelofibrosis with myeloid metaplasia: Diagnostic definition and prognostic classification for clinical studies and treatment guidelines. J Oncol 17:2954–2970, 1999.

29. Tefferi A. Myelofibrosis with myeloid metaplasia. N Engl J Med 341:1255–1265, 2000.

30. Tefferi A, Mesa RA, Schroeder G, Hanson CA, Li CY, Dewald GW. Cytogenetics findings and their clinical relevance in myelofibrosis with myeloid metaplasia. Br J Haematol 113:763–761, 2001.

31. Manoharan A. Idiopathic myelofibrosis: A clinical review. Int J Hematol 68:355–362, 1998.

32. Mesa RA, Hanson CS, Rajkumar V, Schroeder G, Tefferi A. Evaluation and clinical correlations of bone marrow angiogenesis in myelofibrosis with metaplasia. Blood 96:3374–3380, 2000.

33. Reilly JT. Idiopathic myelofibrosis: Pathogenesis, natural history and management. Blood Rev 11:233–242, 1997.

34. Dickstein JI, Vardiman JW. Hematopathologic findings in the myeloproliferative disorders. Semin Oncol 22:355–373, 1995.

35. Spivak JL, Barosi G, Tognoni G, et al. Chronic myeloproliferative disorders. Hematology 1:200–224, 2003.

36. Dupriez B, Morel P, Demory JL, et al. Prognostic factors in agnogenic myeloid metaplasia: A report on 195 cases with a new scoring system. Blood 88:1013–1018, 1996.

37. Tefferi A, Mesa RA, Nagomey DM, Schroeder G, et al. Splenectomy in myelofibrosis with myeloid metaplasia:

A single-institution experience with 223 patients. Blood 95:226–233, 2000.

38. Deeg HJ, Gooley TA, Flowers ME, et al. Allogenetic hematopoietic stem cell transplantation for myelofibrosis. Blood 102:3912–3918, 2003.

39. Cervantes F, Barosi G, Demoray JL, et al. Myelofibrosis with myeloid metaplasia in young individuals: Disease characteristics, prognostic factors and identification of risk groups. Br J Haematol 102:684–690, 1998.

40. Tefferi A, Solberg LA, Silverstein MN. A clinical update in polycythemia vera and essential thrombocythemia. Am J Med 109:141–149, 2000.

41. Nimer S. Essential thrombocythemia: Another "heterogeneous disease" better understood? Blood 93:415–416, 1999.

42. Harrison CN, Gale RE, Machin SJ, Linch DC. A large proportion of patients with a diagnosis of essential thrombocythemia do not have a clonal disorder and may be at lower risk of thrombotic complications. Blood 93:417–424, 1999.

43. Cortelazzo S, Finazzi G, Ruggeri M. Hydroxyurea for patients with essential thrombocythemia and a high risk of thrombosis. N Engl J Med 332:1132–1136, 1995.

44. Ruggeri M, Finazzi G, Tosetro A, et al. No treatment for low-risk thrombocythemia: Results from a prospective study. Br J Haematol 103:772–777, 1998.

45. Fenaux P, Simon M, Caulier MT. Clinical course of essential thrombocythemia in 147 cases. Cancer 66:549–556, 1990.

46. Hehlmann R, Jahn M, Baumann B. Essential thrombocythemia: Clinical characteristics: A study of 61 cases. Cancer 61:2487–2496, 1988.

47. Sterkers Y, Preudhomme C, Lai JL, et al. Acute myeloid leukemia and myelodysplastic syndromes following essential thrombocythemia treated with hydroxyurea. Blood 91:616, 1998.

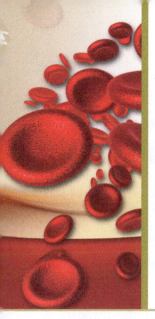

Chapter 13

Lymphoproliferative Disorders and Related Plasma Cell Disorders

Betty Ciesla

Objectives

After completing this chapter, the student will be able to:

1. Define the common features of the chronic lymphoproliferative disorders.

2. Describe the symptoms, peripheral smear morphology, and treatment of individuals with chronic lymphocytic leukemia (CLL).

3. Evaluate the complications of CLL with respect to immunocompetency and bone marrow involvement.

4. Describe pertinent features of hairy cell leukemia, including clinical presentation, peripheral smear, and pertinent cytochemical stains.

5. Define the clinical features of Sézary syndrome.

6. List the morphologic features of the plasma cell.

7. Describe the basic immunoglobulin unit.

8. List the laboratory criteria used to diagnose the monoclonal gammopathies.

9. Differentiate the clinical and laboratory features that distinguish multiple myeloma and Waldenström's macroglobulinemia.

10. List the CD markers used to differentiate B-cell and T-cell disorders.

11. Briefly describe how molecular diagnostics aid in the diagnosis of lymphoid malignancies.

Lymphoproliferative disorders comprise disorders of the B lymphocytes and T lymphocytes that are characterized by a clonal, malignant proliferation of either cell subset. This chapter discusses the malignant lymphoproliferative disorders (with variants) and the plasma cell disorders. There are several common features of each of these groups. They are chronic diseases that primarily affect elderly patients, and they progress slowly. Most complications are related to a compromised immune ability.

Hodgkin's and non-Hodgkin's lymphoma are covered briefly in this chapter. Both diseases have complicated staging systems and are primarily diagnosed with the aid of lymph node biopsy, bone marrow studies, and molecular techniques. Laboratory involvement in these diseases is peripheral at best. Major plasma cell disorders such as multiple myeloma (MM) and Waldenström's macroglobulinemia are also presented. Molecular diagnostic techniques such as flow cytometry and chromosomal analysis with a molecular component provide essential data for diagnosis of malignant disorders. These techniques are mentioned throughout this text.

LYMPHOID MALIGNANCIES

Chronic Lymphocytic Leukemia

Chronic lymphocytic leukemia (CLL) is caused by clonal proliferation of B lymphocytes. It is the most common chronic leukemia, with a predilection for men over women. Most patients are older than 50 years of age.[1] Small lymphocytes begin to accumulate in the spleen, lymph nodes, and bone marrow to a high degree and eventually spill into the peripheral blood. These malignant lymphocytes show CD15, CD19, CD20, and CD22 surface antigen markers and exhibit a low level of surface immunoglobulin (SIg) and CD5, a marker usually reserved for T cells. In greater than 82% of patients, chromosomal abnormalities include chromosomes 11, 12, and 13.[2] Trisomy 12 is reported in almost half of all patients with CLL and is associated with a poor prognosis.[2] The presenting symptoms of this disease (fatigue, pallor, weight loss) are fairly unremarkable, and for this reason, it is often discovered by accident, as a result of other complaints. Lymphadenopathy is the most common initial symptom.[3] WBCs are exaggerated, with many greater than 100×10^9/L. The myeloid:erythroid (M:E) ratio is 10:1 or 20:1, and the bone marrow and peripheral blood present a monotonous tapestry of mature lymphocytes to the exclusion of other normal elements in the blood or bone marrow.

Disease Progression in Chronic Lymphocytic Leukemia

The peripheral blood smear in CLL shows exclusively small lymphocytes intermixed with few lymphoblasts. The lymphocytes show a certain homogeneity in morphology: heavily clumped chromatin combined with a round, sometimes slightly indented nucleus. Figure 13.1 provides a comparison of nucleated red blood cells and lymphocytes in CLL. Smudge cells may be present in the peripheral smear and are visualized as pieces of lymphocyte chromatin splashed across the smear. Because lymphocytes are fragile, smudge cells may arise in the process of making a peripheral smear, where the cytoplasm is disrupted and the nuclear chromatin strands are smudged across the smear in a basket shape or amorphous smudge (Fig. 13.2).

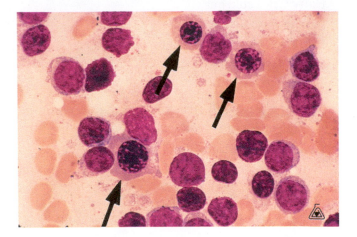

Figure 13.1   Bone marrow view of chronic lymphocytic leukemia. Compare the nucleated red blood cells at the *arrow* with mature lymphocytes.   From the College of American Pathologists, with permission.

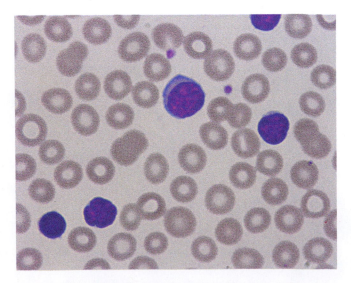

Figure 13.2   Chronic lymphocytic leukemia possible smudge cell lower left.   Courtesy of Kathleen Finnegan, Stony Brook University, New York.

As the disease progresses, a lymphocyte mass accumulates in the bone marrow, and splenomegaly and lymphadenopathy usually develop (Fig. 13.3). Anemia, thrombocytopenia, and neutropenia usually develop in the course of the disease, subsequent to lymphocytic involvement in the bone marrow. Additionally, platelet autoantibodies may cause thrombocytopenia and idiopathic thrombocytopenic purpura (ITP). The altered immune function of the lymphocytes may lead to the complication of **autoimmune hemolytic anemia** in 10% to 30% of individuals with CLL. Spherocytes and nucleated red blood cells that appear in the peripheral smear may be early indicators of the autoimmune hemolytic process. Erythroid hyperplasia is present in the bone marrow, and the **direct antiglobulin test**, which measures antibody coating of the red blood cells, is positive.

Immunologic Function in Chronic Lymphocytic Leukemia and Treatment Options

B lymphocytes in patients with CLL are long-lived and nonproliferating. Programmed cell death, or apoptosis, is a significant feature in most cell line progressions, but 80% of patients with CLL have *BCL2*, an antiapoptosis gene.[4] Therefore, the survival of the dysfunctional B-cell clone is guaranteed. Additionally, the immunologic function of these lymphocytes is compromised, with more than 50% of patients showing a hypogammaglobulinemia. Patients experience bacterial or skin infections, particularly herpes zoster (shingles) and herpes simplex (cold sores), that can be painful and debilitating.[5]

Treatment options for patients with CLL include irradiation for enlarged spleen and lymph nodes as a means of reducing discomfort and related symptoms.[6] The most effective drug for reducing lymphocyte burden is fludarabine, a cytotoxic drug that induces apoptosis.[7] Other therapies include alkylating agents, monoclonal antibodies, and intravenous immunoglobulin (IVIg) therapy. Table 13.1 shows the modified Rai staging system and survival projections. Staging systems are developed to analyze patient data in an attempt to project disease prognosis and risk factors. The Rai staging system was designed by Rai in 1970 and modified in 1987. This system divides patients into risk categories and provides survival statistics.

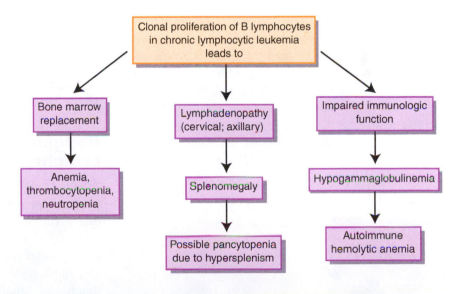

Figure 13.3 Combined effects of B-lymphocyte proliferation.

Table 13.1 ○ Modified Rai Staging for Chronic Lymphocytic Leukemia

Staging	Lymphocytes	Lymph Nodes	Spleen	Platelet Count	Survival (years)
0	Increased				12.5
I	Increased	Enlarged			8.5
II	Increased	Enlarged/some	Enlarged		6
III	Increased	Enlarged/some	Enlarged		1.5
IV	Increased			Decreased	1.5

Hairy Cell Leukemia

Hairy cell leukemia (HCL) is a rare B-cell malignancy in which the key morphologic entity is a fragile-appearing mononuclear cell with hairlike or ruffled projections of the cytoplasm (Fig. 13.4). The nuclear material in these cells is round or dumbbell-shaped with a spongy appearance of the chromatin. Hairy cells represent approximately 50% of cells seen in the peripheral smear. These cells eventually infiltrate the bone marrow and spleen, leading to **pancytopenia** and thrombocytopenia. Most patients are older than 50 years, and more men are affected than women. Abdominal discomfort is a frequent presenting symptom; more than 80% of patients show massive spleens that misplace the stomach. Bleeding, infections, and anemia develop as malignant cells predominate in the bone marrow and peripheral circulation. Neutrophils and monocytes are greatly reduced. Bone marrow aspirates are usually unsuccessful and lead to a "dry tap." Dry taps occur when the normal bone marrow architecture becomes filled with fibrotic material, and liquid marrow cannot be aspirated.

A key item in the diagnosis of HCL is the cytochemical stain known as tartrate-resistant acid phosphatase (TRAP). Most lymphocytes contain many isoenzymes, and isoenzyme 5 is especially abundant in hairy cells.[8] When blood smears from patients with HCL are stained with the acid phosphatase, most cells take up the stain. When tartrate is added, lymphocytes from patients with HCL remain stained, whereas staining in other cells fades. This resistance to tartrate is directly related to the level of isoenzyme 5 activity in hairy cells. CD markers present in hairy cells are CD22, CD11c, CD25, and CD103 (Table 13.2).

Table 13.2 ● CD Markers in Hairy Cell Leukemia
• CD22
• CD11c—membrane adhesion
• CD25
• CD103

Treatment for patients with HCL is individualized according to the progression and course of disease. Therapeutic splenectomy improves cytopenias and hypersplenism as well as physical symptoms such as abdominal fullness and satiety. Treatments with interferon-alfa and 2-chlorodeoxyadenosine (2-CdA) have offered positive remissions.[9]

Prolymphocytic Leukemia

Prolymphocytic leukemia (PLL) is a variant of CLL. In this rare disorder, the peripheral smear of individuals with PLL shows mostly circulating prolymphocytes. These cells of lymphoid origin have more abundant cytoplasm than mature lymphocytes, and their nuclear chromatin appears more mature and coarse. PLL has a poor prognosis, and, in contrast to patients with CLL, patients with PLL have more severe symptoms, such as splenic enlargement, liver involvement, and escalating WBCs. Patients with PLL show strong CD20 markers and SIg activity and are positive for CD19 and CD20.

Hodgkin's and Non-Hodgkin's Lymphoma

Briefly, Hodgkin's lymphoma is a significant lymphoproliferative disorder with a bimodal incidence. It is one of the most common lymphomas in young males 14 to 40 years of age, but it also may be seen in individuals older than 50. Most patients complain of a single lymph node in the cervical region; it is firm to the touch and usually does not disappear. Symptoms of hypermetabolism, such as low-grade fever and weight loss, may be present. Individuals who have had previous exposure to Epstein-Barr virus or who have been exposed to environmental hazards may be more vulnerable to Hodgkin's lymphoma. Diagnosis is based on the cellular features seen on lymph node biopsy specimen, which may feature Reed-Sternberg cells, large multinucleated cells resembling an "owl's eye." Classifications of lymphoma include lymphocyte (5%), nodular (60%), mixed cellularity (20%), and lymphocyte predominant lymphocyte depleted (rare). The

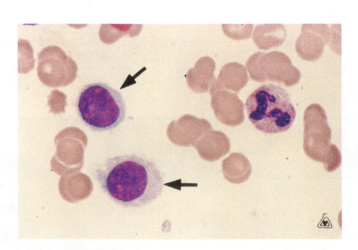

Figure 13.4 Hairy cell leukemia, showing hairlike projections in large mononuclear cells. From The College of American Pathologists, with permission.

disease may spread across the lymphatic system and may involve the liver, spleen, and bone marrow. Prognosis is good, however, with a high cure rate.

Non-Hodgkin's lymphoma is three times more common than Hodgkin's lymphoma and may manifest as painless cervical lymph node involvement. Lymph nodes may be enlarged, and the disease may spread to the gastrointestinal and respiratory systems, skin, liver, and spleen. The range of spread may be more sporadic than that of Hodgkin's lymphoma, and lymphoma cells may be seen in the peripheral blood. Any history of congenital or acquired immunologic disorder may be a predisposing factor in the development of non-Hodgkin's lymphoma. The diagnostic scheme is divided into low grade, intermediate grade, or high grade based on the history of the lymphocytic cells. Radiation and chemotherapy may be successful in obtaining remission, but relapses for non-Hodgkin's lymphoma are frequent.[11]

Sézary Syndrome

T-cell lymphomas may have a cutaneous manifestation in some patients; this is known as mycosis fungoides. Individuals with mycosis fungoides have reddened itchy areas (generalized **erythroderma**) that become thickened, scaly, and pronounced. Skin biopsy specimens of these areas show an infiltration of lymphocytes. As this disease progresses, the spleen, bone marrow, and lymph nodes become involved, presenting the characteristic Sézary syndrome, which is the leukemic phase of T-cell lymphoma. Sézary cells can be identified in the peripheral blood as large cells, approximately 8 to 20 μm, with a convoluted, cerebriform ovoid nucleus. Although they may be mistaken for monocytes, the concentration of chromatin is much thicker and more compact in Sézary cells. Sézary cells are **pathognomonic** for cutaneous T-cell lymphoma; patients who progress to this phase have decreased survival rates. Sézary cells show CD2, CD3, CD4, and CD5 markers (Fig. 13.5).[10]

PLASMA CELL DISORDERS

Normal Plasma Cell Structure and Function

A normal plasma cell evolves as the last stage of a B lymphocyte. In structure and function, this is a unique cellular entity that constitutes less than 5% of the cells in the bone marrow. These cells rarely make an appearance in the peripheral circulation, and when they do, they are responding to infectious, inflammatory conditions or malignant proliferation (Table 13.3). A plasma

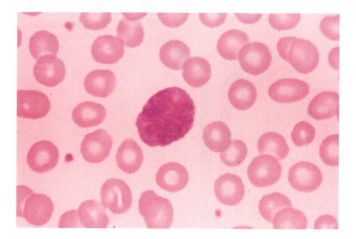

Figure 13.5 Sézary cells. Note the folded or convoluted nuclear membrane that may appear cerebriform. © 1967 American Society of Clinical Pathologists. Reprinted with permission.

Table 13.3 ◉ Increased Plasma Cells in Blood

- Streptococcal infections
- Syphilis
- Epstein-Barr virus
- HIV
- Tuberculosis
- Mumps
- Rubella
- Collagen vascular disease

Adapted from Glassy E. Color Atlas of Hematology: An Illustrated Guide Based on Proficiency Testing. Northfield, IL: College of American Pathologists, 1998.

cell is a medium-sized cell with an eccentric nucleus having a well-defined Golgi apparatus. The color of the cytoplasm, which is a distinct sea blue or cornflower color, is notable. The chromatin, although clumped, is evenly arranged in a pinwheel structure. Plasma cells make immunoglobulins, the basic building blocks of antibody production (see Fig. 13.6). There are five types of immunoglobulin: IgG, IgM, IgD, IgE, and IgA. Each immunoglobulin has the following:

- Four polypeptide chains
- Two H chains (heavy chains)
- Two L chains (light chains)

There are five different types of H chains, as follows:

- Gamma (γ)
- Alpha (α)
- Mu (μ)

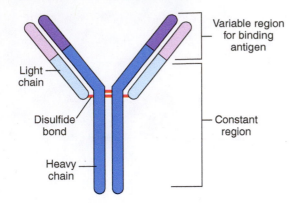

Figure 13.6   Basic immunoglobulin structure.

- Epsilon (ε)
- Delta (δ)

There are two different types of L chains, as follows:

- Kappa (κ)
- Lambda (λ)

Table 13.4 presents the specific function of each immunoglobulin type.

Immunoglobulins are assessed either quantitatively or qualitatively. Serum protein electrophoresis gives a representation of all serum proteins: immunoglobulins, albumins, and some minor proteins (Fig. 13.7). Immunoelectrophoresis separates the specific immunoglobulins by using antibodies directed against each fraction combined with an electrical field and a gel medium.

Multiple Myeloma

One of the premier disorders of plasma cells (Fig. 13.8) is MM. This disorder has a well-defined pathophysiology

Table 13.4 ○ Immunoglobulin and Range of Activity	
Immunoglobulin	**Range of Activity**
IgG	Secondary immune response, precipitating antibodies, hemolysins, virus-neutralizing antibodies
IgA	Secretory antibody, protects airways and gastrointestinal tract
IgM	Primary immune response
IgD	Lymphocyte activator and suppressor
IgE	Antibody found in respiratory and gastrointestinal tract/parasitic infections

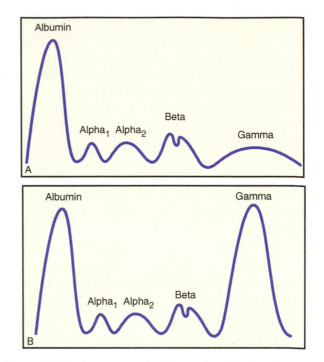

Figure 13.7   Serum protein electrophoresis showing patterns of (A) normal serum and (B) serum from patient with multiple myeloma; note the monoclonal M spike in the gamma region.

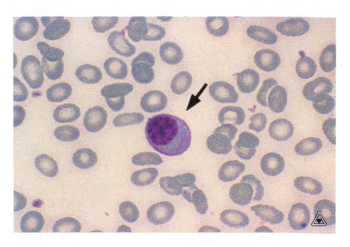

Figure 13.8   Plasma cells. Note basophilic cytoplasm and eccentric nucleus.   From The College of American Pathologists, with permission.

that centers around the accumulation of plasma cells in the bone marrow and other locations. MM occurs in older age groups, affects men more than women, and has greater frequency in African Americans.

Several environmental and occupational factors are thought to contribute to the clonal proliferation of plasma cells, including exposure to atomic radiation; work involving the use of organic solvents; work with toxins within the textile industries; and any occupation that may primarily or secondarily expose individuals to chemicals, pesticides, or herbicides.[12] Additionally, chromosome abnormalities have been defined in 18% to 35% of patients with MM.[13] Aberrations in chromosome 13 have been particularly well-studied and include **monosomy**, deletions, or translocations of the chromosome. MM patients with chromosomal damage have a worse prognosis, a higher rate of disease acceleration, and decreased survival.[14] Screening for chromosomal abnormalities seems a prudent course of action in monitoring disease progress (Table 13.5).

Pathophysiology in Multiple Myeloma

Disease and clinical symptoms in MM follow along three distinct pathways:

1. Acceleration of plasma cells in the bone marrow
2. Activation of bone resorption factors or osteoclasts
3. Production of an abnormal monoclonal protein

Plasma cells accelerate in MM under the direction of the renegade cytokine interleukin (IL)-6. The plasma cells appear in clusters (Fig. 13.9) and may be morphologically normal, or they may appear binucleated and have a bizarre structure. Some cells may develop colorless inclusions called Russell bodies or other crystalline inclusions (Figs. 13.10 and 13.11). Flame cells may also be seen in IgA myelomas and appear as plasma cells with a striking deep pink cytoplasm (Fig. 13.12). Eventually, these clusters or sheets overtake the normal bone marrow structure, leading to the appearance of plasma cells in the peripheral smear and anemias, thrombocytopenia, and neutropenia. Plasma cell tumors may seed to other areas in the body, and plasmacytomas may occur in liver, spleen, gastrointestinal tract, or nasal cavities.

Additionally, the increased plasma cell activity leads to commensurate increased osteoclast activity. Osteoclasts are large multinucleated cells in the bone marrow that absorb bone tissue. With increased activity, bone loss is inevitable, and this pathology usually results in the most frequent complaint from patients

Table 13.5 ⊙ Simplified List of Chromosomal Aberrations in Multiple Myeloma
• 13q14 deletions
• 14q32
• t(11:14)(q13:q32)
• t(4:14)

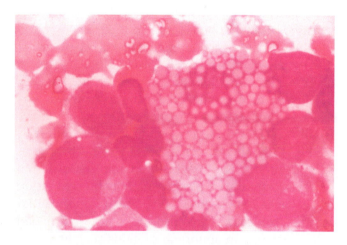

Figure 13.10   Russell bodies. These inclusions are derived from an accumulation of immunoglobulin.   © 1967 American Society of Clinical Pathologists. Reprinted with permission.

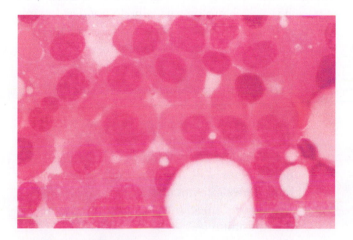

Figure 13.9   Sheets of plasma cells.   © 1967 American Society of Clinical Pathologists. Reprinted with permission.

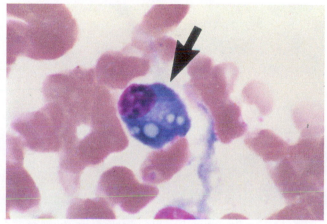

Figure 13.11   Plasma cell with inclusion.   From The College of American Pathologists, with permission.

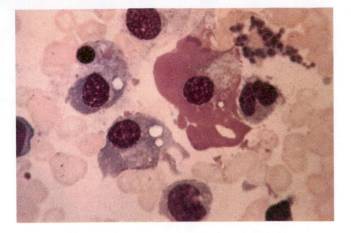

Figure 13.12   Flame cell; a plasma cell with a pink cytoplasm.

with MM—bone pain. Pain usually develops as a result of compressed vertebrae in the back, ribs, or sternum. This compression may lead to loss of sensation, fractures, and paralysis. Serum calcium is also greatly increased because of bone loss, and this event may lead to kidney failure or the formation of kidney stones.

Increased plasma cell production results in increased immunoglobulin production and usually the advent of a monoclonal gammopathy—a purposeless proliferation of one particular antibody, usually IgG. On serum immunoelectrophoresis (see Fig. 13.7), this is seen as an M spike. This excess globulin production may lead to complications from hyperviscosity in the plasma, such as blurred vision or headache. Subsequent laboratory abnormalities such as **rouleaux** may also be seen. Red blood cells circulating in abnormal proteins such as fibrinogen and globulin may cause rouleaux formation

(Fig. 13.13), where red blood cells look like stacks of coins even in the thinner areas of the smear. In contrast to red blood cell agglutination, in which red blood cells are attracted to a specific antibody and appear in clumps, rouleaux formation is a nonspecific binding of red bloods cells where the net negative charge of red blood cells has been neutralized by excess protein (Fig. 13.14). Rouleaux may cause falsely decreased RBC count and falsely increased mean corpuscular volume (MCV) and mean corpuscular hemoglobin content (MCHC). The RBC count appear lower as the doublets and triplets caused by rouleaux pass through the red blood cell–counting aperture of automated equipment as one cell. MCV appears higher because the red blood cell volume is directly measured, and red blood cells showing doublets and triplets are measured as one large cell. The peripheral smear may also show a blue coloration on macroscopic examination because of excess proteins. The erythrocyte sedimentation rate (ESR) (see Chapter 20) is usually elevated because of the increased settling of the red blood cells brought on by the increased globulin content of the plasma (Table 13.6).

Bence Jones protein is a peculiar protein made by some patients with MM as a result of an excess of kappa and lambda light chains. These light chains are small and can be filtered by the kidneys. They appear in the urine and have several unique properties. When urine is heated to 56°C, Bence Jones protein precipitates out, and it redissolves at a higher temperature. As the urine is cooled, precipitates appear again and dissolve on cooling. Bence Jones protein is damaging to the kidneys.

Symptoms and Screening for Multiple Myeloma

Approximately 50,000 Americans are diagnosed with MM each year.[15] Symptoms usually do not develop initially, but as the numbers of plasma cells accelerate, the individual may experience the following:

- Fatigue—caused by anemia
- Excessive thirst and urination—caused by excess calcium
- Nausea—caused by excess calcium
- Bone pain in back and ribs—caused by plasma cell acceleration
- Bone fractures—caused by calcium leeching from bones into circulation
- Unexpected infections—caused by compromised immunity
- Weakness and numbness in the legs—caused by vertebrae compression

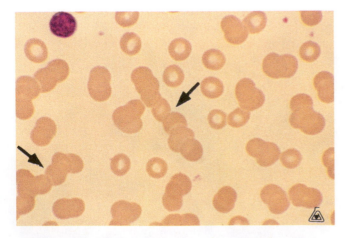

Figure 13.13   Rouleaux. Red blood cells form stacks of "coins" as a reaction to excess protein. Form The College of American Pathologists, with permission

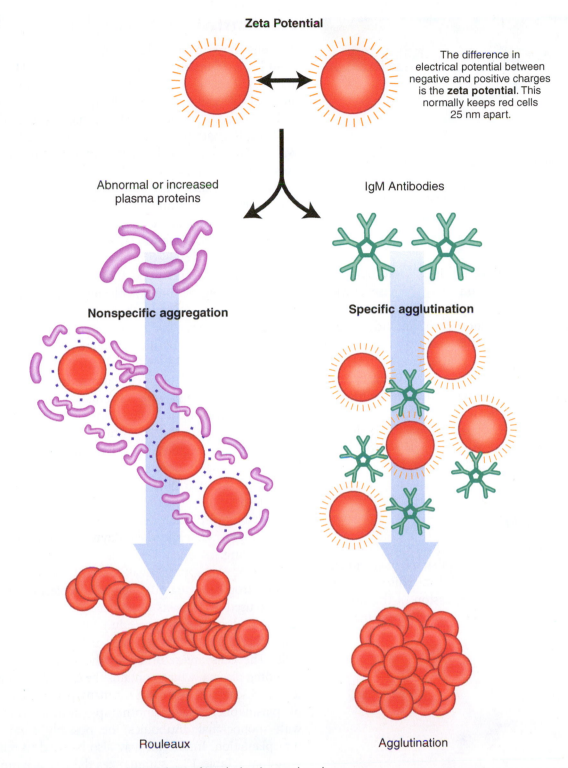

Figure 13.14 Schematic comparison of agglutination and rouleaux. Adapted from Glassy E. Color Atlas of Hematology: An Illustrated Guide Based on Proficiency Testing. Northfield, IL: College of American Pathologists, 1998, with permission.

Screening and diagnosis of patients suspected to have MM include a complete blood count (CBC), possibly a bone marrow, urinalysis, and protein panel. Serum protein electrophoresis (SPE) and beta-microglobulin might also be ordered. Serum beta-microglobulin is a protein produced by the light chains. In the early stages of MM, this protein is at a low level. Levels greater than 6 µg/mL are seen later in the disease and usually indicate higher tumor burden and poor prognosis.

Prognosis and Treatment in Multiple Myeloma

Patients with MM face many difficulties, especially with respect to their skeletal condition. Some patients

Table 13.6 ● Laboratory Findings of Multiple Myeloma

- Pancytopenia
- N/N anemia
- ↑ ESR
- ↑ Calcium
- ↑ Urine protein (Bence Jones protein)
- ↑ Uric acid
- Abnormal serum protein electrophoresis

show punched-out lesions on initial radiographs. Chemotherapy and radiation may be used, with radiation providing some relief in painful bone areas. Agents used in chemotherapy include glucocorticoids and interferon-alfa; survival times from diagnosis are usually 3 to 4 years. A newer therapy involves the use of thalidomide, an antinausea drug of the 1950s. This drug was banned from the market because its use in pregnant women to control nausea led to many birth defects, particularly limb defect. Thalidomide is effective in stalling the growth of myeloma cells, however, and it is used under close supervision.[12]

Plasma Cell Leukemia

Plasma cell leukemia is a complication of MM in which there is an increased number of plasma cells in the circulating blood (Fig. 13.15). This condition is usually seen late in the progression of the disease as plasma cells overtake the normal bone marrow elements.

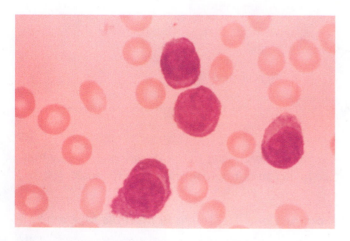

Figure 13.15 Plasma cell leukemia. © 1967 American Society of Clinical Pathologists. Reprinted with permission.

Waldenström's Macroglobulinemia

Waldenström's macroglobulinemia was discovered in 1944 by Waldenström, a Swedish physician. He originally described two patients who had abnormal mucosal bleeding, enlarged lymph nodes, anemia, and thrombocytopenia. No bone pain was evident, and both patients showed an elevated ESR. Waldenström described an abnormal protein that we now know is an overproduction of IgM, which appears as a particular spike on SPE and produces hyperviscosity syndrome. Patients tend to be older, the condition affects men and women equally, and more whites than blacks are affected. The overproduction of globulin is caused by abnormal B lymphocytes that manifest in the bone marrow and peripheral smear as having features of plasma cells—hence the name plasmacytoid lymphocytes. Clinical issues related to hyperviscosity feature largely in the complications experienced by these patients. Because IgM is such a large molecule, overproduction of this macromolecule results in platelet coating, impeding their function, interfering with coagulation factors, and causing potential neurologic or thrombotic complications. Although there is no unique profile of symptoms in these patients, most experience headaches, dizziness, visual problems, and serious coagulation difficulties. The peripheral smear may show rouleaux and plasmacytoid lymphocytes. As a subset of the abnormal IgM protein, cryoglobulins may form in some patients, which leads to **Raynaud's phenomenon** and bleeding.

Chemotherapy is available for patients with Waldenström's macroglobulinemia, and **plasmapheresis** may be used as a means to reduce IgM concentration. In the plasmapheresis procedure, blood is removed from the patient, which separates the plasma from the cells. The cells are returned to the patient, and the offending plasma, which contains the elevated IgM protein, is discarded. Treatment for many patients consists of plasmapheresis, chemotherapy, immunotherapy with monoclonal antibodies, or possibly stem cell transplantation. Interferon may also be used to relieve symptoms. Table 13.7 summarizes the major lymphoproliferative disorders.

● Summary Points

- In lymphoproliferative disorders, there is a clonal malignant proliferation of either B lymphocytes or T lymphocytes.
- Chronic lymphocytic leukemia (CLL) is a clonal proliferation of B lymphocytes that is seen in older patients and often discovered by accident.

Table 13.7 ● Overview of Major Malignant Lymphoproliferative Disorders

	CLL	HCL	HL	NHL	MM	WM
Predominant cell type*	Mature lymphocyte	Hairy cell	Reed-Sternberg cell (in node)	Lymphocyte Lymphocyte variations	Plasma cells in marrow	Plasmacytoid lymphs
Main symptoms	Fatigue Weight loss	Infections Bleeding	Enlarged lymph node	Painless, enlarged lymph node	Bone pain Thirst Fatigue	Bleeding Lymphadenopathy Dizziness Blurred vision
Significant laboratory findings	$\uparrow\uparrow\uparrow$ WBC Peripheral smear shows 90% lymphs	TRAP positive Variable presentations Pancytopenia	Variable presentations	Variable presentation	$\uparrow\uparrow$ Calcium Hyperviscosity ($\uparrow$ ESR) Monoclonal spike IgM	Monoclonal gammopathy (IgM) Rouleaux $\uparrow$ ESR
Organ involvement	Enlarged lymph nodes	$\uparrow\uparrow\uparrow$ Spleen	Possible extranodal sites	Possible extranodal sites	Kidneys Bone marrow	Kidneys Bone marrow
Survival rate	Variable	Good	Good	Poor	Variable	Poor
Immunologic markers	CD15, CD19, CD20, CD22	CD19, CD20, CD22, CD11c, CD25, CD103	CD15	None	CD38	CD19, CD20, CD22

CLL, chronic lymphocytic leukemia; HCL, hairy cell leukemia; HL, Hodgkin's lymphoma; NHL, non-Hodgkin's lymphoma; MM, multiple myeloma; WM, Waldenström's macroglobulinemia; TRAP, tartrate-resistant acid phosphatase stain; ESR, erythrocyte sedimentation rate.

*See text for appearance in bone marrow or peripheral smear.

CONDENSED CASE

Ms. L, a 65-year-old woman, was recently bitten by mosquitoes while she was gardening. This time, her experience with mosquito bites was different than previously. She noticed that despite her normal routine of rubbing alcohol and Calamine lotion on her bites, her bites became suppurative, bumpy, and large. She decided to seek medical attention from her internist. After prescribing steroids and applying a topical antibiotic, the internist ordered a CBC just as a precaution. Two days later, Ms. L was called back into the office. Her results were WBC 65.0×10^9/L, Hct 33%, and platelets 150×10^9/L. A differential was ordered as part of reflex testing and revealed 99% mature lymphocytes.

Are the results of this differential in the normal reference range?

Answer

This is an unexpected case of CLL. Although it is unusual to have a severe cutaneous response to mosquito bites, the fact that the lymphocytic cells in CLL are compromised and unable to provide proper immune response contributes to this unusual presentation. Ms. L will probably do well with little intervention. She will need to be followed as the disease progresses.

• CLL shows an accumulation of mature lymphocytes in the bone marrow and eventually the lymph nodes, spleen, and peripheral blood.

• WBCs in CLL can be extremely elevated, and M:E ratio is 10:1 to 20:1.

• Immune function is compromised in CLL, and 10% to 30% of patients may experience autoimmune hemolytic anemia.

• Hairy cell leukemia (HCL) is a rare B-cell malignancy in which the cells have a lymphoid appearance with hairlike projections in the cytoplasm.

- Pancytopenia, splenomegaly, and dry tap are the key features of HCL.

- Sézary syndrome is the blood equivalent of cutaneous T-cell lymphoma that shows a convoluted, cerebriform, ovoid nucleus.

- Multiple myeloma (MM) is a disorder of plasma cells that leads to a monoclonal gammopathy, bone involvement, and pancytopenia.

- Most abnormal proteins are an accumulation of IgG, which may lead to plasma hyperviscosity and rouleaux in the peripheral smear.

- Serum calcium is elevated in patients with MM because of bone loss and increased distribution of calcium in the peripheral circulation.

- Bence Jones protein may be seen in individuals with MM.

- Plasma cell leukemia is a complication of MM in which mature plasma cells are seen in increasing numbers in the peripheral circulation.

- Waldenström's macroglobulinemia is a rare disorder of plasma cells in which IgM is overproduced.

- Many of the symptoms of Waldenström's macroglobulinemia are related to hyperviscosity of the plasma, which accounts for coagulation abnormalities, rouleaux formation, and bleeding or thrombotic complications.

- Plasmapheresis, the therapeutic removal of plasma, may be used as a treatment to decrease the amount of abnormal IgM protein.

CASE STUDY

A 60-year-old woman complained of gastric pain and vomiting for 2 weeks. She had no fever. A computed tomography (CT) scan was ordered and showed a slightly enlarged spleen. An enlarged lymph node was also discovered. The patient complained of severe itching, redness and scaling of the skin, and pitting edema. A bone marrow showed a hypocellular architecture with increased fat.

Laboratory findings are as follows:

		Differential	
WBC	39.0×10^9/L		
RBC	4.25×10^{12}/L	Segs	29%
Hgb	11.7 g/dL	Lymphs	67%
Hct	38%	Eosinophils	4%
MCV	89 fL	Platelets	Normal
MCH	27.5 pg		
MCHC	30.8%		

Technologist's note: Lymphocytes appear normal with rounded, clefted, folded, or bilobed nucleus; vacuoles in some cells

Considering the patient's symptoms, which are unusual, the increased WBC, and the differential reversal, what are the diagnostic possibilities?

Insights to the Case Study

Relative lymphocytosis is usually reported in conditions such as infectious mononucleosis, hepatitis virus infection, or cytomegalovirus infection. These lymphocytes, however, showed a distinct morphology, with a large cell and a small cell variant. Nuclear clefting or folding may be seen in lymphoma cells, but lymphoma cells rarely have vacuoles. An additional finding is that these cells were very large, some up to 20 µm, and the clefting manifestation is very pronounced. When clinical characteristics are included, the most likely diagnosis in this case is Sézary syndrome, a rare type of T-cell lymphoma. This disorder usually has serious skin manifestations, as shown in our patient, combined with an elevated WBC and increasing lymphocyte count. The abnormal lymphocyte morphology usually causes confusion when performing a differential because of the unusual nuclear manifestations of these cells. Sézary cells are usually confirmed by immunophenotyping and are usually CD4-positive T lymphocytes. The life expectancy for a patient with this condition is around 5 years.

(Adapted from Hematology Problem, November 1981, American Journal of Medical Technology.)

Review Questions

1. What is the most common presenting symptom in patients with chronic lymphocytic leukemia?
   a. Massive spleens
   b. Thrombocytosis
   c. Increased calcium
   d. Enlarged lymph nodes

2. What are the peripheral cell indicators of an autoimmune hemolytic anemia in a patient with CLL?
   a. Nucleated red blood cells and spherocytes
   b. Smudge cells and normal lymphs
   c. Howell-Jolly bodies and siderocytes
   d. Lymphoblasts and prolymphocytes

3. A round-shaped nucleus with fragile, spiny projections similar to cytoplasm best describes
   a. Sézary cells.
   b. lymphoblasts.
   c. hairy cells.
   d. smudge cells.

4. In contrast to most of the other leukemias, which of the following conditions manifests with a pancytopenia?
   a. CLL
   b. HCL
   c. CGL
   d. PV

5. Hypercalcemia in patients with multiple myeloma is the direct result of
   a. increased plasma cell mass.
   b. crystalline inclusions in the plasma cells.
   c. increased osteoclast activity.
   d. hyperviscosity.

6. Plasmapheresis is a possible treatment for
   a. Waldenström's macroglobulinemia.
   b. HCL.
   c. PCL.
   d. CLL.

7. Patients with Waldenström's macroglobulinemia frequently encounter thrombotic complications because of
   a. Increased platelet count.
   b. Increased megakaryocytes in the bone marrow.
   c. Increased plasma cells.
   d. Coating of platelets and clotting by increased IgM.

8. All of the following are consistent with the clinical and pathologic picture of Waldenström's macroglobulinemia *except*
   a. M spike secondary to IgM.
   b. Lymphadenopathy and splenomegaly.
   c. Proliferation of lymphocytes and plasmacytoid lymphocytes.
   d. Destructive bone lesions.

9. A significant feature of hairy cell leukemia not seen in other acute leukemias is
   a. Panmyelosis.
   b. Pancytosis.
   c. Pancytopenia.
   d. Panhyperplasia.

10. What is the most characteristic change seen in the peripheral smear of a patient with multiple myeloma?
    a. Microcytic hypochromic cells
    b. Intracellular inclusion bodies
    c. Rouleaux
    d. Agglutination

⊙ TROUBLESHOOTING

What Do I Do When the Hematology Analyzer Fails to Report a Differential Count?

An 82-year-old man came to the emergency department with altered mental status. His initial WBC through the hematology analyzer was $31.3 \times 10^9/L$, but the instrument voted out the differential and gave a platelet clump warning message. The technologist proceeded with several corrective actions because she was beginning to doubt the reported WBC. She took the following steps:

- She physically checked the specimen for clots; there were none.
- She vortexed the sample because this was the optimal method according to the standard

Continued

operating procedure at this hospital when the platelet clumping flag appeared and there were no visible clots.

The CBC was repeated, and the WBC increased to 39.1×10^9/L and the platelet count was 178.0×10^9/L. The technologist decided to hold the CBC for further study and proceeded to make a differential. When she observed the differential, the WBC appeared much lower, no platelet clumps were observed, but strange, foamy purple blobs were observed. While canvassing the laboratory for other specimens, the technologist noticed that the centrifuged coagulation samples on the same patient contained a 2-cm layer of lipemia, but the rest of the plasma was clear. This is not the typical picture of lipemia. The technologist knew that something was wrong with the plasma, but she could not pinpoint the problem. At this point, the technologist cancelled the CBC and coagulation tests and called the emergency department to inform them of this action and inquire about the patient. Additional patient samples were also requested. The technologist was informed that the patient had Waldenström's macroglobulinemia. The samples were redrawn and run through the hematology analyzer again with a WBC of 12.1×10^9/L. The instrument again gave messages such as platelet clumps and interfering substances. A slide examination was performed, and again the white blood cell estimate appeared lower than the instrument-reported WBC. As a last step, the technologist per formed a *manual* WBC and platelet count. The manual WBC and platelet count were 5.6×10^9/L and 166.0×10^9/L. The technologist left a message for future shifts that a manual WBC and platelet would be necessary for this patient.

This case offers an insight into the level of interference possible with the increased IgM globulin in patients with Waldenström's macroglobulinemia. Because the level of IgM monoclonal antibody is so elevated (paraprotein), it is seen as an interfering substance with significant consequences to the WBC and differential primarily. Many hours of investigation and trying alternatives were spent in obtaining results on this patient. An observant technologist combined with reliable information from the family eventually led to actions that would contribute to the credibility of the patient's hematology samples. The next day, the patient underwent plasmapheresis, and the CBC was run through the instrument with no interferences.

WORD KEY

Autoimmune hemolytic anemia • Process by which cells fail to recognize self and consequently make antibodies that destroy selected red blood cells

Direct antiglobulin test • Laboratory test for the presence of complement or antibodies bound to a patient's red blood cells

Erythroderma • Abnormal widespread redness and scaling of the skin, sometimes involving the entire body

Monosomy • Condition of having only one of a pair of chromosomes, as in Turner's syndrome, where there is only one X chromosome instead of two

Pathognomonic • Indicative of the disease

Raynaud's phenomenon • Intermittent attacks of pallor or cyanosis of the small arteries and arterioles of the fingers as a result of inadequate arterial blood supply

Plasmapheresis • Plasma exchange therapy, involving the removal of plasma from the cellular material that is then returned to the patient

Rouleaux • Group of red blood cells stuck together that look like a stack of coins

Translocations • Alteration of a chromosome through the transfer of a portion of it either to another chromosome or to another portion of the same chromosome

References

1. Cutler SJ, Axtell L, Hesiett H. Ten thousand cases of leukemia 1940-62. J Natl Cancer Inst 39:993, 1967.
2. Dohner H, Stilgenbauer S, Beuner A, et al. Genomic aberrations and survival in chronic lymphocytic leukemia. N Engl J Med 343:1910–1916, 2000.
3. Redaelli A, Laskin BL, Stephens JM, et al. The clinical and epidemiological burden of chronic lymphocytic leukemia. Eur J Cancer Care 13:279–287, 2004.
4. McConkey DJ, Chandra J, Wright S, et al. Apoptosis sensitivity in chronic lymphocytic leukemia is determined by endogenous endonuclease content and related expression of BCL-2 and BAX. J Immunol 156:2624, 1996.
5. Holmer LD, Hamoudi W, Bueso-Ramos CD. Chronic leukemia and related lymphom proliferative disorders. In: Harmening D, ed. Clinical Hematology and Fundamentals of Hemostasis, 4th ed. Philadelphia: FA Davis, 2002; 303.
6. McFarland JT, Kuzma C, Millard FE, et al. Palliative irradiation of the spleen. Am J Clin Oncol 25:178–183, 2003.
7. Rosenwald A, Chuang EY, Dabis RE, et al. Fludarabine treatment of patients with CLL induces a p53-dependent gene expression response. Blood 104:1428–1434, 2004.
8. Bradford C. Cytochemistry. In: Rodak B, ed. Hematology: Clinical Principles and Applications, 2nd ed. Philadelphia: WB Saunders, 2002; 391.

9. Jenn U, Bartl R, Dietzfelbinger H, et al. An update: 12 year follow-up of patients with hairy cell leukemia following treatment with 2-chlorodeoxyadenosine. Leukemia 18:1476–1481, 2004.

10. Turgeon ML. Malignant lymphoid and monocytic disorders and plasma cell dyscrasias. In: Turgeon ML, ed. Clinical Hematology: Theory and Principles, 4th ed. Baltimore: Lippincott Williams & Wilkins, 2005; 287.

11. Manner C. The lymphomas. In: Steine-Martin EA, Lotspeich-Steininger CA, Keopke J, eds. Clinical Hematology: Principles, Procedures, Correlations, 2nd ed. Baltimore: Lippincott Williams & Wilkins, 1998; 490–497.

12. Bergsagel DE, Wong O, Bergsagel PL, et al. Benzene and multiple myeloma: Appraisal of the scientific evidence. Cancer Invest 18:467, 2000.

13. Dewald GW, Kayle RA, Hicks GA, et al. The clinical significance of cytogenetic studies in 100 patients with MM, plasma cell leukemia or amyloidosis. Blood 66:380–390, 1985.

14. Shaughnessy J, Jacobsin J, Sawyer J, et al. Continuous absence of metaphase-defined cytogenetic abnormalities, especially of chromosome 13 and hypodiploidy, ensures long-term survival in multiple myeloma treated with Total Therapy I: Interpretation in the context of global gene expression. Blood 101:3849–3854, 2003.

15. Mayo Clinic. Multiple myeloma. Available at: http://www.mayoclinic. com/health/multiple-myeloma/DS00415. Accessed September 25, 2006.

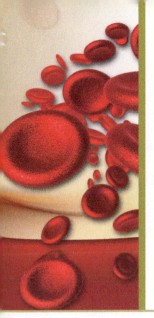

Chapter 14

The Myelodysplastic Syndromes

Betty Ciesla

Objectives

After completing this chapter, the student will be able to:

1. Define the *myelodysplastic syndromes* (MDSs).

2. Outline the possible causes of MDSs.

3. Discuss the major cellular morphologic abnormalities associated with MDSs.

4. Classify MDSs according to the criteria of the World Health Organization (WHO).

5. List the disease indicators that contribute to prognosis of MDSs.

6. Discuss the management of MDSs.

The myelodysplastic syndromes (MDSs) are a group of hematologic disorders that have eluded a firm designation for many decades. These disorders have been known by several other names, including preleukemia, dysmyelopoietic syndrome, oligoblastic leukemia, and refractory anemias. Considerable information has accumulated over 20 years concerning the hematology of these disorders, their molecular biology, and treatment protocols. What began as a group of cases with vague symptoms and morphology has become a recognized entity complete with classification and well-defined characteristics. Presently, 1 in 500 individuals older than 60 years of age have an MDS, making it the most *common* hematologic malignancy in this age group.[1]

Because most patients are older, consideration is always given to preexisting conditions. As more therapeutic options such as stem cell and bone marrow transplants become available, MDS patients are treated far more aggressively, and alternatives such as erythropoietin (EPO), blood products, and growth factors give hope and comfort to these patients.

PATHOPHYSIOLOGY

MDSs are clonal stem cell disorders resulting from stem cell lesions that lead to the formation of neoplasms, abnormal clones of cells. MDSs fall into two categories: de novo (new cases unrelated to any other treatment) and secondary (cases related to prior therapy, usually an **alkylating agent** or radiation). Some populations are more susceptible to MDS, including individuals exposed to benzene and low-dose radiation, petrochemical employees, cigarette smokers, and patients with Fanconi's anemia.[2] Secondary cases often follow immunosuppressive therapy; the transformation to MDS may occur 2 to 5 years after the immunosuppressive agent or agents have been administered.[3] Of all MDS cases, 30% to 40% end in an acute leukemia.[4]

CHROMOSOMAL ABNORMALITIES

Chromosomal abnormalities play a large role in all patients with MDS. Typically, patients exhibit partial or complete absence of certain chromosomes or trisomy of certain chromosomes. The International Prognostic Scoring System provides the following blueprint for MDS risk categories with chromosomal abnormalities:[5]

- Good risk outcome—5 q, del 20q, isolated Y
- Intermediate risk outcome—partial del 11q, trisomy 8
- Poor risk outcome—del 7, trisomy 8

Other abnormalities may include a deletion of 17p.

COMMON FEATURES AND CLINICAL SYMPTOMS

Key features shared by almost all MDS patients include **refractory** macrocytic anemia, cytopenias that affect one or more cell lines, and hypercellular bone marrow. **Organomegaly** occurs infrequently. Depending on which cell line is most affected, clonal abnormalities explain the common symptoms—weakness, infection, and easy bruising. Following is a likely sequence of events:

- Weakness develops from anemia and shortened red blood cell survival.
- Infections develop because of white blood cells with poor microbicidal activity and decreased chemotaxis.
- Bruising develops because of lower platelet levels and abnormally functioning platelets.

A diagnosis of MDS generally is based on the percentage of blasts, the type of dysplasia in the marrow and the peripheral smear, and the presence or absence of ringed sideroblasts (see Chapter 5). Classification into one of the eight MDS subtypes involves gathering all of the information from the marrow, the peripheral smear, cytogenetic studies, and immunologic features.

How to Recognize Dysplasia

By definition, *dysplasia* means "abnormal development of tissue." Because dysplasia in the bone marrow and peripheral smear are hallmark features of MDS, the morphologist must understand the meaning of dysplasia in the context of variations in each cell line. Well-stained and well-distributed peripheral smears and bone marrow preparations are essential ingredients to determining the presence of dysplasia; their importance cannot be underestimated. In the bone marrow, abnormal development may alter the nuclear and cytoplasmic characteristics of precursor cells. Nuclear changes in bone marrow may include multinuclearity, disintegration of the nucleus, asynchrony similar to megaloblastic changes, and nuclear bridging between cells. Cytoplasmic changes in bone marrow include vacuolization or poor granulation. The peripheral smear may show similar changes, such as hypogranulated cells (Fig. 14.1), hypergranulated cells, hyposegmented cells, nuclear material that is too smooth, pseudo–Pelger-Huët cells, and changes in red blood cell size (Fig. 14.2). Platelet abnormalities in the peripheral smear include abnormal size (Fig. 14.3) and megakaryocytic fragments. Degenerating neutrophils (Fig. 14.4) may also be observed. During initial observation of these changes in the peripheral smear,

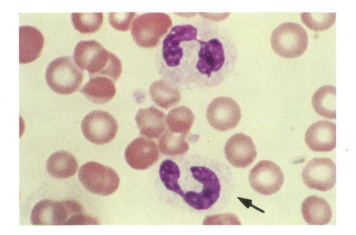

Figure 14.1   Hypogranular band.   From The College of American Pathologists, with permission.

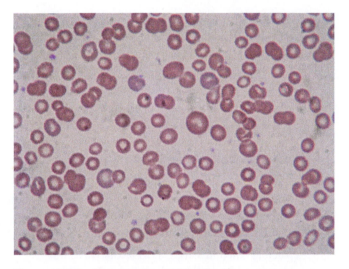

Figure 14.2   Macrocytic red blood cell.   Courtesy of Kathleen Finnegan, Stony Brook University, New York.

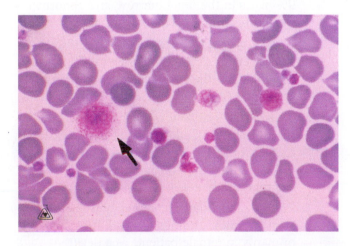

Figure 14.3   Giant platelet.   From The College of American Pathologists, with permission.

technical factors, such as a poorly stained or poorly made smear, usually come to mind. The morphologist, believing that his or her observation is *not* hematologically relevant, may not exercise the index of suspicion.

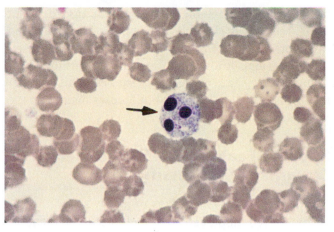

Figure 14.4   Degenerating neutrophil.   From The College of American Pathologists, with permission.

When *10%*[6] of a particular cell line manifests any of the changes noted, that change is significant and usually due to a pathology (Table 14.1).

CLASSIFICATION OF MYELODYSPLASTIC SYNDROMES

In 1981, the French-American-British (FAB) investigative group devised a working classification for MDS based on a study of 50 cases.[6] This classification was groundbreaking work and presented the first formal

Table 14.1 ◉ Dysplastic Changes in MDS

Dysplastic changes of red blood cell: Dyserythropoiesis
- Nuclear budding
- Ringed sideroblasts
- Internuclear bridging
- Dimorphism
- Megaloblastoid asynchrony
- Multinuclearity

Dysplastic changes of white blood cell: Dysgranulopoiesis
- Abnormal staining throughout cytoplasm
- Hyposegmentation
- Hypersegmentation
- Nucleus with little segmentation
- Missing primary granules
- Granules that are poorly stained

Dysplastic changes of platelets: Dysthrombopoiesis
- Micromegakaryocytes
- Abnormal granules
- Giant platelets

body of knowledge on this group of disorders. In 1997, the World Health Organization (WHO) revised this work, developing a classification of MDSs based on additional knowledge gained from molecular, immunologic, and cytogenetic studies. This chapter includes both classifications but focuses mainly on the WHO classification (Table 14.2).[7]

Specific Features of World Health Organization Classification

Refractory anemia (RA) is primarily a disorder of red blood cells that includes a treatment-resistant anemia. The peripheral blood contains no blasts, and the bone marrow contains less than 5% myeloblasts. The marrow shows hyperplasia with megaloblastoid features (e.g., multinuclearity).

Refractory anemia with ringed sideroblasts (RARS) is a refractory anemia in which 15% or more of red blood cell precursors are ringed sideroblasts (Fig. 14.5). The bone marrow shows erythroid hyperplasia and contains less than 5% myeloblasts, and the liver and spleen may show changes related to iron overload.

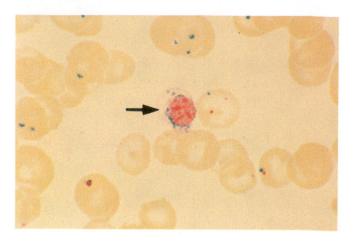

Figure 14.5 Ringed sideroblast. From The College of American Pathologists, with permission.

Refractory cytopenia with multilineage dysplasia (RC-MD) shows bone marrow failure that affects two or more myeloid cell lines. Multiple chromosomal abnormalities, including marked erythroid hyperplasia with nuclear and cytoplasmic dysplastic changes, occur in 50% of patients with MDS. The bone marrow contains less than 5% blasts.

Refractory cytopenia with multinlineage dysplasia and ringed sideroblasts (RCMD/RS) shows more than 10% of myeloid cells with dysplastic changes, abnormal monocytes, and no blasts.

Refractory anemia with excess blasts (RAEB-1) shows anemia, thrombocytopenia, and neutropenia in all myeloid cell lines, 5% to 9% blasts in the bone marrow, and abnormal monocytes in the peripheral smear.

Refractory anemia with excess blasts (RAEB-2) shows generalized cytopenias with 5% to 19% blasts in the bone marrow and possible Auer rods.

Myelodysplastic syndrome unclassifiable (MDS-U) shares features of all MDSs but has no distinct classification. The bone marrow commonly shows neutropenia, thrombocytopenia, and less than 5% blasts.

Deleted 5q chromosomal abnormality is one of the most common findings in MDS. It occurs primarily in female patients as a deletion of the long arm of chromosome 5. Platelet counts are normal or elevated, and there is marked anemia. The peripheral blood shows macrocytes and less than 5% blasts. Deleted 5q chromosomal abnormality is associated with long survival times.

Table 14.2 ● FAB and WHO Classifications of Myelodysplastic Syndromes*	
FAB Classification	**WHO Classification**
Refractory anemia	Refractory anemia
Refractory anemia with ringed sideroblasts	Refractory anemia with ringed sideroblasts
Refractory anemia with excess blasts	Refractory cytopenia with multilineage dysplasia
Chronic myelomonocytic leukemia	Refractory cytopenia with multilineage dysplasia and ringed sideroblasts
Refractory anemia with excess blasts in transformation	Refractory anemia with excess blasts 1
	Refractory anemia with excess blasts 2
	Myelodysplastic syndrome unclassifiable
	5(q) chromosome abnormality

*Table should not be read side by side; WHO classification is greatly extended.

PROGNOSTIC FACTORS AND CLINICAL MANAGEMENT

Progression to an acute leukemia is always a concern for patients with MDSs. Low-grade and unilineage disorders such as RA or RARS have longer survival rates and less tendency to develop into overt acute leukemias. RAEB and the multilineage disorders are life-threatening, however, with much shorter survival rates and a greater incidence of progressing to acute leukemia. Other factors, such as multiple cytogenetic abnormalities (especially chromosome 7 abnormalities), influence prognosis unfavorably (Table 14.3).

Treatment of MDS is difficult to manage, and issues such as quality of life, severe thrombocytopenia, and progression to more advanced disease are serious concerns. Patients with MDSs are classified into low-risk or high-risk categories based on initial WHO designation. Treatment protocols tailored to these designations range from transfusion to EPO and granulocyte colony-stimulating factor (G-CSF), induction chemotherapy, and allogeneic stem cell transplant. Although stem cell transplants offer a potential cure, the morbidity and mortality associated with this procedure require serious consideration.[8] Long-term disease control is only 30% to 50%, even in patients with allogeneic transplants.[9] Most patients receive supportive treatment such as red blood cells, antibiotics, or vitamins, but the anemias are refractory, necessitating more transfusions and possible iron overload. Iron chelating agents are more successful in younger patients. Individuals with iron overload are usually attached to an iron chelating pump that works to clear excess iron while they sleep. Younger patients are generally more compliant than older patients and are better able to cope with the constancy of this procedure. Oral iron chelators such as deferiprone likely would improve iron chelation therapy in this patient group.[10] Patients with cardiopulmonary complications resulting

Table 14.3 ⊙ Factors Indicating Progression to Leukemia in Myelodysplastic Syndromes
• Disease is stable if there is little increase in marrow blast count and original karyotype is unchanged
• Progressive increase in blast count usually indicates transition to acute leukemia
• Sudden change in karyotype that may progress to acute leukemia
• Abnormal karyotype develops without subsequent increase in blasts; acute leukemia may or may not develop

Adapted from Bick RL, Laughlin WR. Myelodysplastic syndromes. Lab Med 11:712–716, 1993.

from progressive anemia require careful management. EPO and G-CSF are important supplementary agents that provide effective short-term measures during difficult episodes of cytopenias.[11] Clinical trials are testing several immunobiologic therapies, such as antithymocyte globulin, anti-CD33 antibody, idarubicin, and fludarabine.[12] Additionally, a new group of therapies, known as **antiangiogenic** therapies, are on the horizon. These agents direct their activities against microenvironmental factors, such as vascular endothelial growth factor (VEGF) and tumor necrosis factor. Increased production of these inflammatory factors likely amplifies ineffective hematopoiesis, fuels the growth of certain premalignant or malignant cells, and suppresses normal hematopoietic progenitor cells. Lenalidomide, a derivative of thalidomide, is an immune modulating agent that shows promise in patients with deleted 5q chromosome abnormality.[13] Therapies for MDSs are likely to improve as the disease mechanisms become more clearly defined.

CONDENSED CASE

A 65-year-old woman visited the nurse practitioner in her assisted living community. She complained of excessive fatigue, rapid heart rate, and bruising. A CBC and differential were performed, and the results suggested a macrocytic anemia with a slightly decreased platelet count. No hypersegmented neutrophils were seen, and no oval macrocytes were observed on the peripheral smear. *What other testing is worth considering in this case?*

Answer

Other causes for a nonmegaloblastic macrocytic anemia include liver disease, reticulocytosis, or hypothyroid conditions. Each of these was ruled out on our patient, and she was referred for a hematology consultation. Bone marrow and cytogenetic studies were ordered. The bone marrow biopsy specimen showed a hypercellular marrow with slightly increased and dysplastic megakaryocytes. Cytogenetic studies show a deleted 5q chromosome. This patient progressed well with transfusion support and has not progressed to acute leukemia.

Summary Points

- Myelodysplastic disorders (MDSs) are a group of clonal disorders characterized by refractory anemias and cytopenias of one or more cell lines.

- The bone marrow and peripheral smear show dysplastic changes in white blood cells, red blood cells, and platelets over time.

- Dyserythropoietic changes include multinucleated red blood cell precursors, bizarre nuclear changes, nuclear bridging, macrocytes, and dimorphism.

- Dysgranulopoietic changes include abnormal granulation of mature cells, hypersegmentation, hyposegmentation, or complete lack of granulation.

- Dysthrombopoietic changes include micromegakaryocytes, abnormal granulation, no granulation, and giant platelets.

- The blast count in MDSs is less than 20% in the bone marrow.

- Weakness, infections, and easy bruising are some of the symptoms that patients with MDSs may manifest.

- According to WHO, there are eight MDS classifications.

CASE STUDY

A 78-year-old man was referred for a hematology consultation after complications from a total knee replacement. After surgery, the patient experienced unexpected bleeding from the operative site. His routine coagulation tests were normal at the time of preoperative review. No organomegaly was noted, and no petechiae were observed. Within 4 weeks, he was readmitted for wound oozing. His CBC and differential on the day of consultation were as follows:

WBC	2.3×10^9/L	Segmented neutrophils 3%
RBC	3.14×10^{12}/L	Bands 4%
Hgb	10.8 g/dL	Metamyelocytes 2%
Hct	31%	Myelocytes 3%
MCV	99 fL	Lymphocytes 60%
MCH	34.3 pg	Monocytes 7%
MCHC	34.8%	Eosinophils 3%
Platelets	15.0×10^9/L	Blasts 18%

Based on the patient's age, clinical presentation, CBC, and differential results, what are some of the diagnostic possibilities?

Insights to the Case Study

The CBC on this patient indicated a low platelet count combined with normocytic, normochromic anemia and differential indicating a left shift. The differential showed a fairly large number of blasts but not enough to qualify as overt acute leukemia (for acute leukemia, 20% or more blasts on the peripheral smear). A bone marrow was requested on this patient. Given the low platelet count, the hematologist was cautious and decided to delay the procedure until the platelet count normalized. The patient received a platelet transfusion to boost his platelet count and was started on prophylactic antibiotics because his WBC was depressed. A preliminary diagnosis of refractory anemia with excess blasts was made pending the bone marrow and cytogenetic studies.

Review Questions

1. Which of the following is the predominant red blood cell morphology in patients with MDSs?
   a. Schistocytes
   b. Macrocytes
   c. Target cells
   d. Bite cells

2. Which MDS group has the best prognosis?
   a. MDS with excess blasts
   b. Refractory anemia with ringed sideroblasts
   c. Refractory anemia
   d. 5q deletion

3. What is considered a significant percentage of ringed sideroblasts in the MDS classification?
   a. 15%
   b. 5%
   c. 10%
   d. 20%

4. Which mechanism accounts for the reticulocytopenia seen in most cases of MDS?
   a. Heavy blast tumor burden in the marrow
   b. Effects of toxins
   c. Marrow aplasia
   d. Ineffective erythropoiesis

5. What is the cutoff blast count used to distinguish a patient with MDS from a patient with acute leukemia?
   a. 50%
   b. 30%
   c. 20%
   d. 15%

6. The most common hematologic malignancy(ies) in adults is(are)
   a. Acute leukemia.
   b. Multiple myeloma.
   c. Myelodysplastic syndromes.
   d. Chronic leukemias.

7. Which of the following bone marrow blast percentages would be consistent with the FAB classification of refractory anemia with excess of blasts (RAEB)?
   a. 5% to 20%
   b. 20% to 30%
   c. Greater than 30%
   d. Less than 5%

8. All of the following are features of MDSs *except*
   a. Anemia.
   b. Organomegaly.
   c. Dysplasia.
   d. Hypercellular marrow.

9. The morphologic classification of anemia in MDSs is
   a. Normocytic, normochromic.
   b. Microcytic, hypochromic.
   c. Macrocytic, normochromic.
   d. Microcytic, normochromic.

10. The most effective means of treating iron overload in MDSs is
    a. Therapeutic phlebotomy.
    b. Limiting iron-containing foods.
    c. Iron chelation therapy.
    d. Fasting.

◉ TROUBLESHOOTING

How Does Patient History Influence Increased MCHC?

A patient had presented to the laboratory for 3 consecutive days with variability in MCH and MCHC. Sometimes MCHC increased to 39%, prompting an investigation. Cold agglutinins, lipemia, or spherocytes can explain an elevated MCHC, but each was eliminated as a reason for the fluctuating MCHC. On day 4, the patient had another CBC, which again showed elevated MCHC.

WBC	16.9×10^9/L
RBC	2.71×10^{12}/L
Hgb	9.0 g/dL
Hct	22.9%
MCV	84.2 fL
MCH	33.2 pg
MCHC	39.3% H
Platelets	52×10^9/L
RDW	15.4

The technologist reviewed the previous results with the comments presented and decided that the patient's history might hold some clues to these variant results. The comments noted that Hgb and Hct had failed the correlation check (Hgb × 3 = Hct ± 2). The technologist discovered that the patient had MDS. MDS has an unknown etiology but may *falsely increase Hgb*,[14] elevating the indices (MCH and MCHC). With this in mind, the technologist decided to apply the laboratory procedure for correcting Hgb values, eliminating tedious manual procedures such as centrifugation, plasma blanks, and pipetting. Hgb concentration is calculated with the following equation, which indicates a ratio of 2.98 between MCV and MCHC:[14]

Hgb (g/L) = MCV × RBC/2.98 × 10 (29.8)
Corrected Hgb/L =
(84.2 × 2.71)/29.8 = 7.7 g/L

Continued

This calculation corrects Hgb. As a result of this new value, MCH and MCHC can be corrected with the new Hgb result.

The CBC now shows:

WBC	16.9×10^9/L
RBC	2.71×10^{12}/L
Hgb	7.7* corrected result
Hct	22.9%
MCV	84.2 fL
MCH	28.4 pg* recalculated result
MCHC	33.4%* recalculated result
Platelets	52×10^9/L
RDW	15.4

MDS is a classification of malignant clonal disorders that show cytopenias, dysplastic-looking cells in the peripheral smear, increasing numbers of blasts in the bone marrow, and a tendency to progress to a leukemic process. This case indicates a corrective action that is *not often used* but appropriate when all other causes of hemoglobin abnormality have been eliminated.

WORD KEY

Alkylating agent • Agent that introduces an alkyl radical into a compound in place of a hydrogen atom; these agents interfere with cell metabolism and growth

Angiogenesis • Development of blood vessels

Organomegaly • Enlargement of any organ

Refractory • Resistant to ordinary treatment

References

1. Hoffman WK, Ottmann OG, Ganser F, et al. Myelopdysplastic syndrome: Clinical features. Semin Hematol 33:177–178, 1996.
2. Willman CL. The biologic basis of myelodysplasia and related leukemias: Cellular and molecular mechanisms. Mod Pathol 12:101–106, 1999.
3. Kjeldsberg CR, ed. Practical Diagnosis of Hematologic Disorders, 3rd ed. Chicago: ASCP Press, 2000: 369–397.
4. Bick RL, Laughlin WR. Myelodysplastic syndromes. Lab Med 11:712–716, 1993.
5. Greenberg P, Cox C, LeBeau MM, et al. International Scoring System for evaluating prognosis in myelodysplastic syndromes. Blood 89:2079–2088, 1997.
6. Bennett HJM, Catovsky D, Daniel MT, et al. Proposals for the classification of the myelodysplastic syndromes. Br J Haematol 51:189–199, 1982.
7. Jaffe ES, Harris NL, Stein H, Vardiman JE, eds. World Health Organization Classification of Tumours. Pathology and Genetics of Tumours of Hematopoietic and Lymphoid Tissues. Lyon: IARC Press, 2001; 63–73.
8. Hellstrom-Lindberg E. Update on supportive care and new therapies: Immunomodulatory drugs, growth factors and epigenetic acting agents. Hematology Am Soc Hematol Educ Program 161–166, 2005.
9. Giralt S. Bone marrow transplant in myelodysplastic syndromes: New technologies, some questions. Curr Hematol Rep 3:165–172, 2004.
10. Hoffbrand VA. Deferiprone therapy for transfusional iron overload. Best Pract Res Clin Haematol 18:299–317, 2005.
11. Negrin RS, Haeuber DH, Nagler A, et al. Maintenance treatment of patients with myelodysplastic syndromes using recombinant human granulocyte colony stimulating factor. Blood 76:36–43, 1990.
12. Appelbaum FR. Immunobiologic therapies for myelodysplastic syndromes. Best Pract Res Clinc Haematol 4:653–661, 2004.
13. Williams JL. The myelodysplastic syndromes and myeloproliferative disorders. Clin Lab Sci 17:227, 2004.
14. Kalache GR, Sartor MM, Hughes WG. The indirect estimation of hemoglobin concentration in whole blood. Pathologist 23:117, 1991.

Part IV

Hemostasis and Disorders of Coagulation

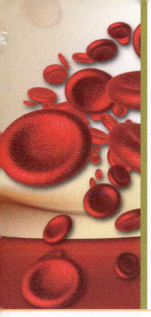

Chapter 15

Overview of Hemostasis and Platelet Physiology

Donna Castellone

Objectives

After completing this chapter, the student will be able to:

1. Describe the systems involved in hemostasis.

2. Describe the interaction of the vascular system and platelets as it relates to activation, adhesion, and vasoconstriction.

3. Identify the process involved in the coagulation cascade, from activation to stable clot formation.

4. Describe the role of platelets in hemostasis with respect to platelet glycoproteins, platelet biochemistry, and platelet function.

5. Define the difference between primary and secondary hemostasis.

6. Outline the intrinsic and extrinsic pathways, the factors involved in each, and their role in the coagulation system.

7. List the coagulation factors, their common names, and function.

8. Explain the interaction between prothrombin time, activated partial thromboplastin time, and factor assays.

9. Identify the relationship of the kinin and complement systems to coagulation.

10. Identify the inhibitors of the coagulation and the fibrinolytic systems and their role in hemostasis.

HISTORY OF BLOOD COAGULATION

The study of blood coagulation can be traced to about 400 BC, when Hippocrates, the father of medicine, observed that the blood of a wounded soldier congealed as it cooled. He also noticed that bleeding from a small wound stopped when skin covered the blood; when the skin was removed, bleeding started again. Aristotle noted that blood cooled when removed from the body and that cooled blood initiated decay that resulted in congealment of the blood. If fibers were removed, there was no clotting. This was known as the cooling theory, or blood coagulation.

It was not until 1627 that Mercurialis observed clots in veins at body temperature. In 1770, Hewson challenged the cooling theory, believing that air and lack of motion were important in the initiation of clotting. Hewson described the clotting process and demonstrated that the clot comes from the liquid portion of blood—the coagulable lymph—and not from the cells, disproving the cooling theory. Morawitz assembled coagulation factors into the scheme of coagulation in 1905. He also demonstrated that in the presence of calcium and thromboplastin, prothrombin (factor II) was converted to thrombin, which converted fibrinogen (factor I) into a fibrin clot. These facts persisted for 40 years.

Factor VIII was identified as the cause of classic hemophilia in 1936–1937. In 1944, Owren discovered factor V after observing a bleeding patient who defied the four-factor concept of clotting. Owren also observed a cofactor that participated in the conversion of prothrombin to thrombin; in 1952, Loeliger named this factor VII. In 1947, Pavlovsky reported that the blood from some hemophiliac patients corrected the abnormal clotting time in others; in 1952, this was called Christmas disease (factor IX), named for the family in which it was discovered. Factor XI deficiency was described in 1953 as a milder bleeding tendency, and in 1955, Ratnoff and Colopy identified a patient, John Hageman, with a factor XII deficiency. Hageman died of a stroke—a thrombotic episode, not a bleeding disease. Factor X deficiency was described in 1957 in a woman named Prower and a man named Stuart. In 1960, Duckert described patients with a bleeding disorder and characteristically delayed wound healing; he called this fibrin-stabilizing factor (factor XIII). Prekallikrein was discovered in four siblings from the Fletcher family who demonstrated no bleeding tendencies (1965) and high-molecular-weight kininogen was identified in (1975). These were both identified as contact activation cofactors that participated in the activation of factor XI by factor XII.[1]

Testing of blood plasma factors and platelets depended on seeing the clotting process directly or microscopically. The first whole blood clotting time was conducted in 1780 by William Hewson, who noted that blood drawn from healthy people clotted in 7 minutes compared with 15 minutes to 1.5 hours in some disease states.

In 1897, Brodie and Russell began observing the clotting process on a glass slide, placing a drop of blood on a glass cone in a temperature-controlled glass chamber agitated by an air jet. Blood no longer moved microscopically but clotted in 3 minutes and was completed at 8 minutes. In 1905, Golhorm used a wire loop attached to a glass tube. In 1910, Kottman observed increased **viscosity** in clotting blood in a *Koaguloviskosimeter,* which rotated blood 12 to 15 times per minute at 20 degrees. In 1936, Baldes and Nygaard added photoelectric tracings called a coagulogram, depicting shape change by light transmittance.

In the 1960s, Baltimore Biologics Laboratory (now Becton Dickinson) introduced the fibrometer, an instrument that provided mechanical registration of clots and allowed more reproducible timing and an expression of the clotting process.[2]

OVERVIEW OF COAGULATION

Coagulation is a complex network of interactions involving vessels, platelets, and factors. The ability to form and remove a clot depends on many synergistic forces. Similar to a balance scale, hemostasis relies on a system of checks and balances between thrombosis and hemorrhage that includes procoagulants and **anticoagulants**. This scale needs to be kept in balance (Fig. 15.1). Thrombosis indicates an inappropriate activation of the hemostatic system. Thrombi formed in this fashion are pathologic and beyond the normal capabilities of the hemostatic mechanism. When physiologic anticoagulants decrease in the circulation, a clot forms. If procoagulants or clotting factors decrease, the scale tips toward bleeding. Hemorrhage or excessive bleeding may result from blood vessel disease, rupture, platelet abnormalities, and acquired or congenital abnormalities. Hemostasis arrests bleeding from a vessel wall defect and simultaneously maintains fluidity within the circulation. Under physiologic conditions, the anticoagulant, profibrinolytic, and antiplatelet properties of the normal endothelium maintain fluidity.[3]

Coagulation is divided into two major systems: primary and secondary systems of hemostasis. The

The Balance of Hemostasis

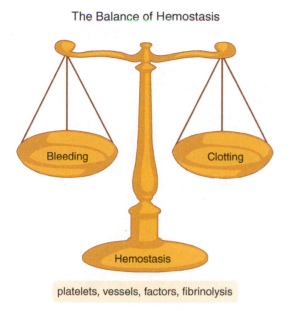

Figure 15.1 The balance scale in hemostasis.

primary hemostatic system comprises platelet function and **vasoconstriction**. The secondary system comprises coagulation proteins, platelet phospholipids, and substrates in a series of delicately balanced enzymatic reactions that culminate in fibrin formation and reinforce platelet plug formation until healing is complete. The conversion of soluble fibrinogen into an insoluble fibrin clot is accomplished by the action of thrombin, a powerful coagulant formed by prothrombin, a precursor circulating protein. Dissolution of the platelet plug and the fibrin clot meshwork is achieved by the fibrinolytic (fibrin lysing) process.

VASCULAR SYSTEM

Overview

The vascular system prevents bleeding by contracting vessels, diverting blood flow from damaged vessels, initiating contact activation of platelets with aggregation, and activating the coagulation system.[4] The vessel wall contains varying amounts of fibrous tissue, such as collagen and elastin, smooth muscle cells and fibroblasts. Arteries are the vessels that take blood away from the heart; they have the thickest walls of the vascular system. Veins that return blood to the heart are larger than the arteries and have a more irregular **lumen**. Veins are thin-walled, however, and elastic fibers are found only in larger veins. Arterioles are a smaller subdivision of arteries, and venules are smaller subdivisions of veins. Capillaries, the most numerous of the blood vessels, have the thinnest walls,

comprising only one cell layer of endothelium, and permit a rapid rate of transporting materials between blood and tissue.[5]

Mechanism of Vasoconstriction

The coagulation process begins with injury to a vessel. The first response of a cut vessel is vasoconstriction, a narrowing of the lumen of the arterioles that minimizes the flow of blood from the wound site. Ordinarily, blood is exposed only to the endothelial cell lining of the vasculature. Endothelial cells lining the lumen of the blood vessel are the principal regulators of vascular functions. Physiologically, the surface of endothelial cells is negatively charged and repels circulating proteins and platelets, which are also negatively charged.[6] This is called thromboresistance. When the endothelial layer is invaded, the exposed deeper layers of the blood vessel become targets for cellular and plasma components. Vasoconstriction, which occurs immediately and lasts only briefly, allows increased contact between the damaged vessel wall, blood platelets, and coagulation factors. Several regulatory molecules, including serotonin and thromboxane A_2, interact with receptors on the surface of cells of the blood vessel wall and promote this necessary activity. Vasoconstriction effectively prevents bleeding in small blood vessels, but it cannot prevent bleeding in larger vessels. Other systems are required for this task.

Endothelium

The endothelium contains connective tissue such as collagen and elastin. This matrix regulates the permeability of the inner vessel wall and provides the principal stimuli to thrombosis after injury to a blood vessel. Circulating platelets recognize and bind to insoluble subendothelial connective tissue molecules, a process that depends on molecules in plasma and on platelets. Two factors, von Willebrand factor (vWF) and fibrinogen, participate in the formation of the platelet plug and the insoluble protein clot, resulting in the activation of the coagulation proteins. Blood flows out through the wall and comes in contact with collagen, an insoluble fibrous protein that accounts for much of the body's connective tissue. Vessel injury leads to the stimulation of platelets, specifically the glycoproteins— GPIb, GPIIb, and GPIIIa. Platelets contain more contractile protein actomyosin than any cells other than muscle cells, giving them the ability to contract. Basically, platelets adhere to collagen, and other platelets adhere to them, building a plug. The ability of platelets to contract further compacts the mass.[7]

In forming the initial plug, platelets build a template on a lipoprotein surface, which activates tissue factor and tilts the balance between coagulation proteins and anticoagulants toward coagulation. This process accelerates vasoconstriction, platelet plug development, and formation of cross-linked fibrin clot (Fig. 15.2).

Events After Vascular Injury

1. Thromboresistant properties of a blood vessel maintain blood in a fluid state.
2. After vascular injury, subendothelial components of collagen induce platelet adhesion and aggregation, which is mediated by vWF and platelet receptor GPIb.
3. Further platelet recruitment occurs after fibrinogen binds to its platelet receptor, GPIIb/IIIa.
4. Tissue factor generates thrombin, which results in cross-linked fibrin strands that reinforce the platelet plug.
5. Platelet actomyosin mediates platelet retraction to compact the platelet mass.[8]

PRIMARY HEMOSTASIS

Platelets: Overview

In 1882, Bizzozero recognized the platelet as a cell structure different from red blood cells and white blood cells. It was not until 1970, however, that scientists recognized the relationship of platelets to hemostasis and thrombosis as significant and extensive.[9] Every cubic millimeter of healthy blood contains 250 million platelets, resulting in approximately 1 trillion platelets in the blood of an average woman. Each platelet makes 14,000 trips through the bloodstream during its life span of 7 to 10 days.[7]

Platelet Development

Platelets, or thrombocytes, are small (0.5 to 3.0 μm) discoid cells that are synthesized in the bone marrow and stimulated by the hormone thrombopoietin. They are developed through a pluripotent stem cell that has been influenced by colony-stimulating factors (CSFs) produced by macrophages, fibroblasts, T lymphocytes, and stimulated endothelial cells. The parent cells of platelets are called megakaryocytes (Fig. 15.3). These large (80 to 150 μm) cells are found in the bone marrow. Megakaryocytes do not undergo complete cellular division but rather undergo a process called endomitosis, or endoreduplication, which creates a cell with a multilobed nucleus. Each megakaryocyte produces about 2,000 platelets. Thrombopoietin is responsible for stimulating maturation and platelet release. This hormone is generated primarily by the kidney and partly by the spleen and liver.[10] The bone marrow contains no reserve of platelets—80% are in the circulation and 20% are in the red pulp of the spleen. Although platelets lack a nucleus, they do have granules: alpha granules and dense granules. These granules are secreted during the platelet release reaction and contain many biochemically active components, such as serotonin, adenosine diphosphate (ADP), and ATP. They are destroyed by the reticuloendothelial system (RES).

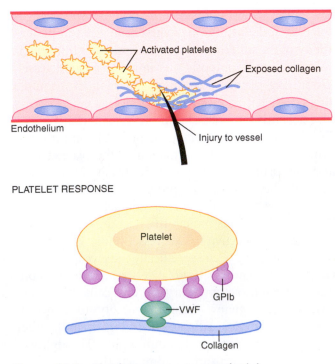

INJURY TO VESSEL

Activated platelets

Exposed collagen

Endothelium

Injury to vessel

PLATELET RESPONSE

Platelet

GPIb

VWF

Collagen

Figure 15.2 Platelet response to vascular injury.

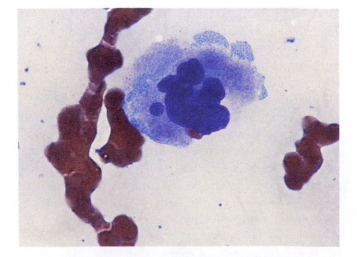

Figure 15.3 Megakaryocyte, the platelet parent cell.
From The College of American Pathologists, with permission.

Platelet development occurs in the following sequence:

1. The *megakaryoblast* is the most immature cell (10 to 15 μm), with a high nuclear:cytoplasmic ratio and two to six nucleoli.
2. The *promegakaryocyte* is a large cell (80 μm) containing dense alpha and lysosomal granules.
3. The *basophilic megakaryocyte* shows evidence of cytoplasmic fragments containing membranes, cytotubules, and several glycoprotein receptors.
4. The *megakaryocyte* is composed of cytoplasmic fragments that are released by a process called the budding of platelets.

Platelet Structure and Biochemistry

Platelets have a complex structure comprising four zones: peripheral, sol gel, organelle, and membrane system (Table 15.1). Figure 15.4 is a diagram of platelet morphology.

Platelet Function and Kinetics

Platelets play an important role in the formation of a primary plug and the coagulation cascade. The formation of a plug at the site of a cut vessel serves as the initial mechanical barrier. The lumen of the vessel is lined with endothelial cells, and a break in this lining initiates a series of reactions (see Chapter 16).

Platelet function includes four reactions:

- *Reaction 1 (adhesion)*: Platelets adhere to collagen, changing shape from disk to spiny sphere. GPIb and vWF aid adhesion. This primary aggregation is reversible. This reaction is mediated by the release of platelet granules.

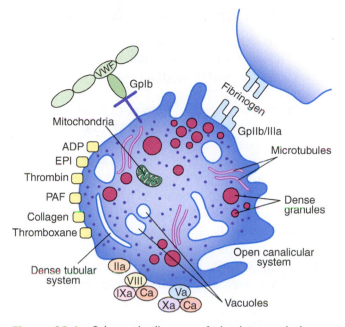

Figure 15.4   Schematic diagram of platelet morphology.

- *Reaction 2 (aggregation)*: Chemical changes lead to platelet aggregation in which platelets adhere to other platelets. Platelet shape change occurs, and platelets form spiny projections that make them more adhesive to other platelets.
- *Reaction 3 (release)*: Platelets release the contents of their dense granules, resulting in a secondary and irreversible aggregation. Platelets release thromboxane A_2, which promotes vasoconstriction. ADP amplifies the process.
- *Reaction 4 (clot stabilization)*: This reaction is responsible for thrombus (clot) formation. The adherent and aggregated platelets release factor V and expose platelet factor 3, accelerating the coagulation cascade, promoting activation of clotting factors, and ultimately stabilizing the platelet plug with a fibrin clot.

The platelet membrane contains important receptors (glycoproteins) on the platelet surface. Further interactions are mediated by plasma protein receptors of vWF and fibrinogen. Other platelet activators are thrombin, ADP, thromboxane A_2, serotonin, epinephrine, and arachidonic acid.

The receptor for vWF is GPIb-IX, whereas GPIIb/IIIa is the receptor for **fibronectin**, vWF, fibrinogen, and factors V and VIII. This interaction recruits more platelets to interact with each other.[11] Activated platelets release ADP and synthesized thromboxane A_2, which mediate activation of additional platelets, resulting in the formation of a platelet plug.[12]

Table 15.1 ○ Four Functional Platelet Zones

1. Peripheral zone is associated with platelet adhesion and aggregation
2. Sol gel zone provides a cytoskeletal system for platelets and contact when the platelets are stimulated
3. Organelle zone contains three types of granules: alpha, dense bodies, and lysosomes
4. Membrane system contains a dense tubular system in which the enzymatic system for the production of prostaglandin synthesis is found

Platelet Aggregation Principle

Aggregation defines the ability of platelets to attach to one another. The formation of aggregates is observed with a platelet aggregometer, a photo-optic instrument connected to a chart recorder. Light transmittance through the platelet-rich plasma (PRP) sample is increased and converted into electronic signals as platelets aggregate, causing the plasma sample to transmit more light (PPP), which is amplified and recorded. Each aggregating agent forms a characteristic curve. Primary aggregation, the first wave, is preceded by a shape change except when platelets are stimulated with epinephrine (Fig. 15.5). Primary aggregation is a reversible process. Secondary aggregation, which occurs when platelet granule contents are secreted, is irreversible. Epinephrine (EPI), collagen, ADP, and arachidonic acid are the aggregating agents most frequently used in clinical platelet aggregation.

1. *EPI*: When added to PRP, EPI stimulates platelet aggregation. Normal platelets respond by releasing endogenous ADP from their granules. Primary and secondary aggregation occurs. An abnormal response is due to an absent or decreased release of nucleotides from dense granules.

2. *ADP*: When added to PRP, ADP stimulates platelets to change their shape and aggregate. High-dose (20 μmol/L) exogenous ADP induces aggregation. The primary and secondary wave aggregations are indistinguishable. Reversible aggregation may occur because of an inadequate release of nucleotides. Lack of a secondary wave indicates defective thromboxane production or a defective granule pool, or both.

3. *Collagen*: When added to PRP, the platelets adhere to the collagen, change their shape, and release endogenous ADP, leading to aggregation. An abnormal response to collagen can occur if thromboxane production is deficient. Aggregation is slower and less complex, resulting in a decreased response.

4. *Arachidonic acid* (AA): AA is a fatty acid present in membranes of human platelets and liberated from phospholipids. In the presence of the enzyme cyclooxygenase, oxygen is incorporated to form the endoperoxide prostaglandin G_2 (PGG_2), which converts to

Platelet Aggregation Tracings

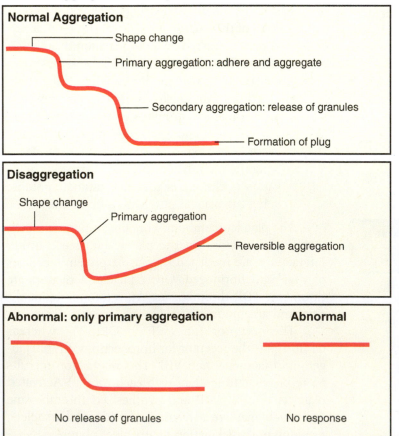

Figure 15.5 Platelet aggregation. Note the stages of aggregation, which include primary and secondary aggregation as well as shape change and plug formation.

thromboxane A_2, a potent inducer of platelet aggregation. Aspirin consumption disrupts this biochemical pathway for the life of the platelet.

SECONDARY HEMOSTASIS

Overview

Secondary hemostasis involves a series of reactions through a cascadelike process that concludes with the formation of an insoluble fibrin clot. This system involves multiple enzymes and several cofactors and inhibitors to keep the system in balance. When the factors are in a precursor form, the enzyme or zymogen is converted to an active enzyme or a protease.

Clotting is initiated with the activation of two enzymatic pathways that ultimately lead to fibrin formation: the intrinsic and extrinsic pathways. Both pathways are necessary for fibrin formation, but their activating factors are different. Intrinsic activation occurs after trauma within the vascular system, such as exposed endothelium. Approximately 10 minutes can elapse from the platelet plug to fibrin formation. This system is slower than the extrinsic pathway but more important. Initiation of the extrinsic pathway occurs tissue factor is released.

Classification of Coagulation Factors

Coagulation factors are categorized into substrates, cofactors, and enzymes. Substrates are the substances on which enzymes act. Fibrinogen is the main substrate. Cofactors accelerate the activities of enzymes that participate in the coagulation cascade. Cofactors include tissue factor, factor V, factor VIII, and Fitzgerald factor. All of the enzymes are serine proteases except factor XIII, which is a **transaminase**.[13]

Coagulation factors can be classified into three groups, as follows:

1. The *fibrinogen* group (factors I, V, VIII, and XIII) is consumed during coagulation. Factors V and VIII are labile and increase during pregnancy and inflammation.
2. The *prothrombin* group (factors II, VII, IX, and X) is dependent on vitamin K during synthesis. The carboxylation of glutamic acid residues is dependent on vitamin K for the addition of calcium. This group is stable and remains preserved in stored plasma.
3. The *contact* group (factor XI, factor XII, prekallikrein, and high-molecular-weight kininogen [HMWK]) participates in the intrinsic pathway. This group is moderately stable and not consumed during coagulation.[5]

Table 15.2 summarizes the coagulation factors, their half-life, clinical symptoms if deficient, likely screening tests, and actions.

Factor I (Fibrinogen)

The substrate for thrombin and precursor of fibrin, factor I is a large globulin protein. Its function is to be converted into an insoluble protein and then back to soluble components. When exposed to thrombin, two peptides split from the fibrinogen molecule, leaving a fibrin monomer to form a **polymerized** clot.

Factor II (Prothrombin)

Precursor to thrombin, in the presence of Ca^{2+} factor II, is converted to thrombin (IIa), which stimulates platelet aggregation and activates cofactors protein C and factor XIII. Prothrombin is vitamin K–dependent.

Factor III (Thromboplastin)

Factor III or tissue factor activates factor VII when blood is exposed to tissue fluids.

Factor IV (Ionized Calcium)

Factor IV is an active form of calcium that is required for the activation of thromboplastin and for conversion of prothrombin to thrombin.

Factor V (Proaccelerin, or Labile Factor)

Factor V is consumed during clotting and accelerates the transformation of prothrombin to thrombin. A vitamin K–dependent factor, 20% of factor V is found on platelets.

Factor VI (Nonexistent)

Factor VI is nonexistent.

Factor VII (Proconvertin, or Stable Factor)

Factor VII is activated by tissue thromboplastin, which activates factor X. It is vitamin K–dependent.

Factor VIII (Antihemophilic)

Factor VIII participates in the cleavage of factor X-Xa by IXa. Factor VIII is described as follows:

- VIII/vWF
- VIII:C, the active portion, which is measured by clotting and is deficient in hemophilia A
- VIII:Ag, the antigenic portion
- vWF:Ag, which measures antigen that binds to endothelium for platelet function

Table 15.2 ● Factor Facts

Factor	Inheritance	Half-life (hours)	Clinical Picture If Deficient	Factor for Hemostasis	Screening Tests
I	Autosomal dominant	64–96	Bleed with trauma, stress, mucosal, umbilical stump, intracranial, gastrointestinal	40–50 mg/dL	↑PT and aPTT
II	Autosomal recessive	48	Severe bleed, mucous membrane, spontaneous	20%–30%	↑ PT and aPTT
V	Autosomal recessive	12	Moderate-severe bleed, mucosal, large ecchymoses	10%–15%	↑ PT and aPTT
VII	Autosomal recessive	4–6	Intra-articular bleed, severe mucosal, epistaxis, hemarthrosis, genitourinary, gastrointestinal, intrapulmonary	10%–15%	↑ PT
VIII	Sex-linked recessive	15–20	Severity based on levels, hematuria, hemarthrosis, intra-articular, intracranial	Greater than 10%	↑ aPTT
IX	Sex-linked recessive	24	Severe mucous membrane, deep tissue, intramuscular	Greater than 10%	↑ aPTT
X	Autosomal recessive	32	Mucous membrane, skin hemorrhages	10%–15%	↑ PT and aPTT
XI	Autosomal recessive	60–80	Severity of bleeds vary, not proportional to factor level	30%	↑ aPTT
XII	Autosomal recessive and dominant	50–70	Hemorrhage is rare, risk for thrombosis	?	↑ aPTT
XIII	Autosomal recessive	40–50	Only homozygotes bleed, deep tissue muscle, intracranial bleed	10%	Normal PT and aPTT

Factor IX (Plasma Thromboplastin Component)

A component of the thromboplastin generating system, factor IX is deficient in hemophilia B, also known as Christmas disease. It is sex-linked and vitamin K–dependent.

Factor X (Stuart-Prower)

This common pathway factor merges to form conversion of prothrombin to thrombin, activity also related to factors VII and IX. It is vitamin K–dependent and can be independently activated by Russell's viper venom.

Factor XI (Plasma Thromboplastin Antecedent)

Essential to intrinsic thromboplastin generating of the cascade, factor XI occurs more frequently in the Jewish population. Bleeding tendencies vary, but there is the risk of postoperative hemorrhage.

Factor XII (Hageman Factor)

Factor XII is a surface contact factor that is activated by collagen. Patients do not bleed but have a tendency toward thrombosis.

Factor XIII (Fibrin-Stabilizing Factor)

In the presence of calcium, factor XIII, a transaminase, stabilizes polymerized fibrin monomers in the initial clot. This is the only factor not measured by PT or aPTT.

High-Molecular-Weight Kininogen (Fitzgerald Factor)

HMWK is a surface contact factor that is activated by kallikrein.

Prekallikrein (Fletcher Factor)

Prekallikrein is a surface contact activator, in which 75% is bound to HMWK.

Physiologic Coagulation (In Vivo)

The original coagulation theory was a cascade or waterfall theory. This description depicted thrombin generation by the soluble coagulation factors and the initiation of coagulation. This theory identified two starting points for thrombin generation: the initiation of the intrinsic pathway with factor XII and surface contact and the extrinsic pathway with factor VIIa and tissue factor. These two pathways meet at the common pathway, where they both generate factor Xa from X, leading to a common pathway of thrombin from prothrombin and the conversion of fibrinogen to fibrin. This process holds true under laboratory conditions (Fig. 15.6). Tissue factor pathway inhibitor (TFPI), a naturally occurring inhibitor of hemostasis, blocks the activity of the tissue factor VIIa complex soon after it becomes active.[14]

Laboratory Model of Coagulation

Laboratory testing looks at the in vitro effect of the coagulation process, which is measured by prothrombin time (PT), activated partial thromboplastin time (aPTT), thrombin time (TT), fibrin degradation products (FDPs), and D-dimer. This section focuses on PT and aPTT; Chapter 20 focuses on the other routine tests mentioned. Although the coagulation cascade does not reflect what occurs in vivo, it does provide a model in which the laboratory relates to testing. The coagulation cascade, however, reflects the mechanisms that the laboratory uses for results. The screening tests provide the physician with a tremendous amount of information. They can be performed quickly and accurately (Fig. 15.7).

Extrinsic Pathway

The extrinsic pathway is initiated with the release of tissue thromboplastin that has been expressed after

In Vitro Coagulation Cascade

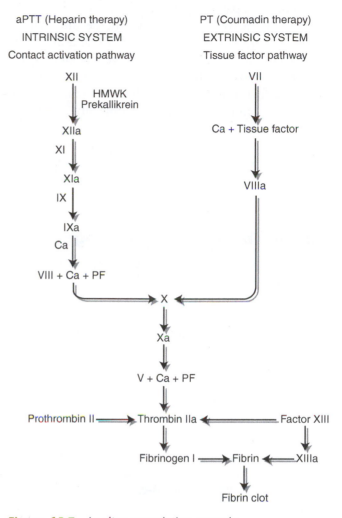

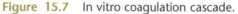

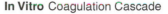

Figure 15.7   In vitro coagulation cascade.

damage to a vessel. The complex formed by factor VII, tissue thromboplastin, and calcium converts factors X and Xa, which convert prothrombin to thrombin. Thrombin converts fibrinogen to fibrin. This entire process takes between 10 and 15 seconds.

Intrinsic Pathway

Vascular trauma induces changes that initiate a cascading sequence of contact activation. Factor XII autoactivates to factor XIIa in the presence of the protein prekallikrein, and activation of factor XI to factor XIa requires the presence of another protein, a cofactor of HMWK. Factor XIa activates factor IX to factor IXa, which converts factor X to factor Xa in the presence of factor VIIIa and PF3, a platelet phospholipid. Rapid activation of factor X also requires calcium. The reaction then enters the common pathway.

Revised Coagulation Cascade: **In Vivo**

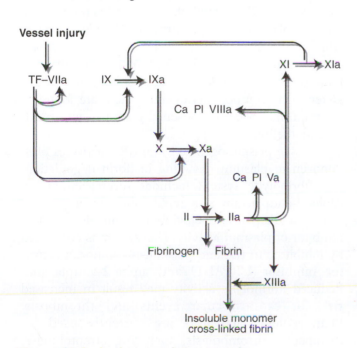

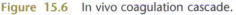

Figure 15.6   In vivo coagulation cascade.

Common Pathway

The common pathway is the point at which the intrinsic and extrinsic pathways merge and where factors I, II, V, and X are measured. PT and aPTT do not detect qualitative or quantitative platelet disorders or factor XIII deficiency. Factor XIII, the fibrin-stabilizing factor, is responsible for stabilizing a soluble fibrin monomer into an insoluble fibrin clot. A patient with factor XIII deficiency cannot stabilize a clot, and bleeding occurs later. Factor XIII is measured by a 5 mol/L urea test that not only examines clot formation but also determines whether the clot lyses after 24 hours.

Role of Thrombin in Fibrinogen

The activation of plasma fibrinogen by thrombin, a protease enzyme, results in a stable fibrin clot, visible proof of fibrin formation. Thrombin also participates in factor XIII-XIIIa activation, which occurs when thrombin cleaves a peptide bond from each of two alpha chains. Combined with Ca^{2+} ions, inactive factor XIII enables factor XIII to dissociate to factor XIIIa. If thrombin were allowed to circulate in its active form (factor Ia), uncontrollable clotting would occur. Thrombin, therefore, circulates in its inactive form, prothrombin (factor II). Thrombin cleaves fibrinogen (factor I), which results in a fibrin monomer and fibrinogen peptides A and B. These initial monomers polymerize end-to-end because of hydrogen bonding.

Fibrin formation occurs in three phases:

1. *Proteolysis* occurs when protease enzyme thrombin cleaves fibrinogen, resulting in a fibrin monomer, A and B fibrinopeptide.
2. *Polymerization* occurs spontaneously when fibrin monomers line up end-to-end because of hydrogen bonding.
3. *Stabilization* occurs when factor XIIIa covalently links fibrin monomers into fibrin polymers, forming an insoluble fibrin clot.

Feedback Inhibition in Clot Formation

Some activated factors have the ability to destroy other factors in the cascade. Thrombin can temporarily activate factors V and VIII, but as it increases, it destroys factors V and VIII by proteolysis. Although factor Xa enhances factor VII, it prevents further activation of factor X by factor VIIa and tissue factor through a reaction with the tissue factor pathway inhibitor (TFPI). These enzymes self-limit their ability to activate the coagulation cascade at different intervals.

Thrombin feedback activation of factor IX might explain how intrinsic coagulation could occur in the absence of contact factors. Tissue factor is expressed after an injury, forming a complex with factor VIIa and then activating factors X and IX. TFPI prevents further activation of factor X. Factors V, VIII, and XI further amplify thrombin formation by leading to activation of the intrinsic pathway. This feedback theory helps to enforce why patients with contact factor abnormalities (factors XI and XII) do not bleed.[8] Figure 15-8 is a diagram of feedback inhibition.

Fibrinolysis

The fibrinolytic system dissolves clots. Fibrin clots are not intended to be permanent. Rather, the purpose of the clot is to stop the flow of blood until the damaged vessel can be repaired. The presence or absence of hemorrhage or thrombosis depends on a balance between the procoagulant and the fibrinolytic system. The key components of the system are plasminogen, plasminogen activators, plasmin, fibrin, fibrin/FDP, and inhibitors of plasminogen activators and plasmin.[6] Fibrinolysis is the process by which the hydrolytic enzyme plasmin digests fibrin and fibrinogen, resulting in progressively reduced clots. This system is activated in response to initiation of the contact factor activation. Plasmin is capable of digesting fibrin or fibrinogen and other factors in the cascade (factors V, VIII, IX, and XI). Normal plasma contains the inactive form of plasmin in a precursor called plasminogen, which remains dormant until it is activated by proteolytic enzymes, the kinases, or plasminogen activators. Fibrinolysis is controlled by the plasminogen activator system. The components of this system are found in tissues, urine, plasma, lysosomal granules, and vascular endothelium.

Tissue plasminogen activator (tPA) activates plasminogen to plasmin, resulting in fibrin degradation. The fibrinolytic system includes several inhibitors. Alpha-2-antiplasmin is a rapid inhibitor of plasmin activity, and alpha-2-macroglobulin is an effective slow inhibitor of plasmin activity. This system is controlled by inhibitors to tPA and plasmin-plasminogen activator inhibitor 1 (PAI-1) and alpha-2-antiplasmin. Reduced fibrinolytic activity may result in increased risk for cardiovascular events and thrombosis. Pharmacologic activators are currently used for therapeutic **thrombolysis**, including streptokinase,

Feedback Inhibition:

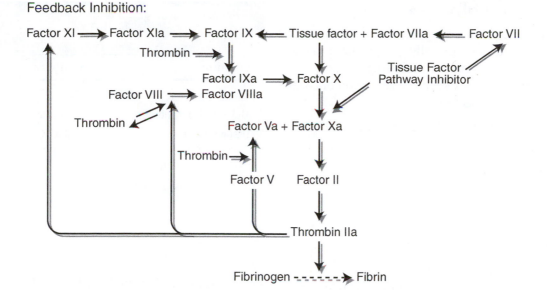

Figure 15.8 Feedback inhibition. Note the role of thrombin in the activation and deactivation of coagulation factors.

urokinase, and tPA. Urokinase directly activates plasminogen into plasmin, and streptokinase forms a streptokinase plasminogen complex, which then converts plasminogen into plasmin.[16]

Screening Tests for Coagulation

Developed by Quick in 1935, the *prothrombin time* (PT) measures the extrinsic and common system of coagulation. It requires the addition of calcium chloride, tissue factor, and platelet phospholipid. Thromboplastin is lipoprotein extracted from rabbit brain and lung.[1]

PT uses citrate anticoagulated plasma. Following the addition of an optimal concentration of calcium and an excess of thromboplastin, an automated device measures clot detection, and the result is reported in seconds. PT is exclusively sensitive for factor VII deficiency, but this test is also sensitive to decreases in the common pathway factors. If a patient presents with a prolonged PT but no other clinical abnormality or medication, the patient most likely has factor VII deficiency. PT is also used to monitor oral anticoagulation or warfarin therapy employed to treat and prevent blood clots. In many instances, patients are placed on lifelong therapy; the dosage is monitored by the PT test and the calculated international normalized ratio (INR) (which is discussed in greater detail in Chapter 19). Anticoagulant therapy attempts to impede thrombus formation in individuals who have predisposing factors for clot formation or who are predisposed by virtue of a medical event without the threat of **morbidity** or **mortality** from hemorrhage.

Warfarin is an oral anticoagulant, which means it must be ingested. It was discovered accidentally at the University of Wisconsin in 1939 after a farmer found that his cattle were hemorrhaging to death for no apparent reason. The cattle grazed in a field of sweet clover, which contains dicumarol (actually, bishydroxycoumarin), causing the cattle to bleed.[6]

There are several compounds of Coumadin: dicumarol, indanedione, and warfarin. Dicumarol works too slowly, and indanedione has too many side effects. Warfarin, or 4-oxycoumarin, is the most commonly used oral anticoagulant. Warfarin (Coumadin) works by inhibiting the y-carboxylation step of clotting and the vitamin K–dependent factors.[15] Chapter 19 discusses laboratory monitoring of oral anticoagulation therapy using INR.

Activated Partial Thromboplastin Time

aPTT measures the intrinsic and common pathway. The test consists of recalcifying plasma in the presence of a standardized amount of plateletlike phospholipid and an activator of the contact factors. It detects abnormalities in factors VIII, IX, XI, and XII and common pathway factors. aPTT is also used to monitor heparin therapy. Heparin is an anticoagulant used to treat or prevent acute thrombotic events, such as deep vein thrombosis (DVT), pulmonary embolism (PE), or acute coronary syndromes. The action of heparin inactivates factors XII, XI, and IX in the presence of antithrombin. Chapter 19 discusses laboratory monitoring of heparin therapy.

Coagulation Inhibitors

Inhibitors are soluble plasma proteins that are *natural* anticoagulants and are normally present in plasma. They prevent the initiation of the clotting cascade. Two major inhibitors in plasma keep the activation of coagulation under control, as follows:

1. Protease inhibitors: Inhibitors of coagulation factors, including
   - Antithrombin
   - Heparin cofactor II
   - TFPI
   - Alpha-2-antiplasmin
   - C1
2. Protein C pathway: Inactivation of activated cofactors, including factors V and VIII

Chapter 19 discusses these inhibitors. Table 15.3 summarizes the inhibitors and their target reaction sites.

Minor Systems Related to Hemostasis

Kinin System

Another plasma protein system in coagulation is the kinin system. This system is capable of increasing vascular permeability leading to hypotension, shock, and end-organ damage.[16] The kinins are peptides of 9 to 11 amino acids activated by factor XII. Factor XIIa (Hageman factor) converts prekallikrein (Fletcher factor) into kallikrein, and kallikrein converts kininogens into kinins. The most important kinin is bradykinin (BK), which participates in vascular permeability and chemical pain mediation. BK can reproduce many characteristics of an inflammatory state, including changes in blood pressure, edema, and pain, resulting in vasodilation and increased microvessel permeability.[13]

Complement System

The complement system participates in inflammation and the immune system and important thrombohemorrhagic disorders, such as disseminated intravascular coagulation (DIC). Activated complement fragments can bind and damage self-tissues. Regulators of complement activation are expressed on cell surfaces, where they protect the cell from the effects of cell-bound complement fragments. If this regulation process is abnormal, it may contribute to the pathogenesis of autoimmune disease and inflammatory disorders. The complement system includes 22 serum proteins that play a role in mediating immune and allergic reactions and cell lysis secondary to

Table 15.3 ● Serine Protease Inhibitors	
Inhibitor	**Specificity**
Antithrombin (AT)	IIa, Xa, IXa
Alpha-2-macroglobulin	Nonspecific
Tissue factor pathway inhibitor	Xa, VIIa/TF complex inhibitor
Heparin cofactor II	IIa
Alpha-2 protease inhibitor	XIa, elastase
CI inhibitor	XIIa, kallikrein, XIa, CI (complement system)

production of membrane attack complex (MAC). The lysis and disruption of red blood cells and platelets lead to the release of procoagulant material. The complement system is a sequential activation pathway. Plasmin activates complement by cleaving C3 into C3a and C3b. C3 causes increased vascular permeability, and because of the degranulation or lysis of mast cells, which results in histamine release, C3b causes immune adherence.[13]

The interrelationship between the complement, kinin, and coagulation systems is complex and revealing. Coagulation and the elements that contribute to the success of the hemostatic system are multifactorial, and more knowledge about this versatile system is continually becoming available. Figure 15.9 illustrates the important interrelationships between the coagulation, fibrinolytic, complement, and kinin systems.

○ *Summary Points*

- Hemostasis depends on a system of checks and balances between thrombosis and hemorrhage that involve procoagulants and anticoagulants.
- The systems involved in hemostasis are the vascular system, platelets, coagulation system, and fibrinolytic system.
- Primary hemostasis consists of platelet function and vasoconstriction.
- Secondary hemostasis includes fibrin clot formation and fibrin clot lysis.
- Platelet aggregation is mediated by von Willebrand factor (vWF) and platelet glycoprotein Ib (GPIb).
- Platelets are small discoid cell fragments that are synthesized in the bone marrow and stimulated by the hormone thrombopoietin.
- There are four phases to platelet function at the site of injury: platelet adherence to collagen, platelet

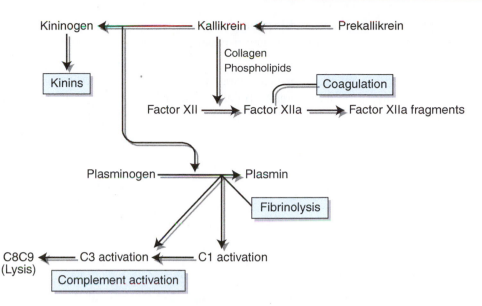

Figure 15.9 Interrelationships between coagulation, fibrinolytic, complement, and kinin systems.

CONDENSED CASE

A 35-year-old woman needs to have an ovarian cyst removed. She had one uneventful delivery. Her mother has a history of bleeding after tooth extraction. The physician needs to determine if there is a bleeding disorder. The coagulation test results are as follows:

PT	12.5 seconds (reference range 10.5 to 13.3 seconds)
aPTT	32.1 seconds (reference range 28.7 to 35.5 seconds)
Platelets	320,000/mm³ (reference range 150,000 to 400,000/mm³)
Bleeding time	11 minutes (reference 8 minutes)

What is the most significant abnormal result in the coagulation panel?

Answer

The bleeding time is the only abnormal test because it is greater than 8 minutes. This suggests a disorder of primary hemostasis. Prolonged bleeding time can be caused by any platelet disorder, such as von Willebrand disease, or a problem secondary to platelet secretion, or it can be caused by several medications. Tests to rule out von Willebrand disease include factor VIII assay, vWF antigen and activity, and platelet aggregation testing. On performing a platelet aggregation, there was only a primary wave for epinephrine and no response for arachidonic acid. The patient was taking 81 µmg of aspirin a day as a preventive measure, and this resulted in a prolonged bleeding time. The patient was removed from aspirin, and the bleeding time returned to normal.

---

aggregation, platelet granule release, and stabilization of the clot.

- Coagulation factors are produced in the liver, with the exception of a portion of factor VIII, which is produced in the endothelial cells.

- The traditional coagulation pathway is divided into the intrinsic, extrinsic, and common pathways.

- The extrinsic pathway is monitored by prothrombin time, whereas the intrinsic pathway is monitored by partial thromboplastin time.

- The intrinsic pathway is initiated by factor XII and surface contact with the endothelial cells.

- Tissue factor pathway inhibitor (TFPI) can block the activity of the tissue factor–factor VII complex soon after it becomes active.

- Thrombin-activated plasma fibrinogen results in a stable fibrin clot.

- Fibrinolysis is the process by which plasmin digests fibrinogen and fibrin, dissolving the clot.

- The key components of the fibrinolytic system are plasminogen, plasminogen activators, plasmin, fibrin, fibrin degradation products, and inhibitors of plasminogen and plasmin.

- Streptokinase, urokinase, and tissue plasminogen activator are activators of the plasmin-plasminogen system.
- Tissue plasminogen activator is available as a pharmacologic product to break up pathologically formed clots.
- Serine protease inhibitors and the protein C pathway are the major physiologic inhibitors of coagulation.
- The kinin system is activated by factor XII and contributes to vascular permeability.
- The activated complement system may contribute to the release of procoagulant material.

CASE STUDY

A 15-year-old boy with chronic strep throat has presented with excessive bruising. His coagulation results were as follows:

PT	15.5 seconds (reference range 10.8 to 13.5 seconds)
aPTT	42.1 seconds (reference range 28.5 to 35.5 seconds)
Platelets	325,000/mm^3 (reference range 150,000 to 400,000/mm^3)
Bleeding	5 minutes (reference 8 minutes)

Which coagulation tests are abnormal, and how should the physician proceed in treating this patient?

Insights to the Case Study

In this case, two parameters, the PT and the aPTT, are elevated. The patient is not bleeding, but he shows a history of recent bruising. Because both the PT and the aPTT are affected, one can assume the problem is in the common pathway, specifically factors I, II, V, and X. Factor assays could be performed to assess the level of activity of each of these clotting factors; however, a closer examination of the patient's history might reveal an additional feature. Because this patient has had chronic strep throat, it is logical to assume that he has been on long-term antibiotics. Antibiotics may deplete the normal flora, a source of vitamin K synthesis. Factors II, VII, IX, and X are vitamin K–dependent factors. Vitamin K is the essential cofactor for the gamma carboxyglutamic acid residues necessary to activate these factors. When vitamin K is in short supply or depleted, these factors fail to function properly. In our patient, vitamin K given by mouth would resume normal coagulation and correct bruising.

Review Questions

1. The factor with the longest half-life is
   a. I.
   b. V.
   c. VII.
   d. X.

2. If a patient has a prolonged PT, the patient most likely is deficient in factor
   a. VIII.
   b. II.
   c. VII.
   d. X.

3. Receptors found on the platelets are called
   a. Glycoproteins.
   b. Vwf.
   c. Fibrinogen.
   b. Beta-thromboglobulin.

4. Vasoconstriction is caused by several regulatory molecules, which include
   a. Fibrinogen and vWF.
   b. ADP and EPI.
   c. Thromboxane A$_2$ and serotonin.
   d. Collagen and actomyosin.

5. The vitamin K–dependent factors are
   a. I, II, V, and X.
   b. II, VII, IX, and X.
   c. I, VII, V, and VIII.
   d. II, IX, XI, and X.

6. The life span of a platelet is
   a. 5 to 8 days.
   b. 7 to 10 days.
   c. 6 to 9 days.
   d. 9 to 12 days.

7. Alpha granules are found in
   a. The peripheral zone.
   b. The sol gel zone.
   c. Organelles.
   d. Membranes.

8. If a patient has a prolonged aPTT only, the patient may be deficient in the following factors:
   a. VIII, X, II, and I
   b. VIII, IX, XI, and XII
   c. VIII, X, XI, and XII
   d. VIII, XI, II, and XII

9. The factor that is responsible for stabilizing a soluble fibrin monomer into an insoluble clot is
   a. II.
   b. X.
   c. XII.
   d. XIII.

10. An inhibitor of plasmin activity is
    a. tPA.
    b. PAI-1.
    c. Alpha-2-antiplasmin.
    d. Plasminogen.

11. Protein C and its cofactor protein S inactivate factors
    a. VIIa and Xa.
    b. Va and VIIIa.
    c. IXa and VIIa.
    d. VIIIa and XIIa.

○ TROUBLESHOOTING

What Do I Do When the Coagulation Sample Is Drawn Incorrectly?

Preanalytic variables represent important sources of error in patient testing and accuracy of results. In hemostasis testing, sample integrity is paramount. Areas in which sample integrity are most affected are in phlebotomy practices, transport and handling of specimens, choice of coagulation tubes, and patient variables.

Phlebotomy Practices

The sample must be provided from an atraumatic draw on a properly identified patient, and the tube must be inverted three to four times for proper mixing of anticoagulant. The order of draw in coagulation testing is important to avoid contamination of the sample with tissue thromboplastin. If multiple tubes are drawn, the coagulation tube should be last. If only a coagulation sample is requested and the sample is drawn through a butterfly, a discard tube should be drawn first. If a syringe is needed for phlebotomy, a 12- to 19-gauge needle is optimal. Additionally, the tubes must be filled to 90% capacity to preserve a 1:9 anticoagulant:blood ratio.

Transport and Handling of Specimens

Several coagulation proteins are labile. Factors V and VIII are labile, with a short half-life. The activity of these factors is lost if the sample is not tested in an appropriate time span. For maximum activity, testing should be performed within 4 hours for aPTT and up to 24 hours for PT. Plasma can be removed from the sample and stored at $-20°C$ for 2 weeks. Additionally, samples must be centrifuged for a period of time that enables them to become platelet-poor plasma, defined as having a platelet count of less than $10.0 \times 10^9/L$, which depends on proper centrifugation. If samples are not platelet-poor, falsely shortened results may occur because of activation of platelet factor 4. Activation of platelet factor 4 may also occur in heparinized samples that are allowed to sit on red blood cells for longer than 4 hours, and the platelet factor 4 may inactivate heparin, giving a falsely shortened PTT result.

Which Tubes to Use?

Most facilities use blue top tubes, which contain 3.2% sodium citrate. There are many reasons for this practice, including the fact that this concentration provides a closer osmolality to plasma, has less binding of calcium, and provides a more favorable environment for heparinized samples.

Patient Variables

Many variables affect coagulation results, including medication, physical and emotional stress, and patient age and personal habits. The laboratory cannot control

Continued

these factors. The laboratory can adjust for a patient's hematocrit, however, when drawing a coagulation sample. For patients who have hematocrits that are greater than 60% (neonates, patients with polycythemia), falsely prolonged results occur if the anticoagulant is not adjusted because there is too much anticoagulant for plasma. For patients who have hematocrits less than 22%, results are falsely decreased as a result of too little anticoagulant because of increasing plasma volume. The standard formula for adjusting the volume of anticoagulant is

$$\text{New volume of sodium citrate} = (1.85 \times 10)^{-3} \times (100 - \text{Hct}) \times \text{volume of sample}$$

WORD KEY

Anticoagulant • Delaying or preventing blood coagulation

Fibronectin • Protein involved in wound healing and cell adhesion

Lumen • Space within an artery, vein, or intestine or tube

Morbidity • State of being diseased

Mortality • Death

Polymerize • Process by which a simple chemical substance or substances are changed into a substance of a much higher molecular weight but with the same proportions

Thrombolysis • Breaking up of a clot

Transaminase • Aminotransferase (an enzyme)

Vasoconstriction • Decrease in the diameter of the blood vessels that decreases the blood flow

Viscosity • State of being sticky or gummy

References

1. Owen CA. A History of Blood Coagulation. Rochester, MN: Mayo Foundation for Medical Education and Research, 2001.
2. Hougie C. Fundamentals of Blood Coagulation in Clinical Medicine. New York: McGraw-Hill, 1963.
3. Schetz M. Coagulation disorder in acute renal failure. Kidney Int S53(suppl 66):96–101, 1998.
4. Harmening D. Clinical Hematology and Fundamentals of Hemostasis, 3rd ed. Philadelphia: FA Davis, 1997.
5. Turgeon ML. Clinical Hematology, Theory and Procedures, 2nd ed. Boston: Little, Brown, 1993.
6. McKenzie SB. Textbook of Hematology. Baltimore: Williams & Wilkins, 1996.
7. Zucker M. The functioning of blood platelets. Sci Am 242:86–89, 1980.
8. Kjeldsberg C. Practical Diagnosis of Hematologic Disorders, 2nd ed. Chicago: ASCP Press, 1995.
9. Plaut D. Platelet function tests. ADVANCE for the Administrators of the Laboratory, July 2003.
10. Southern D, Leclair S. Platelet maturation and unction. In: Rodak B, ed. Diagnostic Hematology. Philadelphia: WB Saunders, 1995.
11. Kolde H-J. Haemostasis. Pentapharm Ltd. Basel: 2001.
12. Rodgers G. Hemostasis Case Studies. Chicago: ASCP Press, 2000.
13. Ogedegbe HO. An overview of hemostasis. Lab Med 12(1):948–953, 2002.
14. Fass D. Overview of hemostasis. Mayo Clinic Coagulation Conference, Mayo Clinic, August 2004.
15. Kandrotis RJ. Pharmacology and pharmacokinetics of antithrombotic agents. Clin Appl Thromb Hemost 3:157–163, 1997.
16. Bick R. Disorders of Thrombosis and Hemostasis. Chicago: ASCP Press, 1991.

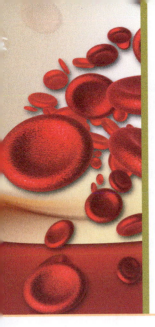

Chapter 16

Quantitative and Qualitative Platelet Disorders

Betty Ciesla

Objectives

After completing this chapter, the student will be able to:

1. Define *quantitative platelet disorders*.

2. Identify the types of bleeding that are seen in platelet disorders.

3. List four laboratory tests that are helpful in evaluating platelet disorders.

4. State how preanalytic variables may affect the platelet count.

5. Describe three characteristics of the qualitative platelet disorders von Willebrand's disease, Bernard-Soulier syndrome, and Glanzmann's thrombasthenia.

6. Identify drugs that are implicated in immune thrombocytopenia.

7. Evaluate conditions that may cause thrombocytosis.

8. Compare and contrast acute versus chronic idiopathic thrombocytopenic purpura in regard to pathophysiology, clinical symptoms, and treatment.

9. Define hemolytic uremic syndrome in terms of pathophysiology, key clinical features, and patient management.

10. Define thrombotic thrombocytopenic purpura in terms of pathophysiology, key clinical features, and severity.

11. Describe platelet abnormalities caused by acquired defects—drug-induced, nonimmune, or vascular.

QUANTITATIVE DISORDERS OF PLATELETS

A normal platelet count is 150 to 450 × 10⁹/L. In this range, an individual has enough platelets to assist in the coagulation process by creating a platelet plug and stimulating the formation of a solid fibrin clot. A decreased platelet count causes bleeding from the mucous membranes of the gums (gingival bleeding) or nose (epistaxis) and extensive bruising (ecchymoses) or petechiae (pinpoint hemorrhages). A patient with a platelet count of 60.0 × 10⁹/L bleeds in surgery, and a patient with a platelet count of 30.0 × 10⁹/L may have petechial bleeding. When the platelet count decreases to less than 5.0 × 10⁹/L, bleeding in the central nervous system may be evident. Laboratory tests that are helpful in determining platelet function include the bleeding time test (or similar platelet function tests), platelet aggregation by one of several methods, or other methods that assess platelet function and aggregation. Several factors cause thrombocytopenia, or decreased platelet count. Decreased production or increased destruction of platelets usually accounts for the pathophysiology of most *quantitative* defects in platelets. Additionally, sample-related conditions or preanalytic variables (Table 16.1) may result in falsely decreased platelet counts.

Thrombocytopenia Related to Sample Integrity and Preanalytic Variables

Coagulation samples are drawn into blue top tubes containing sodium citrate, which prevents coagulation of a specimen by binding calcium in a 9:1 blood:anticoagulant ratio. Sample tubes must be at least 90% full, and the phlebotomy must be nontraumatic. To ensure proper mixing of the anticoagulant, the blue top tube must be inverted at least six times. Without this action, small clots may form at the top of the tube.

Table 16.1 ○ Preanalytic Variables Related to Coagulation Samples

Blood:anticoagulant ratio 9:1

3.2% sodium citrate

No hemolyzed samples

Samples inverted six times

Platelet-poor plasma is optimal

Platelet satellitism is another sample-related condition that may give a falsely decreased platelet count. First reported in 1963,[1] this condition is an in vitro phenomenon in which platelets rosette around segmented neutrophils, monocytes, and bands. This phenomenon occurs only in ethylenediaminetetraacetic acid (EDTA) samples and produces a pseudothrombocytopenia unrelated to medication or any other disease state (see Chapter 10 and Fig. 10.19). If platelet satellitism is observed on the peripheral smear, the sample should be redrawn in sodium citrate and cycled through the automated hematology counter for a more accurate platelet count. The volume of additives in the tube makes it is necessary to multiply this count by 1.11 to determine the platelet count.

Thrombocytopenia Related to Decreased Production

Any condition that leads to bone marrow aplasia, or lack of megakaryocytes, the platelet-forming cells, results in thrombocytopenia. Most patients with leukemia exhibit thrombocytopenia as a result of blast cell infiltration of the bone marrow. Blasts of any cellular origin crowd out normal bone marrow elements, leading to thrombocytopenia. Defects in platelet synthesis can occur in megaloblastic anemias that show pancytopenia, a decrease in all cell lines. **Cytotoxic** agents or chemotherapy usually interferes with the cell cycle, reducing the number of active platelets. Patients undergoing chemotherapy are carefully monitored for platelet count and may require platelet support if the count drops too far below 20.0 × 10⁹/L.

Megakaryocytic function is usually impaired during the infectious process. Infections with several viral agents, such as cytomegalovirus, Epstein-Barr virus, varicella, and rubella, and certain bacterial infections may cause thrombocytopenia. The mechanism at work in viral infections is thought to be megakaryocytic suppression; in bacteria, the mechanism is direct toxicity of circulating platelets.[2]

Thrombocytopenia Related to Altered Distribution of Platelets

The normal spleen holds one-third of the body's platelet volume. The pathologic process of several hematologic conditions, including myeloproliferative disorders, extramedullary hematopoiesis, and hemolytic anemias, may result in an enlarged spleen. As the spleen enlarges, pooling blood withholds platelets from the peripheral circulation. If the organ is removed, numerous platelets may spill into the circulation, causing possible thrombotic complications.[3] Another scenario marked by altered platelet distribution is massive transfusion. When the total blood volume (10 U) has been replaced with two or three volume exchanges, the platelet and the coagulation factors become diluted, leading to transient thrombocytopenia.[4]

Thrombocytopenia Related to Immune Effect of Specific Drugs or Antibody Formation

Drug-induced immune thrombocytopenia produces a reduced platelet count that can be severe and dangerous. Several drug classifications are particularly relevant, including quinines, nonsteroidal anti-inflammatory drugs (NSAIDs), sulfonamides, amoxicillin, and diuretics.[5] The mechanism for thrombocytopenia is twofold. Ingestion of the drug results in antidrug antibody formation that binds to a glycoprotein on the platelet surface and is removed by the reticuloendothelial system (RES). The second mechanism involves the drug combining with a larger carrier protein to form an antigen that triggers an antibody response and subsequent platelet destruction, potentially in the spleen. The incidence of drug-induced thrombocytopenia is 10 cases per 1 million.[5]

Additionally, two rare conditions may cause dramatic thrombocytopenia post-transfusion purpura (PTP). PTP develops when the recipient's blood has an antibody that reacts against a transfusion containing the primary platelet antigen, HPA-1a. The antibody's action on HPA-1a coats the platelets, which are then removed by the spleen. The resultant thrombocytopenia is quite long-lasting, and treatment is directed toward delaying antibody production. Neonatal alloimmune thrombocytopenia (NAIT) occurs as a result of maternal antibody made against a previous exposure to platelet antigens from an earlier pregnancy. The antibody is usually directed against the HPA-1a platelet. Because this antibody can cross the placenta, it can coat the fetus' platelets in utero. Infants born to mothers carrying these antibodies often have normal platelets initially, but within days they develop petechiae and skin hemorrhages, with decreasingly low platelet counts. Infants are carefully observed, and treatment is begun only when there is a risk of central nervous system hemorrhage.[2]

Thrombocytopenia Related to Consumption of Platelets

Hematologic conditions related to platelet consumption usually include idiopathic (immune) thrombocytopenia purpura (ITP), thrombotic thrombocytopenic purpura (TTP), and hemolytic uremic syndrome (HUS). Excessive clot formation throughout the body results in consumed platelets. These conditions are serious and can produce significant life-altering complications.

Idiopathic (Immune) Thrombocytopenic Purpura

Patients with ITP have a decreased platelet count, likely resulting from immune destruction of platelets. In 66% of cases, the culprit antibody is an autoantibody directed against specific sites on a glycoprotein, GPIIb-IIIa or GPIb-IX. Additionally, poorly functioning megakaryocytes may increase in the marrow.[2] There are two types of ITP: chronic and acute. Patients with acute ITP are usually children 2 to 6 years old who have just recovered from a viral illness.[2] Their platelet counts may decrease precipitously, sometimes as low as $20 \times 10^9/L$. In this range, a child usually shows bruising, nosebleeds, or petechiae but not life-threatening hemorrhage. This low platelet count usually resolves in less than 6 weeks as the child fully recovers from the viral illness. Treatment, if necessary, may consist of intravenous immunoglobulin (IVIg or WinRho, anti-D immune globulin), splenectomy, or platelet transfusion.[2]

Patients with chronic ITP are usually 20 to 50 years old, with a platelet count between $30 \times 10^9/L$ and $60 \times 10^9/L$. Patients with chronic ITP produce an IgG antibody that coats the platelets, causing them to be sequestered and subsequently destroyed in the spleen. Common physical symptoms include splenomegaly, epistaxis, and ecchymoses. Most patients are treated with prednisone, which suppresses the antibody response, increases the platelet count, and decreases the hemorrhagic episodes. Patients who are nonresponsive to prednisone may receive anti-CD20, or rituximab, which provides a sustained platelet response.[6] Splenectomy is a therapeutic option, but it must be carefully considered. More recent studies have investigated immune thrombocytopenia related to infections. Patients infected with HIV, hepatitis C, and *Helicobacter pylori* show thrombocytopenia at some point during their disease. The precise mechanism, thought to be immune derived, is under study.[7] Antibiotic treatment improved platelet counts in greater than 85% of patients with *H. pylori*.[7] Table 16.2 compares acute and chronic ITP.

Thrombotic Thrombocytopenic Purpura

TTP is a devastating platelet disorder, described by Moschowitz in 1925, that is acute and nonpredictable. More prevalent in women than in men, TTP can occur in postpartum women or in women near delivery[8]

Table 16.2 ● Chronic and Acute Idiopathic Thrombocytopenic Purpura		
	Acute Idiopathic Thrombocytopenic Purpura	Chronic Idiopathic Thrombocytopenic Purpura
Age	Young children	Adults
Prior infection	History of rubella, rubeola, or chickenpox	No prior history
Platelet count	<20,000	30,000–80,000
Duration	2–6 weeks	Months to years
Therapy	None	Steroids, splenectomy

who have had other immune disorders such as systemic lupus erythematosus (SLE). It also occurs in patients with previous viral infections or gastric carcinomas. Platelet counts are less than 20×10^9/L, but other coagulation tests such as prothrombin time (PT) and partial thromboplastin time (PTT) are within reference range. Platelet thrombi disperse throughout the arterioles and capillaries subsequent to the accumulation of large von Willebrand multimers produced by the endothelial cells and platelets. The etiology for this pathologic accumulation of multimers and subsequent thrombocytopenia is thought to be related to a deficiency of ADAMTS-13, a large metalloprotease.[9,10] This protein is responsible for cleaving large von Willebrand factor (vWF) multimers into smaller proteins. Compared with smaller vWF portions, large vWF multimers have increased binding sites for platelets. Excessive platelet clots may be formed if large vWF multimers are not cleaved and allowed to circulate. Schistocytes are seen in the peripheral smear and are directly related to shear stress as fragments of red blood cells are removed when the cells try to sweep past the thrombi. Patients experience severe anemia and a high level of hemolysis, with increased lactate dehydrogenase (LDH). Some of the hemolysis may be intravascular with hemoglobinuria. Decreased haptoglobin may be seen. **Microangiopathic** hemolytic anemia (MHA) describes this process of severe anemia combined with schistocytes (Fig. 16.1). Patients often present with neurologic complications, visual impairment, and intense headache that can escalate to more severe presentations such as coma and **paresthesias**. Renal dysfunction may occur, and patients with renal impairment experience increased levels of protein and possibly some blood in the urine. Treatment for patients with TTP presents a dilemma for most physicians as they watch their patients spiral rapidly downhill. Diagnosis is difficult and is made by exclusion. When a diagnosis is determined, the patient's

condition has usually worsened dramatically. Corticosteroids are often used in conjunction with plasma exchange, a dramatic procedure performed over a 3- to 5-day period in which the patient's plasma volume is removed and replaced by ABO-matched fresh frozen plasma that is **cryoprecipitate** poor (lacking fibrinogen and vWF). Plasma exchange has dramatically improved the survival rate from 3% before 1960 to 82% presently.[11] Few hospital facilities provide in-house plasma exchange capabilities. Specialty teams of medical professionals using equipment designed for plasmapheresis are usually called on. Timing is essential to the patient's welfare and long-term recovery. Recovery for patients with TTP has improved in the past decade; currently, more than 80% survive.[11]

Hemolytic Uremic Syndrome

HUS frequently occurs in children between the ages of 6 months and 4 years. This clinical condition mimics TTP except that renal damage is more severe. The kidney is the primary site of damage by the toxin *Escherichia coli* O157:H7 or the Shiga toxin.[11] The

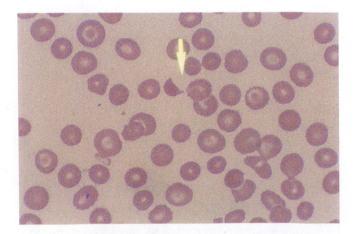

Figure 16.1   Schistocyte.

enterotoxin produced by this particular strain of *E. coli* inevitably leads to cell death, particularly in the renal environment, where platelet thrombi predominate.[12] A child may initially present with bloody diarrhea and vomiting; hemolytic anemia, thrombocytopenia, and renal failure soon follow. Patients may also experience fever and abdominal pain. The hemolytic anemia is microangiopathic with schistocytes present. The illness in children is usually self-limiting when the toxin is eliminated from the body; however, there have been reports of patients relapsing. Children with acute renal failure may require renal dialysis. Most children make a complete recovery, but some have residual kidney problems into adulthood. HUS may occur in adults, but it is more similar to TTP in disease course (Table 16.3).

Disorders such as heparin-induced thrombocytopenia and disseminated intravascular coagulation (DIC) also lead to thrombocytopenia. These are discussed in subsequent chapters.

Thrombocytosis

Thrombocytosis is defined as a platelet count greater than 450×10^9/L. The cause of an increased platelet count may be primary or secondary. Primary thrombocytosis is seen in myeloproliferative disorders (see Chapter 12), in which case platelets are high in number but have an impaired function. Of all of the myeloproliferative disorders, essential thrombocythemia has the highest platelet count, at times exceeding 1 million platelets. Secondary causes of thrombocytosis include acute and chronic blood loss, chronic inflammatory diseases, postsplenectomy, and iron deficiency anemia. In these cases, the platelet function is normal, although the increase in platelet numbers may last days to weeks. In severe iron deficiency anemia, the platelet count may increase to 2 million as a result of marrow stimulation.[13] The platelet count usually returns to normal after initiation of iron therapy.

INHERITED QUALITATIVE DISORDERS OF PLATELETS

Inherited qualitative platelet disorders are disorders in which platelet function is impaired, usually secondary to an intrinsic defect of platelets. Many of these disorders (with the exception of von Willebrand's disease [vWD]) are rare, and in most cases the bleeding time is prolonged. Often, the qualitative defects are separated into disorders of adhesion and platelet release or storage pool defects.

Disorders of Adhesion

von Willebrand's Disease

The most important disease of platelet adhesion is vWD. Discovered in 1926 by von Willebrand, vWD is the most prevalent inherited bleeding disorder worldwide, affecting 1% to 3% of the world population by conservative estimates. In random studies of children investigated for epistaxis and women investigated for **menorrhagia**, vWD was the most frequent cause of bleeding.[14,15] von Willebrand initially described a family of 12 children of whom 10 had excessive nosebleeds, gum bleeds, and menorrhagia. One of the youngest girls died at age 13 from uncontrollable bleeding during her fourth menstrual cycle. vWD is an autosomal dominant disorder marked by easy bruising,

Table 16.3 ⊙ Hemolytic Uremic Syndrome Versus Thrombotic Thrombocytopenic Purpura		
	Hemolytic Uremic Syndrome	**Thrombotic Thrombocytopenic Purpura**
Platelet count	<20,000	<20,000
Organ(s) affected	Kidney	Neurologic manifestations
		Kidney
Age group	Children	Adults (more women than men)
Symptoms	Fever, bloody diarrhea	Fever, headaches
	MHA with schistocytes	Visual impairment, coma
		MHA with schistocytes
Treatment	Renal dialysis, blood transfusions	Plasmapheresis

MHA, microangiopathic hemolytic anemia.

nosebleeds, heavy menses, and excessive bleeding after tooth extraction or dental procedures. Type O individuals have a *lower* plasma concentration of vWF than individuals with other blood types. For many patients, the variations of clinical symptoms and laboratory presentations have contributed to the underdiagnosis of this disorder. Women may represent a significant yet underserved subset of individuals affected by vWD because menorrhagia is a frequent presenting feature of this disease. Lusher[16] observed that vWD may be the underlying cause in 9% to 11% of cases of menorrhagia, but obstetricians and gynecologists often do not consider it as a possible diagnosis.

As a disease entity, vWD is complex with few clear-cut and consistent diagnostic clues. The basic pathophysiology in vWD is a qualitative or quantitative defect in vWF, a large multimeric glycoprotein derived from two sources: endothelial cells and megakaryocytes. vWF is coded by chromosome 12 and carried into plasma circulation by factor VIII, one of the clotting factors. vWF serves as an intermediary for platelet adhesion, providing a receptor molecule for GPIb of the platelets and the subendothelium. With this platform in place, injury-activated platelets adhere to the subendothelium and form a platelet plug that recruits more platelets to the site of injury and eventually leads to platelet aggregation and the formation of an insoluble fibrin clot. Without a fully functioning vWF, platelet adhesion is impaired. There are three *primary* levels of vWD: type 1, type 2, and type 3. Of all individuals with vWD, 70% have the type 1 disorders, characterized by abnormal bleeding time and increased PTT in most patients. Type 2 vWD results from a qualitative defect of wVF. Type 3, the rarest type, is characterized by a total absence of vWF multimers and is autosomal recessive in its presentation. Type 2 vWD has many subtypes: type 2A, type 2B,

type 2M, and type 2N. Table 16-4 describes vWD and its variants. The vWF protein can be measured by several methods, including those that assess its role in adhesion, its secondary role in aggregation, and its role in clotting factor activity. Ristocetin cofactor activity is the best predictive assay[17] and relies on the use of reagent platelets rather than the patient's platelets during ristocetin-induced aggregation studies. Table 16.5 presents a typical testing profile for vWD.

Treatment is usually tailored to the particular type or subtype of vWD. Some products that may be considered are desmopressin acetate (DDAVP), which causes the release of endothelial vWF. DDAVP may be given as an injectable agent or as a nasal spray, which makes it portable and convenient. For nonresponsive patients, vWF can be increased by giving high-purity factor VIII products that contain a sufficient amount of vWF.

Bernard-Soulier Syndrome

Bernard-Soulier syndrome (BSS) is a rare platelet adhesion defect that involves the GPIb-IX complex. After an injury, vWF acts as a medium through which the platelet membrane GPIb has a receptor that allows its binding to collagen. As indicated in Chapter 15, platelet glycoproteins play a significant role in hemostasis. The receptor for vWF is GPIb-IX, a complex that serves as a binding site for thrombin and regulates platelet shape and reactivity.[18] GPIIb and GPIIIa are receptors for fibronectin (an adhesive protein for platelets), vWF, fibrinogen, and factors V and VIII. BSS is inherited as an autosomal recessive disorder, with near-normal amounts of GPIb in heterozygotes. Moderate or severe bleeding may occur if the disorder is inherited homozygously, however. Epistaxis, gingival bleeding, menorrhagia, and purpura are the usual bleeding manifestations. Additionally, thrombocytopenia

---

Table 16.4 ◉ Primary von Willebrand's Disease Derivatives*

	Type 1	Type 2	Type 3
	70%–80%	15%–20%	Rare
Genetics	Autosomal dominant	Autosomal dominant	Autosomal recessive
Bleeding time	↑ or N	↑	↑
PTT	↑ or N	↑ or N	↑
RIPA	Variable	Variable	Absent
vWF antigen	↓	↓	Absent

*Secondary vWD variants include types 2A, 2B, 2M, and 2N (not discussed).
RIPA, ristocetin-induced platelet aggregation.

Table 16.5 ● Basic Test Profile for von Willebrand's Disease

- Platelet count—measured by automated methods
- PTT—measures anticoagulant portion of the factor VIII molecule
- Bleeding time—measures adhesion of platelets to site of injury
- vWF activity—measured by ristocetin-induced platelet aggregation (RIPA)
- vWF antigen—measured by immunoassay

Note: Most patients have variable test results. It is recommended that this test profile be performed multiple times within a time period to aid in diagnosis.

with giant platelets can be observed on the peripheral smear. Ristocetin-induced platelet aggregation is absent in patients with BSS because they lack receptors to bind to vWF, a key ingredient in ristocetin-induced platelet aggregation. Platelet aggregation appears normal with other agents, such as epinephrine, thrombin, and collagen. The bleeding time test is prolonged.

Platelet transfusion is the preferred treatment for active bleeding, but transfusions should be used prudently to prevent the stimulation of platelet antibodies. To date, more than 30 mutations of the glycoproteins involved in the GPIb-IX complex have been described.[19]

Glanzmann's Thrombasthenia

First described in 1918, Glanzmann's thrombasthenia (GT) is an autosomal recessive disorder, associated most frequently with **consanguinity**. Homozygous individuals may experience variable bleeding patterns. When bleeding does occur, it is usually from birth as umbilical cord or circumcisional bleeding, and it may proceed to gingival bleeding, purpura, or prolonged bleeding from minor cuts or childhood injuries. The defect in GT is a deficiency or abnormality of GPIIb and GPIIIa. These glycoproteins serve as the intermediary for fibrinogen binding to platelets, a necessary step in platelet aggregation. Aggregation cannot occur without GPIIb/IIIa, fibrinogen, or calcium.[20] Patients with GT have a prolonged bleeding time, normal platelet count and morphology, and abnormal aggregation with all aggregating agents except ristocetin. Ristocetin-induced aggregation depends on the interaction of vWF and platelet GPIb. The GPIIb/IIIa complex does not play a role in this type of aggregation. Treatment

of GT depends on the severity of the bleeding episode. Platelet transfusions may be considered, but **HLA**-matched or ABO-matched transfusion may reduce the possibilities of platelet **alloimmunization**. Oral contraceptives may be used to control menorrhagia, and agents such as epsilon-aminocaproic acid (EACA) are effective topical thrombin-inducing agents for procedures such as tooth extractions.[21]

Platelet Release Defects

When platelets adhere to an injured surface, the contents of the platelets are released. Platelets contain alpha and dense granules, which are highly metabolic substances containing procoagulant materials, vasoconstrictors ATP and ADP. The disorders that are subsequently described are inherited, usually have abnormal secondary phases of platelet aggregation, and are associated with postoperative bleeding combined with menorrhagia and easy bruisability. In most of these disorders, the bleeding time is abnormal, but the platelet count may be normal.

Hermansky-Pudlak syndrome: An autosomal recessive disorder characterized by a severe deficiency of dense granules. Patients have albinism and may have hemorrhagic events.

Chédiak-Higashi syndrome: An autosomal recessive disorder, in which patients have albinism and giant lysosomal granules in neutrophils. Not only are the white blood cells in these patients qualitatively flawed, but also platelet release is impaired. Patients have frequent infections because of impaired phagocytic ability, and death usually occurs in childhood. Patients manifest thrombocytopenia and hepatosplenomegaly..

Wiskott-Aldrich syndrome: An X-linked recessive disorder in which patients have severe eczema, recurrent infections, immune defects, and thrombocytopenia.

Thrombocytopenia with absent radii (TAR): A rare disorder of the skeletal system in which patients have no radial bones and have other skeletal and cardiac abnormalities. Most patients have thrombocytopenia.

Gray platelet syndrome: A disorder in which platelets lack alpha granules and are noted in the peripheral smear as larger and gray or blue-gray in color. Patients may have thrombocytopenia, bleeding tendencies, and bruisability.

ACQUIRED DEFECTS OF PLATELET FUNCTION

Acquired defects of platelet function include factors that are external to the platelet and nonimmune, such as drug-related platelet abnormalities, extrinsic platelet abnormalities, or a sequela to an underlying disorder. Aspirin is the most commonly used of all drugs that affect platelet function. Ingestion of aspirin irreversibly restrains cyclooxygenase (COX-1) inhibitors by blocking the formation of prostaglandin synthesis. Both chemicals are necessary for the production of thromboxane A_2, a potent platelet aggregator. Without the proper amount of thromboxane A_2, platelet aggregation is impaired. This effect lasts 7 to 10 days, the entire life span of the platelet, and patients taking aspirin have a prolonged bleeding time. To avoid any unexpected bleeding complications, patients should be questioned about their use of aspirin and aspirin-containing products before any elective or nonelective surgical procedure. The effect of aspirin on platelets is rapid, occurring 45 minutes after ingestion.[22] Additionally, aspirin is used as an antiplatelet agent to prevent strokes, heart attacks, or other cardiovascular events in susceptible patients. Other drugs, including NSAIDs and COX-2 inhibitors such as naproxen and ibuprofen, may affect platelet function. Certain antiplatelet agents, such as ticlopidine and clopidogrel, inhibit fibrinogen from binding to GPIIb and GPIIIa. Dextran, a platelet expander, also alters platelet function. Coating platelets with dextran produces an antiplatelet effect by inhibiting the action of the platelet membrane and its surface receptors.

Platelet function may also be impaired by plasma conditions that are unfavorable to the platelet. In most cases, platelet disorders are secondary to the main disorder but may not be present in the initial presentation. Conditions that may lead to disturbed platelet function include uremia secondary to renal disease and the paraproteinemias such as multiple myeloma and Waldenström's macroglobulinemia. The pathophysiology of the platelet defect in these acquired disorders is not clear-cut. Patients with renal disease are known to exhibit purpura (Fig. 16.2), epistaxis, and hemorrhage sometimes. Some factors involved in platelet dysfunction in uremia include decreased thromboxane synthesis, decreased adhesion, decreased platelet release, and decreased aggregation. Most of these patients undergo peritoneal dialysis or hemodialysis, which usually improves platelet function.

Multiple myeloma and Waldenström's macroglobulinemia are part of a group of plasma cell disorders characterized by excessive production of normal

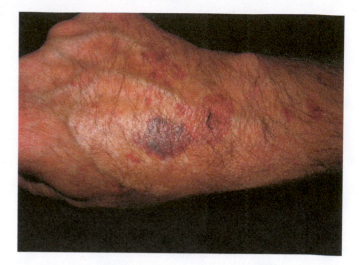

Figure 16.2   Purpura.

immunoglobulin, leading to **hyperviscosity** syndrome and paraproteinemia. Platelets circulating in abnormal amounts of protein cannot fully participate in the activation of coagulation factors and in formation of fibrin. Patients have a prolonged bleeding time and may have postoperative bleeding and ecchymoses. Table 16.6 lists drugs that affect platelet function.

VASCULAR DISORDERS LEADING TO PLATELET DYSFUNCTION

Skin, collagen, and blood vessels are essential elements in the hemostatic system. Any inherited or acquired abnormality in any one of these components of the vascular system leads to mucosal bleeding such as purpura, petechia, ecchymosis, or **telangiectasia** (Fig. 16.3). Tests for platelet function and platelet count

Table 16.6 ◉ Modified List of Drugs That Affect Platelet Function

- Penicillin
- Ampicillin
- Carbenicillin
- Cephalosporin
- Ticlopidine
- Clopidogrel (Plavix)
- Ibuprofen
- Aspirin
- Nitroglycerin
- Propranolol
- Nitroprusside

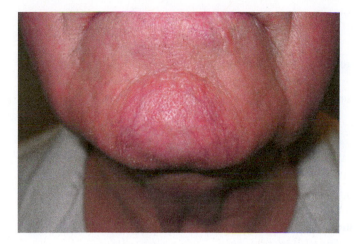

Figure 16.3   Telangiectasia.

are normal. Senile purpura is a condition of aging in which skin loses its elasticity. Older patients with this condition often bruise more easily and more prominently. Allergic purpura occurs in rare childhood disorders such as Henoch-Schönlein purpura, an immune complex disease involving the skin, gastrointestinal tract, heart, and central nervous system. The purpura is often seen in the lower extremities. Purpura may occur because of infectious agents such as meningococcemia, Rocky Mountain spotted fever, staphylococcal infections, or streptococcal infections.[23] Conditions such as amyloidosis, vitamin C deficiency (scurvy), or Cushing syndrome may result in purpura.

Collagen disorders that provoke the formation of purpuric lesions (telangiectasia) include hereditary hemorrhagic telangiectasia (Osler-Weber-Rendu disease), an autosomal dominant disorder of the blood vessels. In this condition, small pinpoint hemorrhagic lesions occur on the tongue, roof of the mouth, palate, face, and hands.[23] Nosebleeds are prominent, and the lesions generally become more fragile with age. Kasabach-Merritt syndrome is a rare congenital disorder featuring giant **hemangiomas**,[23] bleeding, and thrombocytopenia. Hemangiomas may be found on the liver, skin, or spleen, and they are deep and bleed easily and profusely. DIC may develop if thromboplastic substances are released when the blood vessels burst.

○ *Summary Points*

- A normal platelet count is 150 to 450 × 10⁹/L.
- Decreased platelet counts lead to bleeding of mucosal membranes, such as gingival bleeding, epistaxis, purpura, and petechiae.
- Preanalytic variables that may lead to thrombocytopenia include improper mixing of tubes, improper anticoagulant used, and inadequate amount of sample collected.
- Acute idiopathic thrombocytopenia purpura often occurs in children who have a dramatically reduced platelet count while recovering from viral illness.
- Chronic idiopathic thrombocytopenia purpura occurs in adults as a result of IgG antibody produced against platelets.
- Thrombotic thrombocytopenic purpura (TTP) and hemolytic uremic syndrome (HUS) are consumptive disorders of platelets.
- Individuals with TTP present with fever, a microangiopathic hemolytic anemia, neurologic complications, thrombocytopenia, and renal failure.
- Individuals with HUS are predominantly children and present with fever, bloody diarrhea, microangiopathic hemolytic anemia, thrombocytopenia, and renal failure.
- von Willebrand's disease (vWD) is a platelet adhesion disorder characterized by decreased or absent von Willebrand factor.
- vWD is the most common inherited qualitative platelet disorder, affecting 1% to 3% of the world's population.
- There are three primary types of vWD: type 1, type 2, and type 3.
- Bernard-Soulier syndrome is a platelet adhesion defect characterized by decreased or absent GPIb.
- Glanzmann's thrombasthenia is a defect of platelet aggregation characterized by an absence of GPIIb/IIIa.
- Platelets from patients with vWD and Bernard-Soulier syndrome do *not* aggregate with ristocetin.
- Aspirin impairs platelet function by interfering with the synthesis of thromboxane A₂, a potent platelet-aggregating agent.
- The platelet release function is impaired in inherited disorders including Chédiak-Higashi syndrome, Hermansky-Pudlak syndrome, Wiskott-Aldrich syndrome, gray platelet syndrome, and thrombocytopenia with absent radii.
- External conditions that alter platelet function include drugs, paraproteinemias, uremia, and the use of plasma expanders such as dextran.
- Skin, collagen, and blood vessels are essential elements in the hemostatic system.
- Any inherited or acquired abnormality in any one of these components of the vascular system leads to mucosal bleeding, such as purpura, petechiae, ecchymosis, or telangiectasia.

CONDENSED CASE

A 14-year-old girl had a tooth extracted and was noted to have unexpected bleeding after extraction. She bled for 24 hours before the bleeding could be stopped. The dentist recommended that she have a hematology evaluation for the unexpected bleeding. *What questions concerning family history should be asked, and what baseline coagulation tests should be considered?*

Answer

This patient is exhibiting signs of mucosal bleeding, the type of bleeding seen in platelet adhesion defects such as vWD and BSS. The patient's family should be asked about the bleeding history of family members, such as umbilical cord bleeding, circumcision bleeding, bleeding from minor cuts and abrasions, or gum or nose bleeding. The patient's mother revealed that her sibling had serious bleeding after a tonsillectomy procedure. This fact points to an autosomal defect. Routine studies that should be ordered are bleeding time (platelet function assay), PT, and aPTT. Factor assay should be considered if the PT or PTT are prolonged.

CASE STUDY

A 24-year-old woman was evaluated by her gynecologist for menorrhagia. She gave a history of excessive menses since age 12. CBC revealed a microcytic anemia, and she began a course of ferrous sulfate therapy. She had a follow-up visit 3 months later. Although her anemia was being corrected, she still complained of excessive menses. Her physician recommended a hematology consultation. When asked about her family history, she revealed that her brother and mother had recurrent epistaxis and that her first cousin had a postpartum hemorrhage. The consulting physician ordered a CBC, PT, PTT, platelet aggregation studies, and bleeding time. *Based on this patient's history, what is the most likely outcome of this testing, and what additional tests should be considered?*

Insights to the Case Study

This patient has a strong family history of mucosal bleeding. Although no member of her family has been diagnosed with a bleeding disorder, it seems likely that she and some of her relatives may have von Willebrand's disease, an autosomal dominant disorder. The patient's CBC and platelet count are normal; however, the PTT is slightly prolonged at 42 seconds. Factor assays for factors VIII and IX should be considered. Aggregation studies with collagen, ADP, and epinephrine were normal. Ristocetin aggregation was absent, and the bleeding time test was abnormal, with a result of 12 minutes (reference range 3 to 9 minutes). A preliminary diagnosis of type 1 von Willebrand's disease was made pending the result of the vWF:AG by immunoassay. The hematologist recommended contraceptives as a way to control the patient's menstrual bleeding, and the patient was counseled on therapy alternatives such as DDAVP should she need dental extractions or minor surgery.

Review Questions

1. Which of the following are defects of platelet adhesion?
   a. Hermansky-Pudlak syndrome
   b. Glanzmann's thrombasthenia
   c. Bernard-Soulier syndrome
   d. Wiskott-Aldrich syndrome

2. Which one of the following conditions would produce a thrombocytopenia due to an altered distribution of platelets?
   a. Platelet satellitism
   b. Iron deficiency anemia
   c. Splenomegaly
   d. Chemotherapy

3. One of the main differences between TTP and HUS is
   a. Neurologic involvement.
   b. Kidney failure.
   c. Thrombocytopenia.
   d. Microangiopathic hemolytic anemia.

4. Nose bleeding, deep bruising, and gum bleeding are usually manifestations of which type of coagulation disorder?
   a. Clotting factor disorder
   b. Platelet defect
   c. Thrombosis
   d. Vascular disorder

5. The presence of thrombocytopenia and giant platelets best describes
   a. Classic von Willebrand's disease.
   b. Wiskott-Aldrich syndrome.
   c. Glanzmann's thrombasthenia.
   d. Bernard-Soulier syndrome.

6. Chronic idiopathic thrombocytopenia purpura (ITP)
   a. Is found in children.
   b. Usually remits spontaneously within several weeks.
   c. Affects males more commonly than females.
   d. Involves the immune destruction of platelets.

7. Aspirin prevents platelet aggregation by inhibiting the action of
   a. PF 3.
   b. GPII.
   c. TXA_2.
   d. GPIb.

8. Several hours after birth, a newborn develops symptoms of petechiae, purpura, and hemorrhage, and laboratory results show a platelet count of 18.0×10^9/L. The most likely explanation is
   a. Drug-induced thrombocytopenia.
   b. Secondary thrombocytopenia.
   c. Isoimmune neonatal thrombocytopenia.
   d. Neonatal DIC.

9. Which the following test results is normal in a patient with classic von Willebrand's disease?
   a. Bleeding time
   b. Activated partial thromboplastin time
   c. Platelet count
   d. Factor VIII:C and vWF levels

10. The autoantibody generated in ITP is directed against
    a. vWF.
    b. Collagen.
    c. GP IIb/IIIa and GPIb-IX.
    d. Fibrinopeptides A and B.

○ TROUBLESHOOTING

What Do I Do When Preoperative Coagulation Studies Are Abnormal?

Preoperative testing was ordered on a 43-year-old woman scheduled for an elective hysterectomy. She has experienced dysfunctional uterine bleeding for 6 months. Rather than go to the hospital setting, she went to a physician office laboratory that accepted her insurance. Her surgeon ordered a CBC with platelet count and PT and PTT. Her CBC was within reference range, but the results of her PT and aPTT were:

PT	10.6 seconds (reference range 10 to 14 seconds)
aPTT	53 seconds (reference range 28 to 38 seconds)

The elevated PTT was an unexpected result. Possibilities for an elevated PTT include a factor deficiency, the presence of a circulating anticoagulant, or a patient on heparin. Heparin was eliminated as a possible contributor to the prolonged PTT because there was no patient history of anticoagulation therapy. Mixing studies are familiar screening tests in the clinical laboratory, used to determine factor deficiency or a circulating anticoagulant. The technologist decided to perform mixing studies on this patient and proceeded with the laboratory protocol. In mixing studies, the patient's plasma is mixed with pooled normal plasma in a 1:1 ratio, and the elevated test is repeated. Pooled normal plasma contains all clotting factors. Technologists use normal quality control material as the source of pooled plasma. If the result of a repeated test returns to the normal range, it is assumed that the source of aPTT elevation was a clotting factor deficiency, and factor assay tests on the plasma should be ordered. If the

Continued

repeated test does not return to the reference range, it is assumed that the patient's plasma contains a circulating anticoagulant. As an additional screening procedure, the aPTT test was incubated for 1 to 2 hours. The rationale behind this additional step is to determine if there is a weak or time-dependent circulating inhibitor.

Certain inhibitors such as factor VIII inhibitor have a stronger inhibitory effect with prolonged incubation. The patient's mixing study was *not* corrected, and her plasma was sent to a special coagulation laboratory for workup of an inhibitor. These pathologic circulating inhibitors are thoroughly discussed in Chapter 19.

WORD KEY

Alloimmunization • Antibodies that occur as a result of antigens introduced to the body through blood and tissue

Consanguinity • Relationships among close blood relatives

Cryoprecipitate • Product derived from fresh frozen plasma that is rich in factor VIII, von Willebrand factor, and fibrinogen

Cytotoxic • Antibody or toxin that attacks the cells of particular organs

Hemangiomas • Benign tumors of dilated blood vessels

HLA • Human leukocyte antigens, which are found in white blood cells and are part of the major histocompatibility complex

Hyperviscosity • Excessive resistance to the flow of liquids

Menorrhagia • Excessive menstrual bleeding

Microangiopathic • Related to pathology of small blood vessels

Paresthesias • Abnormal sensation that results from an injury to one or more nerves, described as numbness or prickly or tingling feeling

Telangiectasia • Vascular lesion formed by dilation of a group of small blood vessels, most frequently seen on the face and thighs

References

1. Glassy E, ed. Color Atlas of Hematology: An Illustrated Field Guide Based on Proficiency Testing. Chicago: Chicago College of American Pathologists, 1998: 206.
2. Bruce L. Quantitative disorders of platelets. In: Rodak B, ed. Hematology: Clinical Principles and Applications, 2nd ed. Philadelphia: WB Saunders, 2002: 686.
3. Wolf BC, Neiman RS. Disorders of the Spleen. Philadelphia: WB Saunders, 1989: 22.
4. Blaney KD, Howard PR. Basic and Applied Concepts of Immunohematology. Boston: Mosby, 2000: 304.
5. vanden Bent PM, Meyboom PH, Egberts AC. Drug induced thrombocytopenia. Drug Saf 27:1243–1252, 2004.
6. Bengston K, Skinner M, Ware R. Successful use of anti-CD20 (Rituximab) in severe life threatening childhood ITP. J Pediatr 143:670–673, 2003.
7. Stevens W, Koene H, Zwaginga JJ, et al. Chronic idiopathic thrombocytopenic purpura: Present strategy, guidelines and new insights. Neth J Med 64:356–362, 2006.
8. Ezra Y, Rose M, Eldor H. Therapy and prevention of thrombotic thrombocytopenia purpura during pregnancy: A clinical study of 16 pregnancies. Am J Hematol 51:1–6, 1996.
9. Zheng X, Chung D, Tekayama TK, et al. Structure of von Willebrand factor cleaving protease (ADAMS-13), a metalloprotease involved in thrombotic thrombocytopenic purpura. J Biol Chem 270:41059–41063, 2001.
10. Levy GC, Nicolas WC, Lian EC, et al. Mutations in a member of the ADAMTS gene family causing thrombotic thrombocytopenic purpura. Nature 413:488–494, 2001.
11. Kwaan HC, Soff GA. Management of thrombotic thrombocytopenic purpura and hemolytic uremic syndrome. Semin Hematol 34:159–166, 1997.
12. Bell A. Extracorpuscular defects leading to increased erythrocyte destruction: Nonimmune causes. In: Rodak B, ed. Hematology: Clinical Principles and Applications, 2nd ed Philadelphia: WB Saunders, 2002: 67.
13. Bruce L. Quantitative disorders of platelets. In Rodak B, ed. Hematology: Clinical Principles and Applications, 2nd ed. Philadelphia: WB Saunders, 2002: 697.
14. Sondoval C, Dong S, Visintainer P. Clinical and laboratory features of 178 children with recurrent epistaxis. J Pediatr Hematol 24:47–49, 2002.
15. Saxena R, Gupta M, Gupta PC. Inherited bleeding disorders in Indian women with menorrhagia. Hemophilia 9:193–196, 2003.
16. Lusher J. An underlying cause of menorrhagia. Mod Med 63:30–31, 1995.
17. Philips MD, Santhouse A. von Willebrand disease: Recent advances in pathophysiology and treatment. Am J Med Sci August:77–86, 1998.
18. Liles DK, Knupp CL. Quantitative and qualitative platelet disorders and vascular disorders. In: Harmening D, ed. Clinical Hematology and Fundamentals of Hemostasis. Philadelphia: FA Davis, 2002: 481.
19. Kunishima S, Kamiya T, Saito H. Genetic abnormalities of Bernard-Soulier syndrome. Int J Hematol 76:319–327, 2002.
20. Rogers RL, Lazarchick J. Identifying Glanzmann's thrombasthenia. Lab Med 27:579–581, 1996.
21. Paper R, Kelley LA. A Guide to Living With von Willebrand Disease. Pennsylvania: Aventis Bering, 2002: 53.
22. Castellone D. Down and Dirty Coagulation: Practical Solutions and Answers. ASCP Workshop, May 7, 2004, Abstract 5799, Baltimore.
23. Bick RL, Scates SM. Qualitative platelet defects. Lab Med 23:95–103, 1992.

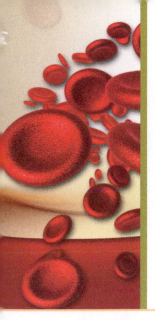

Chapter 17

Defects of Plasma Clotting Factors

Betty Ciesla

Objectives

After completing this chapter, the student will be able to:

1. Describe the variable types of bleeding found in patients with clotting factor deficiencies versus platelet disorders.

2. Define the factor VIII molecule.

3. Outline the genetics of the hemophilia disorders.

4. Describe the symptoms of an individual with hemophilia A and B.

5. Define the laboratory results in an individual with hemophilia A and B.

6. Describe the management and treatment of an individual with hemophilia A and B.

7. Distinguish the clotting factor disorders with little or no bleeding.

8. Distinguish the acquired factor disorders with regard to symptoms and treatment.

EVALUATION OF A BLEEDING DISORDER AND TYPES OF BLEEDING

Patients who experience recurrent bleeding require evaluation for the source of their bleeding disorder. Bleeding may occur because of an inherited clotting factor defect or an acquired deficiency that is secondary to some other cause. Factors to consider in evaluating a bleeding disorder include patient history, physical examination, laboratory testing, and family bleeding history. Patients often do not perceive their bleeding as abnormal because that is all that they have ever known. Questions regarding the types and frequency of bleeding must be extremely specific and nonthreatening. Bleeding comes under two main categories: open bleeds and closed bleeds.

Open bleeds include tongue bleeding, tonsil bleeding, gum bleeding, epistaxis, menorrhagia, umbilical cord bleeding, and circumcisional bleeding. Closed bleeds include soft tissue bleeds; genitourinary bleeding; gastrointestinal bleeding; and bleeding into muscle, joints, skin, bone, or skull. Not every patient experiences all types of bleeding, and some patients with clotting factor deficiencies never experience a bleeding episode. It is prudent, however, to gather as much information as possible to assess an individual with a history of bleeding.

Plasma clotting factors are inactive enzymes that circulate in plasma awaiting activation when injury occurs. They represent a significant ingredient to the proper clotting mechanism. Clotting factors that are poorly synthesized, inactivated by inhibitors, consumed by a rogue clotting process, mutated, or functionally impaired lead to faulty hemostasis.

CLASSIC HEMOPHILIAS

For most individuals, the word *hemophilia* is at least a recognizable term. Many negative perceptions arise with this bleeding disorder, including deep dark family secrets, profuse bleeding from small wounds, excruciating pain, and early death. By definition, *hemophilias* represent *any* of a group of disorders in which a particular clotting factor is decreased. With 13 clotting factors necessary for clot formation, there should be a wide range of hemophilias. Classically, however, only two disorders are characterized as *hemophilias*: hemophilia A (factor VIII deficiency) and hemophilia B (factor IX deficiency). Both varieties are sex-linked recessive disorders, meaning that the mother carries the abnormal gene and passes the gene to her sons. Not every male child is affected, only those who inherit the abnormal gene. Likewise, if daughters inherit the

abnormal gene, they are obligatory carriers. History is rich with accounts of hemophilia, ranging from the Talmud to the British monarchy. Queen Victoria carried the abnormal gene and passed it through her offspring (nine births, five living children) into the Russian royal family, the Spanish dynasty, and the German royal family (Fig. 17.1). Victoria herself had no family history of hemophilia, so her abnormal gene was acquired by spontaneous mutation, which occurs in 30% of cases.

Factor VIII Molecule

Factor VIII is the only clotting factor that is not synthesized exclusively by the liver. It is unique among clotting factors for two reasons. Factor VIII is genetically controlled by the X chromosome (it is sex-linked), and it forms a complex with von Willebrand factor (vWF), which transports the factor into the circulation and is coded by an autosomal chromosome (Fig. 17.2). This clotting factor is also labile and unstable in stored plasma. The vWF level is normal in individuals with hemophilia A, so bleeding time is normal; however, the activated partial thromboplastin time (aPTT) is abnormal because of the reduced level of factor VIII.

Symptoms in Hemophilia A Patients

Clotting factors are measured in terms of their percent activity and their function in coagulation tests. Most clotting factors need to be available in the body at a minimum of 30% to achieve hemostasis. Bleeding manifestation in individuals with hemophilia A relates to the level of factor VIII. There are three levels of clotting factor activity in hemophilia:

- Severe: less than 1%
- Moderate: 1% to 5%
- Mild: 6% to 24%

Patients with severe hemophilia A show early bleeding manifestations such as circumcisional bleeds or umbilical cord bleeding. As these children become more mobile, ordinary activities such as crawling, walking, or running may present challenges. It is common to see a child with severe hemophilia in protective gear (knee pads, ankle pads, helmet) for outside play. Bleeding may occur in other areas, such as the gastrointestinal tract, the kidneys (hematuria), or gums, or in **hematomas**. It is inaccurate to say that individuals with hemophilia bleed more profusely. Rather, bleeding continues for a longer time because of the decreased level of clotting factor. Platelet counts are normal, and blood vessel function is adequate. Perhaps

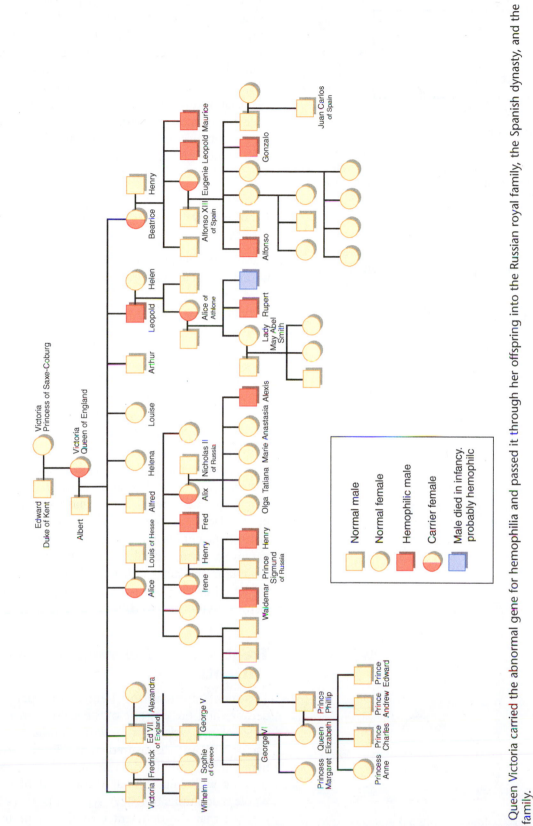

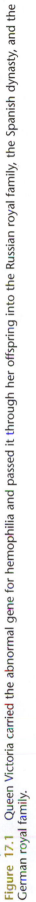

Figure 17.1 Queen Victoria carried the abnormal gene for hemophilia and passed it through her offspring into the Russian royal family, the Spanish dynasty, and the German royal family.

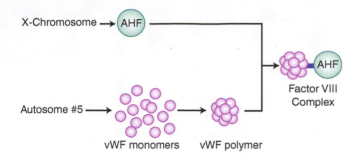

Figure 17.2 Factor VIII complex is controlled by the X chromosome and an autosomal chromosome. This complex transports factor VIII into the circulation. AHF, antihemophilic factor; vWF, von Willebrand factor.

the most debilitating bleeds are muscle bleeds or joint bleeds, which have the potential for causing long-term disability, reduced range of motion, and intense pain. Joints become painful, swollen, and engorged with blood. **Hemarthrosis** occurs in the joints as pooled blood damages the surrounding tissue while a clot eventually forms. The joint become less and less

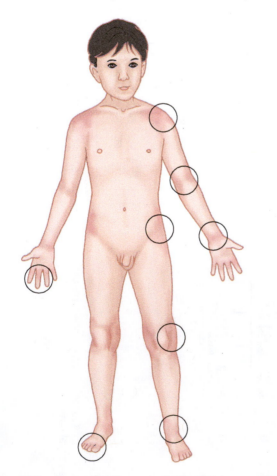

Figure 17.3 Hemarthrosis occurs in the joints as pooled blood damages the surrounding tissues.

mobile, limiting physical activity (Fig. 17.3). Internal hemorrhages into the muscles and deep soft tissues may compress and damage nerves. Intracranial bleeding is a leading cause of death in individuals with hemophilia A, and other complications such as paralysis, coma, memory loss, or stroke may precede an eventual fatality. Female carriers of the hemophilia gene rarely have symptoms, but occasionally carriers may become symptomatic. The union of an individual with hemophilia and a female carrier is likely to produce a symptomatic female.

Laboratory Diagnosis of Hemophilia Patients

Laboratory diagnosis of hemophilia patients is fairly uncomplicated. Laboratory tests include bleeding time, prothrombin time (PT), aPTT, and factor assays. In hemophilia, the bleeding time test is normal, PT is normal, and aPTT is elevated because of reduced factor VIII. Single factor assays provide a means of assessing the percent activity of a clotting factor. These assays are performed using the aPTT. A standard curve is created using serial dilutions of normal plasma of known factor levels and assigning a 1:10 dilution of normal plasma as 100% activity. Commercially prepared factor-deficient plasma is mixed with a 1:10 dilution of patient plasma, and the aPTT is performed. An aPTT that is abnormal when mixed with a specific factor-deficient plasma suggests that the patient lacks the same clotting factor as that specific factor-deficient plasma. If the patient and deficient plasma give a normal result, the patient supplied the factor missing in the factor-deficient plasma. The aPTT result is plotted on the factor-activity curve, and the level of factor activity is derived from the standard curve.

Treatment for Hemophilia A Patients

Treatment options for hemophilia patients span decades and present one of the saddest treatment histories of any patient group with an inherited disorder. Factor VIII was discovered in 1937 and termed antihemophilic globulin. In the early days, treatment of patients with hemophilia A consisted of transfusing whole blood units to relieve symptoms. In 1957, it was realized that the deficient coagulation protein was a component of the plasma portion of blood. Cryoprecipitate, a plasma derivative discovered in 1964, is produced as an insoluble precipitate that results when a unit of fresh frozen plasma is thawed in a standard blood bank refrigerator. Cryoprecipitate contains fibrinogen, factor VIII, and vWF. This product is extracted from plasma and usually pooled before it is given to the patient according to weight and level of factor VIII. Cryoprecipitate presented a major breakthrough for hemophilia patients because it was an easily transfusable product that afforded individuals with the maximum level of factor.

Clotting factor products came next in the chronology of treatment products for hemophilia. These freeze-dried products were developed in the early 1970s. The products were lyophilized and freeze-dried and could be reconstituted and infused at home. This treatment offered hemophilia patients an independence they had not experienced previously. Finally, these individuals were in control because they could self-infuse when necessary and provide themselves with prompt care when a bleeding episode developed. A dark cloud, however, loomed over the bleeding community. Approximately 80% to 90% of hemophilia A patients treated with factor concentrates became infected with the HIV virus. Factor concentrates were made from pooled plasma from a donor pool that was not adequately screened. Additionally, manufacturing companies were less than stringent with sterilization methods, and blood banks did not screen for HIV until 1985. When each of these factors is brought to bear, the tragedy to the bleeding community is easily understood. According to the National Hemophilia Foundation (2005),[2] there are 17,000 to 18,000 hemophilia patients (hemophilia A and hemophilia B) in the United States, of whom 4,200 are infected with HIV/AIDS. No statistics are available for wives or children who might have been secondarily infected.

Recombinant products, which became available in 1989, represent the highest purity product because they are not derived from humans. Recombinant technology uses genetic engineering to insert a clone of the factor VIII gene into mammalian cells, which express the gene characteristic. Production expenses for this product are very costly, and manufacturers pass these costs on to potential users.

As a treatment alternative, gene therapy continues to provide hope for hemophilia patients. The idea here is to insert a copy of the factor VIII or factor IX gene into a virus vector, which lodges in the body and begins producing normal amounts of the necessary circulating factor. Complications from rejection of the virus vector in humans have proved to be a delicate issue, but researchers are optimistic that gene therapy for hemophilia patients can eventually succeed.

Quality-of-Life Issues for Hemophilia A Patients

Having a child with severe hemophilia A or hemophilia B presents special challenges to parents and the family unit. The threat of hospitalization, limited mobility, mainstreaming in schools, and the child's drive for independence all present potentially stressful environments. Added to this is the cost of recombinant or high-purity infusible factor product. Costs can reach $50,000/year if a patient has several bleeding episodes that require hospitalization. Individuals with a chronic condition face many anxieties and may struggle with feelings of isolation, anger, and disappointment (Table 17.1). The United States has hemophilia treatment centers that offer a network of needed services, and many states have local chapters of the National Hemophilia Foundation.[2] Prophylaxis with factor concentrates limits bleeding episodes, and the use of magnetic resonance imaging offers physicians a more effective means of evaluating joint damage.[3] Issues concerning medical insurance coverage continue to plague hemophilia patients.

Factor VIII Inhibitors

Factor VIII inhibitors develop in 15% to 20% of all individuals with hemophilia A.[4] These inhibitors are autoantibodies against factor VIII that are time-dependent and temperature-dependent and capable of neutralizing the coagulant portion of factor VIII. Treatment for patients who develop inhibitors is difficult, and treatment protocols follow various paths. When the inhibitor is low-titered or the individual is a low responder, physicians may infuse an appropriate level of factor VIII in an attempt to neutralize the

Table 17.1 ● Quality-of-Life Issues for Hemophilia A and B Patients

- Joint damage
- Reduced mobility
- Hemorrhage
- Fear
- Physical restrictions
- HIV/AIDS
- Hepatitis C
- Future insurability

inhibitor.[4] If this infusion is ineffective, patients must be treated with a factor substitute, usually **porcine** factor VIII or alternative therapies such as anti-inhibitor coagulant complex.[5]

Hemophilia B (Christmas Disease)

Individuals with hemophilia B lack factor IX clotting factor. Hemophilia B accounts for only 10% of individuals with hemophilia. All of the conditions concerning inheritance, clinical symptoms, laboratory diagnosis, and complications are the same for patients with severe hemophilia B as for patients with severe hemophilia A. Patients with hemophilia B have a prolonged aPTT and decreased factor assay activity. Treatment of hemophilia B consists of factor IX concentrates or prothrombin complex that is a mixture of factors II, VII, IX, and X.

Congenital Factor Deficiencies With Bleeding Manifestations

Deficiencies of factors II, V, VII, and X are rare and usually result from consanguinity. Most of these disorders are autosomal recessive and affect both males and females. Types of bleeding include skin and mucous membrane bleeding. Joint and knee bleeding is unusual except in factor VII–deficient patients, who may experience joint hemorrhages and epistaxis. A survey of the 225 hemophilia treatment centers in the United States determined that 7% of patients have a rare bleeding disorder.[6] Among these, factor VII was the most common. Abnormal preoperative screenings led to the diagnosis of most of these patients, but only half of them required therapy when bleeding occurred.[6] Individuals who inherit these deficiencies heterozygously tend to have few bleeding manifestations because they have one-half of factor activity. Treatment of patients with inherited deficiencies of factors II, VII, and X consists of prothrombin complex concentrates. Because factor VII clears rapidly from the plasma, booster doses are usually necessary to maintain clotting. Two gene mutations discovered more recently are especially pertinent to this discussion.

A prothrombin, factor II deficiency may occur as a result of a dysfunctional protein or diminished production of factor II. A structural defect in the protein is termed *dysproteinemia,* and individuals with this particular deficiency may bleed. Additionally, a specific mutation in the prothrombin gene has been recognized since 1996. Located on chromosome 11, a single substitution of guanine to adenine at position 20210 of the prothrombin gene produces prothrombin G20210A. This mutation increases the prothrombin level and predisposes an individual to venous thrombosis.[7] Individuals should be screened for this mutation if any of the following are part of their patient history: a history of venous thrombosis at any age, venous thrombosis in unusual sites, a history of venous thrombosis during pregnancy, and a first episode of thrombosis before age 50.[8]

Another more recently discovered (1993) mutation is factor V Leiden. This mutation is produced by substituting arginine with glutamine at position 506 of the factor V gene. The new gene product is factor V Leiden. In the normal coagulation scheme, activated protein C works to inactivate factors V and VIII, inhibiting the clotting mechanism. The mutated gene, factor V Leiden, impedes the degradation of factor V by protein C, causing activated protein C resistance. This condition accounts for increased clot formation with the subsequent development of deep vein thrombosis or other hypercoagulability conditions (see Chapter 19).

Congenital Factor Deficiencies in Which Bleeding Is Mild or Absent

Congenital factor deficiencies in which bleeding is mild or absent include deficiencies concerned with contact activation and clot stabilization. Factors XI, XII, Fletcher, and Fitzgerald are each synthesized by the liver and are involved early in the coagulation cascade in vitro. They become responsive when they contact surfaces such as glass in test tubes or ellagic acid in testing reagents.

Factor XI deficiency, or hemophilia C, is an autosomal recessive trait that occurs predominantly in the Ashkenazi Jewish and Basque populations in southern France. The heterozygous frequency of this gene in this population group is 1:8.[9] Bleeding is unlikely unless trauma or surgery occurs, and there is little correlation between the level of factor XI activity and the severity of bleeding episodes.

Factor XII deficiency is an autosomal recessive trait characterized by prolonged PTT in laboratory testing. Individuals with this deficiency do not bleed, however, and they are more prone to pathologic clot formation.

Fletcher factor, or prekallikrein deficiency, manifests as an autosomal dominant and recessive trait. Patients experience thrombotic events such as myocardial infarction or pulmonary embolism. An initially prolonged aPTT shortens after prolonged incubation with kaolin reagents.

Fitzgerald factor deficiency, also called high-molecular-weight kininogen deficiency, is a rare autosomal recessive trait featuring deep vein thrombosis and pulmonary embolism.[10]

Factor XIII Deficiency

Factor XIII is unique because it is a transglutaminase rather than a protease, as are most of the other coagulation factors. During coagulation, factor XIII stabilizes the fibrin clot by cross-linking fibrin polymers. Proper levels of factor XIII are essential for effective wound healing, hemostasis, and the maintenance of pregnancy. Because traditional coagulation tests such as PT, aPTT, thrombin time, or bleeding time do not screen for factor XIII, they are normal in a patient with factor XIII disorder. Screening for factor XIII deficiency is accomplished through the 5 mol/L urea test, a primitive test that measures the stability or firmness of a clot after 24 hours in a 5 mol/L urea solution. If factor XIII decreases, the clot is stringy and loose compared with the firm clot of stable hemostasis. Additionally, quantitative assays for factor XIII are available. Congenital deficiencies of factor XIII are rare autosomal recessive disorders. Deficiencies have been linked to poor wound healing, **keloid** formation, spontaneous abortion, and recurrent hematomas. Approximately one-half of patients have a family bleeding history, and large keloid scar formation appears to be a consistent finding in these patients.[11] Treatment for inherited disorders includes fresh frozen plasma or cryoprecipitate, a source of factor XIII. Acquired deficiencies of this factor may be associated with **Crohn's disease**, leukemias, disseminated intravascular coagulation (DIC), and ulcerative colitis. Table 17.2 provides a composite chart of factors, testing, and bleeding.

Bleeding Secondary to a Chronic Disease Process

Liver disease, renal disease, and autoimmune processes may lead to deficiencies in clotting factors that can cause bleeding. Because almost all procoagulants and inhibitors are synthesized by the liver, conditions such as alcoholic cirrhosis, biliary cancer, congenital liver defects, obstructive liver disease, and hepatitis can each negatively affect clotting factor production and clotting factor function. Factors with a short half-life, such as factor VII and the vitamin K–dependent factors (II, VII, IX, and X), are particularly vulnerable. Liver disease brings myriad potential problems regarding coagulation capability. In addition to poor production and function of clotting factors, there is weak clearance of activated clotting factors and the accumulation of plasminogen activators. Highly activated plasmin stimulates excessive clot lysis, and DIC and hemorrhaging may result. Unexpectedly elevated prothrombin times in a previously healthy patient may signal the advent of liver disease and indicate that the patient should be carefully monitored. Patients with liver disease who are bleeding receive fresh frozen plasma, a source of all clotting factors and natural inhibitors. Administration of 15 mL of plasma can increase clotting factor activity by 15% to 25%.[12]

Table 17.2 ● Preliminary Test Results and Bleeding in Inherited Clotting Factor Defects

Clotting Factor	PT	PTT	Types of Bleeding or Other
Factor II	Increased	Increased	Skin, mucous membrane disorder
Factor V	Increased	Increased	Infrequent bleeding
Factor VII	Increased	Negative	Infrequent bleeding
Factor VIII	Normal	Increased	Hemarthrosis, circumcisional bleeds, hematomas, intracranial bleeds
Factor IX	Normal	Increased	As above
Factor X	Increased	Increased	Infrequent bleeding
Factor XI	Normal	Increased	Infrequent bleeding
Factor XII	Normal	Increased	Thrombotic episodes
Factor XIII*	Normal	Negative	Poor wound healing, keloids, spontaneuous abortion
Fletcher factor	Normal	Increased	Thrombotic episodes
Fitzgerald factor	Normal	Increased	Thrombotic episodes

*5 M urea may be used.

Renal disease, especially nephrotic syndrome, usually leads to poor renal filtration and the presence of low-molecular-weight coagulation proteins in the urine of about 25% of patients with these disorders. Impaired platelet function is a feature of renal disease, and patients with renal disorders are cautioned against taking aspirin or other platelet inhibitors.

Role of Vitamin K in Hemostasis

Vitamin K is fat-soluble and necessary for the activation of factors II, VII, IX, and X. Provided mostly through diet in the form of green leafy vegetables, fish, and liver, vitamin K is also synthesized in small amounts by the intestinal bacterium *Bacteroides fragilis* and some strains of *Escherichia coli.* Because newborns are usually vitamin K–deficient because of the sterile environment of the small intestine, their levels of factors II, VII, IX, and X are low. In premature infants, the levels of vitamin K–dependent factors are 20% to 30%.[13] Since the 1960s, all newborns are given vitamin K to avoid hemorrhagic disease.

The vitamin K–dependent factors are low-molecular-weight proteins, with gamma-carboxyl residues at their terminal ends. In coagulation, activation and participation of such factors require a second carboxyl group through the action of the enzyme gamma glutamyl carboxylase (Fig. 17.4). This reaction requires vitamin K. Once this reaction is accomplished, these factors can bind to calcium and then to phospholipids for full participation in coagulation pathways.

Vitamin K Deficiency and Subsequent Treatment

Several mechanisms can deplete vitamin K. Because body stores of vitamin K are extremely limited, dietary sources are important. Dietary deficiency is likely to develop in patients who have prolonged hospitalizations with only parenteral nutrition, and such patient may require supplementation. Long-term antibiotic therapy that disrupts normal flora, a source of vitamin K synthesis, may lead to vitamin K deficiency and subsequent bleeding. Additionally, vitamin K depletion may occur with long-term antibiotic therapy supported by parenteral nutrition. Chronic diarrhea, biliary **atresia**, or other severe liver problems may lead to vitamin K synthesis because proper absorption of vitamin K requires bile salts. Coumadin or warfarin oral anticoagulant therapy provides anticoagulant activity because this substance is a vitamin K antagonist that prevents gamma carboxylation of factors II, VII, IX, and X. Patients receiving oral anticoagulant therapy require careful monitoring by anticoagulant clinics, and their diet must be modified to compensate for the loss of vitamin K activity. Additionally, numerous drugs may interfere with vitamin K activity and subsequent hemostasis (Table 17.3).

Patients with vitamin K depletion are likely to show elevated PT and aPTT, but normal plasma can correct this imbalance. Factor assays of the specific vitamin K factors reveal depressed activity. Factor VII, with the shortest half-life, is depleted first, within 2 days; the other factors take 3 to 10 days to reach low hemostatic levels. With mild bleeding, oral administration of vitamin K provides hemostatic recovery within a couple of hours. More emergent bleeding situations may result in parenteral administration of vitamin K, blood products, or infusion of prothrombin concentrate complex. An interesting side note involves reports of patients who have used Coumadin as an agent of suicide.[14]

Chapter 19 discusses acquired inhibitors of coagulation.

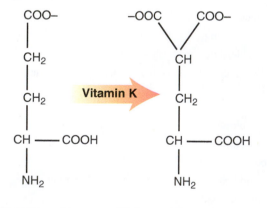

Glutamic acid　　　　Gamma-carboxyglutamic acid

Figure 17.4 The carboxylation of the enzyme glutamic acid. This reaction requires vitamin K.

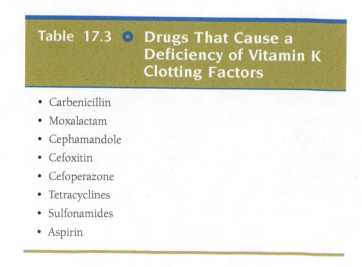

Table 17.3 ● Drugs That Cause a Deficiency of Vitamin K Clotting Factors
• Carbenicillin
• Moxalactam
• Cephamandole
• Cefoxitin
• Cefoperazone
• Tetracyclines
• Sulfonamides
• Aspirin

CONDENSED CASE

A 7-year-old child fell from a piece of playground equipment. After 24 hours, he developed a deep hematoma in his right thigh, and his parents brought him to the emergency department for evaluation. His family history did not indicate any previous bleeding from birth or otherwise. *What tests should be ordered to rule out a coagulation defect?*

Answer

Although his family history does not indicate a clotting factor abnormality, preliminary clotting tests should include a bleeding time, PT, and aPTT. This patient has a normal PT but an aPTT of 50 seconds (reference range 20 to 38 seconds). A factor assay was performed and indicated a mild factor VIII activity of 40% with a reference range of 50% to 150% activity. The patient was diagnosed with mild hemophilia A. This accident revealed a previously undiagnosed condition and added important information to this patient's personal and medical history. Future surgeries or traumas will require careful monitoring.

● *Summary Points*

- Patients with recurrent bleeding episodes must be evaluated for an inherited bleeding disorder.
- Bleeding falls into two main categories: open bleeds or closed bleeds.
- Plasma clotting factors need to maintain approximately 30% activity to achieve adequate clotting.
- The factor VIII molecule is carried into plasma by vWF.
- Hemophilia A and hemophilia B are generally acquired, sex-linked, recessive disorders.
- In hemophilia A, factor VIII is deficient; in hemophilia B, factor IX is deficient.
- Women are carriers of the defective hemophilia gene.
- Individuals with hemophilia experience prolonged bleeding from minor wounds.
- Individuals with hemophilia may experience many types of bleeding, including joint bleeding leading to hemarthrosis, hematomas, umbilical cord bleeding, or mucosal bleeds.
- The bleeding time is normal in patients with hemophilia A and hemophilia B; the aPTT is elevated.
- Current treatment for hemophilia consists of recombinant factor products.
- In the United States, most individuals with hemophilia use factor concentrates prophylactically.
- Prophylactic infusion of factor concentrates minimizes the physical disabilities that may occur from unexpected bleeding episodes.
- Of individuals with hemophilia, 10% to 30% develop factor VIII inhibitors.
- Individuals with factor II, V, VII, and X deficiencies may have minimal bleeding.
- Prothrombin complex concentrate is used to correct deficiencies of factors II, VII, IX, and X.
- Prothrombin G20210A is a mutation of the prothrombin molecule.
- Factor V Leiden is a genetic mutation of the factor V molecule that predisposes to clotting episodes.
- Deficiencies of factors XI, XII, Fletcher, and Fitzgerald usually lead to increased thrombotic events.
- Factor XIII is unique among clotting factors because it is a transglutaminase; the other clotting factors are proteases.
- An inherited deficiency of factor XIII may lead to poor wound healing and spontaneous abortions.
- Liver disease, renal disease, and autoimmune processes may lead to deficiencies in clotting factors that cause bleeding.
- Vitamin K is a fat-soluble vitamin necessary for the activation of factors II, VII, IX, and X.
- Vitamin K is available through the diet; small amounts are synthesized by normal intestinal flora.
- Newborns are vitamin K–deficient and are given vitamin K at birth to avoid hemorrhagic disease of the newborn.
- Vitamin K depletion results in prolonged PT and PTT.
- Coumarin, or warfarin, a therapeutic anticoagulant, is a vitamin K antagonist.

CASE STUDY

A 54-year-old woman was admitted to the hospital with hematuria, anemia, easy bruising, and progressive weakness. She gave no previous bleeding history or family history of bleeding even though she had multiple surgeries in the past, including knee replacement. During this admission, she complained of a deep bruise in her right upper thigh and hematuria. Her admitting laboratory data included:

WBC	6.0×10^9/L
Hgb	6.8 g/dL
Hct	20.2%
Platelets	321×10^9/L
PT	12.5 seconds (reference range 10.5 to 12.4 seconds)
aPTT	67.6 seconds (reference range less than 40 seconds)
Mixing studies: Immediate mixing and repeat PTT	39.6 seconds
aPTT after 1 hour	54.2 seconds
Factor VIII	4% (reference range 50% to 150%)

What is your initial impression?

Insights to the Case Study

This patient's family history is helpful in eliminating a congenital hemostatic defect as a source of her hematuria. She has undergone surgical procedures successfully in the past but now has hematuria and deep bruising. An elevated aPTT value can be seen in anticoagulant therapy (particularly heparin) in clotting factor defects and if a circulating inhibitor is present. Mixing studies in this patient show variable results, with initial correction of the patient's aPTT and subsequent prolongation on incubation. A factor VIII inhibitor was considered a likely explanation for the laboratory results and the low factor VIII assay value. Inhibitors or autoantibodies against factor VIII may develop in people other than patients with hemophilia A, of whom 10% to 30% develop these types of inhibitors. These inhibitors are directed against a portion of the factor VIII molecule and are time-dependent and temperature-dependent. Once identified, the inhibitor should be quantitated using the Bethesda titer. In this procedure, equal volumes of pooled normal plasma that is platelet-poor are mixed with patient platelet-poor plasma at pH 7.4. The mixture is incubated for 2 hours, and the PTT is repeated. If the patient plasma has anti–factor VIII activity, some of the active factor VIII in the normal plasma will be affected. The level of inhibitor is seen as a percentage of the normal activity of the factor compared with the control plasma; 1 Bethesda unit is equivalent to the inhibitor in which 50% factor activity will remain.

Review Questions

1. Which of the clotting factors is not a protease?
   a. Factor II
   b. Factor VII
   c. Factor XIII
   d. Factor IX

2. Why is the bleeding time normal in individuals with hemophilia A?
   a. Because of an increase in factor XIII
   b. Because the clotting problem is a factor VIII problem
   c. Because vWF is normal
   d. Because the clotting problem is a factor IX problem

3. The purest treatment product for hemophilia A patients is
   a. Cryoprecipitate.
   b. Fresh frozen plasma.
   c. Prothrombin complex concentrate.
   d. Recombinant factor VIII.

4. A fatal bleed in a hemophilia patient involves
   a. Intracranial bleeding.
   b. Mucosal bleeding.
   c. Joint bleeding.
   d. Epistaxis.

5. Which clotting factor deficiency is associated with poor wound healing?
   a. Factor II
   b. Factor X
   c. Factor XII
   d. Factor XIII

6. The following laboratory results have been obtained for a 40-year-old woman: PT 20 seconds (reference 11 to 15 seconds), aPTT 50 seconds (reference 22 to 40 seconds). What is the most probable diagnosis?
   a. Factor VII deficiency
   b. Factor VIII deficiency
   c. Factor X deficiency
   d. Factor XIII deficiency

7. Which of the following is the most prevalent inherited bleeding disorder?
   a. von Willebrand's disease
   b. Hemophilia A
   c. Factor VII deficiency
   d. Factor XII deficiency

8. A man with hemophilia A and an unaffected woman can produce a:
   a. Female carrier
   b. Male carrier
   c. Male with hemophilia A
   d. Normal female

9. A prolonged aPTT is corrected with factor VIII–deficient plasma but not with factor IX–deficient plasma. What factor is deficient?
   a. IX
   b. VIII
   c. V
   d. X

10. Which result is normal in a patient with dysfibrinogenemia?
    a. Thrombin time
    b. Activated partial thromboplastin time
    c. Immunologic fibrinogen level
    d. Protein electrophoresis

○ TROUBLESHOOTING

What Do I Do When Laboratory Results Are Inconsistent With the Patient's Physical Presentation?

A 74-year-old woman arrived in the emergency department with bruising over most of her extremities. She gave no family or personal history of bleeding but did indicate that she had delivered eight children. Her bleeding time was slightly abnormal at 9 minutes (reference less than 8 minutes), but her PT and aPTT were within normal range. Factor assays of factors VIII and IX were normal, and platelet aggregation studies were normal. What are the possibilities for the incongruities in this patient workup?

This patient presented a diagnostic dilemma. Quality control was verified at all levels on all pieces of equipment used. A repeat bleeding time, PT, and aPTT were performed and fell within ranges similar to the original. Factor assays were not repeated. These results stumped the coagulation staff. After carefully reviewing the testing target, they considered the possibility of a factor XIII deficiency. Factor XIII is necessary for clot stabilization and wound healing. A 5 mol/L urea test produced abnormal results. An inherited deficiency of factor XIII is the rarest of all of the bleeding disorders, presenting as autosomal recessive. Our patient has a history of multiple pregnancies and successful deliveries, so an inherited coagulation deficiency was not considered. A thorough medication check revealed that the patient was on cardiac medication, which potentially could have caused an inhibitory effect on factor XIII because all other factor-related assays were normal. Cryoprecipitate was infused to prevent any future bleeding complication. The patient's cardiac medication was discontinued, and the patient was given an appropriate alternative medication for her cardiac condition.

(Many thanks to D. Castellone for the resource material for this case.)

WORD KEY

Atresia • As in biliary atresia, congenital closure, or absence of some or all, of the major bile ducts

Crohn's disease • Inflammatory bowel disease marked by patchy areas of inflammation from the mouth to the anus

Hemarthrosis • Bloody effusion inside the joint

Hematoma • Swelling composed of a mass of clotted blood confined to an organ, tissue, or space or caused by a break in the blood vessel

Keloid • Scar that forms at the site of injury that appears to have a rubbery consistency and shiny surface

Porcine • Of or relating to swine (pigs)

References

1. Corriveau DM. Major elements of hemostasis. In: Corriveau DM, Fritsma GA, eds. Hemostasis and Thrombosis in the Clinical Laboratory. Philadelphia: JB Lippincott, 1988: 6.
2. National Hemophilia Foundation. Available at: www.hemophilia.org. Accessed June 14, 2005.
3. Berntrop E, Michiels JJ. A healthy hemophilic patient without arthropathy: From concept to clinical reality. Semin Thromb Hemost 29:5–10, 2003.
4. Fritsma G. Hemorrhagic coagulation disorders. In: Rodak B, ed. Hematology: Clinical Principles and Applications, 2nd ed. Philadelphia: WB Saunders, 2002: 639–640.
5. Kleinman MB. Anti-inhibitor coagulant complex for the rescue therapy of acquired inhibitors to factor VIII: Case report and review of literature. Hemophilia 8:694–697, 2002.
6. Acharya SS, Coughlin A, Dimichele DM, et al. Rare Bleeding Disorder Registry: Deficiencies of II, V, X, fibrinogen and dysfibrinogenemia. J Thromb Hasemost 2:248–256, 2004.
7. Jensen R. Screening and molecular diagnosis in hemostasis. Clin Hemost Rev 13:12, 1999.
8. McGlennen RC, Key NS. Clinical laboratory management of the prothrombin G20210A mutation. Arch Pathol Lab Med 126:1319–1325, 2002.
9. Seligsohn U. High frequency of factor XI (PTA) deficiency in Ashkenazi Jews. Blood 51:1223, 1978.
10. Cheung PP, et al. Total kininogen deficiency (Williams trait) is due to an argstop mutation in exon 5 of the human kininogen gene. Blood 78:3919, 1991.
11. Al-Sharif FZ, Aljurf MD, Al-Momen AM, et al. Clinical and laboratory features of congenital F XIII deficiency. Saudi Med J 23:552–554, 2002.
12. Weiss AE. Acquired coagulation disorders. In: Corriveau DM, Fritsma GA, eds. Hemostasis and Thrombosis in the Clinical Laboratory. Philadelphia: JB Lippincott, 1988: 176.
13. Zipursky A, Desa D, Hsu E, et al. Clinical and laboratory diagnosis of hemostatic disorders in newborn infants. Am J Pediatr Hematol Oncol 1:217–226, 1979.
14. Fritsma GA. Hemorrhagic coagulation disorders. In: Rodak B, ed. Hematology: Clinical Principles and Applications. Philadelphia: WB Saunders, 2002: 173.

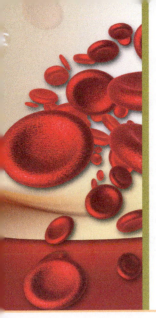

Chapter 18

Fibrinogen, Thrombin, and the Fibrinolytic System

Betty Ciesla

Role of Fibrinogen in Hemostasis

Disorders of Fibrinogen

    Afibrinogenemia

    Hypofibrinogenemia

    Dysfibrinogenemia

Unique Role of Thrombin in Hemostasis

    Physiologic Activators of Fibrinolysis

    Naturally Occurring Inhibitors of Fibrinolysis

    Measurable Products of the Fibrinolytic System

Disseminated Intravascular Coagulation

    Mechanism of Acute Disseminated Intravascular Coagulation

    Primary Fibrinolysis

    Clinical Symptoms and Laboratory Results in Acute Disseminated Intravascular Coagulation

    Treatment in Acute Disseminated Intravascular Coagulation

Objectives

After completing this chapter, the student will be able to:

1. Identify the components of the fibrinolytic system.

2. Recall the role of fibrinogen in the coagulation and fibrinolytic systems.

3. Describe plasmin in terms of activation and inhibition.

4. Differentiate the role of thrombin in the coagulation and fibrinolytic systems.

5. Outline the inherited disorders of fibrinogen.

6. Describe the laboratory tests for fibrinolytic disorders.

7. Define conditions that may precipitate disseminated intravascular coagulation (DIC) states.

8. Describe the laboratory testing and management of patients with DIC.

ROLE OF FIBRINOGEN IN HEMOSTASIS

Fibrinogen is the principal substrate of the coagulation and fibrinolytic systems. This clotting factor has the highest molecular weight of all of the clotting factors, and it is the substrate on which the coagulation system centers. Fibrinogen is heat-labile but stable in storage. When fibrinogen is transformed into fibrin under the influence of thrombin, it marks the onset of solid clot formation. Fibrin formation occurs within minutes, partly as a result of a positive feedback mechanism within the hemostasis system. Following activation, clotting factors accelerate the activity of the next factor, pushing the reaction to conclusion. Negative feedback occurs when reaction activity is delayed, a role played by naturally occurring inhibitors within the hemostatic system (e.g., alpha-2 antiplasmin).

Cross-linked fibrin stabilizes the fibrinogen molecule with the assistance of factor XIII and thrombin. Within hours, the fibrinolytic system swoops in to dissolve clots and restore blood flow. The creation of cross-linked fibrin is an orderly process by which thrombin cleaves fibrinogen into fibrinopeptides A and B. Fibrinogen consists of three pairs of polypeptide chains: alpha, beta, and gamma. Thrombin generation cleaves small portions of the alpha and beta chains, creating fibrinopeptides A and B; the remaining portions of the alpha and beta chains remain attached to the fibrinogen molecule. With fibrinopeptides A and B cleaved, the fibrin monomer is created. These monomers spontaneously polymerize by hydrogen bonding to form a loose and soluble fibrin network. Thrombin activates factor XIII and calcium and then catalyzes the formation of peptide bonds between monomers, forming fibrin polymers that lead to an insoluble and resistant clot (Fig. 18.1).[1]

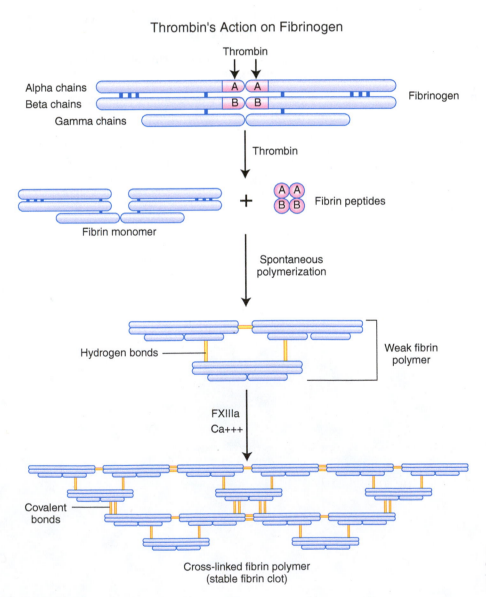

Thrombin's Action on Fibrinogen

Figure 18.1 Activity of thrombin on fibrinogen, from fibrin monomer to fibrin polymer.

Balance between the coagulation and fibrinolytic systems is crucial for maintaining circulation and for repairing injury. An imbalance in the coagulation system could cause excess clotting; an imbalance of the fibrinolytic system could cause hemorrhagic events. Several other components may play a role in hemostatic balance. Early studies suggested that decreased plasmin generation might decrease fibrinolytic activity in individuals with a high concentration of lipoprotein A. Because cholesterol and triglycerides are fatty components of lipoproteins, it is conceivable that reduced plasmin-generating activity in individuals with increased levels of lipoprotein might lead to less clot dissolution, leaving clots available for a pathologic outcome.[2]

DISORDERS OF FIBRINOGEN

Appropriate levels of fibrinogen are necessary to maintain hemostasis and induce platelet aggregation. The reference range for fibrinogen is 200 to 400 mg/dL. Fibrinogen is an acute-phase reactant, meaning that fibrinogen increases transiently during inflammation, pregnancy, stress, and diabetes and when a woman takes oral contraceptives. Evaluating a problem involving fibrinogen requires a careful patient history. For the most part, decreased fibrinogen is due to *acquired* disorders, such as acute liver disease, acute renal disease, or disseminated intravascular coagulation (DIC). Acquired increases in fibrinogen may be apparent in hepatitis patients, pregnant patients, or individuals with atherosclerosis.[3] Inherited fibrinogen disorders include afibrinogenemia, hypofibrinogenemia, and dysfibrinogenemia. These conditions are rare and, depending on severity, are marked by hematomas, hemorrhage, and ecchymoses.

Afibrinogenemia

With afibrinogenemia, a homozygous autosomal recessive disorder, there is less than 10 mg/dL of fibrinogen in the plasma. This small amount of fibrinogen is usually not demonstrable by traditional methods. Infants with afibrinogenemia exhibit bleeding from the umbilical stump. Poor wound healing and spontaneous abortion are also features of this disorder. Laboratory results show elevated prothrombin time (PT), activated partial thromboplastin time (aPTT), **thrombin time** (TT), and **reptilase time** and abnormal platelet aggregation with most aggregating agents and elongated bleeding time. Cryoprecipitate and fresh frozen plasma are the replacement products used for medical management of bleeds in patients with afibrinogenemia.

Hypofibrinogenemia

Hypofibrinogenemia is the heterozygous form of afibrinogenemia. This disorder is autosomal recessive, and patients exhibit 20 to 100 mg/dL fibrinogen in their plasma. Patients with hypofibrinogenemia may have mild spontaneous bleeding and severe postoperative bleeding. Results of laboratory coagulation testing, whether prolonged or normal, depend on the amount of fibrinogen present.

Dysfibrinogenemia

Dysfibrinogenemia refers to fibrinogen disorders that are autosomal dominant and are inherited homozygously and heterozygously. Dysfibrinogenemias produce a qualitative disorder of fibrinogen in which an amino acid substitution produces a functionally abnormal fibrinogen molecule. Although these disorders are an academic curiosity, they are infrequently associated with a bleeding tendency. A few dysfibrinogenemias are associated with thrombosis.[4] Approximately 40 abnormal fibrinogens have been discovered. Because the abnormal fibrinogen molecule in dysfibrinogenemia affects fibrin formation, most of the usual laboratory assessments for fibrinogen are abnormal. Although an **immunologic assay** of fibrinogen that measures the antigenic level of fibrinogen is usually normal, PT, aPTT, TT, and reptilase time increase. The clottable assay for quantitative fibrinogen is abnormal because this assay depends on the proper amount and proper functioning of fibrinogen.

UNIQUE ROLE OF THROMBIN IN HEMOSTASIS

Thrombin holds a respected place in the coagulation mechanism because of its multiplicity of function and the numerous reactions it mediates. The impact of thrombin is far-reaching, from the initial activation of the platelet system to the initiation of the fibrinolytic system and subsequent tissue repair. Prothrombin is the precursor to thrombin and can be converted only by the action of factor X, factor V, platelet factor 3, and calcium. Thrombin is generated in small concentrations through injury to the endothelial cells and proceeds to initiate a more enhanced coagulation mechanism. When generated, thrombin participates in the platelet release reaction and platelet aggregation. Secondarily, thrombin stimulates platelets to produce the platelet inhibitor, prostacyclin (PGI_2). With the coagulation system alerted, thrombin activates factors V and VIII, key cofactors in thrombus formation. Thrombin also activates protein C, a naturally occurring inhibitor to coagulation. Thrombomodulin, an additional product secreted by endothelial cells, amplifies protein C activity when complexed with thrombin.[5] With respect to fibrinogen degradation, thrombin plays a key role in negative feedback by converting plasminogen to plasmin, which digests the soluble fibrin clot. This interplay of thrombin disposition and thrombin initiation of clot disposal is part of the biologic control of hemostasis. After the clot is dissolved, thrombin plays a role in repairing tissue and wounds (Fig. 18.2).

Physiologic Activators of Fibrinolysis

A crucial link in the chain of hemostasis is the dissolution of fibrin clots, which usually occurs several hours after the stable clot is formed. Blood flow is restored at the local levels, and tissue healing is precipitated. The body provides naturally occurring or physiologic activators that initiate this process. The key component in this reaction is plasminogen, a plasma enzyme synthesized in the liver with a half-life of 48 hours. Plasminogen is converted to plasmin, chiefly through the action of tissue plasminogen activator (tPA), a substance released through the activity of endothelial cell damage and the production of thrombin. Additional plasminogen activators include factor XIIa, kallikrein, and high-molecular-weight kininogen (HMWK). Once produced, plasmin, a potent enzyme, does not distinguish between fibrin and fibrinogen and works to digest both. Plasmin also hydrolyzes factors V and VIII, and if it circulates in the plasma as pathologic free plasmin, the damage to the coagulation system is significant because clots are dissolved indiscriminately.

tPA has been synthesized by **recombinant** technology and is presently used as a pharmaceutical product during stroke episodes for fibrinolytic therapy. As a "clot-busting" drug, tPA has been effective in thrombotic strokes; if injected within 3 hours, it can prevent serious side effects of stroke. Another plasminogen activator is urokinase, a protease present in the urine and produced by the kidneys. The physiologic effect of urokinase is minimal in clot dissolution; however, similar to tPA, it is a valuable commercial product, used in **thrombolytic therapy** for patients with heart attacks, strokes, and other thrombotic episodes.[6] Streptokinase, an exogenous fibrinolytic agent, is produced when a bacterial cell product forms a complex with plasminogen, a pairing that converts plasminogen to plasmin. This toxic product results from infection with beta-hemolytic streptococci and is a dangerous by-product if this bacterial strain develops into a systemic infection. It has the most activity on fibrinogen.

Naturally Occurring Inhibitors of Fibrinolysis

Products that restrain fibrinolytic activity aid the balance of hemostasis. These products, plasminogen activator inhibitor 1 (PAI-1) and alpha-2 antiplasmin, act on different substrates in the fibrinolytic system. Endothelial cells secrete PAI-1 during injury and suppress the function of tPA in the plasminogen-plasmin complex. Plasmin as a substrate is directly inhibited by alpha-2 antiplasmin in a 1:1 ratio at the target area. This inhibitor prevents plasmin binding to fibrin in an orderly fashion and is the most important inhibitor of the fibrinolytic system. Inherited deficiencies of this inhibitor invariably lead to hemorrhagic episodes. Secondary agents that can inhibit fibrinolysis include alpha-2 macroglobulin, C1 inactivator, and alpha-1 antitrypsin. As protease inhibitors, these substances act on thrombin formation. Because thrombin is one of the initiators of plasmin generation, the secondary effect on the fibrinolytic system is unavoidable.

Measurable Products of the Fibrinolytic System

Physiologic fibrinolysis occurs in an orderly fashion, producing measurable products that can be captured by laboratory assays. Specifically, the by-products of an orderly fibrinolytic system are fibrin split/degradation products (FSPs/FDPs) composed of fibrin fragments labeled as X, Y, D, and E and the D-dimers, D-D (Fig. 18.3).

The accurate and precise measurement of these products provides the basis for therapeutic decisions once pathologic clot formation and lysing has begun. FSPs/FDPs form as a result of plasmin action on fibrin

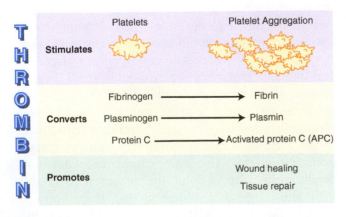

Figure 18.2 Multiple roles of thrombin in hemostasis.

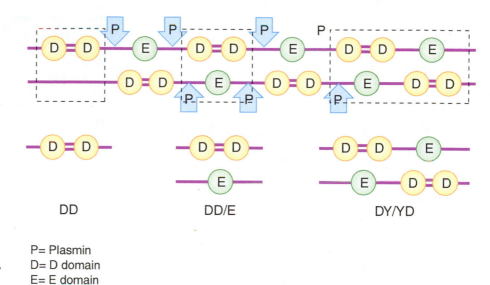

Figure 18.3 Formation of D-dimer and fibrin degradation products. P, plasmin; D, D domain; E, E domain.

P= Plasmin
D= D domain
E= E domain

and fibrinogen. As plasmin degrades the fibrinogen molecule, different fragments split off, leading to early and late degradation products. Normal levels of FDPs are eliminated through the reticuloendothelial system (RES) and usually measure less than 40 µg/mL. Individuals with an intact and operational hemostatic system have normal FDPs. These products are measured semiquantitatively through direct latex agglutination of a thrombin-clotted sample. Latex particles are coated with **monoclonal** antibodies to the human fibrinogen fragments D and E. The test is performed on serum using two dilutions, 1:15 and 1:20. It does not distinguish between the lysis of fibrinogen and fibrin. Pathologic levels of FDPs interfere with thrombin formation and platelet aggregation. Elevated levels may be seen in DIC, pulmonary embolism (PE), obstetric complications, and other conditions (Table 18.1).[7]

Once fibrin has been cross-linked and stabilized by factor XIII, a stable clot has been formed. When this clot is dissolved by plasmin, D-dimers are released. D-dimers suggest a breakdown of fibrin clot and indirectly indicate that clots have formed at the site of injury, at the local level. Excess D-dimers indicate a breakdown of fibrin products within the circulating blood. D-dimers can be assayed semiquantitatively and quantitatively. The semiquantitative assay is a simple agglutination test that uses monoclonal antibodies specific for this domain, mixing undiluted patient plasma with a latex solution. Noticeable agglutination is a positive test that indicates deep vein thrombosis (DVT), pulmonary embolism (PE), or DIC. Quantitative D-dimer tests are automated and use an enzyme-linked immunosorbent assay (ELISA). The advantage of this procedure is its ability to detect low levels of D-dimer and provide specific information regarding pathologic clotting, especially in DVT or PE. D-dimer assays are particularly useful in monitoring thrombolytic therapy.[8]

DISSEMINATED INTRAVASCULAR COAGULATION

The words "the patient has DIC" usually strike fear into the hearts of attending physicians, laboratorians, and nursing staff. An acute DIC event is almost always unanticipated and dramatic. Fatal outcomes occur. DIC is triggered by an underlying pathologic circumstance occurring in the body (Fig. 18.4). As a result, the hemostatic system becomes unbalanced, hyperactivating the coagulation or the fibrinolytic system and or both. This systemic process leads to excessive disposition of thrombi, excessive hemorrhage. Additionally, the process is consumptive, destroying clotting factors and platelets as soon as they are activated for coagulation. The decrease in

Table 18.1 ● Conditions That May Elevate Fibrin Degradation Products

- Disseminated intravascular coagulation
- Pulmonary embolism
- Abruptio placentae
- Preeclampsia
- Eclampsia
- Fetal death in utero
- Postpartum hemorrhage
- Polycystic kidney disease
- Malignancies
- Lupus nephritis
- Thrombolytic therapy

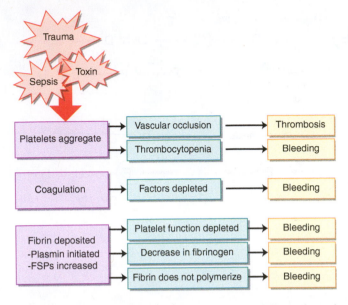

Figure 18.4 Conditions that may precipitate disseminated intravascular coagulation (DIC). Note the multiple pathways. FSPs, fibrin split products.

clotting factors usually overpowers the increase in lysis. In broad terms, DIC is associated with obstetric complications, malignancy, massive trauma, bacterial sepsis, asplenia, or necrotic tissue. Table 18-2 shows other pathologic possibilities for the initiation of a DIC event. Although most DIC events occur as acute, explosive episodes, some conditions may lead to a chronic compensated DIC state. These conditions are much more difficult to diagnose because the bone marrow and liver perform an excellent job of maintaining equilibrium between the coagulation and the fibrinolytic system. Laboratory results may be minimally abnormal, but an acute DIC episode is likely when the underlying pathology intensifies.[9]

Mechanism of Acute Disseminated Intravascular Coagulation

As is customary in normal hemostasis, the coagulation system and the fibrinolytic system are activated in parallel. DIC lacks the negative feedback mechanism that holds the systems in balance, however. Table 18.2 is a composite of events in the DIC cycle:

- The release of excess thromboplastin triggers the excessive generation of thrombin.
- Simultaneous enzymatic conversion of fibrinogen to fibrin occurs.
- Plasmin generation simultaneously degrades fibrinogen/fibrin into FDPs; excess FDPs are formed.
- FDPs have affinity for fibrin monomers but fail to polymerize properly; excess FDPs have an anticoagulant effect.

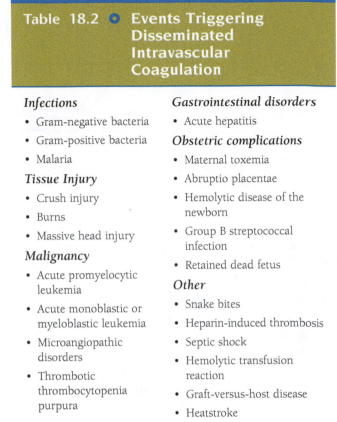

Table 18.2 ○ Events Triggering Disseminated Intravascular Coagulation

Infections	*Gastrointestinal disorders*
• Gram-negative bacteria	• Acute hepatitis
• Gram-positive bacteria	*Obstetric complications*
• Malaria	• Maternal toxemia
Tissue Injury	• Abruptio placentae
• Crush injury	• Hemolytic disease of the newborn
• Burns	• Group B streptococcal infection
• Massive head injury	• Retained dead fetus
Malignancy	*Other*
• Acute promyelocytic leukemia	• Snake bites
• Acute monoblastic or myeloblastic leukemia	• Heparin-induced thrombosis
• Microangiopathic disorders	• Septic shock
• Thrombotic thrombocytopenia purpura	• Hemolytic transfusion reaction
	• Graft-versus-host disease
	• Heatstroke

- Plasmin causes inactivation of factors V, VIII, XI, and XII.
- Hemorrhage occurs as soluble fibrin monomers are formed but degraded by excess FDPs; platelets and clotting factors are inactivated as both are coated by the soluble monomers.
- Clots that are formed are unstable.

Although the body attempts to minimize damage when a DIC event occurs, physiologic inhibitors such as protein C, protein S, and thrombomodulin are each inactivated.

Primary Fibrinolysis

Primary fibrinolysis is a DIC-related disorder in which plasmin within the circulation is activated by sources other than thrombin. In this rare condition, plasmin acts indiscriminately on fibrinogen and fibrin, making hemorrhage inevitable. Because thrombin is bypassed, the platelet count is normal, in contrast to the platelet count in DIC. All other parts of the coagulation profile in DIC are abnormal, however. There is controversy as to whether primary fibrinolysis is a disease entity or just a continuum in the vicious DIC cycle.

Clinical Symptoms and Laboratory Results in Acute Disseminated Intravascular Coagulation

In hemorrhagic episodes, most patients have extensive skin and mucous membrane bleeding, including ecchymosis, epistaxis, and petechiae. Because entry sites such as surgical incisions, catheters, or venipuncture may ooze, they must be carefully observed. In thrombotic episodes, patients may exhibit **acrocyanosis**, hypotension, or shock. Microthrombi may occur in the nose, genitalia, or digits or in major organs such as the kidneys, liver, or brain.

Acute DIC is a medical emergency. The entire basic coagulation profile in DIC is abnormal (Table 18.3). PT and PTT are prolonged, fibrinogen and platelets are decreased, and FDPs and D-dimers are dramatically increased. D-dimer results are an essential piece of data in patients with emerging DIC; however, other pathologies, such as inflammation, renal disease, or local clot, may elevate the result.[10] For this reason, all laboratory data must be carefully reviewed in concert with clinical symptoms before reaching the diagnosis. Not all patients with DIC have decreased fibrinogen levels. Studies have shown that clinical outcomes are much poorer for patients exhibiting DIC but near-normal fibrinogen, resulting in severe organ failure.[11] Recovering patients should be monitored over time using the same initial profile for comparison and evaluation of their coagulation status. Patients develop a microangiopathic hemolytic anemia secondary to microthrombi disposition in the small vessels. Schistocytes are observed as a morphologic marker for this process.

Table 18.3 ● Disseminated Intravascular Coagulation Laboratory Profile

- PT ↑
- aPTT ↑
- Platelets ↓
- Fibrinogen ↓
- D-dimer ↑

Treatment in Acute Disseminated Intravascular Coagulation

Identifying the precipitating event that led to DIC usually results in successful treatment that resolves this pathology. Surgery for obstetric complications or widespread use of antibiotics for septicemia may stem the bleeding episode. Because many clinicians are perplexed about the root cause of the precipitating events, however, blood products can be used judiciously to stop the bleeding. Fresh frozen plasma is a source of all of the clotting factors; packed red blood cells restore oxygen-carrying capacity; and platelet concentrates enable clot formation. Heparin has been used in DIC cases when combined with antithrombin. Although controversial, this agent may provide needed antithrombotic activity to delay excessive coagulation.

CONDENSED CASE

A 20-year-old woman came to the emergency department with unspecified complaints. A CBC was ordered, and her platelet count was recorded as 17.0×10^9/L. A repeat sample was ordered, and the platelet count was recorded as 6.0×10^9/L. The patient failed to delta-check with her CBC history, revealing an admission 3 weeks prior with a platelet count of 250×10^9/L. The technologist called the physician immediately with the report of the thrombocytopenia and inquired about the patient's history.

What additional steps should the technologist take to ensure the accuracy of this result?

Answer

The first step is to check the specimen for clots. Improperly mixed specimens are notorious for containing small clots. Emergency department personnel may be unaware that lavender top tubes must be inverted at least five times for proper mixing. Light blue top tubes (3.2% Na citrate) are used for coagulation studies, but the platelet count in the aforementioned CBC is almost always done using a lavender top tube (EDTA). This was done, and no clots were observed. Next, the technologist queried the physician as to whether or not this was an expected result. Although the physician was less than cooperative, he did reveal that the patient has undergone a cardiac procedure and that the initial consensus was that the thrombocytopenia was induced by medication. The patient was admitted and transfused with platelet concentrates, and the platelet count increased to 56×10^9/L. No additional history is known at this time.

⊙ *Summary Points*

- Fibrinogen is the key substrate of the coagulation and the fibrinolytic systems.
- Fibrinogen has the highest molecular weight of all of the clotting factors.
- Thrombin acts on fibrinogen, converting it to fibrin.
- Stabilization of fibrin by factor XIII and calcium results in an insoluble clot.
- Plasminogen is converted to plasmin primarily through tissue plasminogen activator and then proceeds to destroy the fibrin clot.
- Afibrinogenemia, hypofibrinogenemia, and dys-fibrinogenemia all are inherited disorders of fibrinogen. Each of these may also be an acquired disorder.
- Streptokinase, an exogenous fibrinolytic agent, is produced when a bacterial cell product forms a complex with plasminogen.

- Naturally occurring inhibitors of fibrinolysis are plasminogen activator inhibitor 1 and alpha-2 antiplasmin.
- The by-products of fibrinolysis are fibrin degradation products (FDPs) and D-dimers.
- Excess FDPs provide anticoagulant activity.
- D-dimers are produced from a cross-linked and stabilized fibrin clot.
- Excess D-dimers indicate excessive lysis.
- DIC is usually triggered by an underlying pathologic event.
- Patients with DIC excessively clot or excessively bleed, or both.
- Laboratory results for a patient with acute DIC show a prolonged PT and PTT, decreased fibrinogen and platelets, and increased FDP and D-dimers.
- Treatment for DIC includes investigating and resolving the cause of the disorder and providing blood bank products as needed.

Review Questions

1. Which of the following is one of the key roles of thrombin with respect to fibrinogen?
   a. Changes fibrinogen into plasmin
   b. Releases fibrin split products
   c. Converts fibrinogen into fibrin
   d. Activates factors V and VIII

2. Which of the following laboratory assays is *normal* in a patient with dysfibrinogenemia?
   a. Immunologic assay for fibrinogen
   b. Reptilase time
   c. Thrombin time
   d. PT and PTT

3. What is the primary purpose of the fibrinolytic system?
   a. To form a stable fibrin clot
   b. To activate the complement system
   c. To restore blood flow at the local level
   d. To inhibit coagulation

4. Which bacterial cell product would precipitate a DIC event?
   a. Neuraminidase
   b. Streptokinase
   c. Urokinase
   d. tPA

5. Which of the following is the best possible treatment for a patient with DIC?
   a. Provide supporting blood products
   b. Give the patient tPA if there is excessive clotting
   c. Resolve the underlying cause of the DIC
   d. Give the patient heparin therapy

6. The process of fibrin degradation is called _____ and is controlled by the enzyme _____.
   a. fibrination, plasmin
   b. fibrinolysis, plasmin
   c. fibrination, protease
   d. fibrinolysis, protease

7. A prolonged thrombin time and a normal reptilase time are indicative of
   a. Aspirin therapy.
   b. FDPs.
   c. Heparin therapy.
   d. Warfarin therapy.

8. All of the following are functions of thrombin *except:*
   a. Initiating the platelet release reaction
   b. Stimulating platelets to produce PGI_2
   c. Activating factors V and VIII
   d. Activating thromboplastin

9. D-dimers may be elevated in which of the following conditions?
   a. Sickle cell disease
   b. Glanzmann's thrombasthenia
   c. Deep vein thrombosis
   d. Bernard-Soulier syndrome

10. A primary inhibitor of the fibrinolytic system is:
    a. Alpha-2 antiplasmin.
    b. Alpha-2 macroglobulin.
    c. Antithrombin.
    d. Protein C.

CASE STUDY

A 27-year-old man was brought to the emergency department in serious condition. Earlier in the day, he was hiking and had been bitten on his leg by what he thought was probably a black snake. His leg was swollen, and he was extremely lethargic and barely conscious. Additionally, he was bleeding from the site of the wound. When blood was drawn, the venipuncture site bled profusely. His laboratory results follow:

Platelets	27.0×10^9/L (reference range 150 to 450×10^9/L)
PFA (platelet function assay	Not performed
PT	21.2 seconds (reference range 11.8 to 14.5 seconds)
PTT	53.7 seconds (reference range 23.0 to 35.0 seconds)
Fibrinogen	110 mg/dL (reference range 200 to 400 mg/dL)
D-dimer	3170 ng/mL D-dimer units (reference range 0 to 200 ng/mL D-dimer units)

Given these laboratory results, what is the most likely diagnosis? How can you account for his laboratory results?

Insights to the Case Study

The patient's basic coagulation profile was abnormal. His PT and PTT were markedly prolonged, his platelet count was markedly decreased, his fibrinogen was decreased, and his D-dimer was abnormal. DIC was triggered by the snake bite. Because the venom of poisonous snakes directly activates factor X or factor II, clotting occurs at an accelerated rate within the vessels, consuming all of the clotting factors. The D-dimer result is extremely elevated. D-dimer is the smallest breakdown product of fibrin. When elevated, it is indicative of cross-linked fibrin within the circulating blood, rather than locally at the site of injury. The patient was given antivenin and supported by blood products until his condition stabilized.

(Case submitted by Wendy Sutula, MS, MT(ASCP), SH, Washington Hospital Center.)

⊙ TROUBLESHOOTING

What Do I Do When the Patient Is Scheduled for Surgery and the PTT Is Abnormal, but He Denies Any Bleeding Episodes?

A 24-year-old man had routine preoperative blood work done. Because of the results, he was referred to the hematology service. The man denied any bleeding problems throughout his life and was taking no medications. None of his family members had any bleeding problems. A second sample reproduced the results of the first, which were as follows:

PT   13.9 seconds (reference range 11.8 to 14.5 seconds)

PTT   168.6 seconds (reference range 23.0 to 35.0 seconds)

The patient's PTT is extremely elevated. Three questions come to mind: Is the patient on heparin? Is there a circulating anticoagulant present? Does the patient have a congenital or acquired factor deficiency? A thrombin time was performed in the unlikely event that the patient was somehow receiving heparin (most likely, low-molecular-weight heparin, which can be administered on an outpatient basis). The thrombin time was normal, so the hematologist then ordered a PTT mixing study.

Continued

| Mixing study: Immediate | PTT = 32.9 50:50 mix: | Factor XI | 86% activity (reference range 65% to 135%) |
| 1-Hour incubated 50:50 mix: | PTT = 34.3 | Factor XII | 33% activity (reference range 50% to 150%) |

Based on the mixing study results, one could conclude that the patient has a factor deficiency. Additionally, the incubated mixing study showed that no slow-acting inhibitor is present. Because only the PTT is affected, the most likely factor would be one or more from the intrinsic pathway (factors XII, XI, IX, or VIII; HMWK; or prekallikrein). The hematologist ordered factor assays, with the following results:

| Factor VIII | 109% activity (reference range 55% to 145%) |
| Factor IX | 121% activity (reference range 61% to 140%) |

As can be seen from the laboratory data, this patient was factor XII–deficient. In contrast to deficiencies of factors VIII, IX, and XI, factor XII deficiency does not produce bleeding problems in patients. Factor XII–deficient patients tend to have very long PTTs, however, because the clotting time of a PTT is dependent on the in vitro activation of factor XII. Similar to HMWK and prekallikrein deficiency, factor XII–deficient patients may even have a tendency toward thrombosis. This young man had his surgery with no complications.

(Case submitted by Wendy Sutula, MS, MT(ASCP), SH, Washington Hospital Center.)

WORD KEY

Acrocyanosis • Blue or purple mottled discoloration of the extremities, especially the fingers, toes, and nose

Immunologic assay • Measuring the protein and protein-bound molecules that are concerned with the reaction of the antigen with its specific antibody

Monoclonal • Arising from a single cell

Recombinant • In genetic and molecular biology, pertaining to genetic material combined from different sources

Reptilase time • Coagulation procedure similar to thrombin time except that the clotting is initiated by reptilase, a snake venom; using reptilase, heparin would not affect the assay

Thrombin time • Using thrombin as a substrate, this assay measures the time it takes for fibrinogen to be converted to fibrin

Thrombolytic therapy • Using an agent that causes the breakup of clots

References

1. Loscalzo AD, Schafer AI. Thrombosis and Hemorrhage, 2nd ed. Baltimore: Williams & Wilkins, 1998: 1027–1063.
2. Falco C, Estelles A, Dalmau J, et al. Influence of lipoprotein A levels and isoforms on fibrinolytic activity: Study in families with high lipoprotein A levels. Thromb Haemost 79:818–823, 1998.
3. Liles DK, Knup CL. Disorders of plasma clotting factors. In: Harmening D, ed. Clinical Hematology and Fundamentals of Hemostasis. Philadelphia: FA Davis, 2002: 497.
4. Francis CW, Marder VJ. Physiologic regulation and pathologic disorders of fibrinolysis. In: Colman RW, et al, eds. Hemostasis and Thrombosis: Basic Principles and Clinical Practice, 3rd ed. Philadelphia: JB Lippincott, 1994: 1089.
5. Hosaka Y, Takahashi Y, Ishii H. Thrombomodulin in human plasma contributes to inhibit fibrinolysis through acceleration of thrombin dependent activation of plasma carboxypeptidase. Thromb Haemost 79:371, 1998.
6. Fritsma G. Normal hemostasis and coagulation. In: Rodak B, ed. Hematology: Clinical Principles and Applications, 2nd ed. Philadelphia, WB Saunders, 2002: 625.
7. Jensen R. The diagnostic use of fibrin breakdown products. Clin Hemost Rev 12:1Ð2, 1998.
8. Janssen MC, Sollersheim H, Verbruggen B, et al. Rapid D-dimer assay to exclude deep vein thrombosis and pulmonary embolism: Current status and new developments. Semin Thromb Hemost 24:393–400, 1998.
9. Cunningham VL. A review of disseminated intravascular coagulation: Presentation, laboratory diagnosis and treatment. M L O July:48, 1999.
10. Bick RL, Baker WF. Diagnostic efficacy of the D-dimer assay in disseminated intravascular coagulation (DIC). Thromb Res 65:785–790, 1992.
11. Wada H, Mori Y, Okabayashi K, et al. High plasma fibrinogen levels is associated with poor clinical outcome in DIC patients. Am J Hematol 72:1–7, 2003.

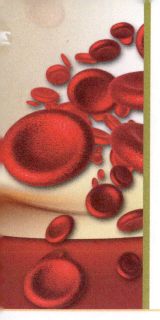

Chapter 19

Introduction to Thrombosis and Anticoagulant Therapy

Mitra Taghizadeh

Objectives

After completing this chapter, the student will be able to:

1. Define thrombophilia and thrombosis.

2. Indicate risk factors associated with inherited and acquired thrombosis.

3. Define hemostatic changes responsible for pathologic thrombosis.

4. Describe antithrombin, protein C, and protein S with regard to properties, mode of action, factors affected, and complications associated with their deficiencies.

5. List inherited risk factors for thrombosis and their frequency of occurrence.

6. Discuss the most commonly acquired risk factors associated with thrombosis.

7. Describe activated protein C resistance with regard to pathophysiology, mode of action, and associated complications.

8. Describe heparin-induced thrombocytopenia with regard to the cause, patient's clinical manifestations, and pathophysiology of the disease.

9. Discuss the laboratory tests and results used for the diagnosis of factor V Leiden and heparin-induced thrombocytopenia.

10. List the types of anticoagulant drugs used for the treatment of thrombotic disorders.

11. Describe the mechanism of action of each anticoagulant drug commonly used for the treatment of thrombotic disorders.

12. Discuss the laboratory test used for monitoring of heparin and Coumadin (warfarin) therapy.

13. Define the anti–factor Xa assay and its clinical application.

14. Name the alternative anticoagulant drugs.

Thrombophilia refers to environmental, inherited, and acquired conditions that alter coagulation and predispose an individual to thrombosis. Thrombosis is the formation of a blood clot in the vasculature. Two types of thrombosis are known: arterial and venous. Arterial thrombi are primarily composed of platelets and small amounts of red blood cells and white blood cells, whereas venous thrombi are composed of fibrin and red blood cells. Thrombosis may result from vascular injury, platelet activation, coagulation activation, defects in the fibrinolytic system, or defects in physiologic inhibitors. Along with complications from thromboembolisms, arterial and venous thrombosis are the most important causes of death in developed countries. More than 800,000 people die annually from myocardial infarction (MI) and thrombotic stroke in the United States.[1] It has also been reported that venous thromboembolic disease is the most common vascular disease after atherosclerotic heart disease and stroke.[1]

This chapter focuses on the physiology and pathology of thrombosis, thrombotic disorders, laboratory diagnosis, and anticoagulant therapy.

PHYSIOLOGIC AND PATHOLOGIC THROMBOSIS

Normal hemostasis refers to the physiologic response of the body to vascular injury. Normal clot formation and clot dissolution are accomplished by interaction among five major hemostatic components: vascular system, platelets, coagulation system, fibrinolytic system, and inhibitors. These components must be functional for normal hemostasis to occur. Imbalance in any of the above components tilts the hemostatic scale in favor of either bleeding or thrombosis. There are two systems of hemostasis: primary and secondary hemostatic systems. Primary hemostasis refers to the process by which the platelet plug is formed at the site of injury, whereas secondary hemostasis refers to the interaction of coagulation factors to generate a cross-linked fibrin clot to stabilize the platelet plug to form physiologic thrombosis.

Physiologic thrombosis results from the natural response of the body to vascular injury. It is localized and formed to prevent excess blood loss. Pathologic thrombosis includes deep venous thrombosis (DVT), arterial thrombosis, and pulmonary embolism (PE). Pathologic thrombosis may be caused by acquired or inherited conditions. Arterial thrombosis is primarily composed of platelets with small amounts of fibrin, red blood cells, and white blood cells. This clot may be also referred to as the "white clot." Complications associated with arterial thrombosis include occlusions of the vascular system leading to infarction of tissues.[1] Factors causing arterial thrombosis include hypertension, hyperviscosity, qualitative platelet abnormalities, and **atherosclerosis**.

Venous thrombosis is composed of large amounts of fibrin and red blood cells resembling the blood clot formed in the test tube. This occlusion is associated with slow blood flow, activation of coagulation, impairment of the fibrinolytic system, and deficiency of physiologic inhibitors. The most serious complication associated with venous thrombosis is demobilization of the clot, which occurs as the clot dislodges from its site of origin and filters out into the pulmonary circulation.

PATHOGENESIS OF THROMBOSIS

Important hemostatic changes in the pathogenesis of thrombosis include vascular injury secondary to the toxic effect of chemotherapy, platelet abnormalities (more important in arterial thrombosis), coagulation abnormalities, fibrinolytic defects, and deficiencies of the antithrombotic factors.

Vascular Injury

Vascular injuries play an important role in arterial thrombosis. Vascular injury initiates platelet adhesion to exposed subendothelium. The adherent platelets release the contents of alpha and dense granules such as adenosine diphosphate (ADP), calcium, and serotonin, causing platelet aggregation and platelet plug formation. In addition, blood coagulation is initiated by tissue factor released from the damaged endothelial cells. The fibrin clot thus formed stabilizes the platelet plug. Vascular endothelial injury may occur by endothelial cell injury, atherosclerosis, hyperhomocysteinemia, or other disorders that may interfere with arterial blood flow. In cancer patients, vascular endothelial cell injury may occur secondary to the toxic effect of chemotherapeutic drugs.

Platelet Abnormalities

Platelets are the main component of arterial thrombosis. As platelets interact with the injured vessels, platelet adhesion and aggregation occur. In normal hemostasis, excess platelet activation is prevented by the antiplatelet activities of endothelial cells such as generation of prostacyclin. In the disease state, excess platelet activation can reflect thromboembolic disease or acceleration of thrombotic episodes.[1]

Coagulation Abnormalities

Risk factors associated with hypercoagulability can be divided into environmental, acquired, or inherited factors (Fig. 19.1).[1,2] Environmental factors are linked to transient conditions that may result from surgery, immobilization, and pregnancy or therapeutic complications associated with oral contraceptives, hormone replacement therapy, chemotherapy, and heparin treatment. Acquired risk factors are associated with conditions that hinder normal hemostasis such as cancer, nephrotic syndrome, **vasculitis**, antiphospholipid antibodies, myeloproliferative disease, hyperviscosity syndrome, and others (Table 19.1).[1] Inherited risk factors are associated with genetic mutations that result in deficiency of naturally occurring inhibitors, such as protein C, protein S, or antithrombin (AT); accumulation of procoagulant factor as in prothrombin G20210A[1,3]; or clotting factor resistance to anticoagulant activities of physiologic inhibitors as in activated protein C resistance (APCR) (Table 19.2). These conditions disturb the hemostatic regulation in favor of increased risk of thrombosis.

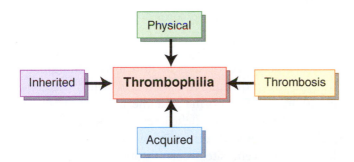

Figure 19.1   Risk factors for thrombosis.

Table 19.1 ● Conditions Associated With Acquired Thrombosis

- Cancer
- Surgery (especially orthopedic surgery)
- Liver disease
- Immobility
- Nephrotic syndrome
- DIC
- Pregnancy
- Antiphospholipid antibodies
- Drugs

Table 19.2 ● Conditions Associated With Inherited Thrombosis

- Antithrombin, protein C and S deficiencies
- Factor XII, Fletcher and Fizgerald factors deficiencies
- Prothrombin G20210A mutation (elevated factor II)
- Elevated factor VIII
- APCR (factor V Leiden)
- Hyperhomocysteinemia

Fibrinolytic Abnormalities

The function of the fibrinolytic system is the breakdown of fibrin clots. A specific group of inhibitors holds this system in balance. Plasmin, an activated form of plasminogen, has a primary role in fibrin breakdown. This enzyme is inhibited primarily by alpha-2 antiplasmin but also by alpha-2 macroglobulin, alpha-1 antitrypsin, AT, and C1 esterase. Plasminogen activation is also inhibited by proteins such as plasminogen activator inhibitors 1, 2, and 3 (PAI-1, PAI-2, and PAI-3).[3] A decrease in fibrinolytic activities, particularly decreased levels of tissue plasminogen activator (tPA) and elevated levels of PAI-1, results in impaired fibrinolysis in vivo, which results in arterial and venous thrombosis.[1]

Antithrombotic Factors (Coagulation Inhibitors)

Antithrombotic factors are circulating plasma proteins that interfere with the clotting factors and prevent thrombin formation and thrombosis. Four types of naturally occurring inhibitors are AT, heparin cofactor II, protein C, and protein S.

Antithrombin

AT is a plasma protein produced in the liver, and it primarily neutralizes the activities of thrombin (IIa) and factor Xa. Other clotting factors inhibited by AT include IXa, XIa, and XIIa. The inhibitory action of AT against clotting factors is slow; however, this activity increases markedly when AT binds to heparin (Fig. 19.2). AT deficiency is associated with thrombosis.[1,2,4]

Heparin Cofactor II

Heparin cofactor II is another coagulation inhibitor. It acts against thrombin, and it is heparin-dependent.

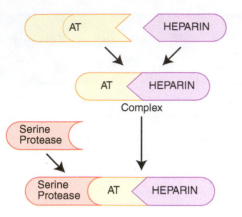

Figure 19.2 Effect of antithrombin (AT) on serine proteases.

Heparin cofactor deficiency alone is not associated with thrombosis.[1]

Protein C and Protein S

Protein C is a vitamin K–dependent protein produced in the liver. Protein C circulates in the form of zymogen, an inactivated protein. It must be activated to a serine protease (activated protein C [APC]) to inhibit the clotting factors. Protein C is activated by the action of the thrombin-thrombomodulin complex with protein S as a cofactor (Fig. 19.3).[1,2,4]

Protein S is a vitamin K–dependent protein produced in the liver and is necessary for activation of protein C. Once protein C is activated, it inhibits the

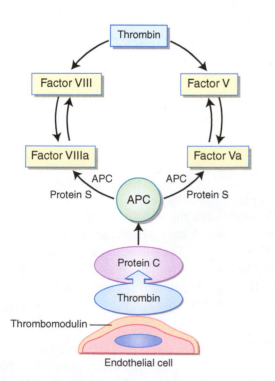

Figure 19.3 Protein C pathway. APC, activated protein C.

activity of cofactors Va and VIIIa to cofactors V and VIII. Deficiencies of protein C and protein S are associated with thrombosis.

THROMBOTIC DISORDERS
Inherited Thrombotic Disorders

Inherited thrombotic disorders occur in young adults and are associated with genetic mutations that result in deficiencies of one or more of the naturally occurring inhibitors or increased or decreased levels of clotting factors. Decreased levels of *inhibitors*, such as AT, protein C, and protein S, and clotting factors, such as factor XII, prekallikrein, and Fitzgerald factor, are associated with thrombosis. Increased levels of clotting factors such as those seen in prothrombin G20210A mutation and elevated factor VIII are associated with thrombosis. Other causes of inherited thrombotic disorders are APCR, particularly factor V Leiden, or an inherited form of hyperhomocysteinemia caused by an enzyme deficiency (see Table 19.2).

Antithrombin Deficiency

First discovered in 1965,[1] AT deficiency is inherited as an autosomal dominant disorder. It has been reported that 1 in 600 people have AT deficiency.[1] There are two types of AT deficiency. Type I is a quantitative disorder characterized by a reduction in the amount of AT. Type II is a qualitative disorder in which the concentration of AT is normal but the molecule is functionally abnormal. AT deficiency is associated with recurrent venous thrombosis, which may include almost every vein site.[1] The thrombotic event may be primary (in the absence of triggering factors) or may be followed by another risk factor, such as pregnancy, surgery, or any other acquired factors. Acquired AT deficiency may be correlated with disseminated intravascular coagulation (DIC), liver disease, nephrotic syndrome, oral contraceptives, and pregnancy.[1]

Heparin Cofactor II Deficiency

Heparin cofactor II was first discovered in 1974[3] and is inherited as an autosomal dominant trait. It is a heparin-dependent factor whose inhibitory effect is primarily against thrombin. Many studies have shown that heparin cofactor deficiency alone is not associated with thrombosis.[1]

Protein C Deficiency

Protein C deficiency is inherited as an autosomal dominant trait. Similar to AT deficiency, there are two types of protein C deficiency: type I (quantitative deficiency) and type II (qualitative deficiency). Type I deficiency is the most common form and is associated with reduction of immunologic and functional activity of protein C to 50% of normal. Type II deficiency is characterized by a normal amount of an abnormal protein.[4] More than 160 different protein C mutations have been reported between the two types.[1,4] Most of the mutations are "nonsense" mutations. Venous thromboembolism (VTE) is the most common complication associated with protein C deficiency in heterozygous adults. Other reported complications include arterial thrombosis, neonatal **purpura fulminans** in homozygous newborns, and warfarin-induced skin **necrosis**.[1]

Many studies show that most patients with protein C deficiency alone are asymptomatic.[1] This finding indicates that some additional inherited or acquired risk factors may provoke thrombotic episodes in these patients. Acquired protein C deficiency may be linked with vitamin K deficiency, liver disease, malnutrition, DIC, and warfarin therapy.[1]

Protein S Deficiency

Discovered in 1984,[1] protein S deficiency is inherited in an autosomal dominant fashion. Protein S circulates in plasma in two forms: free (40%) and bound to C4b-binding protein (60%). The cofactor activity of protein S is carried primarily by free protein S. As with AT and protein C deficiencies, protein S deficiency is divided into two types. Type I is a quantitative disorder in which total protein S (free and bound), free protein S, and protein S activity levels are reduced to about 50% of normal.[1] Type II protein S deficiency is a qualitative disorder and is divided into type IIa and type IIb. In type IIa protein S deficiency, free protein S is reduced, whereas total protein S is normal. In type IIb, free and total protein S levels are normal.[1] Type IIb protein S deficiency has been reported in patients with factor V Leiden. Similar to protein C deficiency, many patients with thrombosis have additional inherited or acquired risk factors.[1] Most patients with protein S deficiency may experience venous thrombosis. However, arterial thrombosis has been reported in 25% of patients with protein S deficiency.[1] Acquired protein S deficiency may be correlated with vitamin K deficiency, liver disease, and DIC.

Activated Protein C Resistance (Factor V Leiden)

APCR is an autosomal dominant disorder that was discovered in 1993.[1,4] APCR was found in 20% to 60% of patients with recurrent thrombosis with no previously recognized inherited thrombotic disorder. Most cases (92%) are inherited and caused by mutation of factor V, Arg506Gln, referred to as factor V Leiden.[1] Factor V Leiden is the most common inherited cause for thrombosis in the Caucasian population of northern and western Europe. In the United States, factor V Leiden is seen in 6% of the Caucasian population.[1] The homozygous form of factor V Leiden has a 80-fold increased risk of thrombosis, whereas heterozygous carriers have a 2-fold to 10-fold increase in thrombosis.[1] Factors V and VIII are inactivated by the protein C–protein S complex. The mutated factor V, factor V Leiden, is not inactivated and leads to excessive clot formation. The thrombotic risks increase further if other inherited or acquired risk factors coexist. The thrombotic complications associated with factor V Leiden are VTE, recurrent miscarriage, and MI. Smoking increases the risk of thrombosis 30-fold in individuals with factor V Leiden.[1] Other causes of APCR (8%) are related to pregnancy, oral contraceptive use, cancer, and other acquired disorders (Fig. 19.4).

Laboratory Diagnosis of Activated Protein C Resistance

APCR may be evaluated by coagulation assays, which include a two-part activated partial thromboplastin time (aPTT) test. The principle of the test is the inhibition of factor Va by APC, which causes prolongation of aPTT. The aPTT test is performed on patient plasma with and without APC. The results are expressed in a ratio:[1]

$$\frac{\text{Patient aPTT} + \text{APC}}{\text{Patient aPTT} - \text{APC}}$$

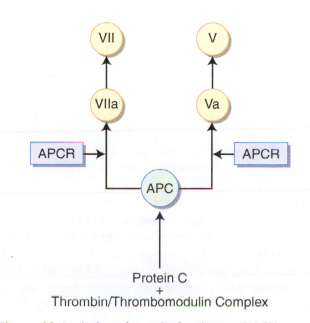

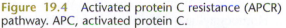

Figure 19.4 Activated protein C resistance (APCR) pathway. APC, activated protein C.

Reference ranges vary from laboratory to laboratory, but the normal ratio generally is 2 or greater. A ratio of less than 2 is diagnostic.

aPTT decreases when APC is added to the normal plasma. Plasma from patients with APCR has a lower ratio than the reference ranges established for normal patients. A DNA test is available to confirm the specific point mutation in patients with factor V Leiden (see Chapter 20 for more coagulation tests).

Prothrombin Mutations

Prothrombin mutation (G20210A) is the second most prevalent cause of an inherited form of hypercoagulability. Caused by a single point mutation, G20210A is an autosomal dominant disorder that causes increased concentration of plasma prothrombin. The risk of VTE increases as the plasma prothrombin level increases to a level greater than 115 IU/dL.[1] As with factor V Leiden, prothrombin mutation tends to follow a geographic and ethnic distribution, with the highest prevalence in Caucasians from southern Europe. About half of the cases reported are from northern Europe.[1] Similar to factor V Leiden, the thrombotic episodes develop early, before the age of 40 years.[1]

Other Inherited Thrombotic Disorders

Elevated activity levels of factor VIII are associated with VTE. If factor VIII activity is greater than 150%, the risk for VTE increases 3-fold; if the activity is greater than 200%, the thrombotic risk increases 11-fold.[1] Factor XII deficiency is also linked to thrombosis.

Factor XII, prekallikrein factor, and Fitzgerald factor, commonly referred to as contact factors, initiate activation of the intrinsic pathway. Patients with deficiencies of these factors have a prolonged aPTT but no bleeding problems. Factor XII plays a major role in the fibrinolytic system and in activating plasminogen to plasmin. Patients with factor XII deficiency have impaired fibrinolysis and are prone to thrombosis.[3]

Dysfibrinogenemia is an inherited abnormality of the fibrinogen molecule with a variable clinical presentation. Arterial or venous thrombosis is the presentation in 20% of cases. Bleeding has been reported in 20% of cases, and 60% of patients may be asymptomatic.[3]

Tissue factor pathway inhibitor (TFPI) deficiency is another marker for thrombosis. TFPI is important in the prevention of clot formation. It inhibits factor Xa and factor VIIa–tissue factor complex.[3] TFPI deficiency is associated with thromboembolic disorder, owing to the excessive activation of the extrinsic pathway.

Hyperhomocysteinemia can be inherited or acquired. Homocysteine is an amino acid formed during the conversion of methionine to cysteine in vitamin B_{12} synthesis. Hyperhomocysteinemia results from deficiencies of either the enzymes necessary for production of homocysteine (inherited form) or vitamin cofactors (vitamin B_6, vitamin B_{12}, and folate) in an acquired form. Increased levels of homocysteine in the blood are reported to be a risk factor for stroke, MI, and thrombotic disorder.[1,3]

Disorders of the fibrinolytic system such as plasminogen deficiency, tPA deficiency, and increased plasminogen activator inhibitor are associated with thrombotic disease.[1]

Acquired Thrombotic Disorders

Many conditions may lead to acquired thrombotic disorders, and they often are linked with underlying conditions, such as cancer, surgery, liver disease, nephrotic syndrome, DIC, pregnancy, and vitamin K deficiency. Drugs such as oral contraceptives or hormone replacement therapy may predispose to thrombosis. The most common causes of acquired thrombotic disorders are antiphospholipid syndrome and heparin-induced thrombocytopenia.

Antiphospholipid Syndrome and Lupus Anticoagulants

Antiphospholipid (aPL) syndrome is an acquired disorder in which patients produce antibodies to phospholipid-binding proteins known as beta-2-glycoprotein I (β_2GPI), prothrombin, or apolipoprotein (apo).[5] Clinical manifestations of aPL antibodies include thrombosis and fetal loss. The IgG2 subtype of aPL usually is associated with thrombosis. Thrombotic episodes include venous and arterial thrombosis and thromboembolism. The usual age at the time of thrombosis is generally about 35 to 45 years. Men and women are equally affected.[5] Thrombosis may occur spontaneously or may be related to other predisposing factors, such as hormone replacement therapy, oral contraceptives, surgery, or trauma. A few patients with aPL antibodies may present with bleeding if there is a concurrent thrombocytopenia or coagulopathy such as hypoprothrombinemia.[5]

The most common forms of aPL antibodies are lupus anticoagulant (LA) and anticardiolipin antibody (ACA). The thrombotic manifestations may be primary (independent autoimmune disorder) or secondary (associated with other autoimmune disorders such as systemic lupus erythematosus [SLE]). In vitro, LA acts against phospholipid-dependent coagulation assays such as aPTT, which are not corrected by a 1:1 mix with normal plasma (see Chapter 20).[4,5] Patients with aPL antibodies may present with thrombosis and fetal loss. Bleeding is uncommon, unless the patient has thrombocytopenia or decreased prothrombin as well.

Laboratory Assays for Antiphospholipid Antibodies

Common tests used to detect LA include aPTT, Kaolin clotting time (KCT), and dilute Russell viper venom test (DRVVT). The prothrombin time (PT) test may be normal or prolonged depending on the titer of the antibodies. For a prolonged aPTT and DRVVT, a mixing study should be performed. In a mixing study, the patient plasma is mixed with normal plasma, and the test is repeated. In the presence of LA, the mixing study does not correct to normal. LA is confirmed by the addition of excess platelets (platelet neutralization test or hexagonal phase phospholipids [DVV Confirm]).[4,6] The International Society of Hemostasis and Thrombosis has recommended four criteria for the diagnosis of LA: (1) prolongation of a phospholipid-dependent test, (2) evidence for the presence of an inhibitor (mixing study), (3) evidence that the inhibitor is directed against phospholipids (confirmatory test), and (4) lack of any other specific inhibitor (Table 19.3). Other factors that are helpful in the diagnosis of LA include the clinical presentation of thrombosis because these patients lack bleeding. LA may coexist with ACA in patients presenting with an acquired thrombosis and fetal loss, and so the test for ACA is recommended as well. ACAs are detected by the enzyme-linked immunosorbent assay (ELISA) method.[6] Other detectable antibodies include anti-β_2GPI.[6]

Heparin-Induced Thrombocytopenia

Heparin-induced thrombocytopenia (HIT) is an immune-mediated complication associated with heparin therapy. HIT may develop in 3% to 5% of patients receiving unfractionated heparin.[1] Thrombocytopenia usually develops 5 to 14 days after heparin therapy. About 36% to 50% of patients with HIT develop life-threatening thrombosis. The thrombotic tendency can last for at least

30 days.[1] Venous thrombosis (extremity venous thrombosis) is more common than arterial thrombosis. Other complications of HIT include thrombocytopenia, heparin-induced skin lesions (10% to 20% of patients), and heparin resistance.[1] The pathogenesis of HIT is that antibodies are produced against heparin–platelet factor 4 complex. This immune complex binds to platelet FC receptors, causing platelet activation, formation of platelet microparticles, thrombocytopenia, and hypercoagulable state (Fig. 19.5).

HIT is independent of dosage or route of administration of heparin and can occur in patients who have had prior exposure via intravenous (IV) or subcutaneous heparin administration. HIT is also known to occur in individuals who have had exposure to an IV heparin flush only. This condition should be suspected in any patient whose platelet count decreases to less than 50% of the baseline value after 5 days of heparin treatment[1] and in patients who develop thrombosis with or without thrombocytopenia during heparin therapy.[1]

Laboratory Diagnosis of Heparin-Induced Thrombocytopenia

Laboratory diagnosis of HIT includes functional assays or immunoassays. Functional assays measure platelet activation or aggregation in the presence of HIT serum and heparin. Functional assays include heparin-induced platelet aggregation, heparin-induced platelet adenosine triphosphate (ATP) release by lumiaggregometry, ^{14}C-serotonin release assay (^{14}C-SRA) by ELISA, and platelet microparticle formation by flow cytometry. Heparin–platelet factor 4 antibodies are detected by ELISA. When HIT is suspected, heparin should be stopped immediately and be replaced by alternative anticoagulant drugs (danaparoid, argatroban).

Table 19.3 ● Criteria for the Diagnosis of Lupus Anticoagulant

- Prolongation of at least one phospholipid-dependent test
- Lack of correction of mixing studies
- Correction of abnormal result with the addition of excess phospholipids
- Lack of any other specific inhibitor

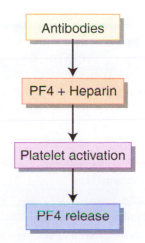

Figure 19.5 Pathophysiology of heparin-induced thrombocytopenia. PF4, platelet factor 4.

Warfarin should be avoided in the acute phase of thrombosis because it may cause venous limb **gangrene**.[1] It is imperative that patients receiving heparin have a baseline platelet count and platelet monitoring every third day between 5 and 14 days.[1]

LABORATORY DIAGNOSIS FOR THROMBOTIC DISORDERS

A wide range of assays is available to evaluate thrombophilia, but these assays are expensive and time-consuming. These laboratory tests should be considered for patients in whom the test results would impact the choice, intensity, and duration of anticoagulant therapy, family planning, and prognosis.[1]

Table 19.4 lists the clinical events that justify laboratory evaluation of thrombophilia. Patients who lack a positive family history should be evaluated for an acquired form of thrombosis such as malignancy, myeloproliferative disorders, and aPL antibodies.[1,7] Laboratory assays should not be done at the time of acute thrombosis or when the patient is receiving any anticoagulant therapy because it may affect the results of the assays.[1] Levels of fibrin degradation products and D-dimer increase in patients with acute VTE. The absence of elevated D-dimer in patients evaluated for acute DVT or PE has an excellent negative predictive value for thrombosis.[1]

Functional tests are preferred over immunologic assays. Table 19.5 summarizes the laboratory screening tests used to evaluate patients suspected to have thrombophilia.

ANTICOAGULANT THERAPY

Thromboembolic diseases are treated with antithrombotic drugs, which include antiplatelet drugs, anticoagulant

---

Table 19.4 ● Conditions That Require Evaluation for Hypercoagulable States

- Recurrent thrombosis in patients younger than 45 years of age
- Patients with a positive family history
- Recurrent spontaneous thromboses
- Thrombosis in unusual sites
- Heparin resistance
- Protein C and protein S deficiency
- Thrombosis associated with pregnancy and estrogen therapy
- Unexplained recurrent pregnancy loss

Table 19.5 ● Screening Laboratory Tests for Thrombophilia

- Activated protein C resistance
- Functional assays for antithrombin, protein C, and protein S
- aPTT, DRVVT, mixing studies, and confirmatory test for lupus anticoagulant
- ELISA for anticardiolipin antibody
- Factor VIII activity

---

drugs, and thrombolytic drugs. Antiplatelet drugs prevent platelet activation and aggregation and are most effective in treating arterial diseases. Anticoagulant drugs inhibit thrombin and fibrin formation and are used commonly for the treatment of venous thrombosis. Thrombolytic drugs are used to break down fibrin clots, restore vascular function, and prevent loss of tissues and organs.

Antiplatelet Drugs

Numerous agents are used against platelets. Aspirin (acetylsalicylic acid) is an antiplatelet drug that irreversibly affects platelet function by inhibiting the cyclooxygenase (COX) enzyme and the formation of thromboxane A_2 (TXA_2). TXA_2 is a potent platelet-activating substance released from activated platelets. Aspirin is rapidly absorbed from the gastrointestinal tract and reaches its peak concentration in plasma 1 hour after ingestion.[1] The effect of aspirin on platelets starts 1 hour after ingestion and lasts for the entire platelet life span (approximately 1 week).[1] Aspirin provides effective treatment of **angina**, acute MI, transient ischemic attack, stroke, arterial **fibrillation**, and thrombi formation due to prostatic heart valve. The minimum effective dosage for these conditions is 75 to 325 mg/day.[1] Aspirin toxicity includes gastrointestinal discomfort, blood loss, and the risk of systemic bleeding. Studies have shown that low-dose aspirin (30 to 75 mg/day) has an antithrombotic effect.[1] Some patients may develop aspirin resistance. Patients who become resistant to aspirin have a higher rate of heart attacks and strokes. Platelet aggregation tests can evaluate aspirin resistance when arachidonic acid reduces aggregation. Other antiplatelet drugs include dipyridamole, thienopyridines, ticlopidine, and clopidogrel.[1]

Anticoagulant Drugs

Anticoagulant drugs are used to prevent and treat thromboembolic disorders. Short-term anticoagulant drugs such as heparin are administered by IV infusion or subcutaneous injection. Long-term anticoagulant drugs such as warfarin (Coumadin) are administered orally.

Unfractionated Heparin Therapy

Heparin is present in human tissue as a naturally occurring, highly sulfated glycosaminoglycan. Commercially unfractionated heparin (UFH) is isolated from bovine lung or porcine intestine. It contains a mixture of polysaccharide chains with a molecular weight of 4,000 to 30,000 daltons.[1] Heparin sulfate is a heparinlike substance made by the vascular endothelium. The anticoagulant activity of heparin is enhanced by binding to AT. Heparin-AT complex inactivates thrombin and factor Xa (see Fig. 19.2). Other clotting factors affected by heparin are factors IXa, XIa, and XIIa.

The half-life of heparin is dose-dependent. Heparin is cleared from the circulation by the reticuloendothelial system and metabolized by the liver.[1] Heparin is given in a weight-adjusted dosage with an initial bolus (5,000 to 10,000 U) followed by continuous low-dose infusion (1,300 U).[8] The therapeutic range of heparin is extremely narrow.

Heparin dosage is monitored by aPTT. The baseline aPTT and platelet count should be performed for each patient before heparin therapy. A prolonged aPTT baseline may be associated with LA or factor deficiencies that could interfere with the laboratory result interpretation.[1,8] During heparin therapy, the aPTT should be repeated every 4 to 6 hours to adjust the dosage to therapeutic level, 1.5 to 2.5 times the mean of the laboratory reference ranges. In addition, the platelet count should be monitored daily. A 40% reduction in platelet count compared with the baseline platelet count is evidence of HIT and requires immediate discontinuation of heparin.

The adverse effects of heparin therapy include bleeding, HIT, and heparin resistance. Heparin resistance may occur as a result of nonspecific binding of heparin to plasma proteins, platelets, and endothelial cells or as a result of AT deficiency.

Monitoring Unfractionated Heparin Therapy

UFH is monitored by aPTT. Because the reagent sensitivity varies among different procedures and lot numbers, the therapeutic values for heparin therapy should be established by each laboratory. The range of therapeutic aPTT values is equivalent to heparin levels of 0.3 to 0.7 U/mL of chromogenic anti–factor Xa.[9] The limitations of using aPTT as a monitoring test include heparin resistance and inflammation associated with

hyperfibrinogenemia. Elevated factor VIII levels tend to shorten the aPTT and make the test less sensitive to heparin therapy. Platelet factor 4 released by activated platelet neutralizes heparin. LA, hypofibrinogenemia, factor deficiency, presence of fibrin degradation products, and paraproteins prolong aPTT independent of heparin therapy.[8] In these situations, chromogenic anti–factor Xa assay can be used to monitor UFH therapy. In anti–factor Xa assay, the concentration of heparin is determined by inhibiting factor Xa by AT. Anti–factor Xa assay uses a reagent with a fixed concentration of factor Xa and AT reagent. Heparin forms a complex with anithrombin and factor Xa reagents. Excess factor Xa combines with the chromogenic substrate to form a colored product; the color intensity is inversely proportional to the concentration of heparin.

Low-Molecular-Weight Heparin Therapy

Low-molecular-weight heparin (LMWH) is derived from UFH via enzymatic digestion to produce smaller low-molecular-weight glycosaminoglycan molecules. The mean weight of LMWH is about 5,000 daltons.[1] LMWH has a longer half-life and low affinity to bind to plasma proteins and endothelial cells.[1,10] The half-life of the drug is not dose-dependent. LMWH is administered subcutaneously once or twice daily based on body weight and does not require monitoring.[1] LMWH has a higher inhibitory effect on factor Xa than on factor IIa.[10] LMWH is cleared by the kidney. The adverse reaction of LMWH includes bleeding, HIT, or sensitivity to LMWH.

Coumadin (Warfarin) Therapy

Coumadin is a vitamin K antagonist drug that inhibits the vitamin K–dependent coagulation factors II, VII, IX, and X. Warfarin is a Coumadin derivative that is widely used in the United States as an oral anticoagulant drug. Warfarin inhibits gamma carboxylation of the vitamin K–dependent clotting factors, reducing their activity, and inhibits vitamin K–dependent anticoagulant proteins such as protein C and protein S. The half-life of warfarin is about 36 hours.[1] Warfarin is given orally as a long-term anticoagulant; the dosage varies from patient to patient and depends on dietary stores of vitamin K, liver function, preexisting medical conditions, and concurrent medications. Warfarin is prescribed prophylactically to prevent thrombosis after trauma or surgery or to prevent strokes in patients with atrial fibrillation. Therapeutic warfarin is used after acute MI to control coagulation. It is also used to prevent recurrence of DVT or PE. The standard warfarin regimen is 5 to 10 mg and varies from patient to patient.[8] The activity of vitamin K–dependent coagulation factors decreases immediately after warfarin therapy. Because of the different half-lives of the vitamin K–dependent clotting factors, however, it takes 4 to 10 days to reach therapeutic levels. Warfarin therapy is monitored by PT and international normalized ratio (INR).

The INR is a method that standardizes PT assays against differences in commercial thromboplastin reagents.[11] The INR was established by the World Health Organization (WHO)[1]; each thromboplastin reagent is calibrated against a WHO reference preparation. The INR is calculated using the following formula: INR = (PT ratio)^{ISI}, where ISI refers to the international sensitivity index, which is calculated for each thromboplastin reagent against a reference thromboplastin reagent.[1]

According to a consensus panel of the American College of Chest Physicians, the therapeutic range of INR is 2.0 to 3.0 for the treatment of VTE. For prosthetic mechanical heart valves and prevention of recurrent MI, a higher dose of warfarin is required to attain an INR of 2.5 to 3.5.[1]

The most common adverse effect of warfarin therapy is bleeding, which is directly dose-related.[11] Patients with an INR of greater than 3.0 are at higher risk of bleeding. Warfarin crosses the placenta and *should be avoided* during pregnancy. Another rare but devastating complication of warfarin therapy is skin necrosis, a phenomenon that mostly occurs in patients who receive high doses of warfarin and may have heterozygous protein C deficiency.[1] Skin necrosis is caused by the rapid decrease in protein C in patients who have preexisting protein C deficiency resulting in a thrombotic state.[1]

Alternative Anticoagulant Drugs

Direct Thrombin Inhibitors

Lepirudin is a recombinant analogue of hirudin. It is used in HIT patients who cannot tolerate UFH or LMWH. A direct thrombin inhibitor (DTI), lepirudin is a large molecule (7,000 daltons) that binds to free thrombin. It is administered intravenously for 2 to 10 days. The half-life of lepirudin is 20 minutes, and it is cleared by the kidneys.[8]

Bivalirudin is a recombinant derivative of hirudin, with molecular weight of 2,180 daltons.[8] It is an alternative drug in patients with HIT. Bivalirudin binds to free and clot-bound thrombin. It is administered intravenously and has a half-life of 25 minutes.

Argatroban is a synthetic arginine derivative with molecular weight of 527 daltons.[8] It is administered intravenously and has a half-life of 51 minutes. Argatroban can be used for prophylaxis, treatment, and anticoagulation during percutaneous coronary procedures in patients with HIT and renal failure who cannot be given hirudin drugs. Direct thrombin inhibitor drugs affect thrombin time (TT), PT, aPTT, and activated clotting time (ACT). aPTT is used to monitor these drugs with the therapeutic range of 1.5 to 3.0 times the mean of the laboratory reference.[8]

Factor Xa Inhibitors

Fondaparinux is a synthetic pentasaccharide that inhibits factor Xa. It binds to AT and enhances its activity to 400-fold. The drug is administered once a day subcutaneously and has a half-life 12 to 17 hours.[8] Fondaparinux is used for surgical prophylaxis and treatment of DVT and PE. aPTT is not sensitive to fondaparinux because it does not react with thrombin. The chromogenic anti–factor Xa assay is used for monitoring therapy for infants, children, pregnant women, and patients who are underweight or overweight. The blood sample is collected 4 hours after injection, and the therapeutic range is 0.14 to 0.19 mg/L.[8]

Thrombolytic Drugs

Thrombolytic drugs are commonly used in acute arterial thrombosis for immediate thrombolysis, restoration of vascular integrity, and prevention of tissue and organ damage. Most fibrinolytic drugs are made by recombinant techniques and are fashioned after tPA and urokinase. tPA binds to fibrin degradation products, activates plasmin, and can cleave fibrinogen with a lesser frequency and severity. Urokinase is not fibrin-specific and causes hypofibrinogenemia by breaking down fibrinogen. Urokinase can be used to treat VTE, MI, and thrombolysis of clotted catheters.[1] Streptokinase is a thrombolytic agent obtained from beta-hemolytic streptococci. Streptokinase is not fibrin-specific, and because it is antigenic, it may cause allergic reactions. Urokinase and streptokinase cause hypofibrinogenemia secondary to fibrinogenolysis; however, the level of hypofibrinogenemia is not clinically significant.

Bleeding is the most common complication associated with thrombolytic drugs. Thrombolytic therapy does not require monitoring. Prior screening tests such as PT, aPTT, TT, fibrinogen, and platelet count may be helpful in predicting patients who are at high risk of bleeding.[3]

CONDENSED CASE

A technical representative for a reference laboratory experienced severe pain in his left knee one day after visiting one of his laboratory accounts. He assumed that the pain may have been related to a recent basketball game. Over the next 24 hours, he had trouble walking, and he noticed that his knee had become swollen, red, and more painful. At this point the patient decided to go to the emergency department for evaluation. *What is your clinical impression?*

Answer

This patient may be experiencing deep vein thrombosis (DVT). On further questioning by the emergency department physician, it was discovered that the patient had done a significant amount of driving during the week while keeping his left knee in a bent position. The laboratory tests revealed that his PT and aPTT results were normal, but the D-dimer result was elevated. The patient was diagnosed with DVT and was treated with LMWH followed by warfarin therapy. His INR was monitored to therapeutic level weekly in an outpatient clinic.

○ *Summary Points*

- Thrombophilia refers to conditions that predispose an individual to thrombosis.
- Risk factors associated with thrombophilia can be divided into environmental, acquired, or inherited risk factors.
- Thrombosis is the formation of blood clots in the vasculature. Thrombosis can be arterial or venous.
- Arterial thrombosis is mainly composed of platelets with small amounts of red blood cells and white blood cells, whereas venous thrombosis is composed of fibrin clots and red blood cells.
- Thrombosis may result from vascular injury, platelet activation, coagulation activation, a defective fibrinolytic system, and defective physiologic inhibitors.
- Physiologic thrombosis results from the body's natural response to vascular injury. It is localized and is formed to prevent excess blood loss.
- Pathologic thrombosis includes DVT, arterial thrombosis, and PE. Pathologic thrombosis may result from acquired or inherited conditions.
- Thromboembolism forms when a clot dislodges from the origination site and is released into the circulation.
- Physiologic anticoagulants including antithrombin (AT), heparin cofactor II, protein C, and protein S are plasma proteins.
- AT is produced in the liver. It inhibits factors IIa, IXa, Xa, XIa, and XIIa. Heparin increases the inhibitory action of AT.

- Protein C is a vitamin K–dependent protein produced in the liver. Protein C is activated by thrombin-thrombomodulin complex. Protein S is a cofactor for protein C activation. Activated protein C deactivates factors Va and VIIIa.
- Inherited risk factors are associated with genetic mutations that result in deficiency of naturally occurring inhibitors such as protein C, protein S, or AT.
- Elevated plasma clotting factors such as prothrombin G20210A or increased factor VIII and fibrinogen are associated with thrombosis.
- Most (92%) cases of activated protein C resistance are inherited and are caused by mutation of factor V Arg506Gln (factor V Leiden).
- Acquired thrombotic disorders are associated with underlying diseases or drugs.
- Antiphospholipid (aPL) syndrome is caused by antibodies against phospholipid-dependent coagulation assays such as aPTT, which are not corrected with 1:1 mix with normal plasma. The most common forms of aPL antibodies are lupus anticoagulant (LA) and anticardiolipin (ACA).
- Laboratory tests for LA include aPTT or DRRVT, mixing studies, and confirmatory studies. ACA are tested by ELISA.
- Heparin-induced thrombocytopenia (HIT) is an immune-mediated thrombotic complication associated with heparin therapy. The antibody is produced against heparin–platelet factor 4 complexes.

- Diagnostic tests for HIT include heparin-dependent platelet activation assays and detection of the antibody by ELISA.

- Antithrombotic drugs include antiplatelet drugs, anticoagulant drugs, and thrombolytic drugs.

- Aspirin is an antiplatelet drug that inhibits the cyclooxygenase (COX) enzyme and prevents formation of thromboxane A_2 (TXA_2). TXA_2 is a potent platelet-activating substance released from the activated platelets.

- Heparin is a short-term anticoagulant drug. It is administered intravenously or intramuscularly.

- Heparin dosage is monitored by aPTT value in the range of 1.5 to 2.5 times the mean of the laboratory reference ranges.

- Coumadin (warfarin) is a vitamin K antagonist drug that inhibits the vitamin K–dependent coagulation factors (II, VII, IX, and X).

- Coumadin is an oral anticoagulant that is administered as a long-term anticoagulant. It is monitored by PT and INR.

- Alternative anticoagulants are used in patients with HIT who cannot tolerate UFH or LMWH.

- Thrombolytic drugs include tPA, urokinase, and streptokinase.

CASE STUDY

A 30-year-old woman was referred to the hospital for evaluation. She presented with a history of multiple spontaneous abortions. She is currently complaining of pain and swelling in her left thigh. Her family history and her past medical history were unremarkable. The patient is currently on oral contraceptives. The patient's laboratory results were as follows:

WBC	8.0×10^9/L (reference range 4.4 to 11.0×10^9/L)
RBC	4.7×10^{12}/L (reference range 4.1 to 5.1×10^{12}/L)
Hgb	14.0 g/dL (reference range 12.3 to 15.3 g/dL)
Hct	43% (reference range 36% to 45%)
Platelets	250×10^9/L (reference range 150 to 400×10^9/L)
PT	13.5 seconds (reference range 10.9 to 12.0 seconds)
aPTT	52 seconds (reference range 34 to 38 seconds)
DRVVT	Prolonged
aPTT 1:1 mixing study	Not corrected immediately and after 2 hours' incubation
DRVVT Confirm	Corrected (with excess phospholipids)
ACA	Present

Insights to the Case Study

The diagnosis of lupus anticoagulant (LA) was made based on physical findings, the patient's history, and laboratory results. Physical findings revealed that the patient had had multiple fetal losses and had pain and swelling in her thigh at the time of medical evaluation. The lack of a positive family history with thrombosis ruled out any inherited thrombotic disorder. Her platelet count was normal, indicating that the thrombotic episodes are not related to any cause of platelet activation.

aPTT and DRVVT were prolonged; however, the patient did not have any bleeding problems. A prolonged aPTT and DRVVT in the absence of bleeding ruled out any clotting factor deficiency. Mixing study with normal plasma differentiated factor deficiency from an inhibitor. The absence of bleeding ruled out factor VIII inhibitor. LA was against in vitro phospholipid-dependent tests. In DRVVT confirmatory tests, excess phospholipids were added to the test system to neutralize the lupus antibodies and correct the prolonged DRVVT initially done.

The platelet neutralization test is another confirmatory test used to confirm LA. This test is used for correction of prolonged aPTT in patients with LA, which belongs to a group of antibodies called antiphospholipid antibodies that also includes anticardiolipin antibodies (ACA). Because LA may coexist with ACA in some patients, it is important to test for both antibodies when LA is suspected.

ACA can be detected by ELISA and was positive in this patient. She was put on warfarin (Coumadin) treatment and monitored by INR.

Review Questions

1. The primary inhibitor of the fibrinolytic system is
   a. antiplasmin.
   b. protein S.
   c. antithrombin.
   d. protein C.

2. Dilute Russell's viper venom test (DRVVT) is helpful in the diagnosis of
   a. HIT.
   b. factor VIII inhibitor.
   c. lupus anticoagulant.
   d. ACA.

3. The lupus anticoagulant is directed against
   a. phospholipid-dependent coagulation tests.
   b. factor VIII.
   c. fibrinogen.
   d. vitamin K–dependent clotting factors.

4. Which statement is correct regarding warfarin (Coumadin)?
   a. It is used to treat bleeding disorders.
   b. It acts on factors IX, X, XI, and XII.
   c. It is used for short-term therapy.
   d. It acts on vitamin K–dependent clotting factors.

5. Which statement is correct regarding protein C?
   a. It is a cofactor to protein S.
   b. Its activity is inhibited by heparin.
   c. It forms a complex with antithrombin.
   d. It is a physiologic inhibitor of coagulation.

6. Activated protein C resistance is associated with
   a. mutation of factor VIII.
   b. deletion of factor VI.
   c. mutation of factor V.
   d. deletion of factor VIII.

7. Thrombin-thrombomodulin complex is necessary for
   a. activation of protein C.
   b. activation of antithrombin.
   c. activation of protein S.
   d. activation of factors V and VIII.

8. Heparin-induced thrombocytopenia is caused by
   a. antibody to platelet factor 4.
   b. antibody to heparin–platelet factor 4 complex.
   c. lupus anticoagulant.
   d. antibody to heparin.

9. Which of the following drugs would put an individual at risk for thrombosis?
   a. Aspirin
   b. Dipyridamole
   c. Streptokinase
   d. Oral contraceptives

10. Which of the following results are correct regarding lupus inhibitors?
    a. Prolonged aPTT on undiluted plasma and 1:1 mix of patient plasma with normal plasma
    b. Corrected aPTT on a 1:1 mix of patient plasma with normal plasma after 2 hours' incubation
    c. Normal undiluted aPTT and prolonged aPTT on a 1:1 mix of patient plasma with normal plasma
    d. Normal undiluted aPTT and 1:1 mix of patient plasma with normal plasma

o PROBLEMSOLVING

What Should Be Done When the Clinical Presentation and Laboratory Results Indicate That the Patient Is Not Responding to Heparin Therapy?

A patient who was in a car accident was admitted to an emergency department with multiple fractures. Routine preoperative laboratory tests were performed, and the results were as follows:

Platelet count	160 × 10⁹/L (reference range 150 to 400 × 10⁹/L)

PT   12 seconds (reference range 10 to 13 seconds)

aPTT   32 seconds (reference range 28 to 37 seconds)

The patient underwent surgery for the fractures and was put on heparin to prevent thrombosis.

The aPTT test was repeated every 4 hours after heparin therapy was initiated to adjust the dosages. After 4 days on heparin therapy, the patient complained of pain and swelling in his leg, his platelet

Continued

count decreased to 80×10^9/L, and his aPTT result was 34 seconds.

The clinical presentations and the lack of response to heparin therapy in this patient indicate HIT. Heparin therapy should be discontinued immediately and replaced by alternative anticoagulant drugs such as danaparoid, argatroban, or other similar drugs. The patient should not be exposed to any other heparin-related treatment, such as intravenous catheter flushes, heparin-coated indwelling catheters, and LMWH. Laboratory tests such as platelet activation assay or heparin–platelet factor 4 antibody detection by ELISA, which tests for the presence of antibodies, should be performed to confirm the diagnosis. Other causes for the lack of response to heparin therapy include antithrombin deficiency; other unreported heparin use, such as heparin flushes; increased plasma fibrinogen; increased factor VIII; and platelet factor 4 released from activated platelets.

WORD KEY

Angina • Oppressive pain or pressure in the chest caused by inadequate blood flow and oxygenation to the heart muscle

Atherosclerosis • Cholesterol-lipid-calcium deposits in the walls of arteries

Fibrillation • Usually refers to a cardiac fluttering caused by faulty electric supply to the heart

Gangrene • Death of tissue usually resulting from deficient or absent blood supply

Necrosis • Death of cells, tissue, or organs

Purpura fulminans • Rapidly progressing form of purpura occurring principally in children; of short duration and frequently fatal

Vasculitis • Inflammation of the blood vessels.

Venogram • Radiograph of the veins

References

1. Deitcher SR, Rodgers GM. Thrombosis and antithrombotic therapy. In: Greer JP, et al, eds. Wintrobe's Clinical Hematology, 11th ed, Vol 2. Philadelphia: Lippincott Williams & Wilkins, 2004: 1714–1750.
2. Goodnight SH, Griffin JH. Hereditary thrombophilia. In: Williams WJ, et al, eds. Hematology, 6th ed. New York: McGraw-Hill, 2001: 1697–1706.
3. Ehsan A, Herrick, JL. Introduction to thrombosis and anticoagulant therapy. In: Harmening D, ed. Clinical Hematology and Fundamentals of Hemostasis, 5th ed. Philadelphia: FA Davis, 2009: 662–689.
4. Bauer KA. Inherited disorders of thrombosis and fibrinolysis. In: Nathan DG, et al, eds. Hematology of Infancy and Childhood, 6th ed, Vol 2. Philadelphia: WB Saunders, 2003: 1583–1659.
5. Rand JH. Lupus anticoagulant and related disorders. In: Williams WJ, et al, eds. Hematology, 6th ed. New York: McGraw-Hill, 2001: 1715–1727.
6. Konkle BA, Palermo C. Laboratory evaluation of the hypercoagulable state. In: Spandofer J, Konkle BA, Merli GJ, eds. Management and Prevention of Thrombosis in Primary Care. New York: Oxford University Press, 2001: 16–25.
7. Bauer KA. Approach to thrombosis. In: Loscalzo J, Schafer AI, eds. Thrombosis and Hemostasis, 3rd ed. Philadelphia: Lippincott Williams & Wilkins, 2003: 330–340.
8. Fritsma GA. Monitoring anticoagulant therapy. In: Rodak BF, Fritsma GA, Doig K, eds. Hematology, Clinical and Application, 3rd ed. Philadelphia: WB Saunders, 2007: 700–711.
9. Haire WD. Deep venous thrombosis and pulmonary embolus. In: Kitchens CS, Alving BM, Kessler CM, eds. Consultative Hemostasis and Thrombosis. Philadelphia: WB Saunders, 2002: 197–221.
10. Merli G. Prophylaxis for deep vein thrombosis and pulmonary embolism in the surgical and medical patient. In: Spandofer J, Konkle BA, Merli GJ, eds. Management and Prevention of Thrombosis in Primary Care. New York: Oxford University Press, 2001: 135–147.
11. Schulman. Oral anticoagulation. In: Williams WJ, et al, eds. Hematology, 6th ed. New York: McGraw-Hill, 2001: 1777–1786.

Part V

Laboratory Procedures

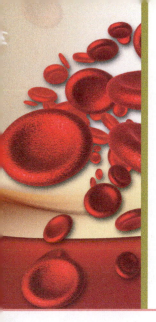

Chapter 20

Basic Procedures in a Hematology Laboratory

Kathleen Finnegan, Betty Ciesla, and Lori Lentowski

Peripheral Smear Procedure

Principle

Reagents and Equipment

Specimen Collection and Storage

Quality Control

Procedure

Limitations

Performing a Manual Differential and Assessing Red Blood Cell Morphology

Principle

Reagents and Equipment

Specimen Collection and Storage

Quality Control

Procedure

Unopette White Blood Cell and Platelet Count

Principle

Reagents and Equipment

Specimen Collection and Storage

Quality Control

Procedure

Cell Counts and Calculations

Normal Ranges

Limitations

Sickle Cell Screening Procedure

Principle

Reagents and Equipment

Specimen Collection and Storage

Quality Control

Procedure

Interpretation of Results and Result Reporting

Limitations

Cerebrospinal Fluid and Body Fluid Cell Count and Differential

Principle

Reagents and Equipment

Specimen Collection and Storage

Quality Control

Procedure

Prothrombin Time and Activated Partial Thromboplastin Time: Automated Procedure

Principle

Reagents and Equipment

Specimen Collection and Storage

Quality Control

Procedure

Results

Limitations

Qualitative D-Dimer Test

Principle

Reagents and Equipment

Specimen Collection and Storage

Quality Control

Procedure

Interpretation

Results

Limitations

Special Testing in Coagulation: An Overview

Mixing Studies

Thrombin Time

Reptilase Time

Dilute Russell's Viper Venom Tests

Hematology Automation: General Principles of Operation

Electrical Impedance

Histograms

Radiofrequency

Opacity

Scatterplot

Optical Scatter

VCS Technology (Volume, Conductivity, and Scatter)

Hydrodynamic Focusing

Flow Cytometry

Instruments

Data Reporting

Quality Assurance and Quality Control

Flow Cytometry Instrumentation

Sample Preparation

Principles of Operation

Fluidics

Optics

Electronics

Analysis

Quality Control

Applications of Flow Cytometry

The following procedures are representative of *basic methods* employed in hematology laboratories and have been written in Standard Operating Procedure (SOP) format. We hope they will provide a ready reference and give students the opportunity to preview how a procedure would be introduced into the clinical setting. In addition to the SOPs, specific manufacturer's instructions on instrumentation and reagents would be strictly followed in a working clinical laboratory.

Information on scatterplots and flow cytometry is presented at the end of this chapter. This information is fairly basic and serves only to kindle students' interest and expose them to this subject matter. No attempt has been made to create comprehensive coverage of these areas.

MICROHEMATOCRIT

Principle

The hematocrit, or packed cell volume, measures the concentration of red blood cells in a given volume of whole blood in a capillary tube. This volume is measured after appropriate centrifugation time and is expressed as a percentage of the total blood sample volume. A whole blood sample in an anticoagulated capillary tube is centrifuged at 10,000 to 13,000 rpm for 5 minutes. Erythrocytes are packed at the bottom of the capillary tube, and the hematocrit is expressed as a measurement of this level compared with the plasma level. A buffy coat composed of leukocytes and platelets marks the interface between plasma and red blood cells. The hematocrit percentage is read below the buffy coat layer. A microhematocrit value can assist in evaluating fluid status, in clarifying various degrees of anemia, and in monitoring acute hemorrhagic conditions.

Reagents and Equipment

1. Microhematocrit centrifuge (Fig. 20.1)
2. Microhematocrit reader disc
3. Capillary tubes (Fig. 20.2)
    a. Plain-blue tip for ethylenediamine-tetraacetic acid (EDTA) tubes
    b. Heparinized-red tip for capillary collection specimens
    Note: Both types of tubes contain self-sealing clay.
4. Mechanical rocker

Specimen Collection and Storage

1. Fresh whole blood collected in EDTA in which the patient tube is at least half full
2. Capillary blood collected in an EDTA Microtainer

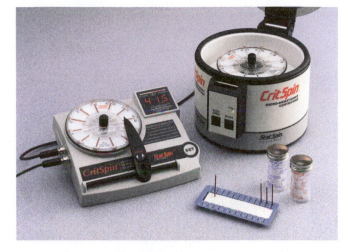

Figure 20.1 Standard microhematocrit centrifuge. Maximum packing time depends on a calibrated centrifuge.

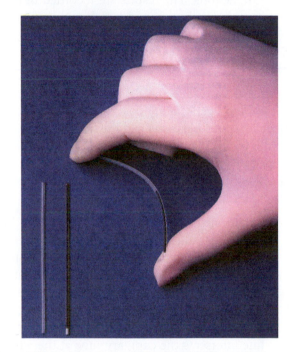

Figure 20.2 Standard and flexible capillary tubes.

3. Capillary blood collected directly into heparinized capillary tubes

Quality Control

Hematocrits are run in duplicate and must agree within ±1%.

Procedure

1. Mix EDTA tube by placing on a mechanical rocker for 3 minutes.
2. After adequate mixing, fill the self-sealing plain capillary tubes two-thirds to three-fourths full. Prepare the tubes in duplicate.

3. Wipe the outside of the capillary tubes with lint-free wipe or gauze.
4. Invert the tube so that the blood runs to sealed end.
5. Place the tubes directly across from each other in the microhematocrit centrifuge, with the sealed ends away from the center of centrifuge.
6. Record the identification and the position number of each patient specimen.
7. Place the head cover and tighten by hand only. Close the outer lid and lock.
8. Centrifuge for 5 minutes, for maximum packing.
9. Remove the tubes from the centrifuge and place in the microhematocrit reader. Read the hematocrit according to the manufacturer's instructions. The results are recorded in percent. The tubes should match within ±1%.

Instructions for the Mechanical Reader

The spun capillary tube should have three visible sections: red blood cells, buffy coat (contains leukocytes and platelets), and plasma. Read the hematocrit results by placing the centrifuged capillary tube in the groove of the plastic indicator reader. The bottom of the red blood cell column should meet with the black line on the plastic indicator (Fig. 20.3).

1. Rotate the bottom plate so that the 100% line is directly beneath the red line on the plastic indicator and hold the bottom plate in this position. With use of the finger hole, rotate the top plate so that the spiral line intersects the capillary tube at the plasma air space.
2. Rotate both discs together until the spiral line intersects the capillary tube at the white blood cell–red blood cell line.
3. The volume of red blood cell is read in percentage from the point on the scale directly beneath the red line of the plastic indicator. The hematocrit percentage is read between the red blood cell column and the clear plasma column.

Notes

- Buffy coats are not included as part of the red blood cell column.
- Repeat procedure if specimen has leaked in the centrifuge.
- Repeat procedure if centrifuge has been stopped manually.
- Repeat if difference between tubes is greater than 1%.

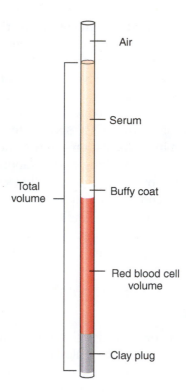

Figure 20.3 Capillary tubes. Note the distinct layers after blood sample has been spun.

Normal Average Values

Newborns: 53% to 65%

Men: 42% to 52%

Women: 37% to 47%

MODIFIED WESTERGREN SEDIMENTATION RATE

Principle

The erythrocyte sedimentation rate (ESR) is a nonspecific screening test that indicates inflammation. It is used as an initial screening tool and as a follow-up test to monitor therapy and progression or remission of disease. This test measures the distance that red blood cells fall in a vertical tube over a given time period. The ESR is directly proportional to red blood cell mass and inversely proportional to its surface area. The ESR is reported in millimeters/hour. Any condition that will increase rouleaux formation will usually increase the settling of red blood cells. Factors affecting the ESR are as follows:

- Red blood cell shape and size: Specimens containing sickle cells, acanthocytes, or spherocytes settle slowly and give a decreased ESR.
- Plasma fibrinogen and globulin levels: Increased fibrinogen or globulin levels cause increased settling and give an increased ESR.

- Mechanical and technical conditions: Surfaces that are not level, influence red blood cell settling. Specimens that are not properly anticoagulated also affect red blood cell settling. EDTA is the recommended anticoagulant.

Reagents and Equipment

1. Sediplast Autozero Westergren ESR system (Fig. 20.4)
   a. Fixed bore pipettes
   b. Sedivials filled with 0.2 mL of 3.8% sodium citrate
   c. Vial holder (rack)
2. Disposable plastic pipettes
3. Rotator/mixer
4. Timer

Specimen Collection and Storage

Specimens are collected in EDTA. Tubes must be at least half full, well mixed, and free of clots and fibrin. ESR can be set up on specimens at room temperature up to 4 hours old. Refrigerated specimens (2 to 8°C) can be set up until 24 hours old.

Quality Control

Commercially prepared controls stored at 2 to 8°C are valid until expiration date. Controls are prepared the same as patients' specimens. Controls are run once daily before setting up patient tests. Do not report out patient results unless controls are in reference range.

Procedure

1. Mix the EDTA tube on the rotator/mixer for a minimum of 5 minutes. If the sample has been refrigerated, allow 30 minutes for the sample to come to room temperature before proceeding.
2. Remove the top of the Sediplast vial, which contains 3.8% sodium citrate. Using a disposable pipette, add blood to the indicated line, return the top, and mix thoroughly.
3. Insert Westergren tube into Sediplast vial with a slight twist, allowing the blood to rise to the zero mark.
4. Place the vial in the rack on a level surface.
5. Set a timer for 1 hour and read at the end of the hour.
6. Record the ESR in millimeters per hour.

Normal Ranges

Men: 0 to 15 mm/hr; 0 to 20 mm/hr if older than 50 years

Women: 0 to 20 mm/hr; 0 to 30 mm/hr if older than 50 years

Limitations

1. Tubes not filled properly yield erroneous results.
2. Refrigerated specimens must come to room temperature for 30 minutes before testing.
3. The ESR rack must be on a level surface and free of vibration. Vibration can cause a falsely increased ESR.
4. Cold agglutinins can cause a falsely elevated ESR. An ESR can be performed at 37°C (incubator) for 60 minutes with no ill effects.
5. Cell size and shape affect ESR, usually resulting in a decreased ESR result.
6. Increased rouleaux formation, excessive globulin, or increased fibrinogen increases the ESR.
7. Specimen must be free of clots and fibrin.
8. A tilted ESR tube gives erroneous results.
9. Hemolyzed samples are unacceptable.
10. Refrigerated specimens older than 24 hours are unacceptable.

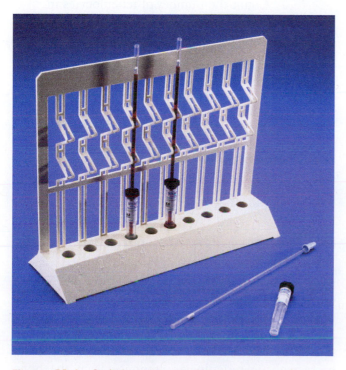

Figure 20.4 Sediplast ESR rack. The sample must be placed on a level surface with no vibration.

Conditions Associated With ...

Increased ESR

1. Kidney disease
2. Pregnancy
3. Rheumatic fever
4. Rheumatoid arthritis
5. Anemia
6. Syphilis
7. Systemic lupus erythematosus
8. Thyroid disease
9. Elevated room temperature

Decreased ESR

1. Congestive heart failure
2. Hyperviscosity
3. Decreased fibrinogen levels
4. Polycythemia
5. Sickle cell anemia

Note: A rapid ESR method (**ESR Stat Plus**) is now available, which gives a result in 3 minutes.

MANUAL RETICULOCYTE PROCEDURE

Principle

The reticulocyte count is an index of bone marrow red blood cell production. The reticulocyte is the cell stage immediately before the mature erythrocyte. This cell spends 2 to 3 days maturing in the bone marrow before it is released into the peripheral circulation, where it spends an additional day of maturation. The reticulocyte count is the most effective measure of erythropoietic activity. Reticulocytes contain RNA and can be observed and quantified using supravital stains such as New Methylene Blue or Brilliant Cresyl Blue. Low reticulocyte counts indicate decreased erythropoietic activity. Increased reticulocyte counts indicate increased erythropoietic activity, usually as the bone marrow compensates in response to anemic stress. Reticulocyte counts are a reflection of bone marrow health or injury. These counts assist physicians in diagnosis, treatment, or monitoring of patients with various anemias.

Reagents and Equipment

1. New Methylene Blue (Supravital Stain)
2. Test tubes
3. Microscope slides with a frosted end
4. Microscope with 100× (oil immersion objective)
5. Transfer pipettes

Specimen Collection and Storage

1. One EDTA tube or EDTA Microtainer
2. Specimens can be stored at room temperature for 8 hours or refrigerated at 2 to 8°C for 24 hours.

Quality Control

Commercially prepared controls are performed each day when reticulocytes are reported manually. Controls are prepared the same as the patient specimens, and the procedure described subsequently for counting reticulocytes is followed. Do not report out patient results until quality control results fall within the acceptable reference range.

Procedure

1. Mix 4 drops of New Methylene Blue with 4 drops of patient's blood. If the specimen is a small amount (such as for a Microtainer), add an equal amount of stain to the Microtainer after the CBC has been completed.
2. Let the specimen mix for 10 to 15 minutes. Make a wedge smear and let it air dry. Label the smears with the patient's name, specimen number, and date.
3. Read under the microscope using 100× oil immersion.
   a. Count the number of reticulocytes in 1,000 cells.
   b. Use the following formula to calculate the percentage of reticulocytes:

Reticulocyte % = number of reticulocytes counted per 1000 cells × 100/1000

Example: 35 × 100/1000 = 3.5%

Normal Ranges

Adults: 0.5% to 2.0%

Infants: 2.0% to 6.0%

Reticulocyte Production Index

Additional information may be gained by reporting the reticulocyte count as the **reticulocyte production index** (RPI). This calculation uses the reticulocyte percentage, the patient's hematocrit, the normal hematocrit (45%), and the reticulocyte maturation time. The calculation is valuable because it gives a more realistic reticulocyte response from the bone marrow factors such as reduced hematocrit. Given the following hematocrits, the reticulocyte maturation time (RMT) is:

If Hct = 45%, RMT = 1 day

If Hct = 24%, RMT = 2.0 days

If Hct = 15%, RMT = 3.0 days

Therefore:

RPI = % reticulocytes × patient hematocrit

Reticulocyte maturation time × 45

Example: RPI = $\dfrac{10\% \times 25\% \div 45\%}{3.0}$ = 1.8

Range = greater than 2.0 to 3.0 indicates hemolytic state

Conditions Associated With ...

Decreased Reticulocyte Count

1. Aplastic anemia
2. Exposure to radiation or radiation therapy
3. Chronic infection
4. Medications such as azathioprine, chloramphenicol, dactinomycin, methotrexate, and other chemotherapy medications
5. Untreated pernicious anemia or megaloblastic anemia

Increased Reticulocyte Count

1. Rapid blood loss
2. High elevation
3. Hemolytic anemias
4. Medications such as levodopa, malarial medications, corticotropin, and fever-reducing medications
5. Pregnancy

Limitations

1. Recent blood transfusion can interfere with accurate reticulocyte results.
2. Mishandling, contamination, or inadequate refrigeration of the sample can cause inaccurate test results.
3. Red blood cell inclusions such as Heinz bodies, siderocytes, and Howell-Jolly bodies can be mistaken for reticulocytes. When counted as reticulocytes, these bodies falsely increase the reticulocyte count. Inclusions should be confirmed with Wright's stain.

RETICULOCYTE PROCEDURE WITH MILLER EYE DISC

Principle

A Miller Eye Disc is placed inside the microscope eyepiece as an aid to counting reticulocytes. This device is a large square with a small square inside. It provides the technologist with the ability to isolate the reticulocytes while counting. Reagent and equipment, quality control, and specimen collection and storage are identical to the manual reticulocyte count.

Procedure

1. Mix 4 drops of New Methylene Blue with 4 drops of patient blood in a test tube. If the specimen amount is small (such as for a Microtainer), add an equal amount of stain to the Microtainer after completing the CBC.
2. Let the specimen incubate for 10 to 15 minutes. Remix the specimen and make an appropriate smear with feathered edges. Label the slides with the patient's name, specimen number, and date.
3. Allow the smear to dry completely and read the slides under the microscope with oil immersion using the Miller Eye Disc (Fig. 20.5).
   a. The Miller Eye Disc is a counting aid that provides a standardized area in which to count red blood cells. Two squares make up the disc. Square 1 is 9× the area of square 2.
   b. Using the disc, count all reticulocytes in the large (1) and small (2) squares. Count only red blood cells in the small square.
   c. Count 111 red blood cells in the small square while counting the number of reticulocytes in the entire square.
   d. Use this formula to calculate the percentage of reticulocytes. See the following example.

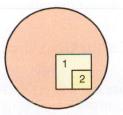

Figure 20.5 Miller Eye Disc. Count red blood cells only in the small square; reticulocytes are counted in both squares.

% Reticulocytes = Total number of reticulocytes counted in large square × 100/Total red blood cells in small square × 9

Example: 40 × 100/999 = 4.0%

Normal Ranges

Adults: 0.5% to 2.0%

Infants: 2.0% to 6.0%

See automated reticulocyte information on page 327.

PERIPHERAL SMEAR PROCEDURE

Principle

When automated differentials do not meet specified criteria programmed into the automated hematology instrument, the technologist/technician must perform a manual differential count from a prepared smear. There are two types of blood smears: wedge smear and spun smear. This procedure discusses the wedge smear. Smears are prepared by placing a drop of blood on a clean glass slide and spreading the drop using another glass slide held at an angle. The slide is then stained and observed microscopically. A well-stained peripheral smear shows the red blood cell background as red-orange. White blood cells appear with blue-purple nuclei and red-purple granules throughout the cytoplasm. A well-prepared, well-distributed peripheral smear has a counting area at the thin portion of the wedge smear, which is approximately 200 red blood cells not touching. A good counting area is an essential ingredient in a peripheral smear for evaluating the numbers of and types of white blood cells present and for evaluating red blood cell and platelet morphology.

Reagents and Equipment

1. Glass slides (frosted)
2. Wooden applicator sticks
3. DIFF-SAFE device (an apparatus designed to avoid removing the tube top)

Specimen Collection and Storage

1. EDTA specimen or EDTA Microtainer
2. Smears are made from EDTA
   a. Microtainers within 1 hour of collection
   b. EDTA blood within 2 to 3 hours
   c. Check all Microtainers for clots with applicator sticks

Quality Control

A random slide is selected after it has been stained and a technologist/technician checks the quality of the stain for white blood cells, red blood cells, platelets, and cell distribution (see Principle).

Procedure

1. Hold the tube in an upright position and insert the DIFF-SAFE dispenser through the stopper.
2. Turn the tube upside down and apply pressure at the frosted end of the slide. Discontinue pressure when the drop of blood appears.
3. Using a second slide (spreader slide), place the edge of the second slide against the surface of the first slide at an angle between 30 degrees and 45 degrees (Fig. 20.6).
4. Bring the spreader slide back into the blood drop until contact is made with the drop of blood.
5. Move the spreader slide forward on the slide and make a smear that is approximately 3 to 4 cm in length. The smear should be half the length of the slide, with no ridges and a "feathered edge" toward the end of the smear.

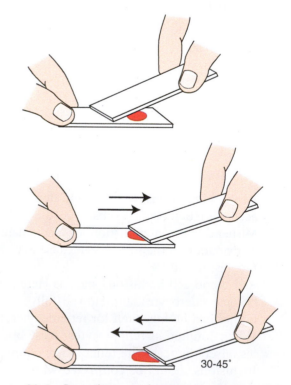

30-45°

Figure 20.6 Preparing a wedge-type smear. Size of drop and angle of spread are important features.

6. Label the frosted end of the slide with the patient's last name and first initial, specimen number, and date.
7. Allow the smear to air dry completely.
8. Proceed with staining. Manual Wright's stain is not found often in the clinical laboratory setting. Most clinical laboratories have an automated staining instrument attached to their automated CBC analyzer. If there is no automated stainer attached to the analyzer, a separate staining instrument may be used for slide staining.

Limitations

1. The angle of the spreader slide depends on the size of the blood drop and viscosity of the blood. The optimal angle is 45 degrees.
2. The larger the drop of blood and smaller the hematocrit, the greater the necessary angle needs to be to ensure that the blood smear is not too long.
3. Blood with a larger hematocrit requires a smaller angle to avoid a smear that is not too short and thick.
4. Glass slides must be clean; otherwise, cell distribution will be imperfect, resulting in improper staining.
5. The smear must be made immediately once the blood drop makes contact with the slide. Otherwise, the blood will clump and dry, resulting in uneven distribution of white blood cells and platelets.

PERFORMING A MANUAL DIFFERENTIAL AND ASSESSING RED BLOOD CELL MORPHOLOGY

Principle

Blood samples evaluated by automated hematology analyzers include automated differentials. Because the institution programs specific criteria pertaining to normal, abnormal, and critical values into the hematology analyzers, differentials that do not meet these criteria require verification. This verification is done by performing manual differentials and evaluating the peripheral smear further. First, a WBC differential is performed to determine the relative number of each type of white blood cell present. Technologists/technicians must recognize and record properly the types of white blood cell observed. Simultaneously, significant red blood cell, white blood cell, and platelet morphology is noted and recorded, and the technologist/technician makes a rough estimate of platelets and WBC to determine whether these numbers generally correlate with the automated hematology analyzer. Technologists/technicians must be proficient at recognizing red blood cell and white blood cell abnormalities, identifying them correctly, and quantifying them.

Reagents and Equipment

1. Microscope
2. Immersion oil
3. Differential cell counter

Specimen Collection and Storage

A well-made stained blood smear should be obtained from a capillary puncture or an EDTA tube at least three-fourths full.

Quality Control

The slide should have three zones: head, body, and tail (Fig. 20.7). Neutrophils and monocytes predominate in the tail area, whereas red blood cells lie singly. Lymphocytes predominate in the body area, and red blood cells overlap to some extent.

1. White blood cells should contain a blue nucleus along with a lighter staining cytoplasm.
2. Red blood cells should have good quality of color ranging from buff pink to orange.
3. Platelets should be blue with granules and no nucleus.

Procedure

Observations Under 10×

1. Place a well-stained slide on the stage of the microscope, smear side up, and focus using the low-power objective (10×).
2. Check for the availability of good counting areas, free of ragged edges and cell clumps.
3. Check the white blood cell distribution over the smear.

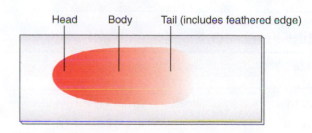

Figure 20.7 Three zones of wedge preparation.

4. Check that the slide is properly stained.
5. Check for the presence of large platelets, platelet clumps, and fibrin strands.

Observations Under 40×: White Blood Cell Estimates

1. Place a drop of immersion oil on the slide and change the objective to 50× oil. (In cases where no 50× is available, use the 40× high dry, with no oil.)
2. Choose a portion of the peripheral smear that has only slight overlapping of red blood cells. Count 10 fields, take the total number of white blood cells and divide by 10, and refer to Table 20.1 to determine the WBC estimate.
3. An alternative technique is to do a white blood cell estimate by taking the average number of white blood cells and multiplying by 2,000.

Observations Under 100×: Platelet Estimates

1. Platelet estimates are done under 100× with the red blood cells barely touching, approximately 200 red blood cells. On average, there are 8 to 20 platelets per field. See Table 20.2.
2. Count 10 fields using the zigzag method, going back and forth lengthwise or sideways (Fig. 20.8).
   Platelets per *oil immersion field* (OIF)
   Fewer than 8 platelets/OIF = decreased
   8 to 20 platelets/OIF = adequate
   More than 20 platelets/OIF = increased
3. After counting the 10 fields, divide the total number of platelets by 10 to get the average. Next, multiply the average number by a factor of 20,000 for wedge preparations. For

Table 20.1 ● Estimated White Blood Cell Count From Peripheral Smear	
White Blood Cells/ High-Power Field	**Estimated WBC**
2–4	4.0–7.0 × 10^9/L
4–6	7.0–10.0 × 10^9/L
6–10	10.0–13.0 × 10^9/L
10–20	13.0–18.0 × 10^9/L

Table 20.2 ● Platelet Estimate From Peripheral Smear	
Average No. Platelets per 100× Field	**Platelet Count Estimate**
0–1	Less than 20,000/L
1–4	20,000–80,000/L
5–8	100,000–160,000/L
10–15	200,000–300,000/L
16–20	320,000–400,000/L
Greater than 21	Greater than 420,000/L

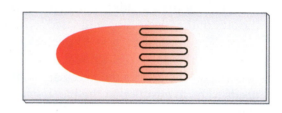
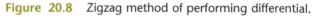

Figure 20.8 Zigzag method of performing differential.

automated monolayer preparations, use a factor of 15,000.

Example: 120 platelets/10 fields = 12 platelets per field

12 × 20,000 = 240,000 platelets

Manual Differential Counts

1. These counts are done in the same area as white blood cell and platelet estimates, with the red blood cells barely touching.
2. The count takes place under 50× or 100× (oil), using the zigzag method previously described in the platelet estimate (see Fig. 20.8).
3. Count 100 white blood cells including all cell lines from immature to mature. Table 20.3 shows normal values for white blood cells.

Observing and Recording Nucleated Red Blood Cells

1. Newer hematology analyzers include a count if nucleated red blood cells are observed. The WBC is automatically corrected. This section is intended as instructional and is useful if the instrument does not include a nucleated red blood cell channel. If nucleated red

Table 20.3 ○ Normal Differential Results in Adults and Infants		
White Blood Cell Type	**Adult**	**Infant**
Segmented neutrophils	50%–70%	20%–44%
Bands	2%–6%	0%–5%
Lymphocytes	20%–44%	48%–78%
Monocytes	2%–9%	2%–11%
Eosinophils	0%–4%	1%–4%
Basophils	0%–2%	0%–2%

blood cells are observed while performing the differential, they need to be reported. These elements in a peripheral smear are indicative of increased erythropoietic activity and usually a pathologic condition. Additionally, the presence of nucleated red blood cells per 100 white blood cells falsely elevates the WBC and is clinically significant.

2. Correct the WBC if the nucleated red blood cell count is greater than 5 nucleated red blood cells/100. *Note:* Some institutions correct the WBC if any nucleated red blood cell is observed. The following formula is applied for correcting nucleated red blood cells:

WBC × 100/nucleated red blood cell + 100

Example: If WBC = 5000 and 10 nucleated red blood cells have been counted

Then

5000 × 100/110 = 4545.50

The corrected WBC is 4.545 × 10^9/L.

Recording Red Blood Cell Morphology

1. Scan area using 50× or 100× (oil immersion).
2. Observe 10 fields.
3. Red blood cells are observed for size, color, hemoglobin content or pallor, and shape.
4. Normal morphology
   a. Normocytic: Normal cell size and shape
   b. Normochromic: Normal hemoglobin content and color
5. Abnormal morphology: Red blood cell morphology is assessed according to size, shape, hemoglobin content, and presence or absence of inclusions. See the following

sample grading system. Red blood cell morphology must be scanned in a good counting area.

Two questions should be asked:

- Is the morphology seen in every field?
- Is the morphology pathologic and not artificially induced?

Table 20.4 represents a system derived to determine a quantitative scale.

a. **Red blood cell size**. *Anisocytosis* is a term meaning variation in the size of the red blood cells. The average size of a red blood cell is 7.2 μm (range 6.8 to 7.5 μm).
   - Normocyte: Normal size of red blood cell
   - Macrocyte: Larger than the normal red blood cell (greater than 8.2 μm)
   - Microcytic: Smaller than the normal red blood cell (less than 7.2 μm)

b. **Shape**. *Poikilocytosis* is the variation in shape from normal mature erythrocytes, which are round, biconcave discs. Variation in red blood cell morphology may be due to pathologic conditions of the red blood cell.
   - Acanthocytes: Thorny projections distributed irregularly around the red blood cell, which lacks central pallor.
   - Burr cells (echinocytes): Short and spikelike projections distributed evenly around the cell membrane.
   - Ovalocyte (elliptocyte): Elongated oval cell.
   - Schistocytes: Red blood cell fragments that are irregular in shape and size. They are usually half the size of the normal red blood cell; therefore, they have a deeper red color.

Table 20.4 ○ Qualitative Grading of Red Blood Cell Morphology	
	Grade Degree of Size and Shape Abnormalities
1–5 cells/10 fields	Slight
6–15 cells/10 fields	Moderate
Greater than 15 cells/ 10 fields	Marked

- Sickle cells: Crescent-shaped cells, usually with one pointed end.
- Spherocytes: Red blood cells that lack central pallor or biconcave discs. They are usually smaller (less than 6 μm) and appear darker from the red blood cell background.
- Stomatocytes: Red blood cells with slitlike central pallor that resembles a mouth.
- Target cells: Red blood cells with a "target" or "bull's-eye" appearance.
- Teardrop: Resembles a tear and usually smaller than the normal red blood cell.

c. **Variation in erythrocyte color**. A normal erythrocyte is pinkish red, with a slightly lighter colored center (central pallor) when stained with a blood stain such as Wright's stain. Erythrocyte color is representative of hemoglobin concentration in the cell. Under normal conditions, when the color, central pallor, and hemoglobin are proportional, the erythrocyte is characterized as normochromic.

   - Hypochromia: Increased central pallor and decreased hemoglobin concentration.
   - Polychromasia: Used to describe erythrocytes that have a faint blue-orange color and erythrocytes that are slightly larger than normal red blood cells.

d. **Inclusions**. Several inclusions can be observed in erythrocytes or white blood cells or both. Use Table 20.5 for grading inclusions. Inclusions are listed in alphabetical order.

   - Auer rods are aggregates of fused primary granules and appear as red needle-like inclusions. Found in myeloblasts, promyelocytes, and monoblasts, they are seen in pathologic conditions.
   - Basophilic stippling appears as tiny round granules distributed evenly throughout the red blood cell. Composed of RNA, these inclusions stain deep blue with Wright's stain.
   - Cabot rings are delicate threadlike inclusions in the red blood cell, thought to be composed of remnants of the mitotic spindle. They appear in various shapes, including ring, figure-of-eight, or twisted.
   - Döhle bodies are composed of ribosomal RNA. They are light blue–staining inclusions found in the cytoplasm of neutrophils.
   - Hemoglobin C crystals are found in hemoglobin C diseases that have at least 50% target cells. The shape of the hemoglobin C crystal is usually oblong in homozygous conditions. In hemoglobin SC disease, the hemoglobin C crystal resembles a gloved hand.
   - Heinz body inclusions can be either round or irregularly shaped and are composed of denatured hemoglobin. Observation of these inclusions is made possible by supravital stains such as Brilliant Cresyl Blue or Crystal Violet. They are *not* observed on Wright's stain.
   - Howell-Jolly bodies are round, dark-staining nuclear remnants of DNA.
   - Pappenheimer bodies (siderocytes) are composed of ferric iron and appear as small, dark blue or purple dots in clusters along the periphery of the red blood cells when using Prussian blue stain. In Wright-stained smears, they appear as pale blue clusters.
   - Toxic granulation is an increased number of primary granules with intensified coloring seen in neutrophils and band forms during acute bacterial infections.

UNOPETTE WHITE BLOOD CELL AND PLATELET COUNT

Principle

The Unopette system consists of prefilled blood dilution vials containing solutions that preserve certain cell types while lysing others. Capillary pipettes are available to draw up different volumes of blood. The dilution is determined by the type of capillary used. Diluted blood is added to a hemacytometer chamber, and cells are counted in a specified area. For this procedure, whole blood is added to ammonium oxalate

Table 20.5 ● Grading Inclusions	
Rare	0–1/high-power field
Few	1–2/high-power field
Moderate	2–4/high-power field
Many	Greater than 5/high-power field

diluent, which lyses the red blood cells while preserving platelets, leukocytes, and reticulocytes.

Reagents and Equipment

1. Unopette reservoirs containing ammonium oxalate diluent at 1:100 dilution. Check expiration dates and do not use expired Unopettes. Protect from sunlight. Storage temperature is 1 to 30°C.
2. Unopette capillary pipette, 20 μL.
3. Hemacytometer: improved Neubauer ruling.
4. Hemacytometer cover slips free of debris.
5. Petri dish lined with filter paper that has been moistened and two applicator sticks to hold the hemacytometer.
6. Microscope with phase contrast.
7. Hand counter.

Specimen Collection and Storage

Specimen of choice is a Microtainer EDTA or EDTA tube, which should be at least half full.

Quality Control

1. All WBCs and platelet counts are done in duplicate. WBCs should agree ±20%. Platelet counts must agree ±10%. If they do not agree, repeat counts.
2. A visual estimate of the WBC and platelets can be done on the peripheral smear. Refer to charts.
3. Laboratory professionals are trained and tested for proficiency. Results are documented in their training file.

Procedure

1. Specimen should be well mixed and left on a rocker at least 5 minutes before using.
2. Check Unopettes for clarity and contents. If the Unopette chambers appear cloudy or the amount of reagent looks questionable, do not use.
3. With the reservoir on a flat surface, puncture the diaphragm of the reservoir using the protective shield of the capillary pipette.
   a. Using a twist action, remove protective shield from the pipette assembly.
   b. Holding the pipette and the tube of blood almost horizontally, touch the tip of the pipette to the blood. The pipette will fill by capillary action and stop automatically when the blood reaches the end of the capillary bore in the neck of the pipette.
   c. Wipe the excess blood from the outside of the capillary pipette. Be careful not to touch the tip of the capillary.
   d. Before entering the reservoir, it is necessary to force some air out of the reservoir. Do not expel any liquid, and maintain pressure on reservoir.
   e. Place an index finger over opening of overflow chamber and position pipette into reservoir neck.
   f. Release pressure on reservoir and then remove finger. The negative pressure will draw blood into pipette.
   g. Rinse the capillary pipette with the diluent by squeezing the reservoir gently two or three times. This forces diluent up into, but not out of, the overflow chamber and releases pressure each time to ensure that the mixture returns to the reservoir.
   h. Return protective shield over upper opening and gently invert several times to mix blood adequately.
   i. Allow the Unopette to stand for 10 minutes to allow red blood cells to hemolyze. Leukocyte counts should be performed within 3 hours.
4. Charge hemacytometer
   a. Mix the dilution by inversion, and convert the Unopette to the dropper assembly.
   b. Gently squeeze Unopette and discard first 3 or 4 drops. This allows proper mixing, with no excess diluent in the tip of the capillary.
   c. Carefully charge hemacytometer with the diluted blood, gently squeezing the reservoir to release contents until chamber is properly filled. Be sure to charge both sides and not to overfill chambers.
5. Place the hemacytometer in the premoistened Petri dish and leave for 15 minutes. This allows the sample to settle evenly.

Cell Counts and Calculations

A WBC is performed with a Neubauer hemacytometer.

1. Using 10× microscope magnification, white blood cells are counted using all nine squares of the counting chamber. Count both sides of the chamber and average the count. Refer to diagram.
2. Do not include cells that touch the extreme lower and the extreme left lines in the count.

3. Use the following formulas to calculate the WBC:

Cells/mm³ = average number of cells × depth factor (10) × dilution factor (100)/area

Example: side 1 = 85 cells

Side 2 = 95 cells

90 cells average/all 9 squares counted

90 × 10 × 100/9 =10,000 white blood cells

Normal Ranges for WBC

Adult: 4,800 to 10,800 white blood cells/mm³

Newborn: 10,000 to 30,000 white blood cells/mm³

Platelet Count

1. Platelet counts are performed with a Neubauer hemacytometer (Fig. 20.9).
   a. Counting is done using a 40× dry phase contrast objective. Platelets will have a faint halo. Count the middle square of the hemacytometer chamber, which contains 25 small squares.
   b. Platelets are counted in all the 25 squares. Take the average of both sides. Refer to diagram (Fig. 20-9)
   c. To calculate platelets, use the following formula:

$$\frac{\text{\# platelets} \times 10 \times 100}{\text{area (1.0 mm)}}$$

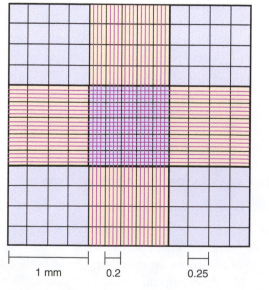

Figure 20.9 Neubauer hemacytometer counting chamber. Note the difference in depth depending on area examined.

1 mm   0.2   0.25

Multiply number of platelets × 1,000 = number of platelets/mm³

Platelets

150,000 to 450,000 platelets/mm³

Limitations

1. Specimen should be properly mixed and have sufficient blood volume so that there is no dilution of anticoagulant.
2. The capillary tube must be filled completely and be free of any air bubbles.
3. After the hemacytometer is charged, place it in a premoistened Petri dish to prevent evaporation while the cells are settling out.
4. The microscope light adjustment is critical. It is important for both white blood cells and platelets, but especially platelets. If the condenser is not in the correct position, it will make the platelets very difficult to see.
5. Debris and bacteria can be mistaken for platelets.
6. Clumped platelets cannot be counted properly; the specimen must be recollected. The preferred anticoagulant for preventing platelet clumping is EDTA.
7. Avoid overloading of hemacytometer chamber.

SICKLE CELL SCREENING PROCEDURE

Principle

The sickle screen kit provides a procedure based on hemoglobin solubility. Hemoglobin S is insoluble when combined with a buffer and a reducing agent. This occurs when the blood is mixed with the buffer and sodium hydrosulfite solution. Cells containing hemoglobin S are insoluble and show a turbid cloudy solution. Normal adult hemoglobin A is soluble and produces a transparent solution. The presence of hemoglobin S in either the heterozygous or the homozygous state produces a cloudy solution. Because this is a qualitative screening procedure, all positive results must be followed up with hemoglobin electrophoresis at alkaline or acid pH or isoelectric focusing.

Reagents and Equipment

1. Sickle cell kit
   a. Phosphate buffer/sodium hydrosulfite solution. Prepare by pouring entire contents of sodium hydrosulfite vial into one phosphate buffer bottle. Cap and mix for 1 to 2 minutes. Once reconstituted, reagent is good for 5 days when stored at 2 to 8°C.
   b. Unmixed reagents are good until expiration date on package when stored at 2 to 8°C.
2. 12-mm × 75-mm test tubes
3. Test tube caps or parafilm
4. 50-μL pipette and tips
5. Reading rack
6. 5-mL pipette (to pipette the buffer)

Specimen Collection and Storage

1. Whole blood obtained in EDTA, heparin, or sodium citrate.
2. Specimens can be refrigerated at 2° to 8°C for 2 weeks before testing.

Quality Control

Commercially prepared negative and positive controls are run along with the patient's blood. Control results must be correct to report patient results.

Procedure

1. Pipette 4 mL of the phosphate buffer/sodium hydrosulfite solution to each test tube (one for each test and each control).
2. Add 50 μL of well-mixed whole blood or control to each labeled tube.
3. Cover each tube with a cap or parafilm, and invert to mix three or four times.
4. Place each tube in the reading rack at room temperature, and let the tubes incubate for 10 to 20 minutes.

Interpretation of Results and Result Reporting

Positive: If hemoglobin S or any other sickling hemoglobin (hemoglobin C Harlem) is present, the solution will be turbid and the lines on the reading rack will be invisible.

Negative: If no sickling hemoglobin is present, the lines on the reading rack will be visible through the solution (Fig. 20.10).

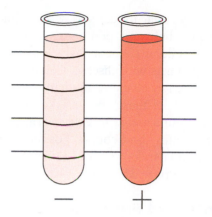

Figure 20.10 Tube solubility screen for hemoglobin S. The procedure simply gives an indication of the presence of hemoglobin S and should be followed up with hemoglobin electrophoresis.

Limitations

1. Severe anemias can cause false-negative results. The sample volume should be doubled (100 μL) if the hemoglobin is less than 8 g/dL.
2. False-negative results can occur with infants younger than 6 months because hemoglobin F is insoluble in the test solution. Therefore, testing should not be done on infants.
3. Patients with multiple myeloma, cryoglobulinemia, and other dysglobulinemias may show false-positive results because the high protein level may affect the test.
4. Some rare hemoglobin variants such as hemoglobin C Harlem or C Georgetown may give false-positive results. These are sickling hemoglobins but do not contain hemoglobin S.
5. Patients who have been recently transfused may give false-positive or false-negative results.
6. Patients who have sickle trait give positive results. These results should be confirmed with hemoglobin electrophoresis.
7. Positive results and questionable results should be confirmed with hemoglobin electrophoresis.

CEREBROSPINAL FLUID AND BODY FLUID CELL COUNT AND DIFFERENTIAL

Principle

Examining the cellular component of body fluids is an important part of total body fluid testing. Cell counts are performed in a counting chamber. Cerebrospinal fluid (CSF), synovial fluids, and serous fluids of the pleural, pericardial, and peritoneal cavities all have characteristic cellular elements, which often change in predictable patterns with disease. Cell counts and cell morphology are key elements in identifying abnormalities within each of these systems. The methods outlined here present a *unique method and calculation reference* for performing fluid counts. For the standard cell counting formula, refer to the Unopette method for manual cell (see page 310).

Reagents and Equipment

1. Saline
2. Slide stainer
3. Phase microscope
4. Neubauer hemacytometer with cover slip
5. Petri dish
6. Pipettes
   a. 0.2 MLA
   b. 0.1 MLA
   c. 1.0 volumetric
   d. 10.0 volumetric
7. 12-mm × 75-mm plastic tubes
8. Cytospin
9. Disposable Cytofunnels with white filter attached
10. Bovine albumin, 22%
11. Hyaluronidase
12. Plain microhematocrit tubes
13. Crystal violet diluent

Specimen Collection and Storage

Cerebrospinal Fluid

1. Cells are collected in numbered sterile plastic tubes from the spinal tray. The laboratory accepts tubes 1 through 3; the hematology department prefers tube 3.
2. Tube 4 is the preferred tube because it is least likely to be contaminated with blood.
3. CSF cell counts should be performed within *1 hour* of receipt in the laboratory because cells lyse on prolonged standing, and accurate counts become impossible.

Synovial and Serous Fluids (Pleural, Pericardial, and Peritoneal)

1. Fluids should be collected in a heparinized tube or EDTA tube.
2. Perform testing within 4 hours.
3. The addition of hyaluronidase to the fluid may reduce the viscosity of synovial fluid.

Quality Control

The College of American Pathologists has removed daily quality control for all body fluids. Each laboratory receives proficiency testing at least two times a year from the proficiency program of the College of American Pathologists.

Procedure

Cell Counting Method

1. Based on the gross appearance of the fluid, dilute the specimen by one of the following methods:
   a. *Method A* (clear or slightly cloudy fluid) Dilute 1:2 with crystal violet diluent (0.2 mL specimen + 0.2 mL diluent)
   b. *Method B* (moderately cloudy fluid) Dilute 1:11 with saline (0.1 mL specimen + 1.0 mL saline) using a volumetric pipette. Then dilute 1:2 with crystal violet diluent (0.2 mL of 1:11 dilution + 0.2 mL diluent)
   c. *Method C* (very cloudy or bloody fluid) Dilute 1:101 with saline (0.1 mL specimen + 10.0 mL saline) using a volumetric pipette. Then dilute 1:2 with crystal violet diluent (0.2 mL of 1:101 dilution + 0.2 diluent)
2. Using a plain microhematocrit tube, fill each side of the hemacytometer with the dilution. Place the hematometer in a premoistened Petri dish. Allow the cells to settle for 3 to 5 minutes in the Petri dish.
   a. Place the hemacytometer on the stage of the phase microscope. Determining the number of squares to be counted depends on the initial viewing of the fluid on the hemacytometer chamber under the microscope. This is the judgment of the technologist/technician.
   b. Using the 40× objective, count the white blood cells and red blood cells on each side. Now enter the WBC and RBC of each dilution in the CSF/body fluid worksheet (see Table 20.7).
   c. Combine the two totals and average the WBC and RBC, which must agree within 20%. If this criterion is not met, reload the chamber and redo the counts.
   d. The gross appearance of non-CSF fluid will determine whether a red blood cell dilution is needed. If the fluid is cloudy

and bloody, the red blood cells are too numerous to count (TNTC); report red blood cells as "TNTC."

e. Tables 20.6 and 20.7 offer a unique calculation reference for fluids. Once a dilution is determined and counts are performed for various fluids, data can be plugged into these ready reference tables for a quick calculation of a final result. For example:

	Dilution (A, B, or C)	No. of Squares Counted	No. of Cells Count 1	Count 2	Average No. of Cells	Calculation	Result
WBC	A	9	90	100	95	95 × 2.2 = 209	209/μL
RBC	A	9	26	30	28	28 × 2.2 = 61.6	62/μL

Table 20.6 ● Reference Factors for Fluid Calculations

Multiplication Factors

Total No. Squares Counted	Method A	Method B	Method C
1	×20	×220	×2,020
2	×10	×110	×1,010
3	×6.7	×73.3	×673.3
4	×5.0	×55	×505
5	×4.0	×44	×404
6	×3.3	×36.7	×336.7
7	×2.9	×31.4	×288.6
8	×2.5	×27.5	×252.5
9	×2.2	×24.4	×224.4
10 small center	×100	×1,100	×10,100
11 small center	×50	×550	×5,050

Table 20.7 ● Fluid Worksheet

	Dilution A, B, or C	No. Squares Counted	No. Cells Count 1	Count 2	Average No. Cells	Calculation	Result
WBC						___ × ___ = ___	/μL
RBC						___ × ___ = ___	/μL
Example							

	Dilution A, B, or C	No. Squares Counted	No. Cells Count 1	Count 2	Average No. Cells	Calculation	Result
WBC	A	9	90	100	95	95 × 2.2 = 209	209/μL
RBC	A	9	26	30	28	28 × 2.2 = 61.6	62/μL

Differential Using Cytospin Method

Figures 20.11, 20.12, and 20.13 represent a variety of cells in body fluids.

1. Prepare slide for the cytospin by first labeling the slide with the patient's name, specimen number, and date.
2. Attach slide for cytospin with the cytocup by the Cytoclip.
3. Add 1 drop of 22% albumin to the bottom of the cytocup.
   a. Clear to slightly cloudy to moderately cloudy fluid: Add 200 µL of specimen.
   b. Very cloudy or bloody fluid: Add 50 to 100 µL of specimen.
4. Place assembled slide/cytocup into one of the positions on the head with a balance in the position opposite to its location.
5. Cover cytospin head with lid and lock in place by pushing center down on the base.

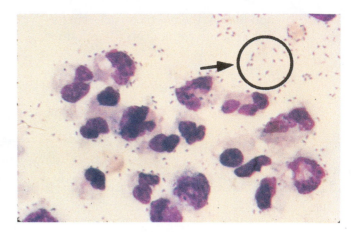

Figure 20.13 Bacteria in cerebrospinal fluid. From The College of American Pathologists, with permission.

6. Program the cytospin for 10 minutes at 700 rpm.
   a. Use "Hi" acceleration for serous and synovial fluids.
   b. Use "Lo" acceleration for CSF.
7. Start the unit. When the cycle completes, remove the sealed head. Remove the clip assembly and hold it in a horizontal position with the funnel facing down.
8. Release the tension clip and remove the sample chamber and filter card. Remove the slide from the clip and allow to air dry completely.
9. Stain the slides in the stainer and allow them to dry completely.
10. Perform a differential count on the stained smear. See Table 20.8 for normal results.
    a. Identify the cells as segmented neutrophils; lymphocytes; monocytes; eosinophils; and others including mesothelial, macrophages, and tumor cells. Table 20.9 includes abnormal cells in CSF.
    b. After completing the differential, a pathologist should review any abnormal cells. Table 20.10 lists abnormal cells in serous fluids, and Table 20.11 lists abnormal cells in synovial fluids. For color and appearance for CSF, (see Table 20.12, page 318).

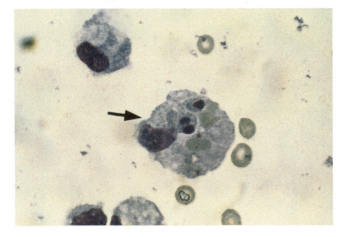

Figure 20.11 Histiocyte in peritoneal fluid. From The College of American Pathologists, with permission.

PROTHROMBIN TIME AND ACTIVATED PARTIAL THROMBOPLASTIN TIME: AUTOMATED PROCEDURE

Principle

Presently, coagulation instruments are fully automated to analyze large volume of samples with a high degree of accuracy. Many of the instruments are capable of

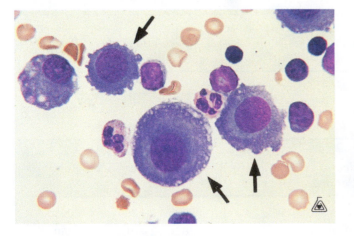

Figure 20.12 Mesothelial cell in pleural fluid. From The College of American Pathologists, with permission.

Table 20.8 ● Normal Body Fluid Results

Descriptive/ Cell Count	Normal CSF Adult	Normal CSF Neonate	Normal Serous Fluid (Pleural, Pericardial, Peritoneal)	Normal Synovial Fluid
Appearance	Clear and colorless	Clear and colorless	Pale yellow and clear	Pale yellow and clear
Red blood cells	$0–1/mm^3$	$0–3/mm^3$	$0–1/mm^3$	$0–1/mm^3$
White blood cells	$0–5/mm^3$	$0–30/mm^3$	$0–200/mm^3$	$0–200/mm^3$
Neutrophils (includes bands)	2%–6%	0%–8%	<25%	<25%
Lymphocytes	40%–80%	5%–35%	<25%	<25%
Monocytes	5%–45%	50%–90%	Included with others	Included with others
Others	Rare	Rare	Monocytes and macrophages 65%–75%	Monocytes and macrophages 65%–75%

See Figures 20.11, 20.12, and 20.13 for body fluid cells.
CSF, cerebrospinal fluid.

Table 20.9 ● Causes of Abnormal Cells in Cerebrospinal Fluid

Abnormal Results	CSF	Abnormal Results	CSF
Increased neutrophils	Acute inflammation	Increased monocytes	Newborn infants
	Early viral meningitis		Recovery phase of meningitis
	Bacterial meningitis (see Fig. 20.13)	Increased macrophages	Siderophages present, indicating a CNS hemorrhage in past 48 hours
Increased lymphocytes	Neurosyphilis		Erythrophages present, indicating active CNS bleed and if siderophages are also present
	Viral and fungal meningitis		
	Alzheimer's disease		
	Multiple sclerosis		Lipophages present in brain abscesses and cerebral infarctions
	Tumors		
	Lymphocytic leukemias and lymphomas	Increased eosinophils	Parasitic infections
			Postmyelogram specimens
	Reactive lymphocytes to include plasma cells in most of the above diseases, particularly in multiple sclerosis and viral meningitis	Tumor/malignant cells	Acute and chronic leukemias
		Others	Primary neurologic tumors
			Choroid plexus and ependymal cells seen in postencephalogram specimens

CNS, central nervous system; CSF, cerebrospinal fluid.

Table 20.10 ● Abnormal Cells in Serous Fluids

Abnormal Results	Serous Fluids (Pleural, Pericardial, and Peritoneal)
↑RBC	Traumatic tap
	Hemorrhage
	Malignancy or infections
↑WBC >1000/mm³	Infections
	Malignancies
	Inflammatory conditions
>50% Neutrophils	Acute inflammatory conditions
	Infectious bacterial processes
>50% Lymphocytes	Tuberculosis
	Carcinomas
	Lymphoproliferative diseases
Increased reactive lymphocytes and plasma cells	Multiple myeloma
	Malignancy and tuberculous effusions
Malignant cells	Diagnostically significant if found on the differential
	Solid tumors and hematologic malignancies shedding cells are usually caused by metastatic adenocarcinoma
<1% Mesothelial	Tuberculous effusions

Table 20.11 ● Abnormal Cells in Synovial Fluids

Abnormal Results	Synovial Fluids
Neutrophils >80%	Septic arthritis
	Later stages of rheumatoid arthritis
Lymphocytes	Early stages of rheumatoid arthritis
Reactive lymphocytes/ plasma	Early stages of rheumatoid arthritis
Monocytes	Viral infections such as hepatitis and rubella arthritis
Eosinophilia	Chronic urticaria and angioedema
	Rheumatic fever
	Parasitic infections
	Metastatic disease
	Rheumatoid arthritis

Table 20.12 ● Color and Appearance of Cerebrospinal Fluid

Color/Appearance	CSF Possible Pathology
Colorless	Normal
Cloudy	Infections
Straw	Excess protein
Yellow	Xanthochromia
Bloody	Traumatic tap
	CNS hemorrhage

CNS, central nervous system; CSF, cerebrospinal fluid.

analyzing samples using clotting, chromogenic, or immunoassay methods. The clot method of photodetection is described here. This method uses light transmission (optical detection method) to determine prothrombin time (PT) and activated partial thromboplastin time (aPTT). The optical detection method detects the change in absorbance as a light-emitting diode recognized as a clot formation. A sensor picks up the light beam and converts it into an electrical signal. The electrical power is signaled and calculated by a microcomputer to determine the coagulation time. Some automated coagulation testing now identifies variables such as lipemia and hemolysis and is still able to present accurate clotting times.

Reagents and Equipment

1. Automated coagulation analyzer that uses optical detection
2. Volumetric pipettes: 1 mL and 10 mL
3. Centrifuge
4. Thromboplastin
   a. Reconstitute with 10 mL of reagent grade deionized water.

b. Immediately recap and mix until contents are completely dissolved.

c. Allow reagent to stand for 15 minutes.

d. Check package insert for stability once reconstituted.

5. Coagulation controls, two levels: Reconstitute according to manufacturer's instructions.

6. Deionized water

7. Calcium chloride solution

8. aPTT reagent

Specimen Collection and Storage

1. Collect whole blood into vacuum tube with 3.2% sodium citrate. This requires a 9:1 dilution of blood to anticoagulant.
   a. 4.5 mL of blood with 0.5 mL of anticoagulant, *or*
   b. 2.7 mL of blood with 0.3 mL of anticoagulant

2. For specimens with hematocrits greater than 60%, see Limitations section.

3. Specimens should not be obtained through a heparin lock or any other heparinized line.

4. Specimens are spun down for 5 minutes at 3,000 rpm to be platelet poor.

5. Coagulation samples are good for 24 hours at room temperature or refrigerated.

Quality Control

1. Coagulation controls are the laboratory's choice. Follow manufacturer's instructions for reconstitution and stability.

2. Coagulation controls are run at the beginning of each shift.

3. If quality control is out, repeat if necessary. If still out, troubleshoot or notify supervisor.

Procedure

PT

1. Prepare reagents and controls.
2. Place reagents and control inside analyzer.
3. Replenish any other materials.
4. Run quality control.
5. Verify quality control; repeat any controls if necessary, and document any abnormal controls.
6. Load centrifuged specimen onto instrument with cap removed.
7. Press "Start."
8. The instrument places 50 µL of the patient's plasma into a cup, incubates the sample for 3 minutes, and adds 100 µL of thromboplastin (Fig. 20.14).

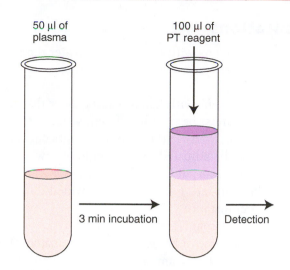
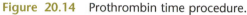

Figure 20.14 Prothrombin time procedure.

aPTT

1. Follow steps 1 through 7 in the PT procedure.

2. The instrument places 50 µL of the patient's plasma into a cup, incubates for 1 minute, adds 50 µL of aPTT reagent, continues with another 3-minute incubation, and adds 50 µL of calcium chloride to the specimen (Fig. 20.15).

Results

1. Reference range: PT 11.0 to 13.0 seconds, international normalized ratio (INR) 2.0 to 3.0

2. Reference range: aPTT 25.0 to 31.0 seconds

3. Critical results
   a. PT greater than 50.00 seconds
   b. INR greater than 4.9
   c. aPTT greater than 100.00 seconds

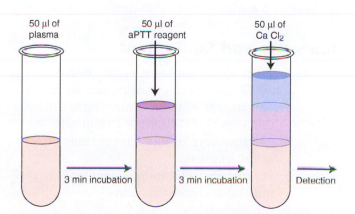

Figure 20.15 Activated partial thromboplastin time procedure.

Limitations

1. Specimens with hematocrits greater than 60% result in falsely prolonged clotting times.
2. Specimens with hematocrits greater than 60% must be drawn differently than ordinary samples. Either the amount of anticoagulant must be adjusted, or the amount of whole blood collected into the sample tube must be adjusted. Formulas are provided for both circumstances.
   a. Anticoagulant adjustment
      Volume of blood $\times$ (100 − hematocrit) $\times$ 0.00185 = amount of anticoagulant to be added
   b. Volume of blood adjustment
      Volume of blood $\times$ (60/100) − hematocrit = mL of whole blood to be collected

QUALITATIVE D-DIMER TEST

Principle

D-dimer is a fibrin fragment that results when plasmin acts on cross-linked fibrin in the presence of factor XIII. D-dimers are produced from an insoluble fibrin clot. Available since the 1990s, this semiquantitative assay provides evidence of normal or abnormal levels of D-dimer. Latex particles are coated with mouse anti–D-dimer monoclonal antibodies. When mixed with plasma containing D-dimers, agglutination occurs. The test plays an important role in detecting and monitoring patients suspected to have thrombotic disorders. Its clinical uses include detecting deep vein thrombosis (DVT), pulmonary embolism (PE), and, in patients with disseminated intravascular coagulation (DIC), postoperative complications or septicemia. Quantitative D-dimer procedures are available, using latex-enhanced turbidimetric methods. The qualitative test is widely used in most coagulation laboratories, however, as a screening test for D-dimers.

Reagents and Equipment

1. D-dimer kit containing reagents (stored at 2 to 8°C), good until expiration date on the kit
   a. Test reagent solution containing red blood cell anti–XL-FDP antibody conjugate
   b. Negative control solution containing 0.9% saline solution
   c. Positive control solution containing purified D-dimer fragment
2. Plastic agglutination trays

3. White plastic stirrers
4. Timer
5. 10-µL pipette with disposable tips

Specimen Collection and Storage

1. Collect venous whole blood into a vacuum tube with 3.2% sodium citrate. Dilution of blood to anticoagulant must be 9:1.
   a. 4.5 mL of blood with 0.5 mL of anticoagulant, *or*
   b. 2.7 mL of blood with 0.3 mL of anticoagulant
2. Collection of venous blood into heparin is acceptable.
3. Store specimens at 18 to 24°C. Specimens should be tested within 4 hours of specimen collection. If testing will take place after 4 hours, specimens must be refrigerated at 2 to 8°C; refrigerated specimens are good up to 24 hours.

Quality Control

1. Quality control is performed under several conditions:
   a. Daily
   b. When opening a new kit
   c. When receiving a new shipment
   d. When a new lot number is put into use
2. A whole blood sample that has a negative D-dimer result is used for quality control.
3. Quality control method
   a. Follow directions in the procedure to do the quality control, steps 1 through 5.
   b. Add 1 drop of positive control to the test well, and proceed with steps 6 through 8b.

Procedure

1. Allow reagents to come to room temperature for at least 20 minutes before use.
2. Specimen should be thoroughly mixed; do not allow cells to settle out.
3. For each sample, pipette 10 µL of whole blood into each reaction well; place wells on a plastic agglutination tray; the first is labeled "negative control well" and the second is labeled "test well."
4. Add 1 drop of the negative control to the negative control well.
5. Add 1 drop of the test reagent to the test well.

6. With a plastic stirrer, mix the contents of each well thoroughly for 3 to 5 seconds, using a different stirrer for each well and spreading the reagent across the entire well surface.
7. To promote agglutination, mix by gentle rocking of the plastic agglutination tray for 2 minutes.
8. At the end of the 2 minutes, observe for the presence of agglutination.
   a. Positive results: Agglutination is present in the test well compared with no agglutination in the negative control well.
   b. If the negative control well agglutinates, the test is invalid.
   c. If the test result is negative, add 1 drop of positive control to the test well and rock the plastic tray. Agglutination should occur within 15 seconds. If agglutination does not occur with the addition of the positive control, the test is invalid.

Interpretation

1. Positive: Agglutination seen in the test well and no agglutination seen in the negative control well.
2. Negative: No agglutination seen in the test well and the negative control well. This would be confirmed by adding the positive control to the test well and observing agglutination.
3. Invalid
   a. Agglutination occurs in the negative control well.
   b. No agglutination occurs with the positive control.

Results

Negative: No agglutination seen in negative agglutination well (less than 0.5 mg/L)

Positive: Agglutination seen in undiluted sample (0.5 to 4.0 mg/L)

Positive samples can be diluted 1:8 or 1:64 to provide more specific semiquantitative data on the amount of D-dimer present.

Limitations

The presence of cold agglutinins in patient samples can cause agglutination in patient blood. This may cause agglutination of the negative control, invalidating the test results.

A quantitative D-dimer test is available, and it is usually performed using a turbidimetric procedure on automated coagulation equipment. The advantage of this method is that it gives an absolute quantity of D-dimer in milligrams per liter, which is an effective tool for determining whether a thrombotic episode has occurred or predicting whether one will occur.

SPECIAL TESTING IN COAGULATION: AN OVERVIEW

Mixing Studies

When a patient has an elevated PTT, the cause of the elevation should be determined. Mix the patient's plasma in a 1:1 ratio with normal pooled plasma and then repeat the test. If the aPTT is corrected, consider a factor deficiency because the normal reagent plasma supplied a missing factor. If the aPTT is uncorrected, consider a patient on heparin or a patient with an inhibitor. An aPTT whose result comes within 10% of the reference range is considered a correction. Mixing studies may be incubated 1 hr if considering factor VIII inhibitors.

Thrombin Time

This procedure uses patient plasma as a source of fibrinogen, and it measures the integrity of the fibrinolytic system. If fibrinogen is available in the plasma, qualitatively and quantitatively, a fibrin clot is established once a standard concentration of thrombin has been added to the plasma. The reference range is 11 to 15 seconds. Thrombin time is elevated in heparin contamination, in samples with increased fibrin degradation products (FDPs), and in patients who have hypofibrinogenemia and dysfibrinogenemia.

Reptilase Time

This test is used to determine whether an elevated thrombin time results from heparin contamination or one of the fibrinogen disorders. Reptilase is a snake venom that is unaffected by heparin; this product acts like thrombin. Thrombin works by hydrolyzing fibrinopeptide A and B, whereas reptilase works by hydrolyzing only fibrinopeptide A. The normal reference range is 11 to 15 seconds. A prolonged reptilase time would suggest increased FDPs, inhibitors, or fibrinogen deficiencies. A normal reptilase time would suggest a patient on heparin.

Dilute Russell's Viper Venom Tests

When a mixing study has been performed and found to be prolonged, testing must be performed to uncover a possible inhibitor. One of the most common inhibitors is the lupus anticoagulant (LA), which is directed against phospholipids. These antibodies are also implicated in thrombosis and fetal loss. Four features must be satisfied:

1. The aPTT mixing study must be prolonged after 1-hour incubation (heparin excluded).
2. The dilute Russell's viper venom time (DRVVT) must be prolonged.
3. A high phospholipid reagent must normalize the prolonged aPTT.
4. Other inhibitors must be excluded.

Procedure

Mix patient plasma with calcium, a small amount of phospholipid, and Russell's viper venom. The venom will directly activate coagulation at factor X and bypass the intrinsic and extrinsic system. If LA is present (or if factor X is deficient), the test will be prolonged. To confirm test results, redo this procedure with a high phospholipid reagent. If corrected, the phospholipid reagent has bound the antibody and normalized the aPTT, confirming LA.

HEMATOLOGY AUTOMATION: GENERAL PRINCIPLES OF OPERATION*

Electrical Impedance

Cells are sized and counted by detecting and measuring changes in electrical resistance when a particle passes through a small aperture. This is called the electrical impedance principle of counting cells. A blood sample is diluted in saline, a good conductor of electrical current, and the cells are pulled through an aperture by creating a vacuum. Two electrodes establish an electrical current. The external electrode is located in the blood cell suspension. The internal electrode is located inside the glass hollow tube, which contains the aperture. Low-frequency electrical current is applied to the external electrode and the internal electrode, and DC current is applied between the two electrodes. Electrical resistance or impedance occurs as the cells pass through the aperture, causing a change in voltage and generating a pulse (Fig. 20.16). The number of pulses is proportional to the number of cells counted. In addition, the size of the voltage pulse is directly proportional to the volume or size of the cell. This principle is also known as the Coulter principle.

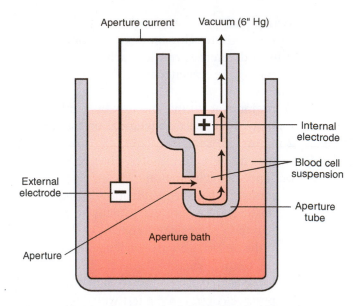

Figure 20.16 Coulter principle of electrical impedance.

Histograms

Histograms are graphic representations of cell frequencies versus size. Pulses are channelized by their height or amplitude, and data are collected and plotted on a volume/frequency distribution histogram. The relative number is on the y-axis, and the size, or volume, is on the x-axis. Histograms are created for the erythrocyte or red blood cell, leukocyte (white blood cell), and platelet populations based on cell volume measure in femtoliters (fL) and relative number. Histograms provide information about red blood cells, white blood cells, and platelet frequency; distribution about the mean; and the presence of subpopulations (Fig. 20.17).

Radiofrequency

Radiofrequency (RF) resistance is a high-voltage electromagnetic current flowing between the electrodes that detects cell size, based on cellular density. RF is a high-frequency pulsating sine wave. Conductivity or RF measurements provide information about the internal characteristics of the cell. When exposed to high-frequency current, the cell wall acts as a conductor. As the current passes through the cell, it detects measurable changes. The cell interior density, or nuclear volume, is directly proportional to pulse size or a change in RF resistance. The nuclear-to-cytoplasmic ratio, nuclear density, and cytoplasmic granulation are determined.

*The author wishes to acknowledge Joyce Feinberg MT (ASCP) of Beckman-Coulter and Kathleen Finnegan, MS, MT (ASCP) SH of the MT Program at Stony Brook, NY, for their assistance with this section.

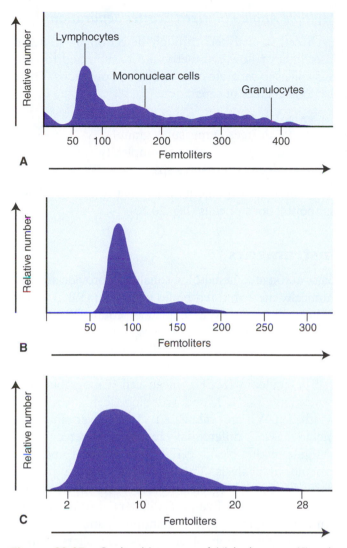

Figure 20.17   Coulter histogram of (A) leukocytes, (B) red blood cells, and (C) platelets.

Opacity

Opacity is a mathematical equation derived from the ratio of RF and DC. Opacity represents conductivity related to cellular density and the internal structure of cells. Nuclear cells have low density. Using the measurement of opacity, cells with a higher nuclear-to-cytoplasmic ratio have low opacity. White blood cells that have more cytoplasm also have higher opacity.

Scatterplot

Scatterplots are graphic representations of two or more measurable characteristics of cells. These three-dimensional plots use conductivity and light scatter to visualize and analyze cell data. The scatterplot provides information about population abnormalities and subpopulations of cells. Prominent cell populations viewed by scatterplots include lymphocytes, granulocytes, and monocytes (Fig. 20.18).

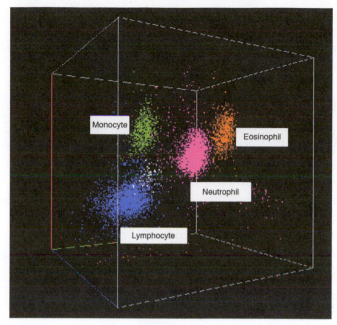

Figure 20.18   Beckman-Coulter scattergram.   Courtesy of Beckman-Coulter.

Optical Scatter

A sample of blood is diluted with an isotonic diluent and then hydrodynamically focused through a quartz flow cell. Cells pass through a flow cell on which a beam of light is focused. The light source is a laser light (i.e., light amplified by stimulated emission of radiation). Laser or monochromatic light is emitted as a single wavelength. As the cell passes through the sensing zone, light scatters in all directions. Photodetectors sense and collect the scattered rays at different angles and then convert the data into an electrical pulse. The number of pulses generated is directly proportional to the number of cells passing through the sensing zone. Optical scatter measures patterns of light at various angles: forward light scatter at 180 degrees and right angle scatter at 90 degrees. Cell counts, size, cell structure, shape, and reflectivity are determined by analyzing scatter light data. Forward angle light scatter (0 degrees) is diffracted light that relates to volume. Forward low-angle light scatter (2 to 3 degrees) relates to cell size or volume. Forward high-angle scatter (5 to 15 degrees) relates to the internal complexity or refractive index of cellular components. Orthogonal light scatter (90 degrees) or side scatter is a combination of reflection and refraction and relates to internal components.

VCS Technology (Volume, Conductivity, and Scatter)

Low-frequency current measures volume, whereas high-frequency current measures changes in conductivity.

Light from the laser bouncing off white blood cells characterizes the surface shape and reflectivity of each cell. This technology differentiates white blood cell characteristics.

Hydrodynamic Focusing

Hydrodynamic focusing is a technique that narrows the stream of cells to single file, eliminating data above and below the focus points. Hydrodynamic focusing allows greater accuracy and resolution of blood cells. Diluted cells are surrounded by a sheath fluid that lines the cells up in a single file as they pass through the detection aperture. Cells are directed away from the back of the aperture. This process eliminates recirculation of cells and the necessity for counting cells twice.

Flow Cytometry

Flow cytometry uses a laser light source to measure the physical or antigenic characteristics of cells as they pass through a beam of laser light. Each cell can be measured for the intensity of scattered light, including cell size and density, nuclear complexity, cell granularity, and the staining capacity of dye in each cell. In addition, flow cytometry can evaluate nuclear DNA content, surface antigens, and cytoplasmic antigens.

Light scatter is measured at a forward light scatter (FALS) of 2 to 10 degrees and orthogonal or side scatter (SSC) at 70 to 90 degrees (Fig. 20.19). FALS evaluates cell size, whereas SCC evaluates cytoplasmic and nuclear complexity. Light scatter signals are amplified and converted to digital signals. FALS and SSC are plotted to form a scattergram that separates the cells into cell clusters. These clusters are separated into granulocytes, monocytes, and lymphocytes (Fig. 20.19). The cells of interest can be selected for specific analysis.

Use of Flow Cells

Flow cells are composed of quartz rather than glass and provide a better atmosphere in which to measure cellular qualities. Light does not bend, and ultraviolet (UV) light can pass through the flow cell. Cell characteristics are then measured. The flow cells measure cell volume; internal content; and cell surface, shape, and reflectivity.

Median Angle Light Scatter

Median angle light scatter (MALS) is defined as the light scatter information that is obtained between the 10-degree and the 70-degree angles. Light scatter in the median angles is proportional to cell size, granularity, surface properties, and reflectance.

Multiple Angle Polarized Scatter Separation

Each cell is analyzed through detection of scattered laser light or flow cytometry and is subjected to various angles to separate cells into cell populations. There are four degrees of separation:

- 90 degrees measures lobularity
- 90 degrees D measures granularity
- 10 degrees measures complexity
- 0 degrees measures size

These measurements can identify the five basic subpopulations of cells (Fig. 20.20).

Instruments

Basic automated hematology analyzers provide an electronically measured red blood cell count (RBC), white blood cell count (WBC), platelet count (Plt), mean platelet volume (MPV), hemoglobin concentration (Hb), and mean red blood cell volume (MCV). From these measured quantities, the hematocrit (Hct), mean cell hemoglobin (MCH), mean cell hemoglobin concentration (MCHC), and red blood cell distribution width (RDW) are calculated. The newer analyzers include WBC differential, relative or percent and absolute white blood cell number, and sometimes reticulocyte analysis. The differential may be a three-part differential (granulocytes, lymphocytes, and monocytes) or a five-part differential (neutrophils, lymphocytes, monocytes, eosinophils, and basophils). The new generation of analyzers also offers a sixth parameter, the enumeration of nucleated red blood cells. State-of-the-art hematology instruments also include verification systems. The verification system reviews past patient results and uses delta checks and instrument flagging, including R flags, population flags, suspect flags, and definitive or quantitative flags.

Data Reporting

Most automated systems report the CBC numerically. The differential is numerically recorded and then graphically displayed. These displays include scatterplots, scattergrams, and histograms. The basic principles behind the graphic displays of these data are fairly universal. Scatterplots and scattergrams place a specific cell on a grid identification system, whereas histograms measure size thresholds of white blood cells, red blood cells, and platelets compared with the normal data for each of these cell groups.

Scatterplots and scattergrams provide colorful imaging of normal and abnormal cells. An operator can immediately notice a particular deviation in numbers

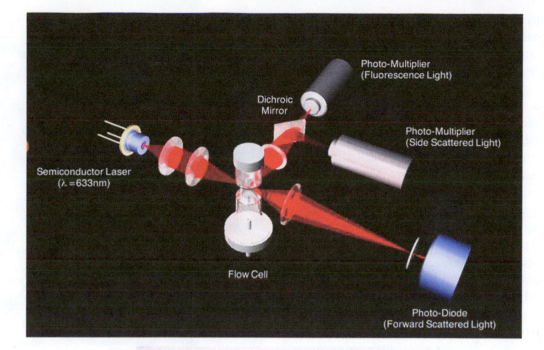

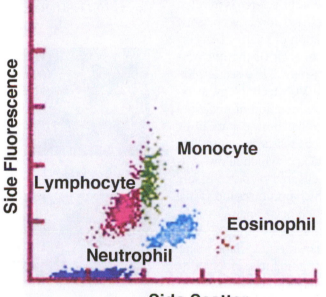

Figure 20.19 Sysmex Flow Technology. *Courtesy of Sysmex.*

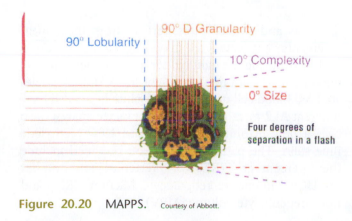

Figure 20.20 MAPPS. *Courtesy of Abbott.*

and distribution of a particular cell line by analyzing scatterplots.

Beckman-Coulter Instrumentation

Coulter GEN S, Coulter LH Series, and the UniCel DxH Coulter Analysis System (http://www.beckmancoulter.com) use VCS technology, which is an acronym for volume (V), conductivity (C), and laser light scatter (S). The simultaneous measurement of cell volume, conductivity, and light scatter provides high statistical accuracy. Cell volume is measured by electrical impedance using low-frequency DC. To ensure accuracy, Coulter has incorporated pulse editing and sweep flow technology. This technology allows cells to line up in a single file, ensuring integrity of size measurement and preventing double counting. The RBC, WBC, and platelet count are obtained by analyzing the number of pulses generated. RBC, WBC, and platelet count data are then plotted in the form of a histogram. The cell number is plotted on the y-axis, and the cell size is plotted on the x-axis. MCV and RDW are derived from the RBC histogram, whereas MPV is derived from the platelet histogram. Hct, MCH, and MCHC are calculated. Hb is measured by the cyanmethemoglobin method.

Conductivity is measured using high-frequency electromagnetic current for nuclear and granular constituents. Conductivity is influenced by the internal structures of the cell, such as the nuclear-to-cytoplasm ratio and the cytoplasmic granular content. A monochromatic helium:neon laser provides the light source for measuring light scatter for surface structure, shape, and granularity. Forward angle light scatter is affected by cell shape, surface characteristics, and cytoplasmic granular content. The enumeration of relative percentage and the absolute number of each (if the five normal white cells) five cells are displayed in a scatterplot.

The LH series is based on VCS technology, a six-part differential that includes enumeration of nucleated red blood cells. VCS technology has been enhanced by the use of Intellikenetics, which assists in controlling environment fluctuations; AccuGate, which allows better separation of white blood cells, red blood cells, and reticulocytes; and AccuFlex, which optimizes individual flagging of cell populations. Reticulocyte analysis is performed by New Methylene Blue stain and the VCS flow cell for analysis. Figure 20.21 shows a three-dimensional scatterplot and parameters of immature reticulocyte fraction (IFR) and mean reticulocyte volume (MRV).

The UniCel DxH800 Coulter Cellular Analysis System incorporates new electronic and mechanical designs with advanced algorithm technology to improve performance. The UniCel DxH800 has four analysis modules, one each for WBC, RBC, Plt, and Hb. These modules use algorithms, a digital count, and size information. The WBC differential methodology has a new flow cell that measures seven distinct parameters, including volume, conductivity, axial light loss (AL2), low angle light scatter (LALS), median angle light scatter (MALS), lower median angle light scatter (LMALS), and upper median angle light scatter (UMALS). Collected information includes cellular size, internal cellular characteristics, and individual cell light scat properties, parameters that define and separate cell populations. Figure 20.22 shows two-dimensional

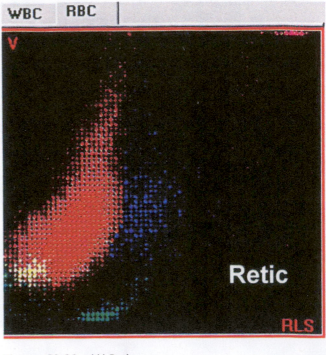

Figure 20.21 LH Retic. Courtesy of Beckman-Coulter.

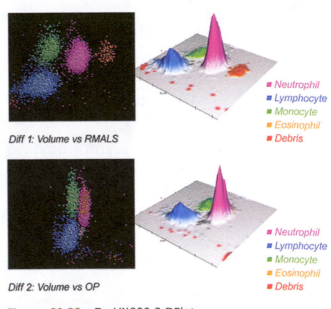

Diff 1: Volume vs RMALS

- ■ Neutrophil
- ■ Lymphocyte
- ■ Monocyte
- ■ Eosinophil
- ■ Debris

Diff 2: Volume vs OP

- ■ Neutrophil
- ■ Lymphocyte
- ■ Monocyte
- ■ Eosinophil
- ■ Debris

Figure 20.22 Dx HX800 2-DPlots. Courtesy of Beckman-Coulter.

dataplots and surface plots derived from these measurements. Nucleated red blood cell enumeration is performed using the light scatter measurement and the measurement from the Axial light loss (AL2). A nucleated red blood cell nucleus and a white blood cell have different AL2 measurements. Reticulocyte analysis also uses a flow cytometric method and New Methylene Blue stain. The parameters that are provided include the percentage (RET%), reticulocyte number (RETIC#), immature reticulocyte fraction (IRF), and mean reticulocyte volume (MRV).

Sysmex Instrumentation

Sysmex Corporation (www.sysmex.com) manufactures a full line of hematology analyzers, including the XT, XS, and XE series that use electronic resistance, hydrodynamic focusing, and fluorescent flow cytometry with light scatter. The XS and XE series provide a full CBC with a five-part differential. The newest analyzers added to the Sysmex line are the XE-2100 and XE-5000, which provide a CBC, five-part differential, and a fully automated reticulocyte count. The XE series measures WBC, RBC, and platelets using DC electrical impedance for counting and sizing cells, hydrodynamic focusing, and automatic discrimination for accuracy and precision. The XE series generates the standard hematology parameters and the added parameters of RDW-SD (red blood cell distribution width by standard deviation), RDW-CV (red blood cell distribution width by coefficient), and MPV (mean platelet volume). Hemoglobin values are determined using a cyanide-free, nontoxic reagent and are measured at 555 nm. The WBC uses a separate channel and uses DC electrical impedance.

The principle for the WBC differential includes simultaneous measurements of RF and DC detection methods for separating white blood cell populations and fluorescent flow cytometry. Leukocytes are sensitized to the two special reagents, stromatolyser-4DL (a surfactant that induces hemolysis of red blood cells and forms a pore in the white blood cell membrane) and Stromatolyser-4DS (a fluorescent dye for staining the nucleic acids and organelles). Cellular signals related to side scatter or internal complexity and side fluorescence or staining intensity are plotted on a scattergram. White blood cells with similar chemical and physical properties form a group or cluster, which is used to differentiate white blood cell populations. Four separate detection channels allow determination of each white blood cell type. The DIFF channel—side scatter plotted on the x-axis and side fluorescence plotted on the y-axis—determines lymphocytes, monocytes, and granulocytes (Fig. 20.23). The WBC/BASO channel enumerates basophils by adding Stromatolyser-FB, which lyses the cells leaving only the basophil. After the sample has been treated with a specific lysing reagent, the cells are flowed by forward and lateral light scatter. The IMI channel is used with a special reagent Stromatolyser-IM for detecting the presence of immature cells by plotting low-frequency DC impedance on the x-axis and high-frequency current RF on the y-axis. This channel also allows for abnormal white blood cell morphology because various types of immature cells react differently to the reagent and appear in different regions (Fig. 20.24).

The nucleated red blood cell chamber uses Stromatolyser-NR to lyse the red blood cells, then removes the cytoplasm of the nucleated red blood cell and leaves the nucleus for examination by fluorescence and forward light scatter. The smaller volume of the nucleated red blood cell nuclei scatters less light and has less fluorescence intensity. Reticulocytes are counted by fluorescence. Red blood cells are stained with the fluorescent dye, and the forward fluorescence scatter is directly proportional to the amount of RNA in each cell. By plotting forward scattered light and side fluorescence, reticulocyte count and reticulocyte maturity can be measured as well as reticulocyte percentage,

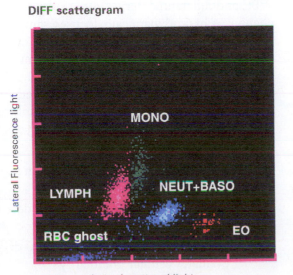

DIFF scattergram

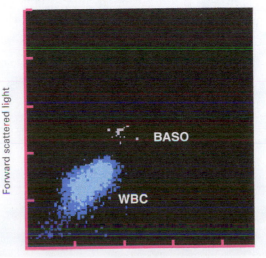

WBC / BASO scattergram

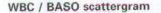

Figure 20.23 Sysmex Diff Channel.

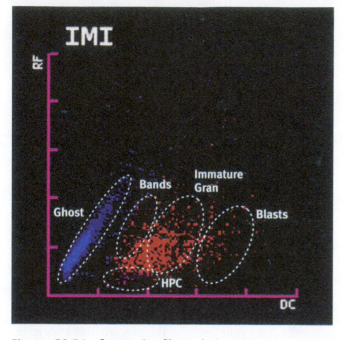

Figure 20.24 Sysmex Im Channel. Courtesy of Sysmex Corporation.

number, and immature reticulocyte fraction (IRF). Platelets can be measured by impedance and by fluorescent optical (PLT-O). The fluorescent count improves accuracy for very low and very high platelet counts (Fig. 20.25).

Figure 20.26 provides an example of a Sysmex report.

The XE-5000 has a body fluid mode that provides a WBC, red blood cell enumeration, and differential

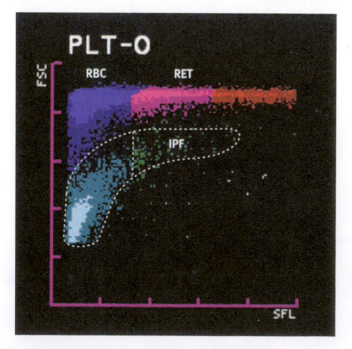

Figure 20.25 Sysmex Fluorescent Optical Platelet. Courtesy of Sysmex Corporation.

including polymorphonuclear and mononuclear count and total count (TC-BF). White blood cells are enumerated by fluorescence flow cytometry, and red blood cells are enumerated by direct current. XE-5000 can also analyze CSF, serous fluid, and synovial fluid. Specimens should be collected in EDTA (Fig. 20.27).

CellaVision Automated Digital Cell Morphology

CellaVision is an automated cell identification technology that locates cells and preclassifies and characterizes white blood cell and red blood cell images. CellaVision DM96 accessorizes an existing automated analyzer to perform manual differential, grouping cells with like cells, preclassifying white blood cells into 18 classes for identification, examining red blood cell morphology, and determining platelet estimations.

CellaVision Competency Software is a digital blood cell program used for management of proficiency and education of the manual differential. Participants perform the differential on a digital case test, then compare the participant's results with the correct result done by an examiner and with other participants.

Cell-Dyn Instrumentation

Manufactured by Abbott Diagnostics Instrumentation (www.abbottdiagnostics.com), the Cell-Dyn System uses three independent measurement technologies, including an optical channel for the WBC and differential, an impedance channel for the RBC and platelets, and a hemoglobin channel for hemoglobin determination.

Cell-Dyn has designed a unique technology of multiangle polarized scatter separation (MAPSS). The WBC and differential derive from this patented optical channel. A hydrodynamically focused sample stream is directed through a high-resolution flow cytometer. A cell suspension is prepared with a diluent that maintains white blood cells in their native state. The suspension then passes through an air-cooled Argon ion laser. Scattered light is measured at multiple angles:

Low-angle forward light scatter (1 to 3 degrees) represents the cell size.

Wide-angle forward light (3 to 11 degrees) measures the cell complexity.

Orthogonal light scatter (90 degrees) determines cell lobularity.

90 degrees depolarized light scatter (90 degrees D) evaluates cellular granularity.

Various combinations of these four angle measurements are used to differentiate white blood cell

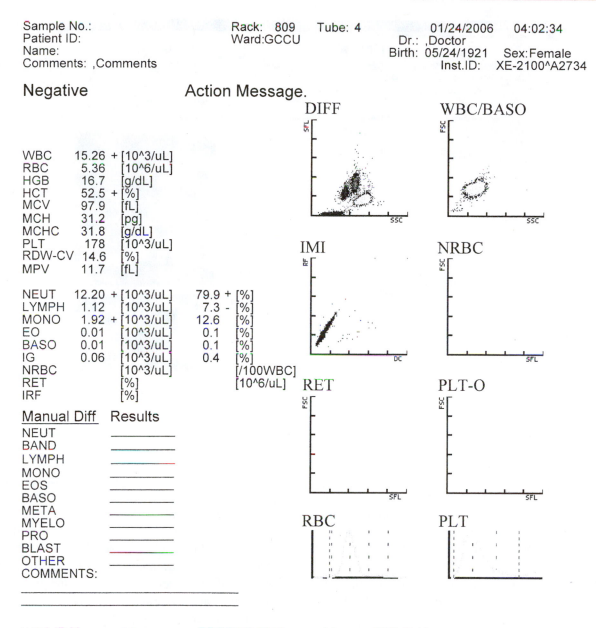

Sample No.:   Rack: 809   Tube: 4   01/24/2006   04:02:34
Patient ID: Ward:GCCU   Dr.: ,Doctor
Name: Birth: 05/24/1921   Sex:Female
Comments: ,Comments   Inst.ID: XE-2100^A2734

Negative   Action Message.

DIFF   WBC/BASO

WBC	15.26	+	[10^3/uL]		
RBC	5.36		[10^6/uL]		
HGB	16.7		[g/dL]		
HCT	52.5	+	[%]		
MCV	97.9		[fL]		
MCH	31.2		[pg]		
MCHC	31.8		[g/dL]		
PLT	178		[10^3/uL]		
RDW-CV	14.6		[%]		
MPV	11.7		[fL]		
NEUT	12.20	+	[10^3/uL]	79.9 +	[%]
LYMPH	1.12		[10^3/uL]	7.3 -	[%]
MONO	1.92	+	[10^3/uL]	12.6	[%]
EO	0.01		[10^3/uL]	0.1	[%]
BASO	0.01		[10^3/uL]	0.1	[%]
IG	0.06		[10^3/uL]	0.4	[%]
NRBC			[10^3/uL]		[/100WBC]
RET			[%]		[10^6/uL]
IRF			[%]		

IMI   NRBC

RET   PLT-O

Manual Diff   Results

NEUT	_____
BAND	_____
LYMPH	_____
MONO	_____
EOS	_____
BASO	_____
META	_____
MYELO	_____
PRO	_____
BLAST	_____
OTHER	_____
COMMENTS:	

RBC   PLT

_____

_____

WBC IP Message(s)   RBC/RET IP Message(s)   PLT IP Message(s)

Figure 20.26 Sysmex report.

populations. Neutrophils and eosinophils can be separated from mononuclear cells by plotting 90-degree light scatter data on the y-axis and wide-angle forward light scatter data on the x-axis. The ability of eosinophils to depolarize the polarized light scatter separates them from the neutrophil population. Lymphocytes, monocytes, and basophils can be separated by plotting low-angle forward light scatter on the y-axis and wide-angle forward light scatter on the x-axis. Information from the four channels then constructs a five-part WBC differential (Fig. 20.28).

Cell-Dyn Ruby is a multiparameter hematology analyzer. This instrument uses MAPSS technology for a five-part WBC differential. The most widely used plot, size versus complexity (0 degrees/10 degrees), separates lymphocytes from monocytes, granulocytes from monocytes, and neutrophils from eosinophils. Granularity versus lobularity (90 degrees D/90 degrees) views the separation of neutrophils and eosinophils. Platelets are enumerated by dual-angle optical analysis. Red blood cells are counted by using three angles of light scatter. The reticulocyte count is accomplished with thiazine New Methylene Blue, which is used to stain the RNA before introducing it to the 0-degree, 10-degree, and 90-degree angles. Data generated by this process are used to differentiate mature red blood cells from reticulocytes and platelet clumps.

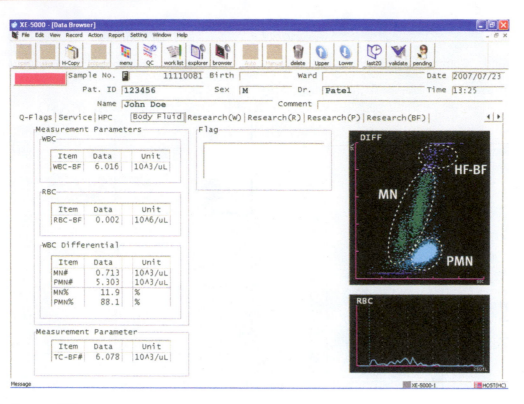

Figure 20.27   Sysmex CSR.   Courtesy of Sysmex Corporation.

Cell-Dyn Sapphire is a high-volume multiparameter analyzer that also uses MAPSS technology plus three-color fluorescence. The instrument uses the flow cytometric measurements of multiangle light scatter. This technology identifies white blood cells and their subpopulations, abnormal cell populations, nucleated red blood cells, and platelet clumps (Fig. 20.29). MAPSS plus fluorescent analysis consists of light scatter information from axial light loss (AxLL) or 0 degrees, intermediate angle scatter (IAS) or 7 degrees, polarized side scatter (PSS) or 90 degrees, and depolarized side scatter (DSS) or 90 degrees D. Along with these angles of measurement, the technology also introduces three-color fluorescence—FL1 (green), Fl 2(orange), and FL 3 (red). The measurements AxLL, IAS, and PSS determine size, complexity, and lobularity. For nucleated red blood cells, the AxLL, IAS, and FL 3 measurements are used for the absolute number and number per 100 white blood cells. Reticulocytes are measured by fluorescence that separates the reticulocytes from mature red blood cells and provides the immature reticulocyte fraction (IRM). The

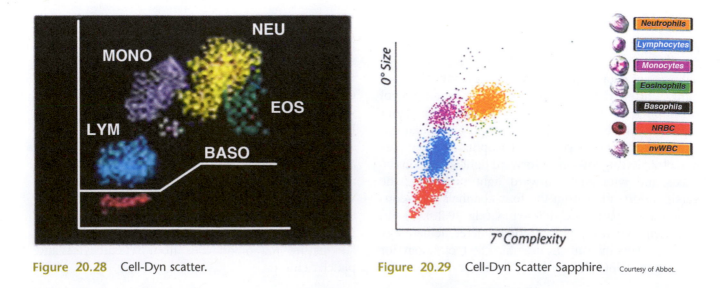

Figure 20.28   Cell-Dyn scatter.

Figure 20.29   Cell-Dyn Scatter Sapphire.   Courtesy of Abbot.

platelet count uses a dual-angle optical scatter and additional impedance count.

Advia Instrumentation

The ADVIA 120/2120 hematology analyzer is a whole blood cell analyzer from Siemens HealthCare Diagnostics (www.medical.siems.com) that uses Unifluidics technology, which consists of an eight-layer acrylic block Unifluidics uses flow cytometry to measure total WBC and differential cluster analysis to identify each cell by size and absorption. This technology of the ADVIA 120 has evolved from the Technicon H systems. Pathways for the fluids and air flow are machined within the acrylic layers for blood analysis, eliminating most tubing and pinch values. The analyzer has five reaction chambers: a hemoglobin chamber, a basophil-lobularity (BASO) chamber, an RBC/PLT chamber, a reticulocyte chamber, and a peroxidase (PEROX) chamber. The ADVIA 120/2120 analyzer uses flow cytometry for the analysis of cells. Aperture impedance counting is not used in this analyzer. The only parameter not derived from flow cytometry is hemoglobin, which is determined by the classic colorimetric method and is read at 546 nm. The ADVIA 120/2120 incorporates two independent flow cytometers: a laser-diode crystal that measures red blood cells and platelets and a tungsten halogen lamp for staining white blood cells and performing the WBC differential. Both cytometers operate simultaneously for forward light scatter and absorption for the counting and sorting of cells.

The RBC/PLT channel measures the RBC, red blood cell indices, hemoglobin concentration, and platelet count. Red blood cell analysis involves an isovolumetric sphering that eliminates the variability of cell shape. The specimen passes through low-angle light scatter (2 to 3 degrees), which correlates to cell volume and size, and high-angle (5 to 15 degrees) light scatter, which correlate with internal complexity. The analyzer generates a scatterplot, placing the high-angle scatter on the x-axis (hemoglobin concentration) and the low-angle scatter on the y-axis (red blood cell volume). The red blood cell erythrogram can provide nine areas of identification based on volume and hemoglobin content. Independent histograms for red blood cell volume and hemoglobin concentration are plotted. The red blood cell histogram provides the MCV and RDW measurements. Hematocrit, MCH, and MCH are calculated.

The system analyzes platelets using a two-dimensional analysis that measures the volume (size) and refractive index (density) of each platelet. The ADVIA 120/2120 generates a platelet scatterplot that includes cell volume and refractive index.

Hemoglobin concentration is measured by the cyanmethemoglobin method. The MCHC is derived from the colorimetrically measured hemoglobin concentration, the RBC, and the MCV. The cell hemoglobin concentration mean (CHCM) derives from the directly measured red blood cell hemoglobin concentration histogram. Interferences in the hemoglobin colorimetric method, such as lipemia or icterus, affect the calculated MCHC but do not interfere with the CHCM parameter.

WBC is measured from two reaction chambers, the peroxidase channel and BASO lobularity channel, using cytochemistry or myeloperoxidase activity and light scatter. In the peroxidase chamber, white blood cells are stained for myeloperoxidase activity and then pass through an optical chamber that measures light scatter or cell size and light absorption or stain intensity. These two measurements allow enumeration and classification of leukocytes into neutrophils, monocytes, lymphocytes, and eosinophils. Only cells with peroxidase activity are stained. Neutrophils and eosinophils contain the most peroxidase. Monocytes stain weakly. Lymphocytes, basophils, and large unstained cells (LUCs) contain no peroxidase staining. LUCs include activated lymphocytes, plasma cells, hairy cells, or blast cells that are negative for peroxidase reaction. Each cell passing the focused beam is counted, and the light absorbed relates to peroxidase staining. Light scatter in the forward direction (1 to 3 degrees) relates to size (Fig. 20.30).

The BASO/lobularity channel strips the leukocytes of their cytoplasm, with exception of basophils, which are counted along with the total WBC and the lobularity index (LI). The LI measures the difference between the positions of two cell populations. Basophils are identifiable by their large low-angle scatter. The BASO cytogram identifies and counts the cells and nuclei based on position, density, and location.

The reticulocyte reaction chamber measures low-angle and high-angle scatter and cell absorption. The absorption data are used to classify reticulocytes or mature red blood cells. Low-angle scatter and high-angle scatter are proportional to cell size and hemoglobin concentration, and light absorption is proportional to RNA content. The reticulocyte hemoglobin concentration (CHr) is a parameter that can be used for early detection of functional iron deficiency and anemia.

Cerebrospinal Fluid Analysis on the Advia 120/2120

Red blood cells and white blood cells are enumerated by direct cytometry in CSF. The cells are enumerated and differentiated by three measurements: low-angle

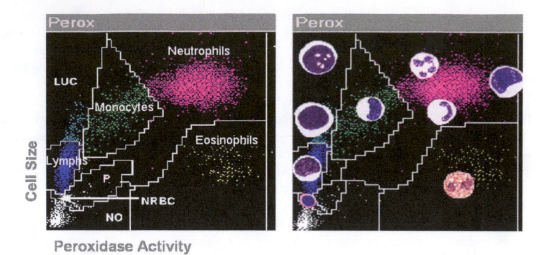

Figure 20.30 Advia peroxidase chamber. Courtesy of Siemens Healthcare Diagnostics.

scatter, high-angle scatter, and absorbance. A cytogram is constructed (Fig. 20.31). Results include RBC, WBC, and mononuclear and polymorphonuclear values in percent and absolute. These cells are then differentiated into monocytes, lymphocytes, and neutrophils.

Quality Assurance and Quality Control

All automated methods require the use of quality assurance procedures. The Clinical Laboratory and Standards Institute (CLSI) provides performance goal standards for hematology analyzers. These standards provide guidelines for instrument calibration, calibration verification, instrument validation, and quality control. Calibration procedures are established by the manufacturer to ensure accuracy and precision. Calibration must be performed at initial installation and should be verified every 6 months, and calibration

verification should be performed after part replacement or instrument repair. Commercial calibration kits are available.

Quality control for hematology analyzers involves the use of stabilized control material with established values to verify that the instrument is running properly. The running of controls ensures the accuracy and precision of the instrument. This analysis monitors and checks the analyzer's performance. All laboratories should establish or verify the manufacturer means or "true value" before using that lot of control material. Usually three levels of controls are run on each shift or every 8 hours of every day before patient testing is performed and reported. Quality control results should be evaluated daily for acceptability. The use of quality control materials ensures that the instrument is in good working order and validates patient results before they are reported. If the value of the

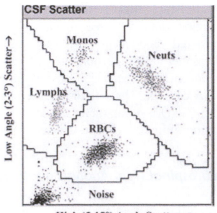

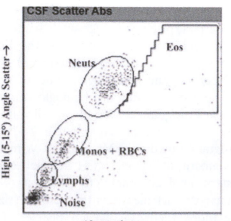

Figure 20.31 Advia CSF. Courtesy of Siemens Healthcare Diagnostics.

control is not within the predetermined acceptable range, patient results cannot be reported. The procedure must be reviewed for potential error. Once the error has been corrected, testing must be repeated when the control value falls within the established acceptable range patient samples can be run. The laboratory must always ensure reliable results. Quality control should be run when the reagent lot number has been changed, after calibration, after an unusual shift or trend in patient results, and after maintenance.

What Knowledge Is Necessary for the Operator of an Automated Instrument?

Operating automated cell counting instrumentation requires many skills. The operator must:

1. Know normal reference ranges.
2. Be familiar with normal scatterplots and histograms for the particular piece of equipment.
3. Be familiar with the flagging criteria determined by the particular laboratory information system (LIS).
   - Reference ranges will be preset according to the LIS; specimens that fall out of the reference range are *flagged*.
4. Be familiar with delta checks.
   - Delta checks are historical checks of test results from the patient's previous samples.
5. Be familiar with reflex testing.
   - Reflex testing represents additional testing, such as manual slide reviews, which must be accomplished before test results can be released. Operators make decisions on which reflex tests to perform.
6. Notify the appropriate personnel of critical results.
   - Critical results are results that exceed or are markedly decreased from the reference range or the patient history of results.
7. Be familiar with daily maintenance procedures.
8. Be familiar with specimen handling and appropriate specimen requirements.

Sample Case Using Coulter VCS Technology

An approach to verifying and sending test results follows (this approach can be used for each automated system explained in this section).

1. The CBC results look normal (Fig. 20.32).
2. When we preview the results, we can see that the eosinophil count is extremely high on the differential report.

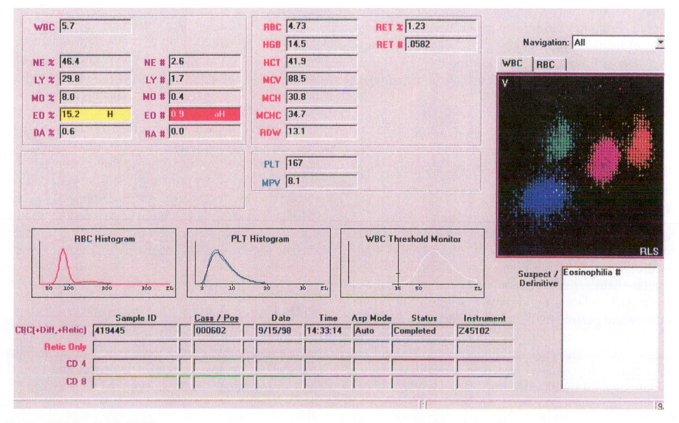

Figure 20.32 Coulter VCS.

3. We also notice that the eosinophil area on the scatterplot is particularly bright.
4. The eosinophil result on the differential is flagged.
5. Delta check revealed that the patient sample had been run on the instrument 4 days before with normal results in all categories.
6. Because the abnormal results have been flagged, reflex testing demands that the best course of action is to do a manual smear review and verify the large number of eosinophils.
7. Once this is accomplished, the results can be reported.

FLOW CYTOMETRY INSTRUMENTATION†

Flow cytometry is a technology that measures the physical characteristics, chemical properties, and phenotype of cells and defines the maturation of cell stages. This methodology uses principles of light scatter, light excitation, and emission of fluorochrome to generate specific data from cells or particles. The data obtained allow the measurement of quantity, size, morphology, and internal and external structure of cells in question. These applications are used for the diagnosis, prognosis, and monitoring of disease. Fluorescent signals emitted by dyes that are bound to specific monoclonal antibodies have many applications in the diagnosis of hematologic malignancies (Table 20.13). Flow cytometry offers an improved method over cytochemistry and morphology for the diagnosis of hematologic malignancies.

Flow cytometers consist of three systems: fluidics or transport system, optics for the detection of light scatter and fluorescent light signals, and electronics to monitor and control the operation and storage of data.

Sample Preparation

Specimens that are used for analysis include bone marrow cores, peripheral blood, CSF, pleural fluid, fine-needle aspirates, lymph nodes, and solid tumors. The cellular characteristics that are measured include granularity, cell surface area, and internal complexity. Bone marrow and peripheral blood are collected in K2 or K3 EDTA. The specimens are stored at room temperature and should be analyzed within 24 hours after collection. Lymphoid tissue is placed in a sterile container containing cold tissue medium.

Table 20.13 ⊙ Application of Flow Cytometry
Immunophenotyping
Diagnosis and staging of leukemia/lymphoma
Lymphocyte screening panel: AIDS patients
DNA content analysis
RNA content
Enzyme studies
Fetal cell enumeration

Principles of Operation

Flow cytometry uses the principle of hydrodynamic focusing, which allows the cell to enter the center of sheath flow or carrier fluid one cell at a time. Single cells scatter light as they enter one or more of the light sources for excitation. Fluorochromes are excited to a high-energy source. Optical detectors convert scattered and emitted light from the cells into electronic pulses. Light is sent to different detectors using optical filters. These electronic pulses or signals are processed for analysis, classification, sorting, or separation of cells and data storage.

Fluidics

The fluidics system is a pumping system that transports cells from a three-dimensional sample suspension to a single file single cell suspension at a very high speed. As the cell enters the flow chamber, the sheath fluid, usually phosphate-buffered saline, hydrodynamically (single cell fluid stream) focuses the fluid to a single file for excitation of cells or particles (Fig. 20.33). The sample in an isotonic fluid is forced through the flow cell at a constant pressure that is surrounded by another isotonic fluid to produce a laminar flow. The hydrodynamic properties cause the cells to line up in a single file for interrogation by the laser. This focusing increases accuracy for better interrogation and sorting of the cells.

Optics

Optics provide illumination of stained or unstained particles and detect light scatter and fluorescent light signals. Flow cytometers use laser sources and optical filters to quantitate intrinsic cellular parameters and

†The author wishes to acknowledge Candace Breen Golightly, MS, MT (ASCP), and Mark Golightly, PhD, for their assistance with this section.

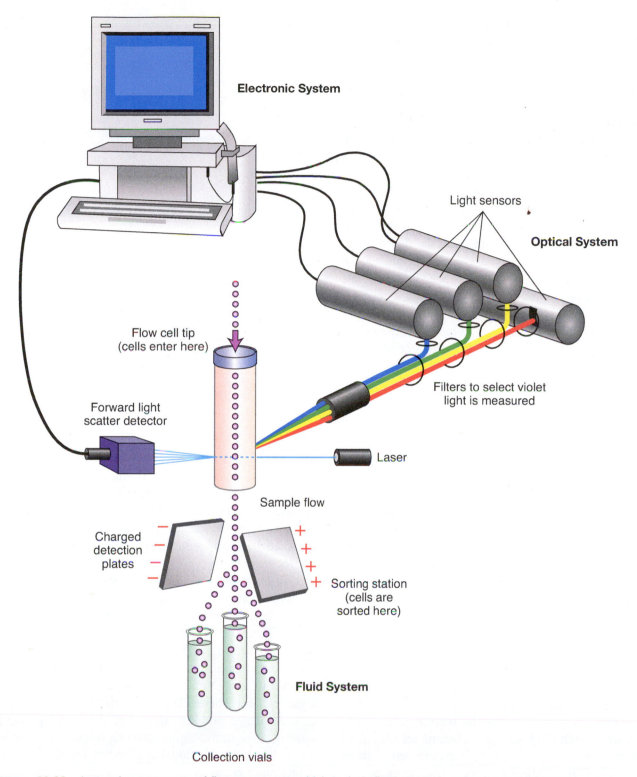

Figure 20.33 Internal components of flow cytometer, which include fluid, optical, and electronic systems.

extrinsic cell properties by cell excitation and emission. Laser lights are monochromic or single wavelength. Light scattering or emission occurs when excitation light is absorbed and then reradiated with no change in wavelength. Different fluorescent molecules have different excitation and emission. Every cell has a unique fluorescent profile or scatter pattern. The

information from light scatter and emission of the fluorescent light is separated and directed to photomultiplier tubes (PMT). Light scatter is strongest in the forward direction (FLS). Fluorescence occurs when a molecule excited by light of one wavelength returns to a lower state by emitting light of a longer wavelength. Cellular constituents can be measured simultaneously by using several excitation sources. With the addition of fluorescent dyes, four-colored analysis can be performed.

Electronics

The electronics of the flow cytometer involve the control, acquisition, and analysis of data and the storage of that data. Light signals collected by PMT detectors are converted to digital signals by the system's computer. Instrument electronics are controlled by a personal computer or Macintosh-type computer, which controls the function of the instrument, stores data, and provides software for data analysis. The signals generated are digitized and are proportional to the amount of scatter light or fluorescence. These signals are stored. Several parameters of the data are generated for each cell that is interrogated.

Results received from flow cytometry are quantitative in absolute numbers and fluorescence intensity. Most analyzers are capable of analyzing 10,000 events per second. Rare and unusual cells can be analyzed in great detail.

Analysis

Data collected from the flow cytometer are analyzed to determine the light-scattering properties of the cells, which determine what population of cells requires further examination. Light is scattered in all directions but is collected along the axis of the laser beam or forward angle light scatter and at a 90-degree angle or side angle light scatter. Fluorescent emissions are collected at the 90-degree angle. Forward angle light scatter (FALS) is related to the size of the cells: The higher the FALS, the larger the cell. Side angle light scatter is related to the internal cellular complexity, including cell density and granularity. The greater the side light scatter signal, the more internally complex is the cell. The photodiode collects forward scatter light, and PMTs collect side scatter light and fluorescent emissions. Filters define the wavelength of light that reaches each PMT. Cell populations are identified by plotting the two light-scattering parameters along the x- and y-axes. Mature monocytes, lymphocytes, and granulocytes are identified through their light-scattering properties (Fig. 20.34). Next, a population of cells is identified for further analysis by fluorescence. This process is called gating, which refers to identifying and enumerating subsets of cells to analyze a specific cell population.

Analysis of the fluorescent properties is performed by fluorescent-labeled monoclonal antibody markers. Fluorochromes are dyes that absorb light of

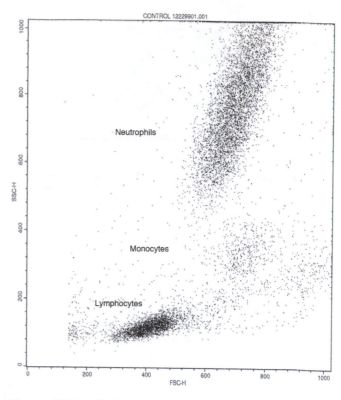

Figure 20.34 Light scatter.

one wavelength and then emit light of a different or higher wavelength. Fluorochromes by themselves or coupled with monoclonal antibodies are used to assess viability, immunophenotype, and nucleic acid content. The list of fluorochromes has increased over the years. Table 20.14 shows some commonly used hematologic fluorochromes.

Fluorochrome analysis involves the attachment of a fluorochrome to a monoclonal antibody. The staining of specific cells helps to identify, characterize, and enumerate normal and abnormal cell populations. Cluster of differentiation (CD) is defined as a cluster of antibodies recognizing the same antigen. These are referred to as CD markers. Table 20.15 lists hematologic markers. These CD markers define characteristics of cell lineage and function and the developmental stage of cells. Immunophenotyping refers to the use of monoclonal or polyclonal antibodies for the specific detection of antigens.

Most flow cytometric instruments use four different monoclonal antibody markers, each labeled with a different fluorochrome; this is called multiple color analysis. The fluorescent data can be examined for absolute number or percent of cells that are positive and fluorescent intensity, which is related to antigen density. This fluorescent intensity or antigen density helps identify the maturational stages and phenotypes of the cells and helps define criteria for diagnosis and prognosis.

Table 20.14 ◉ Commonly Used Fluorochromes

Probe	Excitation Wavelength (nm)	Emission Wavelength (nm)
Reactive and Conjugated		
Fluorescein (FITC)	495	519
Phycoerythrin (PE)	565	575
PE-carbocyanina-5 (PE-Cy 5)	565	670
PE-Cy 5.5	565	695
PE-Cy7	565	770
Per-Cp	490	670
Cy5	650	665
APC-Cy7	650	770
Alexa Fluors		
Alexa 350	350	445
Alexa 430	435	445
Alexa 488	500	520
Alexa 700	700	720
DNA Content		
DAPI	360	460
Acridine Orange	495	535
Propidium Iodide (PI)	535	620
7-AAD	545	650

Table 20.15 ◉ Cluster of Differentiation

Immature	
CD34	Stem cell
CD38	Hematopoietic
CD117	Stem cells, mast
TdT	Precursor lymph
HLA-DR	Hematopoietic
B Cell	
CD10	Precursor B
CD19	Precursor and mature B
CD20	B-cell activation
CD22	B cell with cytoplasmic activation
Kappa	B cell with Fc receptor
Lambda	
FMC7	B cell
T Cell	
CD2	Early
CD3	Pan-T cell
CD4	T-cell subset
CD5	T cell
CD7	Early
CD8	T cell
CD56	T-cell subset
Erythroid	
CD36	
CD71	
Glycophorin A	
Megakaryocyte	
CD31	
CD41	GP IIb/IIa
CD42	
CD61	GP IIb/IIIa
Granulocytic	
CD13	Pan myeloid
CD33	Pan myeloid
CD15	Promyelocyte
CD11b	Myelocyte
MPO	Myeloid
Monocytic	
CD11b	Granulocytic and monocytic
CD13	Early monocyte
CD14	Mature monocytes
CD33	Granulocytic and monocytic
HLA-DR	Monocytic maturation

CD, cluster designation; GP, glycoprotein; HLA, human leukocyte antigen; MPO, myeloperoxidase; TdT, terminal deoxynucleotidyl transferase.

The data that are generated can be displayed in a single-parameter or two-parameter histogram. In the single-parameter histogram, the x-axis is the fluorescence intensity, and the number of events is displaced onto the y-axis (Fig. 20.35). The two-parameter histogram can be displayed in several ways. A dot plot displays each cell on the graph as a single event. The contour plot shows different cell densities. Two parameter plots are divided into four quadrants or regions that generate statistics on the subpopulations. The data these quadrants relay are negative, positive, or double positive cells. Percentages of positive cells are calculated based on the number of events within each quadrant. Events in the upper right (UR) quadrant are double positive for the two selected CD markers, and events in the lower left (LL) quadrant are negative for the two markers. The upper left (UL) and lower right (LR) quadrants show single positive CD populations (see Fig. 20.35).

Fluorescence intensity can also be measured. This measurement represents the fluorescence per cell in a gated population (Fig. 20.36).

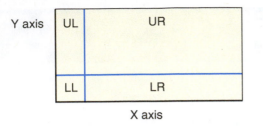

Figure 20.35 How flow cytometry data are graphed. LL, cells negative for both *x*-axis and *y*-axis. UR, cells positive for both *x*-axis and *y*-axis. UL, cells positive for *y*-axis and negative for *x*-axis. LR, cells positive for *x*-axis and negative for *y*-axis. Different CD antibodies are placed on the *x*- and *y*-axes.

In disease diagnosis, the data generated can help characterize and aid treatment of various types of leukemias and lymphomas. Total cell count, population percentages, and brightness of fluorescent differences between populations can be analyzed for better treatment.

Quality Control

Quality control in flow cytometry is divided into an internal quality control and external quality control. Internal quality control ensures that the instrument, reagents, and laboratory staff are performing within the testing limits set by the individual laboratory. Quality control of the instrument involves checking the performance of the lasers, PMTs, optical filters, and amplifiers. A daily start-up of the instrument is very important, as is using the appropriate reference material. The calibration of the fluorescence channels should be within established tolerance levels. Normal controls must be tested daily to ensure accurate sample processing and proper performance of the analyzer. Controls are commercially available with defined ranges. External quality control involves running distributed control samples,

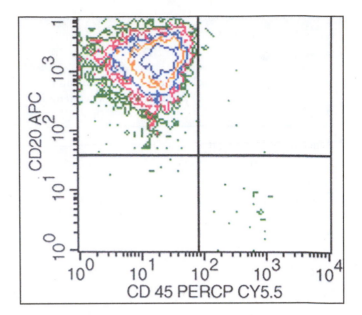

Figure 20.36 Contour plot.

either fresh or reconstituted lyophilized specimens; this provides a means of comparing the performance of one laboratory with the performance of others. This method facilitates direct comparisons, performance assessments, and method validation.

Applications of Flow Cytometry

Flow cytometry adds an additional piece of supporting information to the diagnosis of leukemia and lymphoma. Bone marrow aspirate smears, blood smear interpretation, CBC results, patient's symptoms, cytogenetics, cytochemical staining, and flow cytometry all play a role in the patient's diagnosis. Immunophenotyping is helpful in distinguishing between lymphoid and myeloid acute leukemias, the subclassification of the lymphoid and myeloid leukemias (Table 20.16),

Table 20.16 ○ Immunophenotype

Myeloid

AML	CD33	CD34	HLA-DR	CD11b	CD13	CD14	Glyco A	CD61
M0	+	+	+	−	+	−	−	−
M1	+	+	+	+/−	+	−	−	−
M2	+	+	+	+/−	+	−	−	−
M3	+	−	−	−	+	−	−	−
M4	+	−	+	+	+	+	−	−
M5	+	−	+	+	+	+	−	−
M6	+/−	−	+/−	−	−	−	+	−
M7	+/−	−	+	−	−	−	−	+

Table 20.16 ⚬ Immunophenotype—cont'd

Lymphoid

ALL	CD10	CD20	CD19	CD2	CD5	CD7	CIg	SIg	TdT
Early pre-B	+	−	+	−	−	−	−	−	+
Pre-B	+	+	+	−	−	−	+	−	+
Mature B	+/−	+	+	−	−	−	−	+	−
Precursor T	−	−	−	+	+	+	−	−	+

ALL, acute lymphoblastic leukemia; AML, acute myelogenous leukemia; CD, cluster designation.

classification of lymphomas, evaluation of therapeutic responses, and detection of minimal residual disease after treatment.

Other applications of flow cytometry involve the diagnosis of immunodeficiency disorders that include enumeration of lymphocytes subsets seen in HIV, evaluation of neutrophil function helpful in the diagnosis of chronic granulomatous disease (CGD), hyper-IgM syndrome, leukocyte adhesion deficiency, and paroxysmal nocturnal hemoglobinuria (PNH). Clinical applications in organ transplantation include monitoring patients receiving antirejection therapy, detection of HLA alloantibody, and enumeration of CD34 stem and progenitor cells. Additionally, this technique has clinical application in transfusion medicine, including the detection of fetal hemoglobin and fetomaternal hemorrhage and measuring residual white blood cells in leukocyte-reduced blood.

Flow cytometry is a diagnostic tool with many applications under development that will ultimately lead to better patient care. Figure 20.37 presents a case example of use of flow cytometry.

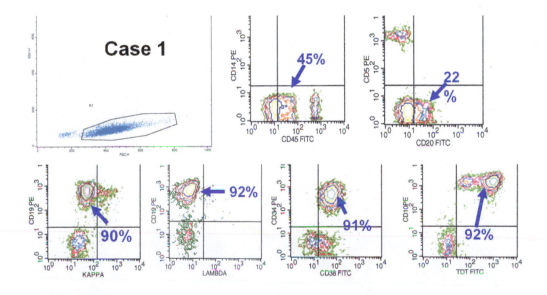

Case 1- Patient's light scatter demonstrates intermediate to large sized cells. Gated population is positive for CD45, CD10, CD19, CD38, CD34, TdT, and HLA-DR, with dual CD38/CD34, and CD10/TdT. Kappa negative, with some CD20.

Figure 20.37 Flow case.

References
Suggested Reading

Adams C. Autocrit II Centrifuge and Adams Microhematocrit II Centrifuge, Becton, Dickinson and Company, 1976.

CAP, 2005 Surveys and Anatomic Pathology Education Programs, Hematology, Clinical Microscopy, and Body Fluids Glossary.

Ciesla BE, Simpson P. Evaluation of cell morphology and evaluation of white cell and platelet morphology. In: Harmening DH, ed. Clinical Hematology Theory and Fundamentals of Hemostasis, 4th ed. Philadelphia: FA Davis, 2002: 95–97.

Davidsohn I, Henry JB. Clinical Diagnosis and Management by Laboratory Methods, 16th ed. Philadelphia: WB Saunders, 1979.

Kjeldsberg C, Knight J. Body Fluids. Chicago: ASCP Press, 1982.

NCCLS. Collection, Transport, and Processing of Blood Specimens for Testing Plasma-Based Coagulation Assays Approved Guideline, 4th ed. Wayne, PA: NCCLS, 2003: NCCLS document H21-A4.

Sysmex Corporation. Sysmex Ca-1500 System Operators Manual. Kobe, Japan: Sysmex Corporation, 2001.

Turgeon ML. Clinical Hematology Theory and Procedures, 3rd ed. Philadelphia: Lippincott Williams & Wilkins, 1999.

Wooldridge-King M. Determination of Microhematocrit via Centrifuge. AACN Procedure Manual for Critical Care, 4th ed. Philadelphia: WB Saunders, 2000.

Wyrick GJ, Hughes VC. Routine hematology methods. In: Harmening DH, ed. Clinical Hematology and Fundamentals of Hemostasis, 4th ed. Philadelphia: FA Davis, 2002: 571–573.

Hematology Automation

Beckman Coulter Higher Performance: With You in Mind The Coulter LH 780 Hematology Systems. 2006.

Beckman Coulter Transforming the Hematology Laboratory: Unicel DxH 800 Coulter Cellular Analysis System. 2008.

Sysmex Corporation: XE-500 Automated Hematology System, Advanced Technology. 2007.

Sysmex Corporation: The Cell Analysis Center, Scientific Bulletin No. 1, Principle of Flow Cytometry. 2008.

Sysmex Corporation: The Cell Analysis Center, Scientific Bulletin No. 4, Principle for Automated Leukocyte Differentiation. 2008.

Abbott: Cell-Dyn Ruby Casebook "Principles and Practice." 2008.

Siemens Healthcare Diagnostics Inc: Advia 2110 Hematology System.

Flow Cytometry

Dako: Flow Cytometry Educational Guide, 2nd ed. 2005.

Henel G, Schmitz J. Basic theory and clinical applications of flow cytometry. LabMedicine 38, 2007.

King D. Flow cytometry: An overview. MLO 2007.

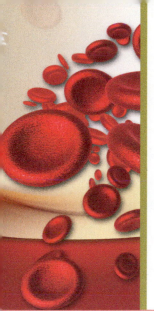

Appendix A

Answers to Review Questions

CHAPTER 1
1. B
2. C
3. A
4. D
5. C/A
6. D
7. C
8. B
9. A
10. A

CHAPTER 2
1. C
2. A
3. A
4. B
5. B
6. B
7. C
8. B
9. A
10. B

CHAPTER 3
1. C
2. B
3. D
4. B
5. C
6. B
7. D
8. B
9. C
10. A

CHAPTER 4
1. B
2. C
3. A
4. C
5. C
6. B
7. B
8. C
9. A
10. B

CHAPTER 5
1. C
2. B
3. D
4. A
5. C
6. A
7. C
8. D
9. C
10. B

CHAPTER 6
1. C
2. A
3. B
4. C
5. C
6. D
7. A
8. B
9. C
10. C

CHAPTER 7
1. D
2. B
3. C
4. C
5. B
6. A
7. B
8. D
9. B
10. B

CHAPTER 8
1. C
2. D
3. B
4. B
5. A
6. A
7. C
8. D
9. C
10. A

CHAPTER 9
1. C
2. B
3. C
4. D
5. A
6. A
7. D
8. C
9. C
10. A

CHAPTER 10

1. C
2. A
3. B
4. B
5. C
6. B
7. B
8. A
9. C
10. D

CHAPTER 11

1. C
2. B
3. A
4. D
5. C
6. A
7. C
8. D
9. C
10. A

CHAPTER 12

1. D
2. B
3. B
4. C
5. A
6. B
7. C
8. C
9. D
10. B

CHAPTER 13

1. D
2. A
3. C
4. B
5. C
6. A
7. D
8. D
9. C
10. C

CHAPTER 14

1. B
2. C
3. A
4. C
5. C
6. C
7. A
8. B
9. C
10. C

CHAPTER 15

1. A
2. C
3. A
4. C
5. B
6. B
7. C
8. B
9. D
10. C
11. B

CHAPTER 16

1. C
2. C
3. A
4. B
5. D
6. D
7. C
8. C
9. C
10. C

CHAPTER 17

1. C
2. B
3. D
4. A
5. D
6. C
7. A
8. A
9. A
10. C

CHAPTER 18

1. C
2. A
3. C
4. B
5. C
6. B
7. C
8. D
9. C
10. A

CHAPTER 19

1. A
2. C
3. A
4. D
5. D
6. C
7. A
8. B
9. D
10. A

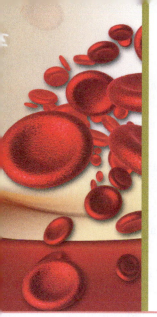

Appendix B

List of Abbreviations

AA	arachidonic acid
ACTH	adrenocorticotropic hormone
ADP	adenosine diphosphate
AIDS	acquired immunodeficiency syndrome
ALL	acute lymphoblastic leukemia
AML	acute myelogenous leukemia
APL	acute promyelocytic leukemia
aPTT	activated partial thromboplastin time
AS	ankylosing spondylitis
ASD	atrial septal defect
ATP	adenosine triphosphate
AxLL	axial light loss
BASO	basophil
BK	bradykinin
BSS	Bernard-Soulier syndrome
Ca^{2+}	calcium ion
CBC	complete blood count
CBFB	core binding factor beta subunit
CD	cluster of differentiation
2-CdA	2-chlorodeoxyadenosine
CEL	chronic eosinophilic leukemia
CFU-GEMM	colony-forming unit granulocyte, erythrocyte, monocyte, myelocyte
CFU-S	colony-forming unit spleen
CGD	chronic granulomatous disease
CHAD	cold hemagglutinin disease

CHr	reticulocyte hemoglobin concentration
Cl	chloride
CLL	chronic lymphocytic leukemia
CML	chronic myelogenous leukemia
CMPD	chronic myeloproliferative disorder
CMV	cytomegalovirus
CNL	chronic neutrophilic leukemia
CNS	central nervous system
CNSHA	congenital nonspherocytic hemolytic anemia
COX	cyclooxygenase inhibitor
CSF	colony-stimulating factor, cerebrospinal fluid
CSSCD	Cooperative Study of Sickle Cell Disease
CV	coefficient of variation
DDAVP	desmopressin acetate
DIC	disseminated intravascular coagulation
DNA	deoxyribonucleic acid
2,3-DPG	2,3-diphosphoglycerate
DSS	depolarized side scatter
DVT	deep vein thrombosis
EACA	epsilon-aminocaproic acid
EBV	Epstein-Barr virus
EDTA	ethylenediaminetetraacetic acid
ELISA	enzyme-linked immunosorbent assay
EPI	epinephrine

EPO	erythropoietin
ESR	erythrocyte sedimentation rate
ET	essential thrombocythemia
FAB	French-American-British investigative group
FALS	forward light scatter
FDP	fibrin degradation product
FITC	fluorescein
fL	femtoliter
FLAER	fluorescent-labeled aerolysin
FLT3	fms-related tyrosine kinase 3
FSP/FDP	fibrin split product/fibrin degradation product
G-CSF	granulocyte colony-stimulating factor
GI	gastrointestinal
GM	granulocyte-monocyte
GM-CSF	granulocyte-macrophage colony-stimulating factor
GP	glycoprotein
GPI	glycosylphosphatidylinositol
GT	Glanzmann's thrombasthenia
GVHD	graft-versus-host disease
HCO_3	bicarbonate
Hct	hematocrit
HES	hypereosinophilic syndrome
HGA	human granulocytic anaplasmosis
Hgb	hemoglobin
HH	hereditary hemochromatosis
HLA	human leukocyte antigen
HME	human monocytic ehrlichiosis
HMWK	high-molecular-weight kininogen
H_2O	water
HUS	hemolytic uremic syndrome
ILS	intermediate light scatter
IDA	iron deficiency anemia
IEF	isoelectric focusing
IgG	immunoglobulin G
IL	interleukin
IMF	idiopathic myelofibrosis
INR	international normalized ratio
IRF	immature reticulocyte fraction
ISC	irreversibly sickled cell

ITP	idiopathic (immune) thrombocytopenic purpura
IVIg	intravenous immunoglobulin
K^+	potassium ion
LA	lupus anticoagulant
LALS	low-angle light scatter
LAP	leukocyte alkaline phosphatase
LDH	lactate dehydrogenase
LI	lobularity index
LIS	laboratory information system
LMALS	lower median angle light scatter
LSC	lymphocytic committed cell
MAC	membrane attack complex
MALS	median angle light scatter
MAPSS	multiangle polarized scatter separation
MCH	mean corpuscular hemoglobin
MCHC	mean corpuscular hemoglobin content
MCV	mean corpuscular volume
MDS	myelodysplastic syndrome
MDS-U	myelodysplastic syndrome unclassifiable
M:E	myeloid:erythroid ratio
MHA	microangiopathic hemolytic anemia
MPN	myeloproliferative neoplasm
MPO	myeloperoxidase
MPV	mean platelet volume
MRV	mean reticulocyte volume
NA	aperture number
Na^+	sodium ion
NAD	nicotinamide adenine
NADPH	nicotinamide adenine dinucleotide phosphate
NAITP	neonatal isoimmune thrombocytopenia
N:C	nucleus:cytoplasm ratio
NK	natural killer
NOS	not otherwise specified
NPM1	nucleophosmin
nRBC	nucleated red blood cell
NSAID	nonsteroidal anti-inflammatory drug

NSE	nonspecific esterase		RES	reticuloendothelial system
OD	oxygen dissociation		RETIC#	reticulocyte number
OPSI	overwhelming postsplenectomy infections		RF	radiofrequency
PAI-1	plasmin-plasminogen activator inhibitor 1		r-HuEPO	recombinant human erythropoietin
PCH	paroxysmal cold hemoglobinuria		RIPA	ristocetin-induced platelet aggregation
PDGF	platelet-derived growth factor		RNA	ribonucleic acid
PE	pulmonary embolism		RPI	reticulocyte production index
PEROX	peroxidase		SBB	Sudan black B
PGG_2	prostaglandin G_2		SD	standard deviation
PGI_2	prostacyclin		SGOT	serum glutamic oxaloacetic transaminase
PIGA	phosphatidylinositol glycan class A		SIg	surface immunoglobulin
PK	pyruvate kinase deficiency		SLE	systemic lupus erythematosus
Plt	platelet		SOP	standard operating procedure
PMT	photomultiplier tube		sTfR	serum transferrin receptor
PNH	paroxysmal nocturnal hemoglobinuria		TAR	thrombocytopenia with absent radii
PPE	personal protective equipment		TdT	terminal deoxynucleotidyltransferase
PPP	platelet-poor plasma			
PRP	platelet-rich plasma		TFPI	tissue factor pathway inhibitor
PSC	pluripotent stem cell		TGF	transforming growth factor
PSS	polarized side scatter		TIBC	total iron binding capacity
PT	prothrombin time		TNTC	too numerous to count
PTP	post-transfusion purpura		tPA	tissue plasminogen activator
PV	polycythemia vera		TRAP	tartrate-resistant acid phosphatase
PVSG	Polycythemia Vera Study Group		TT	thrombin time
RA	refractory anemia		TTP	thrombotic thrombocytopenic purpura
RAEB-1	refractory anemia with excess blasts			
RAEB-2	refractory anemia with excess blasts 2		UMALS	upper median angle light scatter
			VCS	volume, conductivity, and scatter
RARS	refractory anemia with ringed sideroblasts		VEGF	vascular endothelial growth factor
RBC	red blood cell count		vWF	von Willebrand factor
RCM	red blood cell mass		WBC	white blood cell count
RCMD	refractory cytopenia with multilineage dysplasia		WHO	World Health Organization
RCMD/RS	refractory cytopenia with multilineage dysplasia and ringed sideroblasts			
RDW	red blood cell distribution width			
REAL	Revised European-American Lymphoma Classification			

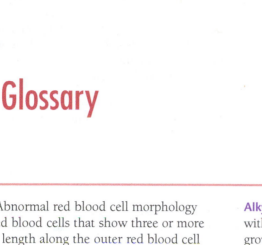

Glossary

Acanthocyte • Abnormal red blood cell morphology characterized by red blood cells that show three or more spicules of uneven length along the outer red blood cell membrane; associated with abetalipoproteinemia, neonatal hepatitis, postsplenectomy, and liver cirrhosis

Accuracy • Closest measurement of a result when compared with the true value

Achlorhydria • Lack of hydrochloric acid in the stomach

Acidosis • Increased acidity of blood (e.g., diabetic acidosis) caused by excessive loss of bicarbonate (as in renal disease)

Acrocyanosis • Blue or purple mottled discoloration of the fingers, toes, nose, or all three

Activated protein C resistance (APCR) • Autosomal dominant thrombotic disorder caused by mutation of factor V; most common inherited cause of thrombosis; referred to as factor V Leiden

Acute lymphoblastic leukemia (ALL) • Malignant disease of the bone marrow, with proliferation of lymphoblasts in intramedullary and extramedullary sites

Acute myeloblastic leukemia (AML) • Malignant disease of bone marrow associated with rapid proliferation of blasts in the bone marrow, peripheral blood, and other tissues. Depending on the subtype of AML, the blasts may include myeloblasts, monoblasts, and (rarely) pronormoblasts or megakaryoblasts, or any combination

Afibrinogenemia • Autosomal recessive bleeding disorder associated with less than 10 mg/dL of fibrinogen

Albinism • Partial or total absence of pigment in the hair, skin, and eyes

Alder's anomaly (Alder-Reilly anomaly) • Rare inherited disorder associated with the presence of coarse dark granules in neutrophils, lymphocytes, and monocytes

Alkalosis • Increased blood alkalinity caused by an accumulation of alkali or reduction of acids

Alkylating agent • Agent that replaces a hydrogen atom with an alkyl radical, interfering with cell metabolism and growth

Alloimmunization • Immune response to antigens on blood or tissue cells received from a donor of the same species

Allosteric • Change in shape and activity of a protein, resulting from combination with another substance at a point other than the chemically active site

Alpha-2 antiplasmin • Important inhibitor of fibrinolysis that suppresses plasmin binding to fibrin

Alpha thalassemia • Four possible hematologic conditions resulting from deletion of one or more alpha genes, causing decreased alpha-globin production and subsequent excess of beta chains in adults and excess gamma chains in newborns; variable degree of microcytic, hypochromic anemia depending on the number of affected alpha-globin alleles

Amino acid • One of a large group of organic compounds marked by the presence of both an amino group (NH_2) and a carboxyl group (COOH); the building blocks of protein and the end products of protein digestion

Anaerobic • Able to live without oxygen

Angina • Severe and crushing chest pain caused by inadequate blood flow and oxygenation to the heart muscle

Angina pectoris • Oppressive pain or pressure in the chest, caused by inadequate blood flow and oxygenation to the heart muscles; usually produced by atherosclerosis of the coronary arteries

Angiogenesis • Development of blood vessels

Ankyrin • Structural protein in red blood cells that binds cell membrane transport molecules to spectrin

Anticoagulant • Agent that prevents or delays blood coagulation

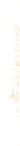

Antiglobulin test • Test used to determine the presence of red blood cell coating by antibodies (immunoglobulin G [IgG]) or complement, or both

Antiphospholipid (aPL) syndrome • Acquired thrombotic disorder associated with antibody production against the phospholipids binding protein beta-2-glycoprotein 1 (β_2GPI) or apolipoprotein (aPL)

Antithrombin (AT) • Naturally occurring inhibitor that neutralizes the action of thrombin, IXa, Xa, XIa, and XIIa, inhibiting coagulation; activity increases markedly when AT binds to heparin

Arteriosclerosis • Disease of the arterial vessels marked by thickening, hardening, and loss of elasticity in the arterial walls

Asynchrony • In hematology, when nuclear age and cytoplasmic age do not correspond

Atherosclerosis • Most common form of arteriosclerosis, marked by cholesterol-lipid-calcium deposits in the walls of arteries that may restrict blood flow

Atresia • As in biliary atresia, congenital closure, or absence of some or all of the major bile ducts

Auer rods • Elliptical, spindlelike inclusions composed of fused azurophilic granules that may be present in myeloblasts, monoblasts, or promyelocytes in various acute myeloblastic leukemias

Autoimmune hemolytic anemia • Process by which cells fail to recognize self and consequently make antibodies that destroy selected red blood cells

Autosomal • Non–sex-linked chromosomal pattern of inheritance

Band neutrophil • Leukocyte stage; size = 9 to 15 μm; coarsely clumped and band-shaped nuclear chromatin lacking filaments; cytoplasm with fine blue-staining and pink-staining secondary granules

Bart's hydrops fetalis • Clinical condition in infants with cardiac decompensation and hepatosplenomegaly; respiratory and circulatory distress; caused by absence of alpha chains, resulting in the most severe state of alpha thalassemia and unstable tetramers (β4); most infants with hydrops fetalis are stillborn at birth, and infants who are born alive die shortly after birth

Basophilic stippling • Diffuse, small, or coarse intracellular red blood cell inclusions seen on Wright-Giemsa stain; composed of RNA and mitochondrial remnants; present in accelerated erythropoiesis and lead poisoning

Bernard-Soulier syndrome • Rare autosomal recessive platelet adhesion disorder involving glycoprotein IB/IX complex (which is also the receptor for von Willebrand factor), thrombocytopenia, giant platelets, and absent ristocetin-induced platelet aggregation

Beta thalassemia • Inheritance of defective beta genes in a homozygous or heterozygous pattern; severity depends on the type of mutation; associated with a range of mild to severe microcytic, hypochromic anemia.

Burr cells (echinocytes) • Abnormal red blood cell morphology with red blood cells that demonstrate 10 to 30 even membrane spicules along the outer red blood cell membrane; associated with various anemias, renal insufficiency, uremia, gastric carcinoma, peptic ulcers, and pyruvate kinase deficiency

Cervical • Relating to the neck

Chédiak-Higashi syndrome • Lethal metabolic disorder in which neutrophils contain peroxidase-positive inclusion bodies; inherited as an autosomal recessive trait

Chelation • Therapy that removes heavy metals from the body

Chemotherapy • Drug therapy used to treat infections, cancers, and other diseases and conditions

Cholelithiasis • Presence or formation of gallstones

Clonal • Arising from a single cell

Cluster of designation (CD) • Monoclonal antibodies manufactured to identify and differentiate cell surface antigens that appear at various stages of hematopoietic and lymphopoietic development

Chronic lymphocytic leukemia (CLL) • Leukemia caused by clonal proliferation of B lymphocytes; associated with markedly increased mature lymphocytes and smudge cells in the peripheral blood, lymphadenopathy, and splenomegaly

Chronic myelogenous leukemia (CML) • Proliferative bone marrow disease characterized by marked leukocytosis; overall myeloid hyperplasia; increased number of mature band and segmented neutrophils, myelocytes, promyelocytes, and myeloblasts; hepatosplenomegaly; and presence of Philadelphia chromosome

Coefficient of variation (CV) • Standard deviation expressed as a percentage; a low CV indicates better precision

Cold agglutinin syndrome • Hemolytic disorder associated with IgM-mediated complement fixation, red blood cell agglutination, and subsequent intravascular hemolysis

Collagen vascular disease • Disorder that primarily affects the joints and mobility

Complement • Group of proteins in the blood that play a vital role in the body's immune defenses through a cascade of interaction

Consanguinity • Relationships among close blood relatives

Convalescence • Period of recovery after disease or surgery

Coumadin • Vitamin K antagonist compound that inhibits coagulation by acting against vitamin K–dependent coagulation factors; monitored by prothrombin time test and international normalized ratio

Crenation • Conversion of normally round red corpuscles into shrunken, knobbed, starry forms observed on a peripheral smear

Critical result • Laboratory result outside the reference range (critical high or low value), requiring immediate notification of a patient's physician or designee to avert significant patient morbidity or mortality

Critical test • Test that always requires rapid communication of results to the physician, even if the result is normal

Crohn's disease • Inflammatory bowel disease characterized by patchy areas of inflammation anywhere in the gastrointestinal tract, from the mouth to the anus

Cryoprecipitate • Product derived from fresh-frozen plasma that is rich in factor VIII, von Willebrand factor, and fibrinogen

Cyanosis • Blue tinge of lips and extremities (fingers, toes)

Cytochemistry • Chemistry of the living cell, involving special stains and usually performed on bone marrow samples that are examined microscopically to identify enzymes, lipids, or other chemical constituents within the blast population of cells in acute leukemia

Cytokines • Cell-produced substances that promote communication between cells and are responsible for immune modulation (i.e., interleukins, interferons, colony-stimulating factors)

Cytoskeleton • Network of protein filaments and microtubules in the cytoplasm that controls cell shape, maintains intracellular organization, and is involved in cell movement

Cytoxin • Antibody or toxin that attacks the cells of particular organs

Deep vein thrombosis • Formation of a blood clot in the deep veins of the legs, arms, or pelvis

Delta check • Comparison of current laboratory result with historical data; each institution sets the delta check time period and percent change considered significant for each analyte

2,3-Diphosphoglycerate (2,3-DPG) • A red blood cell phosphate produced by the action of the Embden-Meyerhof pathway, which controls the affinity of hemoglobin for oxygen

Direct antiglobulin test • Laboratory test for the presence of complement or antibodies bound to a patient's red blood cells

Disseminated intravascular coagulation (DIC) • Condition triggered by many pathologic events in which the coagulation pathways are hyperstimulated by either excessive fibrin disposition or excess fibrinolysis; patients with DIC clot, bleed, or both

Döhle bodies • Large, blue-staining cytoplasmic inclusions in the periphery of a neutrophilic cytoplasm and rarely in monocytes of nondiagnostic significance

Dysfibrinogenemia • Autosomal dominant fibrinogen disorder associated with abnormal fibrinogen molecule and abnormal clottable assay for qualitative fibrinogen

Dysplasia • Abnormal maturation of cells in the bone marrow

Dyspnea • Shortness of breath

Ecchymosis • Bruising

Elliptocyte • Abnormal red blood cell morphology present in marked amounts in patient with hereditary elliptocytosis and in smaller amounts in patients with iron deficiency anemia, idiopathic myelofibrosis, and other disorders; associated with abnormal red blood cell membrane proteins spectrin and protein 4.1 component

Embden-Meyerhof pathway • Red blood cell metabolic pathway that provides 90% of cellular adenosine triphosphate (ATP) and generates the oxidized form of nicotinamide adenine dinucleotide (NAD$^+$) from the reduced form of NAD (NADH), which is then available to form 2, 3-diphosphoglycerate

Embolism • Occlusion of a blood vessel by debris

Erythrocyte sedimentation rate (ESR) • Rate at which red blood cells settle out in a tube of blood under standardized conditions in a nonspecific screening test that monitors inflammatory processes or disease progression, or both; common methods include Wintrobe and Westergren

Erythroderma • Abnormal widespread redness and scaling of the skin, sometimes involving the entire body

Erythroid hyperplasia • Increased proliferation of red blood cell precursors in the bone marrow, resulting in a decreased myeloid:erythroid (M:E) ratio; normal ratio = 3:1 to 4:1; erythroid hyperplasia may result in M:E ratio of 1:1 or 1:2

Essential thrombocythemia (ET) • Clonal proliferative disorder characterized by increased production of platelets, megakaryocytic hyperplasia, megakaryocytic fragments in peripheral blood and bone marrow, and abnormal platelet function

Extramedullary hematopoiesis • Hematopoiesis outside of the bone marrow, primarily in the liver and spleen

Extravascular hemolysis • Red blood cell destruction occurring outside the vasculature in the spleen, liver, lymph nodes, and bone marrow, resulting in increased serum bilirubin, lactate dehydrogenase, and decreased hemoglobin, hematocrit, and haptoglobin; may also be associated with splenomegaly

Fanconi's anemia • Rare autosomal recessive disorder resulting in red blood cell aplasia; often manifests with a macrocytic process and thrombocytopenia and leukopenia; frequently associated with the development of leukemia and other cancers

Favism • Disorder found in individuals with glucose-6-phosphate dehydrogenase deficiency; characterized by hemolytic reaction to consumption of young fava beans or broad beans

Fibrillation • Usually refers to cardiac fluttering resulting from faulty electrical supply to the heart

Fibrinolysis • Hemostatic process involving enzymes, activators, and inhibitors, resulting in plasmin digestion of fibrin and fibrinogen and subsequent clot dissolution and restoration of blood flow

Fibronectin • Protein involved in wound healing and cell adhesion

Gangrene • Tissue death, usually resulting from deficient or absent blood supply

Gastrectomy • Removal of a portion of the stomach

Gaucher's disease • Rare lipid storage disorder associated with distinctive cells in the bone marrow that appear as large cells with "crinkled tissue paper" cytoplasm

Gingival hyperplasia • Swelling of the gingival tissues (gums); in leukemia, this is due to leukemic cell infiltration of gum tissues

Glanzmann's thrombasthenia • Rare autosomal recessive bleeding disorder involving defective glycoprotein IIb/IIIa and abnormal platelet aggregation with all platelet-aggregating agents except ristocetin

Glucose-6-phosphate dehydrogenase (G6PD) deficiency • Silent deficiency of the enzyme glucose-6-phosphate dehydrogenase (G6PD), with five possible genotypes having hemolytic manifestations that become moderate to severe (depending on the variant) on exposure to certain drugs, fava beans or fava bean residue.

Glycoprotein (GP) Ib • Platelet receptor in platelet adhesion

Glycoprotein (GP) IIB/IIIa • Receptor for fibronectin, von Willebrand factor, fibrinogen, and factors V and VIII

Gout • Arthritic disorder marked by crystal formation (usually uric acid) in the joints or tissues

Granulocytes • Granulated leukocytes or white blood cells

Hairy cell leukemia • Rare B-cell leukemia characterized by proliferation of abnormal, mononuclear cells with hair-like cytoplasmic projections and a round or kidney bean–shaped nucleus

Heinz bodies • Large red blood cell inclusions formed from denatured or precipitated globin chains produced in individuals with glucose-6-phosphate dehydrogenase deficiency after exposure to certain oxidizing drugs

Hemangioma • Benign tumor of dilated blood vessels

Hemarthrosis • Bloody effusion inside the joint

Hematoma • Swelling composed of a mass of clotted blood confined to an organ, tissue, or space or caused by a break in the blood vessel

Hematopoiesis • Production, differentiation, and maturation of blood cells

Hemoglobin C crystals • Intracellular red blood cell crystals shaped like blocks or "bars of gold," found in hemoglobin C disease

Hemoglobin C disease • Condition associated with chronic normocytic/normochromic anemia resulting from substitution of lysine for glutamic acid in the sixth position of N-terminal end of the beta chain ($\alpha_2\beta_2^{6\ glu\ lys}$)

Hemoglobin SC crystals • Intracellular red blood cell crystals that protrude from the red blood cell membrane in a Washington Monument–like or fingerlike projection; associated with hemoglobin SC disease

Hemoglobin SC disease • Condition associated with moderate normocytic/normochromic anemia resulting from the combination of hemoglobin S and hemoglobin C

Hemolytic uremic syndrome (HUS) • Childhood disease associated with platelet counts of less than 20×10^9/L and renal damage caused by toxin from *Escherichia coli* 0157:H7 or *Shigella* toxin

Hemophilia A • Sex-linked recessive bleeding disorder caused by factor VIII deficiency

Hemophilia B • Sex-linked recessive bleeding disorder caused by factor IX deficiency

Heparin • Naturally occurring or commercially manufactured anticoagulant; monitored by activated partial thromboplastin time or anti–factor Xa heparin assay

Heparin cofactor II • Heparin-dependent hemostatic inhibitor enzyme that acts on thrombin

Heparin-induced thrombocytopenia (HIT) • Immune-mediated thrombocytopenia in a subset of patients on heparin therapy or exposed to heparin in catheters or IV flush

Hepatosplenomegaly • Enlargement of liver and spleen

Hereditary elliptocytosis • Autosomal dominant red blood cell disorder caused by deficient spectrin, resulting in elliptocyte formation

Hereditary hemochromatosis • Autosomal recessive, homozygous, or heterozygous iron-loading disorder associated with elevated serum iron, ferritin, and transferrin saturation and multiple organ damage

Hereditary pyropoikilocytosis • Rare recessive red blood cell membrane disorder caused by decreased membrane alpha and beta spectrin and increased susceptibility of spectrin degradation

Hereditary spherocytosis • Autosomal dominant (75%) or autosomal recessive (25%) red blood cell disorder caused by deficiency of the key red blood cell membrane protein spectrin; to a lesser degree, deficiency of the membrane protein ankyrin and minor membrane proteins band 3 and protein 4.2

Hereditary stomatocytosis • Rare autosomal dominant red blood cell disorder associated with deficiency of the membrane protein stomatin, resulting in red blood cell morphology of cells having slits or a barlike area of central pallor in the center of the cell

Hereditary xerocytosis • Rare autosomal dominant condition in which red blood cells have a "puddle" hemoglobin appearance in a patient with moderate to severe anemia

Hexose monophosphate shunt • Red blood cell metabolic pathway that provides 5% to 10% of ATP needed to produce the NADPH necessary to prevent degradation of globin chains

HLA • Human leukocyte antigens, which are found in white blood cells and are part of the major histocompatibility complex

Hodgkin's lymphoma • Lymphoproliferative disease associated with lymphadenopathy and presence of Reed-Sternberg cells in lymph nodes

Howell-Jolly bodies • Red blood cell inclusions composed of DNA remnants that appear as round, deep purple, 1- to 2-m inclusions; may be seen postsplenectomy or under conditions of accelerated erythropoiesis

Humoral • When relating to immunity, antibody formation

Hyperplasia • Excessive proliferation of normal cells in the normal tissue of an organ

Hypersegmented neutrophil • Segmented neutrophil with more than five nuclear lobes, usually associated with a megaloblastic process

Hyperviscosity • Excessive resistance to the flow of liquids

Hypochromia • Red blood cells exhibiting greater than normal degree of central pallor and mean corpuscular hemoglobin concentration less than 32%, as calculated on the complete blood count; may be seen to a variable degree in iron deficiency anemia, thalassemias, and sideroblastic processes

Hypofibrinogenemia • Heterozygous form of afibrinogenemia associated with fibrinogen levels between 20 mg/dL and 100 mg/dL

Hypovolemic • Low blood volume

Hypoxia • Decreased oxygen

Idiopathic myelofibrosis (IMF) • Clonal proliferative bone marrow disorder characterized by marked bone marrow fibrosis, leukoerythroblastic anemia, teardrop red blood cells, and extramedullary hematopoiesis

Idiopathic thrombocytopenic purpura (ITP) • Platelet disorder associated with decreased platelet count resulting from immune destruction of platelets; in two-thirds of cases, related to antibody directed against glycoprotein IIb/IIIa or glycoprotein Ib-IX

Immunologic assay • Measuring the protein and protein-bound molecules concerned with the reaction between an antigen and its specific antibody

Immunophenotyping • Process of using monoclonal antibodies directed against cell surface markers to identify antigens unique to a specific lineage and stage of maturation; flow cytometry or immunohistochemistry technology is used to identify myeloid or lymphoid neoplasm

Infarction • Area of tissue that has been deprived of blood and has lost some of its function

Inguinal • Relating to the groin area

Interleukins • Group of cytokines (proteins) produced by $CD4^+$ helper T lymphocytes, monocytes, macrophages, and endothelial cells that promote the development and differentiation of T cells, B cells, and hematopoietic cells

Intramedullary hematopoiesis • Hematopoiesis within the bone marrow cavity

Intramedullary hemolysis • Premature hemolysis of red blood cell precursors in the bone marrow

Intravascular hemolysis • Red blood cell destruction within the blood vessels, resulting in increased bilirubin, lactate dehydrogenase, and free hemoglobin; decreased hemoglobin, hematocrit, haptoglobin; and, in some cases, hemoglobinuria

Intrinsic factor • Glycoprotein produced by the parietal cells of the stomach; needed for absorption of vitamin B_{12}

Iris diaphragm • Optical microscope element located under the microscope stage that controls the amount of light from the microscope light source

Jaundice • Increase in bilirubin leading to yellow discoloration of the mucous membranes of the eyes and imparting a yellow tone to the skin

Keloid • Thick, shiny, rubbery scar resulting from excessive growth of fibrous tissue

Koilonychia • Also known as spooning of nails, a condition of the nails that may indicate iron deficiency anemia; nails appear abnormally thin and flat or concave in shape

Left shift • Increased numbers of granulocytic precursors in the peripheral blood

Leukemoid reaction • Enhanced response to infection and inflammation; leukocyte count may be 20 to 50 $\times 10^9$/L

Leukocytosis • Increased total leukocyte count

Leukoerythroblastosis • Increased levels of immature granulocytes, immature red blood cells, and possibly platelet abnormalities

Leukopoiesis • Production of leukocytes or white blood cells

Lineage • Referring to one specific cell line

Lumen • Space within an artery, vein, or intestine or tube

Lymphoblast • Lymphocyte maturation stage; size = 10 to 20 μm; nuclear:cytoplasmic ratio = 4:1; nucleus has fine chromatin with one to two nucleoli and basophilic cytoplasm

Lymphocyte • Lymphocyte maturation stage; small lymphocyte size = 7 to 18 μm, nuclear:cytoplasmic ratio = 4:1, scant basophilic cytoplasm, possibly with a few azurophilic granules; large lymphocyte size = 9 to 12 μm, nuclear:cytoplasmic ratio = 3:1, coarsely clumped but less dense chromatin, and abundant cytoplasm, possibly with a few azurophilic granules

Lymphoma • Neoplasm involving abnormal proliferation of cells arising in the lymph nodes; these tumor cells may also metastasize to involve extranodal sites

Macrocyte • Abnormal red blood cell morphology seen to varying degrees in folic acid deficiency, vitamin B₁₂ deficiency, pernicious anemia, alcoholism, liver disease, and as a normal morphology in neonates. Mean corpuscular volume is greater than 100 fL when macrocytes are present in large numbers

Macrocytic/normochromic anemia • Anemia with red blood cells, hemoglobin, and hematocrit less than reference ranges; mean corpuscular volume greater than 100 fL; and normal mean corpuscular hemoglobin content

Macrocytosis • Condition characterized by larger than normal red blood cells with mean corpuscular volume less than 100 fL

May Hegglin anomaly • Inherited disorder associated with thrombocytopenia and giant platelets

Mean corpuscular volume (MCV) • Red blood cell index derived by the following formula:

$$\text{MCV (fL)} = \frac{\text{Hematocrit (\%)} \times 10}{\text{Erythrocyte count}}$$

Mean corpuscular hemoglobin (MCH) • Red blood cell index derived by the following formula:

$$\text{MCH (pg)} = \frac{\text{Hemoglobin (g/dL)} \times 10}{\text{Erythrocyte count}}$$

Mean corpuscular hemoglobin content (MCHC) • Calculation of the average concentration of hemoglobin in a red blood cell:

$$\text{MCHC (\%)} = \frac{\text{Hemoglobin (g/dL)} \times 100}{\text{Hematocrit (\%)}}$$

Megakaryoblast • Platelet maturation stage; size = 10 to 15 μm; nucleus contains two to six nucleoli and has a high nuclear:cytoplasmic ratio; dark blue–staining cytoplasm

Megakaryocyte • Platelet maturation stage; size ranges from 30 to 100 μm; coarse nuclear chromatin present in uninuclear or lobulated nucleus; as megakaryocyte cytoplasm ruptures, the cytoplasmic fragments and platelets are released (thrombopoiesis process)

Megaloblastic anemia • Anemia caused by vitamin B₁₂ or folic acid deficiency, resulting in impaired DNA synthesis and subsequent formation of megaloblastic precursors in the bone marrow and macrocytosis in the peripheral blood

Meningeal leukemia • Leukemic cell proliferation in the central nervous system

Menorrhagia • Excessive menstrual bleeding

Methemoglobin reductase pathway • Red blood cell metabolic pathway that maintains hemoglobin iron in the reduced ferrous state (Fe⁺⁺) and is dependent on reduction of NAD to NADPH

Microangiopathic • Related to pathology of small blood vessels

Microcyte • Red blood cell with mean corpuscular volume less than 70 fL; characterized by large quantities of microcytes in iron deficiency anemia and hemoglobinopathies

Microcytic/hypochromic anemia • Anemia with red blood cells, hemoglobin, and hematocrit less than reference ranges; mean corpuscular volume less than 80 fL; and mean corpuscular hemoglobin content less than 32%

Microcytosis • Condition of smaller than normal red blood cells; mean corpuscular volume less than 80 fL

Monoclonal • Arising from a single cell

Monosomy • Condition of having only one of a pair of chromosomes, as in Turner's syndrome, which has only one X chromosome rather than two

Morbidity • State of being diseased

Mortality • Death

Multiple myeloma • Clonal proliferative bone marrow disease characterized by increased plasma cells in bone marrow, osteoclast activation, production of abnormal monoclonal protein, and pancytopenia

Multipotential stem cells • Primitive stem cells that differentiate into lymphoid or nonlymphoid (hematopoietic) committed precursor cells

Myelin • Fatty substance around a nerve

Myeloblast • Leukocyte maturation stage; size = 12 to 20 μm; nuclear:cytoplasmic ratio = 4:1; two to five nucleoli; fine nuclear chromatin; basophilic cytoplasm

Myelocytic • Stage of leukocyte maturation

Myelodysplasia • Abnormal maturation or differentiation of granulocytes, erythrocytes, monocytes, and platelets

Myelofibrosis • Increased reticulin or fibrotic tissue in the bone marrow

Myeloperoxidase • Stain used to classify blast population lineage in acute leukemia; myeloblasts stain strongly positive, monoblasts stain faintly positive

Myeloproliferative • Abnormal proliferation of normal-appearing hematopoietic cells in the absence of an appropriate stimulus

Myelotoxic • Destructive to white blood cells

Necrosis • Death of cells, tissue, or organs

Niemann-Pick disease • Lipid storage disorder having distinctive cells in the bone marrow that appear as round uniform cells with cytoplasmic globules composed of lipids

Nonspecific esterase (NSE) • Stain used to identify monocytic cells; substrates most often used are alpha-naphthyl butyrate and alpha-naphthyl acetate; macrophages, histiocytes, megakaryoblasts, and some carcinomas also stain positive; sodium fluoride inhibition step is used to differentiate positivity

Normocytic/normochromic anemia • Anemia with red blood cells, hemoglobin, and hematocrit less than reference ranges, with normal mean corpuscular volume and mean corpuscular hemoglobin content

Objective • Part of the microscope responsible for magnification; degree of magnification depends on three factors—magnification number, aperture number, and tube length

Ocular • Optical microscope element that functions as an additional magnification component to the objective magnification

Oncogene • Gene responsible for cancer development

Organomegaly • Enlargement of an organ

Osteosclerosis • Abnormal increase in the thickening or density of bone

Ovalocyte • Abnormal red blood cell morphology represented as oval or egg-shaped erythrocyte; present in varying degrees in thalassemic syndromes, hemoglobinopathies, hereditary ovalocytosis, iron deficiency anemia; macro-ovalocytes are seen in megaloblastic anemias; often used interchangeably with the term elliptocyte; however, these two distinct morphologies have recognizable differences

Palpitation • Sensation of rapid or irregular heartbeat

Pancytopenia • Decreased number of red blood cells, white blood cells, and platelets in the peripheral blood

Pappenheimer bodies • Small clusters of intracellular red blood cell inclusions that stain purple with Prussian blue stain and are composed of iron; present in hereditary hemochromatosis and iron-loading anemias

Paranoia • Mental condition characterized by persistent persecutory delusions or delusional jealousy

Paresthesias • Abnormal sensation resulting from an injury to one or more nerves; described as numbness or a prickly or tingling feeling

Paroxysmal cold hemoglobinuria • Rare hemolytic anemia associated with anti-P antibody that attaches to red blood cells in lower temperatures and then activates complement at warmer temperatures, causing hemolysis and hemoglobinuria

Paroxysmal nocturnal hemoglobinuria • Red blood cell membrane defect associated with increased susceptibility of red blood cells to complement-mediated lysis during night hours; caused by mutation of phosphatidylinositol glycan class in the hematopoietic stem cells

Pathognomonic • Indicative of a disease, especially its characteristic symptoms

Pathology • Study of the nature and cause of disease that involves changes in structure and function of cells or organ systems, or both

Pathophysiology • Study of how normal processes are altered by disease

Pelger-Huët anomaly • High-frequency genetic disorder characterized by hyposegmented band and segmented neutrophils or uninuclear lobulation; type of hyposegmented neutrophils depends on the zygosity inheritance pattern

Periodic acid–Schiff (PAS) • Cytochemical stain used to evaluate the blast population in acute leukemias; however, other cells also stain positive, and lymphoblasts and pronormoblasts stain strongly positive; PAS is most helpful in support of acute lymphoblastic leukemia or erythroleukemia; myeloblasts occasionally show a faint diffuse positive reaction; PAS stains the cellular element glycogen

Pernicious anemia • Subset of megaloblastic anemias resulting from impaired absorption of vitamin B_{12}; most likely caused by immune destruction of intrinsic factor

Photophobia • Unusual intolerance of light

Placebo • Inactive substance or treatment given instead of one that has a proven effect

Plasmapheresis • Plasma exchange therapy involving removal of plasma from cellular material that is then returned to the patient

Plasminogen • Inactive precursor of plasmin synthesized in the liver; converted to plasmin when acted on by thrombin and tissue plasminogen activator

Plasminogen activator inhibitor 1 (PAI-1) • Fibrinolytic inhibitor secreted by endothelial cells that acts to restrain the function of tissue plasminogen activator

Plasmin • Hydrolytic enzyme that digests fibrin and fibrinogen

Plethora • Excess blood volume

Poikilocytosis • Variation in red blood cell shape related to various pathophysiologic processes

Polychromasia • Blue tinge to red blood cells with Wright-Giemsa stain, indicating a younger red blood cell and premature release of the red blood cell from the bone marrow

Polycythemia vera (PV) • Clonal proliferative bone marrow disorder associated with marked increased production of red blood cells and accompanying increase in leukocytes and platelets

Polymerization • Process of changing a simple chemical substance (or substances) into another compound having the same elements, usually in the same proportion but with a higher molecular weight

Porcine • Of or relating to swine (pigs)

Postural hypotension • Low blood pressure occurring in some people when they stand too quickly from a prone or sitting position

Precision • Measure of reproducibility of test samples for a given procedure

Priapism • Persistent painful erection of the penis

Prolymphocyte • Lymphocyte maturation stage; size = 9 to 18 μm; nuclear:cytoplasmic ratio = 3:1; zero to one nucleolus; slightly condensed chromatin; scant amount of basophilic cytoplasm

Promegakaryocyte • Platelet maturation stage; size = 20 to 80 μm; contains a single round, oval, or kidney bean–shaped nucleus with moderately coarse chromatin and zero to one nucleolus; abundant basophilic cytoplasm with pseudopodia; fine alpha and lysosomal granules

Promyelocyte • Leukocyte maturation stage; size = 15 to 21 μm; nuclear:cytoplasmic ratio = 3:1; one to two nucleoli; moderately basophilic cytoplasm having fine to large, blue-staining to purple-staining diffuse, azurophilic, nonspecific granules

Prognostic • Prediction of the chance for recovery

Prophylactic • Preventive

Protein C • Vitamin K–dependent protein that inhibits clotting factors V and VIII when activated by thrombin-thrombomodulin complex

Protein S • Vitamin K–dependent protein that is required for activation of protein C

Prothrombin mutation • Second most common inherited cause of thrombosis; caused by a single-point mutation (G20210A)

Prothrombin time (PT) • Coagulation test that measures the extrinsic system of coagulation and involves the addition of reagent calcium chloride and tissue factor

Protocol • Formal ideas, plans, or schemes concerning patient care, bench work, administration, or research

Pruritus • Itching

Purpura fulminans • Rapidly progressing form of purpura occurring principally in children; of short duration and frequently fatal

Pyknosis • Shrinkage of cells through degeneration

Pyruvate kinase (PK) deficiency • Rare inherited enzyme deficiency of the Embden-Myerhoff red blood cell metabolic pathway resulting in inflexible red blood cells that are sequestered in the spleen and have a moderate hemolysis

Raynaud's phenomenon • Intermittent attacks of pallor or cyanosis of the small arteries and arterioles of the fingers caused by inadequate arterial blood supply

Reactive lymphocytosis • Increase in total number of lymphocytes where lymphocytes have abundant dark blue–staining cytoplasm; often seen with accompanying decrease in neutrophils

Recombinant • In genetic and molecular biology, pertaining to genetic material combined from different sources

Red blood cell distribution width (RDW) • Calculation of the standard deviation of red blood cell volume divided by mean corpuscular volume, multiplied by 100; elevated RDW correlates with the degree of anisocytosis and poikilocytosis

Reference range • Set of values used to interpret results for a given test, usually defined as the values that encompass 95% (or 2 standard deviations) of the population

Refractory • Resistant to ordinary treatment

Refractory anemia (RA) • Treatment-resistant anemia characterized by megaloblastoid bone marrow hyperplasia and less than 5% myeloblasts in the bone marrow

Refractory anemia with multilineage dysplasia • Anemia characterized by erythroid hyperplasia and dysplastic nuclear and cytoplasmic changes involving two or more myeloid cell lines

Refractory anemia with ringed sideroblasts (RARS) • Anemia characterized by erythroid hyperplasia and greater than 15% ringed sideroblasts in the bone marrow

Reptilase time • Coagulation procedure similar to thrombin time except that the clotting is initiated by reptilase, a snake venom; using reptilase, heparin would not affect the assay

Reticuloendothelial system (RES) • Mononuclear phagocytic system

Rhinorrhea • Excessive watery discharge from nose

Ringed sideroblast • Red blood cell precursors with iron deposits surrounding the nucleus in a ring formation

Rouleaux • Group of red blood cells stacked together, resembling a stack of coins

Schistocyte • Abnormal red blood cell morphology formed when the red blood cell membrane has been sheared, causing irregularly shaped red blood cell fragments; associated with hemolytic anemias, disseminated intravascular coagulation, hemolytic uremic syndrome, thrombotic thrombocytopenic purpura, renal transplant, and postsplenectomy

Segmented neutrophil • Leukocyte stage; size = 9 to 15 μm; nuclear chromatin is coarsely clumped; three to five lobes of nucleus connected by thin threadlike nuclear chromatin filaments; cytoplasm with fine blue-staining and pink-staining secondary granules

Sepsis • Systemic inflammatory response to infection from microorganisms; symptoms include fever, hypothermia, and tachycardia

Sézary syndrome • T-cell lymphoma, also known as mycosis fungoides, with malignant cells having a predilection for cutaneous tissues; presence of Sézary cells with morphology of large cells with convoluted cerebriform, ovoid nucleus

Sickle cell • Abnormal red blood cell morphology associated with sickle cell disorders in patients with a high quantity of hemoglobin S; crescent-shaped or sickle-shaped red blood cells; may also be oat-shaped in the reversible state

Sickle cell anemia • Beta chain variant caused by inheritance of hemoglobin S ($\alpha_2\beta_2$ $^{6\ glu\ \to\ val}$), resulting in inflexible sickled cells that obstruct blood vessels and cause hemolysis, infection, and shortened life expectancy

Sideroblastic anemia • Inherited or acquired iron-loading disorder associated with the presence of iron deposits in the red blood cell precursors in the bone marrow called ringed sideroblasts, a dimorphic red blood cell morphology, and increased serum ferritin

Spasticity • Involuntary muscular contractions

Spectrin • Red blood cell membrane protein responsible for deformability properties of the red blood cell

Spherocyte • Abnormal red blood cell shape seen on the peripheral blood smear as dense, deeper red shade, small erythrocyte; when present in large quantities, mean corpuscular hemoglobin content is greater than 36%; found in hereditary spherocytosis where spectrin is abnormal, in autoimmune syndromes as a result of loss of red blood cell membrane from splenic pitting of antibody-coated cells leaving a more compact red blood cell, postsplenectomy; also represents the normal red blood cell morphology as a red blood cell ages

Splenectomy • Removal of the spleen

Splenomegaly • Enlarged spleen

Spooning of nails • See **Koilonychia**

Standard deviation • Measurement that describes the average distance each data point lies from the mean of a given set of data

Standard precautions • Compliance measures employed by health-care workers to prevent disease transmission that might be caused by contact with blood or body fluids; combines principles of handling body substances, safety, and universal precautions; personal protective equipment is an important part of standard precaution measures

Stomatocyte • Abnormal red blood cell shape; red blood cells have a slitlike area of central pallor; associated with alcoholism, hereditary stomatocytosis, liver disease, malignancies, and in small numbers in various other disorders

Subclavian • Situated beneath the clavicle or collarbone

Sudan black B (SBB) • Cytochemistry stain of phospholipids found in the primary (specific) and secondary (nonspecific) granules of neutrophilic and eosinophilic cells and to a lesser extent monocytes and macrophages; used to differentiate acute myeloblastic leukemia (positive) from acute lymphoblastic leukemia (negative); staining intensity increases in later stages of maturation

Syncope • Fainting

Tachycardia • Fast and hard heartbeat

Target cell • Abnormal red blood cell shape where the cell appears as a "bull's eye"–shaped cell with the hemoglobin concentrated in the center and outer edges of the cell membrane; found in increased numbers in iron deficiency anemia, hemoglobinopathies, liver disease, hemolytic anemia, and postsplenectomy

Teardrop erythrocyte • Abnormal red blood cell shaped like a teardrop, frequently seen in myeloproliferative disorders, severe anemias, and postsplenectomy

Telangiectasia • Vascular lesion formed by dilation of a group of small blood vessels; most frequently seen on face and thighs

Therapeutic phlebotomy • Withdrawing blood for a medical purpose

Thoracic • Relating to the chest

Thrombin • Clotting factor (factor IIa) responsible for stimulation of platelet aggregation and activation of cofactors protein C and factor VIII; key protease enzyme of hemostasis that functions to cleave fibrinogen resulting in fibrin monomers, A and B fibrinopeptides; thrombin activates factors V and VIII; as thrombin levels increase, thrombin ultimately destroys factors V and VIII by proteolysis

Thrombin time • Assay that uses thrombin as a substrate to measure the time it takes to convert fibrinogen to fibrin

Thrombocytopenia • Decreased platelet count; condition associated with many disorders

Thrombocytosis • Increase in peripheral blood platelet count

Thrombolysis • Breaking up of a clot

Thrombolytic therapy • Using an agent that causes the breakup of clots

Thrombotic thrombocytopenic purpura (TTP) • Platelet disorder associated with platelet counts of 20 × 10^9/L, platelet microthrombi, and microangiopathic hemolytic anemia; caused by deficiency of the metalloprotease ADAMTS-13 and accumulation of large von Willebrand factor multimers

Thromboxane A$_2$ • Potent inducer of platelet aggregation

Thrombus • Blood clot that obstructs a blood vessel or a cavity of the heart

Thymus • Ductless gland located above the heart that plays a role in immunity

Tissue plasminogen activator (tPA) • Converts plasminogen to plasmin, resulting in fibrin degradation

Toxic granulation • Excessive dark-staining granulation in neutrophils; sometimes seen in myeloid precursors (band neutrophils, metamyelocytes, and rarely, myelocytes), usually in response to infection

Toxic vacuolization • Cytoplasmic vacuoles seen in segmented and band neutrophils in response to sepsis; sometimes seen with prolonged exposure to particular drugs

Transaminase • Aminotransferase (an enzyme)

Transcobalamin II • Carrier protein that forms a complex with vitamin B_{12} and transports vitamin B_{12} into the peripheral blood circulation and then into the liver, bone marrow, and other tissues

Transient ischemic attack (TIA) • Neurologic deficit, having a vascular cause, that produces stroke symptoms that resolve in 24 hours

Translocation • Alteration of a chromosome by transfer of a portion of it either to another chromosome or to another portion of the same chromosome

Trisomy • In genetics, having three homologous chromosomes per cell instead of two

Vasculitis • Inflammation of blood vessels

Vasoconstriction • Decrease in the diameter of the blood vessels that decreases the blood flow and increases blood pressure

Venogram • Radiograph of the veins

Vertigo • Dizziness

Viscosity • Thickness

von Willebrand disease (vWD) • Autosomal dominant bleeding disorder caused by qualitative or quantitative defect in VWF:VWF molecule, resulting in impaired platelet adhesion

von Willebrand factor (vWF) • Large multimeric glycoprotein with two important functions: (1) mediating the adhesion of platelets to sites of vascular injury and (2) binding and stabilizing factor VIII

Waldenström's macroglobulinemia • Rare disorder involving the hyperviscosity syndrome, hepatosplenomegaly, abnormal mucosal bleeding, and overproduction of IgM by abnormal B lymphocytes that manifest in the bone marrow and peripheral blood as having features of plasma cells (plasmacytoid lymphocytes)

White blood cell (WBC) differential count • Automated or manual microscopic classification, reported as a percentage of each leukocyte cell type identified. The manual differential usually includes an evaluation of red blood cell morphology and platelet estimate and morphology

Wiskott-Aldrich syndrome • X-linked recessive disorder associated with severe eczema, recurrent infections, immune defects, and thrombocytopenia

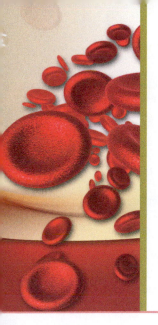

Index

Note: Page numbers followed by "f" and "t" indicate figures and tables, respectively.